NATIONAL ACADEMIES
Sciences
Engineering
Medicine

T0295139

NATIONAL
ACADEMIES
PRESS
Washington, DC

Myopia

Causes, Prevention, and Treatment of an Increasingly Common Disease

Committee on Focus on Myopia: Pathogenesis
and Rising Incidence

Board on Behavioral, Cognitive, and Sensory
Sciences

Division of Behavioral and Social Sciences
and Education

Consensus Study Report

NATIONAL ACADEMIES PRESS 500 Fifth Street, NW Washington, DC 20001

This activity was supported by contracts between the National Academy of Sciences and the American Academy of Optometry; the American Optometric Association; the Health Care Alliance for Patient Safety; the Herbert Wertheim School of Optometry & Vision Science, University of California, Berkeley; Johnson & Johnson Vision; the National Eye Institute (HHSN263201800029I/75N98022F00005); Reality Labs Research; Research to Prevent Blindness; and the Warby Parker Impact Foundation. Any opinions, findings, conclusions, or recommendations expressed in this publication do not necessarily reflect the views of any organization or agency that provided support for the project.

International Standard Book Number-13: 978-0-309-71785-4
International Standard Book Number-10: 0-309-71785-X
Digital Object Identifier: https://doi.org/10.17226/27734

This publication is available from the National Academies Press, 500 Fifth Street, NW, Keck 360, Washington, DC 20001; (800) 624-6242; http://www.nap.edu.

Suggested citation: National Academies of Sciences, Engineering, and Medicine. 2024. *Myopia: Causes, Prevention, and Treatment of an Increasingly Common Disease*. Washington, DC: National Academies Press. https://doi.org/10.17226/27734.

The **National Academy of Sciences** was established in 1863 by an Act of Congress, signed by President Lincoln, as a private, nongovernmental institution to advise the nation on issues related to science and technology. Members are elected by their peers for outstanding contributions to research. Dr. Marcia McNutt is president.

The **National Academy of Engineering** was established in 1964 under the charter of the National Academy of Sciences to bring the practices of engineering to advising the nation. Members are elected by their peers for extraordinary contributions to engineering. Dr. John L. Anderson is president.

The **National Academy of Medicine** (formerly the Institute of Medicine) was established in 1970 under the charter of the National Academy of Sciences to advise the nation on medical and health issues. Members are elected by their peers for distinguished contributions to medicine and health. Dr. Victor J. Dzau is president.

The three Academies work together as the **National Academies of Sciences, Engineering, and Medicine** to provide independent, objective analysis and advice to the nation and conduct other activities to solve complex problems and inform public policy decisions. The National Academies also encourage education and research, recognize outstanding contributions to knowledge, and increase public understanding in matters of science, engineering, and medicine.

Learn more about the National Academies of Sciences, Engineering, and Medicine at **www.nationalacademies.org**.

COMMITTEE ON FOCUS ON MYOPIA: PATHOGENESIS AND RISING INCIDENCE

K. DAVINA FRICK (*Co-Chair*; she/her/hers), Johns Hopkins Carey Business School
TERRI L. YOUNG (*Co-Chair*; she/her/hers), University of Wisconsin–Madison
AFUA O. ASARE (she/her/hers), University of Utah
DAVID BERSON (he/him/his), Brown University
RICHARD T. BORN (he/him/his), Harvard School of Medicine
JING CHEN (she/her/hers), Rice University
JEREMY A. GUGGENHEIM (he/him/his), Cardiff University
ANTHONY N. KUO (he/him/his), Duke University
DAPHNE MAURER (she/her/hers), McMaster University
J. ANTHONY MOVSHON (he/him/his), New York University
DONALD O. MUTTI (he/him/his), The Ohio State University
MACHELLE T. PARDUE (she/her/hers), Emory University
RAMKUMAR SABESAN (he/him/his), University of Washington
JODY ANN SUMMERS (she/her/hers), University of Oklahoma
KATHERINE K. WEISE (she/her/hers), University of Alabama at Birmingham

Study Staff
MOLLY CHECKSFIELD DORRIES (she/her/hers), Study Director
DANIEL J. WEISS (he/him/his), Board Director
TINA M. WINTERS (she/her/hers), Program Officer
J. ASHTON RAY (she/her/hers), Senior Program Assistant

NOTE: See Appendix B, Disclosure of Unavoidable Conflict of Interest.

Reviewers

This Consensus Study Report was reviewed in draft form by individuals chosen for their diverse perspectives and technical expertise. The purpose of this independent review is to provide candid and critical comments that will assist the National Academies of Sciences, Engineering, and Medicine in making each published report as sound as possible and to ensure that it meets the institutional standards for quality, objectivity, evidence, and responsiveness to the study charge. The review comments and draft manuscript remain confidential to protect the integrity of the deliberative process.

We thank the following individuals for their review of this report:

ALLISON G. ABRAHAM, Department of Ophthalmology, School of Medicine, University of Colorado Anschutz Medical Campus

MICHAEL DO, Harvard Medical School and F.M. Kirby Neurobiology Center, Boston Children's Hospital

PATRICE M. HICKS, Department of Ophthalmology and Visual Sciences, Kellogg Eye Center, University of Michigan

ELIZABETH IRVING, School of Optometry and Vision Science, University of Waterloo

MICHELE RUCCI, Brain & Cognitive Sciences, Center for Visual Science, University of Rochester

FRANK SCHAEFFEL, Institute of Ophthalmic Research, Centre for Ophthalmology, University Clinics, Tübingen, Germany

EARL L. SMITH, College of Optometry, University of Houston

BRIAN STAGG, Moran Eye Center, Department of Ophthalmology and Visual Sciences, University of Utah

CHI-HO TO, School of Optometry, The Hong Kong Polytechnic University

GEUNYOUNG YOON, College of Optometry, University of Houston

Although the reviewers listed above provided many constructive comments and suggestions, they were not asked to endorse the conclusions or recommendations of this report nor did they see the final draft before its release. The review of this report was overseen by **THOMAS D. ALBRIGHT,** Salk Institute for Biological Studies, and **EVE J. HIGGINBOTHAM,** Perelman School of Medicine, University of Pennsylvania. They were responsible for making certain that an independent examination of this report was carried out in accordance with the standards of the National Academies and that all review comments were carefully considered. Responsibility for the final content rests entirely with the authoring committee and the National Academies.

Contents

Boxes, Figures, and Tables

BOXES

FIGURES

TABLES

Preface

The committee was charged with assessing the state of knowledge regarding the mechanistic understanding of myopia pathogenesis and identifying the causes of myopia's increased prevalence and the knowledge gaps and barriers to progress. The committee developed a research agenda over the course of the study process. For each of the report's chapters, the committee reviewed relevant areas of empirical research across multiple disciplines related to myopia; for instance, epidemiology, biology, physiology, optics, public health, and technology. The data underscore that the refractive error shift towards myopia noted in multiple global populations has risen to epidemic proportions. The increasing prevalence of myopia seen in urban Asia is now happening in the United States as well, although the United States lacks rigorous data collection on refractive errors. The evidence points strongly to environmental factors as the most influential, but there is also evidence of genetic contributions, particularly those that interact with the environment.

Even though there is existing and ongoing research in this field, the committee identified numerous critical gaps. There is a pressing need to understand the causal mechanisms underlying myopic eye growth in order to develop more effective treatments to slow myopia progression or prevent its onset altogether. In addition, more evidence-based research is needed on what produces sustainable, equitable, nimble ocular health assessment and effective treatments that can be adapted and applied across all communities. In addition to filling the gaps, the committee envisioned an aspirational research agenda that could help facilitate a future line of transformational and groundbreaking work that pushes the field forward in ways it identified as innovative, necessary, and challenging.

Ocular developmental growth can be affected by visual diet (i.e., the various visual stimuli from the environment that enter the eye), so starting intentional (data-based) interventions earlier in life is better. There is a definite need to perform scientific and clinical assessments at an earlier age—ideally, prior to formal schooling. Earlier age of onset of myopia has implications for the likelihood of ocular morbidities associated with myopia and therefore impacts quality of life and lifestyle choices, with economic implications both individually and community-wide, as well as impacts on educational and vocational choices, opportunities, and productivity.

Developing communities will likely experience the most dramatic changes over the next few decades, and the most affected urban areas will experience higher patient concerns of ocular co-morbidities with associated impairment of visual acuity. Based on the evidence stated above, the committee encourages change now with increased outdoor time during daylight for young children and persistent outdoor activity throughout childhood and into young adulthood. With population health concerns, incremental adaptive changes have historically been shown to be the most effective.

Multiple stakeholders and implicated parties should recognize their responsibility and potential impact in affecting intentional and increased change to thwart the trend toward myopic eye growth. There is a need to think big-picture and in nontraditional ways regarding partners to address this issue on multiple levels. The committee suggests greater attention to and offerings of competitive small to large multi-site research grants, and local screening and treatment provision efforts that are coordinated both statewide and nationwide, including collaborations with global health agencies. All efforts and data collection need to be harmonized so true comparisons can be made to detect refractive error and other visual disorder shifts in communities. The committee recommends greater efforts to customize therapies coordinated with evidence-based risk assessments. This will require multidisciplinary teams that might not directly study myopia but would have the tools and varied perspectives to approach the problem differently and more comprehensively.

Myopia, in our opinion, is indisputably a disease, and should be treated as such. At present, especially in the United States, it is generally considered a visual inconvenience. However, the impact on visual function and the risk for blinding complications later in life are significant. The increasing prevalence of myopia is an urgent issue that requires better awareness to attract the funding dollars needed for effective treatments, screening, and research study. Finally, the health impacts of this global myopic epidemic will be experienced unequally between and within countries, with the most vulnerable communities often suffering from the highest impact. Linked to this, inequality is also arguably fueling this crisis.

The committee desires to congratulate the National Academies of Sciences, Engineering, and Medicine's Board on Behavioral, Cognitive, and Sensory Sciences (BBCSS) on recognizing the importance of this subject, as such an effort had not been performed since its 1989 report. Substantial changes in the human condition of myopia have occurred since then, along with substantive research to better understand these changes. A recalibration of our understanding of this ocular disorder and its impacts globally was long overdue.

We would like to thank our generous committee sponsors, the National Eye Institute, the American Academy of Optometry, the American Optometric Association, Health Care Alliance for Patient Safety, the Herbert Wertheim School of Optometry & Vision Science, University of California, Berkeley, Johnson & Johnson Vision, Reality Labs Research, Research to Prevent Blindness, and the Warby Parker Impact Foundation.

Molly Checksfield Dorries, the study director, demonstrated exceptional commitment in keeping the project on track. Tina Winters, program officer, provided guidance on all elements of the project, including ushering the report to publication. We also appreciate the efforts of Ashton Ray for her invaluable support. Special thanks to Kirsten Sampson Snyder for overseeing the review process, Bea Porter for her work on preparing the manuscript files, Marc DeFrancis for his adept editing skills, and Kim Halperin and Doug Sprunger for their strategic guidance on communications and development of dissemination materials.

We appreciate the commissioned paper authors who contributed enlightening and thought-provoking papers to the committee:

- Mark Bullimore, M.C. Optom, Ph.D., University of Houston (*Animal Models of Myopia: Lessons for the Understanding of Human Myopia*)
- Susana Marcos, Ph.D., University of Rochester Medical Center (*Optical and Visual Diet in Myopia*)
- Christopher Hammond, MA, MD, MRCP, FRCO, King's College London and Katie Williams, OD, Ph.D., King's College London (*Perspectives on Genetic and Environmental Factors in Myopia, Its Prediction, and the Future Direction of Research*)

- Joy Harewood, OD, FAAO, Dipl ABO, State University of New York (SUNY) College of Optometry; Melissa Contreras, OD, Marshall B. Ketchum University; Shelby Leach, OD, SUNY Optometry; Kristine Huang, OD, MPH, FAAO, Southern California College of Optometry, Marshall B. Ketchum University; and Jing Wang, PhD, SUNY Optometry (*Access to Myopia: A Scoping Review*)
- Safal Khanal, OD, Ph.D., FAAO, The University of Alabama at Birmingham School of Optometry; Síofra Harrington, Ph.D., Dublin Institute of Technology; Erin Tomiyama, OD, Ph.D., FAAO, Marshall B. Ketchum University (*Treatment of Childhood Myopia*).

This committee is grateful to all workshop presenters who provided the committee with valuable insight and expertise through presentations at public workshops: Martin Banks (University of California, Berkeley), BBCSS board member William Geisler (University of Texas at Austin), David Williams (University of Rochester), David Mackey (University of Western Australia), Daniel Ting (Singapore National Eye Centre), Pie-Chang Wu (Chang Gung University), Andrew Bastawrous (London School of Hygiene & Tropical Medicine & Peek Vision), Priya Morjaria (London School of Hygiene & Tropical Medicine & Peek Vision), Donna Fishman (National Center for Children's Vision and Eye Health), Megan Collins (Johns Hopkins University), and Jessie Mandle (Healthy Schools Campaign).

It is our hope that this consensus study sets forth a research agenda, as directed by the committee's Statement of Task, which states that the committee's final consensus report will "identify and assess the current mechanistic understanding of myopia pathogenesis and the causes of its increased prevalence, to identify knowledge gaps and barriers to progress, and to develop a research agenda aimed at better understanding the biological and environmental factors that could explain its increasing incidence."

K. Davina Frick, *Co-Chair*
Terri L. Young, *Co-Chair*
Committee on Focus on Myopia: Pathogenesis and Rising Incidence

Acronyms and Abbreviations

AACO	American Association of Certified Orthoptists
AAFP	American Academy of Family Physicians
AAO	American Academy of Ophthalmology
AAP	American Academy of Pediatrics
AAPOS	American Association for Pediatric Ophthalmology and Strabismus
AMD	age-related macular degeneration
AREDS2	Age-Related Eye-Disease Study 2
ASD	autism spectrum disorder
AUC	area under the curve
BLINK	Bifocal Lenses in Nearsighted Kids
cCSNB	complete congenital stationary night blindness
CI	confidence interval
CLEERE	Collaborative Longitudinal Evaluation of Ethnicity and Refractive Error
CMS	Center for Medicaid and Medicare Services
COMET	Correction of Myopia Evaluation Trial
COMP	cartilage olimeric matrix protein
CVD	color vision deficiency
D	diopter
DA	dopaminergic amacrine
DAC	dopaminergic amacrine cell
DIMS	defocus-incorporated multiple-segment
ECM	extracellular matrix
EPSDT	Early and Periodic Screening, Diagnostic and Treatment
ERG	electroretinogram, electroretinography
FEM	fixational eye movement
ft	feet (measure)
GAC	glucagonergic amacrine cells
GWAS	Genome-wide association study
IMI	International Myopia Institute
IPL	inner plexiform layer
ipRGCs	intrinsically photosensitive retinal ganglion cells
IRBP	inter-retinoid binding protein
LASIK	laser in situ keratomileusis
LCA	longitudinal chromatic aberration
LIM	lens-induced myopia

m	meter
MRI	magnetic resonance imaging
MTF	modulation transfer function
OCT	optical coherence tomography
Opn	opsin
PRK	photorefractive keratectomy
PSF	point spread function
RCT	randomized controlled trial
RGC	retinal ganglion cell
RGP	rigid gas-permeable
RLRL	repeated low-level red light
RPE	retinal pigment epithelium
SCORM	Singapore Cohort Study of the Risk Factors for Myopia
SMILE	small-incision lenticule extraction
VEHSS	Vision and Eye Health Surveillance System

Summary

Myopia, commonly called nearsightedness, is a refractive error of the eye in which distant objects appear blurred while close objects remain clear. Since the release of the 1989 National Academies of Sciences, Engineering, and Medicine's report, *Myopia: Prevalence and Progression,* the prevalence of myopia has increased globally. At the same time, understanding of myopia has been enhanced by advances in genetics, ocular imaging, epidemiology, and physiology, by new investigations employing animal models, by research on the visual environment, and by clinical trials of intervention strategies. This includes a growing body of evidence suggesting that increased risk of myopia may be associated with deficient outdoor exposure. Spending time outdoors, particularly in natural sunlight, appears to stimulate specific retinal pathways that have a protective effect against myopia development. Other developments since the 1989 report was released include new approaches to measuring the prevalence, prevention, and treatment of myopia. It is clear there is potential for more progress with concomitant research.

The National Academies appointed the Committee on Focus on Myopia: Pathogenesis and Rising Incidence to identify and assess the current mechanistic understanding of myopia pathogenesis and the causes of myopia's increased prevalence, to identify knowledge gaps and barriers to progress, and to develop a research agenda aimed at better understanding the biological and environmental factors that could explain its increasing incidence. Experts in vision science, visual neuroscience, ophthalmology, optometry, physical and physiological optics, experimental methodology, human factors, genetics, computer sciences, psychology, population studies, and healthcare delivery, organization, and financing were considered for committee membership to address the committee charge from a holistic perspective.

To carry out its charge, the committee reviewed the literature on six topics: global data on myopia prevalence, technologies to assess and diagnose myopia, environmental and genetic contributions to myopia onset and progression, the mechanistic causes of myopia pathogenesis, treatment optics for myopia, and barriers to vision care for children with myopia. The major conclusions and recommendations are summarized below.

UNDERSTANDING MYOPIA AND ITS PREVALENCE

Conclusions: The prevalence of myopia appears to be increasing worldwide, including in the United States. Most research comes from international studies, with limited evidence available in the United States due to a lack of standardized definitions of myopia, irregular and inconsistent screening practices locally to nationally, and the use of varied assessment techniques. (Conclusion 3-1)

Recommendations: The Centers for Disease Control and Prevention and state health departments should collect consistent, harmonized data on the prevalence of myopia in the

United States, prioritizing longitudinal surveillance on refractive error prevalence in children using standardized procedures (Recommendation 3-1). Furthermore, the Centers for Disease Control and Prevention should coordinate with the World Health Organization to create consistent, harmonized definitions and monitoring methods that would benefit the global community (Recommendation 3-2).

ASSESSMENT AND DIAGNOSTIC TECHNOLOGIES

Conclusions: There is no consensus as to the mandatory assessment and diagnostic components of a clinical examination of the myopia patient (Conclusion 4-1). Diagnostic technologies sensitive to newly understood biomarkers are under development that may improve diagnostics, management, and understanding of myopia (Conclusion 4-2).

Recommendations: To obtain a consistent retinoscopy/refractive reading, ophthalmologists and optometrists should use cycloplegic eye drops (which temporarily dilate the pupil and prevent the eye's crystalline lens from changing focus) in children (Recommendation 4-1). Researchers and developers of assessment and diagnostic technologies should design assessments and tests to better understand the myopic eye, its development, and its environment (the visual diet). This could lead to better methods to identify myopic eyes and those at risk for myopia (Recommendation 4-2).

ONSET AND PROGRESSION OF MYOPIA

Conclusions: Environmental factors, particularly the protective effect of outdoor time during daylight, appear to play a significant role in myopia development, suggesting a larger influence than genetics (Conclusions 5-1, 5-2). Important gaps in knowledge exist as to the impact on myopic eye growth of "near work" (such as reading, with the eyes focused up close), both with and without electronic devices (Conclusions 5-3, 5-6). While evidence suggests other aspects of the visual diet (like spectra and contrast from different light sources) also affect eye growth, important details are lacking (Conclusions 5-4, 5-5).

Recommendations: The Centers for Disease Control should produce evidence-based guidelines, supported by Departments of Education and healthcare providers, promoting more time outdoors (at least one hour per day) for children (Recommendation 5-1). The National Institutes of Health and other funding agencies should solicit and fund research to investigate novel questions about the genetic and environmental mechanisms in myopia (Recommendation 5-2).

MYOPIA PATHOGENESIS: FROM RETINAL IMAGE TO SCLERAL GROWTH

Conclusions: Retinal images regulate eye growth, with the entire retina (not just fovea) playing a critical role (Conclusion 6-1). The retinal network, which encodes light intensity, provides a mechanistic link between reduced time outdoors and increased incidence of myopia that is supported by multiple lines of evidence (Conclusion 6-2). The specific retinal image properties and mechanisms encoding the retino-scleral signaling cascade for homeostasis of eye growth are currently unknown (Conclusion 6-3). Animal models have provided important insights into potentially conserved processes controlling postnatal eye growth, such as visually driven signaling events in the retina, retinal pigment epithelium, and choroid that regulate the rapid remodeling of the scleral extracellular matrix, thereby changing eye size and refraction (Conclusions 6-4, 6-5).

Recommendations: Funding agencies, including the National Institutes of Health, the National Science Foundation, the Department of Defense, and private foundations, as well as industry, should seek to fund proposals across disciplines for both human and animal studies to investigate the mechanisms of emmetropization and myopia, including candidates for retino-scleral signaling, retinal neurons that detect the sign of defocus, the role of the choroid in regulating eye growth, the changes in the sclera that lead to axial elongation, gene–environment interactions, and the development of in-vitro experimental models (Recommendation 6-1). Furthermore, these funding agencies should target audacious proposals to foster the innovative, multi-disciplinary research that is needed to fully harmonize our understanding of the visual information processing by the retina that leads to changes in scleral remodeling (Recommendation 6-2). The field of myopia research should adopt an approach that considers the whole retina rather than the fovea alone (Recommendation 6-3).

CURRENT AND EMERGING TREATMENT OPTIONS FOR MYOPIA

Conclusions: Treatment options for myopia progression have increased in the last 20 years and include multifocal optical corrections and the sole pharmacological treatment: atropine eye drops (Conclusions 7-1, 7-2). Time outdoors during daylight is an emerging treatment strategy, especially in the younger years (Conclusion 7-3). Further research is needed to understand the mechanism of action of the current treatments that have limited effects and can cause rapid eye growth after cessation of treatment (Conclusions 7-4, 7-5). Safety of myopia treatments is paramount due to the probable need for daily applications (e.g. of atropine) for a decade or more of life (Conclusion 7-8). The current state of knowledge of treatment options reflects our limited understanding of both the fundamental mechanisms of eye length regulation and how treatments act to alter the progression—and perhaps even the onset—of the disease (Conclusion 7-9).

Recommendations: Funding agencies, including the National Institutes of Health, Research to Prevent Blindness, and others, should support research to develop new treatment strategies for myopia as well as to determine the mechanisms underlying current treatments. Progress in this area needs intentionally integrated, multidisciplinary research in basic and clinical vision science to understand the mechanisms by which therapies can control eye growth (Recommendation 7-1). Scientists should develop treatment strategies to minimize short- and long-term side effects and maximize safety (Recommendation 7-2). Funding for multi-center randomized clinical trials should be directed toward longer-term human studies, starting at earlier ages, to determine long-term benefits with respect to ultimate refractive error and ocular health (Recommendation 7-3).

IDENTIFYING CHILDREN WITH MYOPIA AND THE LINKS TO TREATMENT: METHODS AND BARRIERS

Conclusions: Multiple socioeconomic barriers to vision care for children exist, with the most significant being an uneven awareness of the importance of checking children's ocular health, parents' difficulties in gaining access to an eye care professional, and barriers to compliance with prescribed treatments (Conclusion 8-1). Vision screening and referrals are important for identifying children with vision impairment and facilitating access to treatment (Conclusion 8-2).

Recommendations: The U.S. Department of Health and Human Services, in collaboration with departments of education at the state level, should take measures to ensure that children receive a vision screening before first grade and a comprehensive eye exam when needed. (Recommendation 8-1). An integrated, national data surveillance system is needed for collecting state-level data on vision screening, referrals to eye care providers, sociodemographics (age, race/ethnicity, sex, and geographic location) and outcomes of referrals. This data system would not only enhance care integration and communication but also enable monitoring to ensure that follow-up care is received, especially in high-risk populations (Recommendation 8-2).

Myopia is a disease with increasing worldwide prevalence and severity--recognition of the impact of its downstream complications needs to be taken seriously. Importantly, the committee recommends that the Centers for Medicare & Medicaid Services classify myopia as a disease and therefore a medical diagnosis (Recommendation 8-5). This reclassification is to ensure efforts are undertaken not only to treat blurry vision resulting from uncorrected or under-corrected refractive error but also to ensure that stakeholders such as federal and state agencies, professional associations, patients, and caregivers are investing in the prevention and management of myopia. Funding agencies should support innovative, multidisciplinary research to identify mechanisms and novel treatments for myopia. Collaborative efforts involving healthcare providers, policymakers, researchers, and funding agencies are essential to tackle this disease effectively.

1
Introduction

In the past four decades, tremendous increases in the prevalence of myopia (near-sightedness) have been reported worldwide. In the United States, myopia, which affected 25% of the population in 1971–1972, increased in prevalence to affect 42% by 2004 (Vitale et al., 2009). Equivalent figures for some Asian countries are as high as 88% currently (Xiang & Zou, 2020). Along with the overall rise in myopia prevalence, the prevalence of high myopia (in excess of –5.00 diopters [D] myopia) has also climbed; high myopia is commonly associated with earlier onset and prolonged myopia progression. Myopia progression is defined as a clinically meaningful increase in the degree of existing myopia, that is, on the order of –0.50 D, a change sufficient to reduce visual acuity for objects seen at a distance (see Box 2-1 for an explanation of the term diopter).

If current trends continue, there will be 5 billion near-sighted individuals globally by 2050 (Holden et al., 2016). And while increased prevalence may be disconcerting, the negative effects of myopia on the eye, beyond distance blur without glasses, will also increase. As such, the goal of treating myopia is to reduce the risk of vision loss associated with myopia. The benefit of slowing down myopia growth by one diopter is associated with a 40% reduction in risk of myopic maculopathy (Bullimore & Brennan, 2019). While currently available treatments have not been able to slow myopia by more than 0.75 D in two years (Lawrenson et al., 2023), the preponderance of evidence suggests that both myopia and myopia progression should be treated. And, given the risk to ocular health in the myopic eye, these factors lend themselves to calling myopia a disease rather than a simple refractive error.

The National Academies of Sciences, Engineering, and Medicine appointed a committee to address four questions about myopia (see Box 1-1 for the full charge to the committee). This report was prepared by the appointed committee to address this charge. The topics covered in this report include the basic anatomical and physiological development of myopia; the environmental factors that might increase risk (such as near work) or offer protective effects (such as time outdoors); the inconsistent evidence around the effect of electronic devices; treatment options; screening tools and procedures; types of screening options/opportunities; diagnosis; treatment; public policy; and professional practice approaches to promote equitable and continued access to ocular healthcare for diagnosis and treatment.

The project was supported by the National Institutes of Health, specifically the National Eye Institute; the American Academy of Optometry; the American Optometric Association; Health Care Alliance for Patient Safety; the Herbert Wertheim School of Optometry & Vision Science, University of California, Berkeley; Johnson & Johnson Vision; Reality Labs Research; Research to Prevent Blindness; and the Warby Parker Impact Foundation.

BOX 1-1
Committee Charge

The National Academies propose to conduct a consensus study that will consider various aspects related to the global increase in myopia. The goals of the study are to assess the current mechanistic understanding of myopia pathogenesis and causes of its increased prevalence, to identify knowledge gaps and barriers to progress, and to develop a research agenda aimed at better understanding the biological and environmental factors that could explain its increasing incidence. Questions to be addressed include:

- Given the key findings to date from experimental models of emmetropization and myopia, what are the gaps in knowledge and/or barriers to progress in understanding the link between known risk factors for myopia development in children and the cellular and molecular biology controlling eye growth?
- Epidemiological data indicate changes in environmental factors (e.g., amount of time outdoors or near work) explain the rapid increase in myopia prevalence. What are the limits in interpreting these data? What experimental studies can address mechanistic drivers? How can these findings inform preventive and counteractive measures?
- What are the unique characteristics of electronic devices that contribute to the rapid increase in myopia? What additional research is needed to inform potential design changes to make electronic devices safer?
- Despite the existence of effective interventions, uncorrected refractive error (for myopia and hyperopia) is the leading cause of vision impairment. What are the socioeconomic, demographic, and regional barriers to diagnosing refractive correction in underserved populations? What research efforts might lead to innovative and effective methods for mitigating and overcoming these issues?

The committee will develop a final report that will present consensus findings, conclusions, and recommendations. Dissemination will be targeted to the practitioner and scientific community, educational institutions, industry and organization leaders, as well as policymakers and the public in the form of the final report, report briefs targeting distinct audiences, and presentations at professional conferences.

COMMITTEE FORMATION

Conflict-of-interest concerns were salient in this consensus study due to the involvement of industry sponsors and the tight link between industry and basic science in the field of myopia remediation. While a strict prohibition on conflicts of interest was upheld, exceptions were made if deemed unavoidable and publicly disclosed by the National Academy of Sciences. One such exception was made for committee member Donald Mutti from The Ohio State University, whose expertise was deemed essential for addressing all aspects of the committee's statement of task (see Appendix B for additional information about the disclosure of unavoidable conflict of interest).

COMMITTEE FOCUS AND PROCESS

Refractive errors arise when the eye shape hinders light from focusing properly on the retina. While its review encompassed various types of refractive errors, the committee's strongest focus was on addressing myopia. It is crucial to note that all degrees of myopia are associated with a heightened risk of serious eye conditions and morbidities, such as retinal detachment, myopic maculopathy, cataracts, and glaucoma (Haarman et al., 2020). Moreover, this risk escalates with the severity of myopia, consequently increasing the likelihood of visual impairment.

To address all components of its charge, the committee determined it would need to collect information about the factors that contribute to the onset and progression of myopia, what is known about myopia prevalence shifts in the United States and worldwide, myopia pathogenesis, options for diagnosing and treating myopia, and current vision screening and treatment practices with an emphasis on disparities. The committee was also tasked to describe "unique characteristics of electronic device contribution to the rapid increase in myopia." Due to the inconsistent evidence regarding a correlation between the use of electronic devices and myopia incidence, the committee highlighted the need for additional research to better understand this relationship.

Also, the committee underscores the separate influences genetics and environmental factors may have on the onset and progression of myopia, as these factors may lead to potentially different paths of management. Genetics may require less prevention and more management, as compared to the manipulation of environmental factors that could be minimized or altered by introducing likely public health interventions.

The committee identified areas requiring additional expertise, invited supplementary experts to present data, and commissioned papers on selected topics. The committee conducted an intensive literature review and convened a public workshop,[1] which allowed members to learn more about a range of topics related to its statement of task. During the public workshop, experts addressed the rise in myopia, exploring possible contributors and investigating screening practices, policies, and programs. Myopia experts and those adjacent to the field relayed information that helped inform committee deliberations, including presentations on novel international initiatives in Australia, Singapore, and Taiwan. Implications for the development and progression of myopia, and practices, policies, and programs aimed at identifying and reducing myopia in the United States, were also discussed.

Finally, the committee commissioned papers to delve more deeply into five key topics: animal models, genetic versus environmental factors, access to care, treatment of childhood myopia, and the optical and visual diet. Each commissioned paper enhanced the committee's understanding of key issues in this report. They are:

- *Animal Models of Myopia: Lessons for the Understanding of Human Myopia* (Bullimore, 2024);
- *Perspectives on Genetic and Environmental Factors in Myopia, Its Prediction, and the Future Direction of Research* (Hammond & Williams, 2024);

---

[1]The workshop recording is available on the project website: https://www.nationalacademies.org/event/41360_12-2023_workshop-on-the-rise-in-myopia-exploring-possible-contributors-and-investigating-screening-practices-policies-and-programs

- *Access to Myopia Care—A Scoping Review* (Harwood et al., 2024);
- *Treatment of Childhood Myopia* (Khanal et al., 2024); and
- *Optical and Visual Diet in Myopia* (Marcos, 2024).

The committee also reviewed literature related to the statement of task that was addressed in several other reports published by the National Academies, including but not limited to: *Reproducibility and Replicability in Science* (National Academies, 2019); *Making Eye Health a Population Health Imperative: Vision for Tomorrow* (National Academies, 2016); *Relieving Pain in America: A Blueprint for Transforming Prevention, Care, Education, and Research* (Institute of Medicine, 2011); *Reports of the Committee on Vision: 1947–1990* (NRC, 1990); and *Myopia: Prevalence and Progression* (NRC, 1989).

ORGANIZATION OF THE REPORT

With the above guidance in mind, the committee developed a report that addresses the statement of task in the following format:

- A primer on the basic nature of myopia and the human eye (Chapter 2)
- An overview of myopia prevalence data and emerging patterns (Chapter 3)
- Assessment and diagnostic technologies used in screenings and evaluations of myopia (Chapter 4)
- The current state of understanding the genetic and environmental contributions to the onset and progression of myopia (Chapter 5)
- Pathogenesis: Underlying ocular mechanisms responsible for myopia (Chapter 6)
- Treatment options available to individuals with myopia (Chapter 7), and
- Barriers to identifying and treating myopia (Chapter 8).

Chapters 3 through 8 present recommendations tailored to various stakeholders in research, policy, and related domains to advance our comprehension of myopia. Chapter 9 consolidates and organizes these recommendations according to the type of stakeholder, such as researchers/practitioners, policymakers, developers of assessment and diagnostic technologies, and industry leaders. Some chapters will be easier to comprehend for readers with more technical knowledge, but all chapters are written to introduce and conclude in a manner accessible to the breadth of readership. Readers of the entire document will find some repetition, as the Committee anticipates that not everyone will read the entire document and each chapter is written to be self-contained. This categorization aims to provide a framework for guiding interdisciplinary research on myopia, emphasizing the importance of collaboration across different fields.

For the benefit of any reader unfamiliar with the more specialized terms used in the fields of optometry, ophthalmology, and vision science generally, a glossary of terms related to refractive errors (specifically myopia) as well as research related to other subjects discussed in this report is provided in Appendix C.

REFERENCES

Bullimore, M. (2024). [Animal models of myopia: Lessons for the understanding of human myopia]. Commissioned Paper for the Committee on Focus on Myopia: Pathogenesis and Rising Incidence.

Bullimore, M. A., & Brennan, N. A. (2019). Myopia control: Why each diopter matters. *Optometry and Vision Science: Official Publication of the American Academy of Optometry*, *96*(6), 463–465. https://doi.org/10.1097/OPX.0000000000001367

Haarman, A. E. G., Enthoven, C. A., Tideman, J. W. L., Tedja, M. S., Verhoeven, V. J. M., & Klaver, C. C. W. (2020). The complications of myopia: A review and meta-analysis. *Investigative Ophthalmology & Visual Science*, *61*(4), 49. https://doi.org/10.1167/iovs.61.4.49

Hammond, C., & Williams, K. (2024). [Perspectives on genetic and environmental factors in myopia, its prediction, and the future direction of research]. Commissioned Paper for the Committee on Focus on Myopia: Pathogenesis and Rising Incidence.

Harewood, J., Contreras, M., Huang, K., Leach, S., & Wang, J. (2024). [Access to myopia care—A scoping review]. Commissioned Paper for the Committee on Focus on Myopia: Pathogenesis and Rising Incidence.

Holden, B. A., Fricke, T. R., Wilson, D. A., Jong, M., Naidoo, K. S., Sankaridurg, P., Wong, T. Y., Naduvilath, T. J., & Resnikoff, S. (2016). Global prevalence of myopia and high myopia and temporal trends from 2000 through 2050. *Ophthalmology*, *123*(5), 1036–1042. https://doi.org/10.1016/j.ophtha.2016.01.006

Institute of Medicine. (2011). *Relieving pain in America: A blueprint for transforming prevention, care, education, and research*. The National Academies Press. https://doi.org/10.17226/13172

Khanal, S., Harrington, S., & Tomiyama, E. (2024). [Treatment of childhood myopia]. Commissioned Paper for the Committee on Focus on Myopia: Pathogenesis and Rising Incidence.

Macros, S. (2024). [Optical and visual diet in myopia]. Commissioned Paper for the Committee on Focus on Myopia: Pathogenesis and Rising Incidence.

Lawrenson, J. G., Shah, R., Huntjens, B., Downie, L. E., Virgili, G., Dhakal, R., Verkicharla, P. K., Li, D., Mavi, S., Kernohan, A., Li, T., & Walline, J. J. (2023). Interventions for myopia control in children: A living systematic review and network meta-analysis. *The Cochrane Database of Systematic Reviews*, *2*(2), CD014758. https://doi.org/10.1002/14651858.CD014758.pub2

National Academies of Sciences, Engineering, and Medicine (National Academies). (2016). *Making eye health a population health imperative: Vision for tomorrow*. The National Academies Press. https://doi.org/10.17226/23471

___. (2019). *Reproducibility and replicability in science*. The National Academies Press. https://doi.org/10.17226/25303

National Research Council (NRC). (1989). *Myopia: Prevalence and progression*. National Academies Press. https://doi.org/10.17226/1420

___. (1990). *Reports of the committee on vision: 1947–1990*. The National Academies Press. https://doi.org/10.17226/1456

Vitale, S., Sperduto, R. D., & Ferris, F. L., 3rd. (2009). Increased prevalence of myopia in the United States between 1971–1972 and 1999–2004. *Archives of Ophthalmology*, *127*(12), 1632–1639. https://doi.org/10.1001/archophthalmol.2009.303

Xiang, Z. Y., & Zou, H. D. (2020) Recent epidemiology study data of myopia. *Journal of Ophthalmology*, *2020*, 4395278. https://doi.org/10.1155/2020/4395278

2
Myopia and the Human Eye: A Primer

This chapter lays the groundwork for the remainder of the report by providing fundamental information about myopia and the eye. Descriptions and definitions of components of the eye are included here (and also in the Glossary) to assist readers unfamiliar with the eye and/or myopia in understanding the remaining chapters.

The concept of myopia was first described in 350 BCE by Aristotle, who noted that myopic individuals narrowed their eyelids to decrease the aperture of light (de Jong, 2018). Many decades later, squeezing of the eyelids was associated with causing a pinhole effect (stenopeic slit) to elicit a sharper image (de Jong, 2018). The smaller pupillary aperture allows for a narrower beam of light rays to reach the central macular retina rather than stimulating the extra-macular retina with indirect, aberrant rays. The term myopia originates from the Greek word μφϖψ, derived from μωειν (*muein*, to close) and ϖψ (*ops*, the eye), which together means short-sighted (de Jong, 2018). By the 1700s, it was shown that nearsighted eyes are longer in length from front to back (axial length) relative to non-myopic eyes (Glauder, 1751).

Today, much is known about eye growth from birth. The length of the eye can have a strong influence on what is known as refractive error of the eye, with farsighted eyes being too short (hyperopia) and nearsighted eyes being too long (myopia) to allow for all optical component contributions to focus an object of regard on the retinal plane. (The component contributions include corneal curvature and thickness, lens curvature and thickness, and the optical indices of the cornea, lens, and vitreous humor). It is known that while newborns have a wide range of refractive error, including hyperopia and myopia, in general they are hyperopic (Cook & Glasscock, 1951; Mutti et al., 2005; see Figure 2-1). Refractive error due to optical component mismatch causes blurred vision. The infant eye grows to focus light more clearly on the retinal plane, generally starting from a smaller axial length consistent with hyperopia, a refinement process in response to visual blur that is called emmetropization. Myopia develops when the combined optical component powers are too strong for the eye's axial length, focusing the image in front of the retinal plane with a concomitant defocused image on the retina (see Figure 2-2). In common childhood myopia, an excessive increase in axial length appears to be the cause.

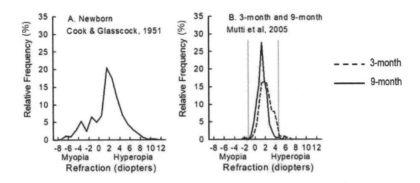

FIGURE 2-1 Relative frequency (%) of refractive errors in newborns and infants. Infants with no refractive error (emmetropia) are plotted at 0.
SOURCE: Committee-generated from data in Cook & Glasscock, 1951, Mutti et al., 2005.

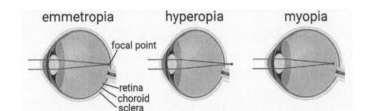

FIGURE 2-2 Relationship between axial length and (de)focus.
NOTE: This figure illustrates how axial length of the eye affects whether what is being viewed is focused on the retina (emmotropia [normal vision]), behind the retina (hyperopia [farsightedness]), or in front of the retina (myopia [nearsightedness]).
SOURCE: Reprinted from Tkatchenko & Tkatchenko, 2019, with permission from Elsevier.

Myopia occurs when the homeostasis between the length and shape of the eye versus its focusing elements fails to occur. Major lines of evidence pinpoint the role of the retina and early visual encoding in regulating eye growth (Rohrer & Stell, 1994). The inability of the optics of the eye to match the elongating eye in myopia suggests that whereas in an emmetrope a coordinated and intricate relationship between the eye's optics and its length/shape is tightly maintained, this coordination is not the case in a myope. However, both the mechanism(s) responsible for this coordinated growth (emmetropization) and those leading to myopia development have remained elusive. (Also, see Box 5-2: Are mechanisms signaling normal eye growth and myopia the same?) What is known is explained in Chapters 5 and 6.

The eyes in most children grow to near-emmetropia or to be slightly farsighted within the first year of life (Mayer et al., 2005; Mutti, 2007; Mutti et al., 2005). However, even after infancy it is theorized that eyes receive "stop" and "go" signals that regulate growth (Rohrer & Stell, 1994). If these refractive growth signals are disrupted or abnormal, the eye can elongate too much. Once an eye is nearsighted, typically it will continue to grow and become progressively more nearsighted (Gwiazda et al., 1993; Norton, 1999; Wildsoet, 1997); wearing a regular pair of glasses or contact lenses does not prevent this further progression (Hou et al., 2018; Walline et al., 2020). Chapter 7 summarizes what is known about the effects of treatment.

The average age of onset of myopia in U.S. children is roughly 11 years old, and onset generally ranges from age 7 to age 16 (Kleinstein, 2012). After the onset, in about half of myopic

U.S. children there is a slow increase in the amount of myopia, a process that stabilizes around age 15. About 75% of myopic eyes are stable by age 18, but 4% may continue to lengthen to age 24 (COMET Group, 2013).

BOX 2-1
What Is a Diopter?

A diopter (D) is the unit of measurement for any focusing lens, such as for a refractive error prescription (spectacles or contact lenses), a telescope or microscope, or the natural lens inside of one's eye. Thus, a higher (stronger) prescription will be indicated by larger D values, whereas a milder prescription will have smaller D values.

There is a reciprocal relationship between refractive error in diopters and the focal length of the spectacle lens (measured in meters) needed to achieve clear vision. For example, a lens with 1 diopter (1 D) strength will bring an object into focus at 1 meter. A lens with a 2 diopter (2 D) strength will have a focal length of 1/2 meter. A lens with a 3 diopter strength (3 D) will have a focal length of 1/3 meter. Thus, a shorter focal length means a stronger focusing power for the lens.

Convex-shaped lenses, such as the natural lens inside the eye, converge the light passing through them, bringing the light to a focal point. By contrast, concave-shaped lenses diverge the light passing through them, spreading the light into a wider optical path (see bottom panel of Figure 2-3). To signify their converging or diverging effect, convex lenses, which are used to correct farsightedness, have a positive D value, whereas concave lenses, which are used to correct nearsightedness, have a minus D value.

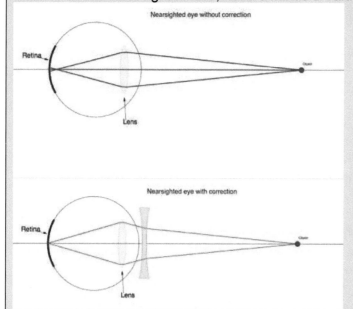

FIGURE 2-3 Correction of nearsighted defocus with a concave-shaped diverging lens.
SOURCE: Reprinted from Keramati, 2019, under a Creative Commons Attribution-NonCommercial-ShareAlike 4.0 International License (https://creativecommons.org/licenses/by-nc-sa/4.0).

MYOPIC BLUR

Light from distant objects enters the eye in parallel rays. The eye has two refractive elements, the cornea and the lens, that transmit the parallel rays through the eye and attempt to converge the light to a perfect point on the retina. When this happens, the eye is in perfect focus and the individual sees clearly.

If the light rays entering the eye focus behind the back of the eye or the retina, the eye is too short compared to its optical power. This condition is known as hyperopia or farsightedness. In children and younger adults, the eye can compensate for mild and moderate amounts of hyperopia by making the crystalline lens more convex, thus converging the light more strongly on the plane of the retina of the short eye. This dynamic focusing process is called accommodation and usually occurs quickly and without conscious effort (although from mid-adulthood, the crystalline lens gradually loses its elasticity and accommodation becomes increasingly difficult).

If the light rays entering the eye focus in front of the retina, the eye is too long for its optical power. This represents the myopic or nearsighted eye. The eye itself cannot do anything to compensate for even the smallest amounts of myopia. The eyelids can squeeze together or squint, which creates a pinhole effect. Such a pinhole momentarily reduces the blurriness of vision when the blur is from refractive error, improving central vision, but peripheral vision is then dramatically reduced, making a pinhole an infeasible management option for myopia in daily life. The options for managing the side effect of blur from the myopic eye are therefore generally centered on optical devices such as glasses or surgical procedures.

ANATOMY OF THE EYE

The human eye is a complex organ with many components that contribute to its functioning. Figure 2-4 shows the components that are mentioned in this report. Each of these components is then briefly described.

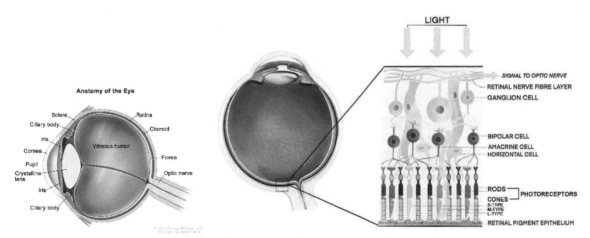

FIGURE 2-4 Components of the eye discussed in this report.
SOURCE: (A) © 2014 Terese Winslow LLC, U.S. Govt. has certain rights (updated from figure appearing in National Cancer Institute, 2008); (B) adapted from Kilduff, 2020, with permission from Gene Vision.

Amacrine cells—A class of retinal neurons that interact with ganglion cells and bipolar cells. Amacrine cells are diverse in their structural and biochemical features, suggesting they perform a variety of functions. For example, the starburst class of amacrine cells plays a role in detecting the direction of a moving image on the retina.

Choroid—A layer of tissue lying beneath the retina that has a very rich blood supply. A key role of the choroid is to provide nutrients and oxygen for the retina.

Ciliary body—The tissue that produces nutrient fluid for the eye and that contains the ciliary muscle, the involuntary smooth muscle that controls the optical power of the crystalline lens by slightly altering its shape.

Cornea—A transparent tissue about half a millimeter thick that allows light to enter the eye. The curved shape of the cornea is responsible for focusing light rays toward the crystalline lens and retina. The cornea is part of the tough, outer shell of the eye.

Crystalline lens—A transparent, biconvex structure situated inside the eye. After passing through the cornea and pupil, light passes through the 3-to-4-millimeter-thick crystalline lens before reaching the retina. The curvature of this lens is altered without conscious effort by the ciliary muscle (see above) to help precisely focus the retinal image, for example steepening in curvature to help focus light from nearby objects, in a process called accommodation. Beyond age 40 years, the crystalline lens gradually loses the flexibility needed to change shape, which leads to difficulty focusing on near objects such as smaller fonts or print—a condition termed presbyopia.

Fovea—The area of the central retina with the highest density of cone photoreceptors, which provides maximum visual acuity.

Iris—A highly pigmented tissue that serves the same function in the eye as an aperture stop in a camera, namely, to control the amount of light that enters the eye. In bright conditions the iris constricts, while in dim conditions the iris dilates. The iris also determines a person's eye color, e.g., blue or brown eyes.

Macula—A round area at the center of the retina, or the back of the eye, that is responsible for central vision, color vision, and fine details. It is about 5 millimeters across and 250 microns thick and contains blood vessels and nerve fibers. The fovea constitutes the central part of the macula.

Optic nerve—A bundle of approximately 1 million nerve fibers that travels from the eye to the brain. The nerve fibers are the axons of retinal ganglion cells; they convey information about the visual image, including its color, whether it is moving, and its level of contrast.

Pupil—A circular opening formed by the iris that controls the level of light entering the eye. The size of the pupil changes reflexively in response to the intensity of incident light. When the pupil constricts, it has an optical effect like a pinhole; this pinhole effect reduces retinal image blurriness in an eye with refractive error.

Retina—A multilayered tissue lining the inner surface of the back half of the eye. The retina is responsible for detecting light, performing the first steps in processing the visual signal and sending neural signals about the visual image to the brain. The neural cells of the retina (see rods and cones, below) perform a diverse range of computations to sense not only color and brightness but also movement, speed/direction, and other image features.

Retinal ganglion cells—The terminal neurons for processing the retinal signal. The axons of the retinal ganglion cells form the optic nerve, which sends visual information to the brain. More than 18 different types of retinal ganglion cells have been identified, depending on the species. Some retinal ganglion cells contain photosensitive pigments and can be directly stimulated by light or through rod and cone pathways, such as intrinsically photosensitive retinal ganglion cells (ipRGCs) that express Opn4 or melanopsin. Other photopigments found in retinal ganglion cells include neuropsin (Opn5) and encephalopsin (Opn3).

Retinal pigment epithelium—A single layer of highly specialized cells, situated between the retinal photoreceptors and the choroid. These cells have many functions that are essential to healthy functioning of the retina.

Rods and cones—Light-sensitive cells in the retina, also known as photoreceptors. Rods are specialized for detecting images under dim illumination and are more abundant in the periphery of the retina than in the central, foveal region. Cones are specialized for detecting light under bright conditions and are much more abundant in the central, foveal region. The human retina contains three types of cones, each most sensitive to either blue (*s*hort wavelength), green (*m*edium wavelength), or red (*l*ong wavelength) light and therefore known as S-, M- and L-cones, for short.

Sclera—An opaque, tough layer of tissue that forms the outer shell of the middle and back of the eye. The tissue of the sclera is continuous with the cornea. The sclera largely determines the size and shape of the eye.

Vitreous—A transparent gel that fills the cavity between the crystalline lens and the retina. By occupying much of the eye's volume, the vitreous acts in concert with the sclera to maintain the shape of the eye. Also known as the vitreous humor.

MYOPIA—MOVING FORWARD

Although refractive error and myopia have been studied for hundreds of years, limited evidence is available to fully understand the progression of myopia and its rising incidence. While lifestyle-related risk factors in people's daily lives may have changed over that time, their effect on eyesight must still operate through basic anatomical and physiological development. This report seeks to use the most current knowledge on the biological regulation of eye growth to understand how changes in modern lifestyle may have made humans more susceptible to the development of myopia.

Having set the foundation for understanding the structural features of the myopic eye and its etiology, the key then is to understand what we know about managing the risk of incidence and the risk of progression, and how these risks play out not just over childhood and adolescence but over a lifetime of risks of eye conditions associated with myopia. To pull all of this together as a societal public health issue rather than simply an individual medical decision-making exercise, this report also explores what is known about disparities in the screening for, diagnosis of, and effective management of myopia over the life course.

REFERENCES

COMET Group. (2013). Myopia stabilization and associated factors among participants in the Correction of Myopia Evaluation Trial (COMET). *Investigative Ophthalmology & Visual Science*, *54*(13), 7871–7884. https://doi.org/10.1167/iovs.13-12403

Cook, R. C., & Glasscock, R. E. (1951). Refractive and ocular findings in the newborn. *American Journal of Ophthalmology*, *34*(10), 1407–1413. https://doi.org/10.1016/0002-9394(51)90481-3

de Jong P. T. V. M. (2018). Myopia: Its historical contexts. *The British Journal of Ophthalmology*, *102*(8), 1021–1027. https://doi.org/10.1136/bjophthalmol-2017-311625

Glauder, G. F. (1751). Hermann Boerhavens Abhandlung von Augenkrankheiten und deroselben Kur. Herman Boerhaaven's treatise on eye diseases and their cure.

Gwiazda, J., Thorn, F., Bauer, J., & Held, R. (1993). Myopic children show insufficient accommodative response to blur. *Investigative Ophthalmology & Visual Science, 34*(3), 690–694. https://pubmed.ncbi.nlm.nih.gov/8449687/

Hou, W., Norton, T. T., Hyman, L., Gwiazda, J., & COMET Group. (2018). Axial elongation in myopic children and its association with myopia progression in the Correction of Myopia Evaluation Trial. *Eye & Contact Lens, 44*(4), 248–259. https://doi.org/10.1097/ICL.0000000000000505

Keramati, B. (2019). *Introduction to physics: An outline of selected topics.* Pressbooks. https://pressbooks.pub/introphys1/

Kilduff, C. (2020). Microscopic view of the cells in the retina. Figure in retina. *Gene Vision.* https://gene.vision/retina/

Kleinstein, R. N., Sinnott, L. T., Jones-Jordan, L. A., Sims, J., Zadnik, K., & Collaborative Longitudinal Evaluation of Ethnicity and Refractive Error Study Group. (2012). New cases of myopia in children. *Archives of Ophthalmology, 130*(10), 1274–1279. https://doi.org/10.1001/archophthalmol.2012.1449

Mayer, D. L., Beiser, A. S., Warner, A. F., Pratt, E. M., Raye, K. N., & Lang, J. M. (1995). Monocular acuity norms for the Teller Acuity Cards between ages one month and four years. *Investigative Ophthalmology & Visual Science, 36*(3), 671–685.

Mutti D. O. (2007). To emmetropize or not to emmetropize? The question for hyperopic development. *Optometry and Vision Science, 84*(2), 97–102. https://doi.org/10.1097/OPX.0b013e318031b079

Mutti, D. O., Mitchell, G. L., Jones, L. A., Friedman, N. E., Frane, S. L., Lin, W. K., Moeschberger, M. L., & Zadnik, K. (2005). Axial growth and changes in lenticular and corneal power during emmetropization in infants. *Investigative Ophthalmology & Visual Science, 46*(9), 3074–3080. https://doi.org/10.1167/iovs.04-1040

National Cancer Institute. (2008). Eye anatomy [Image]. https://visualsonline.cancer.gov/details.cfm?imageid=7161

Norton T. T. (1999). Animal models of myopia: Learning how vision controls the size of the eye. *ILAR Journal, 40*(2), 59–77. https://doi.org/10.1093/ilar.40.2.59

Rohrer, B., & Stell, W. K. (1994). Basic fibroblast growth factor (bFGF) and transforming growth factor beta (TGF-beta) act as stop and go signals to modulate postnatal ocular growth in the chick. *Experimental Eye Research, 58*(5), 553–561. https://doi.org/10.1006/exer.1994.1049

Tkatchenko, T. V., & Tkatchenko, A. V. (2019). Pharmacogenomic approach to antimyopia drug development: Pathways lead the way. *Trends in Pharmacological Sciences, 40*(11), 833–852. https://doi.org/10.1016/j.tips.2019.09.009

Walline, J. J., Walker, M. K., Mutti, D. O., Jones-Jordan, L. A., Sinnott, L. T., Giannoni, A. G., Bickle, K. M., Schulle, K. L., Nixon, A., Pierce, G. E., Berntsen, D. A., & BLINK Study Group. (2020). Effect of high add power, medium add power, or single-vision contact lenses on myopia progression in children: The BLINK randomized clinical trial. *JAMA, 324*(6), 571–580. https://doi.org/10.1001/jama.2020.10834

Wildsoet C. F. (1997). Active emmetropization—Evidence for its existence and ramifications for clinical practice. *Ophthalmic & Physiological Optics, 17*(4), 279–290.

3

Understanding Myopia and Its Prevalence

This chapter establishes the significance of myopia by examining prevalence throughout the world and in the United States. It also examines how myopia is defined and measured, which is fundamental to interpreting the other chapters. Readers will find that the prevalence data on myopia motivate this report and underlie the urgency in determining the mechanisms of the disease's development.

The prevalence of myopia appears to be increasing worldwide (Holden et al., 2016), including in the United States (Tailor et al., 2024; Vitale et al., 2009), and is predicted to continue to increase globally. The Brien Holden Vision Institute has suggested that 50% of the world's population will be nearsighted by 2050, up from 23% in 2000 (Holden et al., 2016). The National Eye Institute predicts that 44.5 million people in the United States will be nearsighted in 2050, with greater increases among African and Hispanic Americans (National Eye Institute, 2020). Although prevalence is clearly high, the exact estimate will depend on the definition of myopia, how myopia is measured, and at what age it is measured.

The measurement of myopia's current prevalence in the United States is only an imperfect estimate. National data are now more than 20 years old, so they precede the widespread use of laptops, tablets, smartphones, and other personal digital devices, as well as the recent indoor quarantine period induced by the COVID-19 pandemic. Most recent population data are limited to specific regions of the country and therefore may be unrepresentative in terms of race/ethnicity, level of education, access to care, and a variety of other factors. Since myopia generally increases in severity with age during childhood, prevalence data vary by the age studied. Finally, myopia (and refractive error in general) can be measured and defined in multiple ways, making comparisons across studies difficult.

This section of the chapter describes the data on prevalence in the United States in the context of worldwide changes in prevalence and using data from specific global locations that are possibly informative about mechanisms. The committee chose to concentrate on rigorous studies with representative samples, studies that use the same method longitudinally or cross-sectionally at a variety of ages. Interestingly, the rate at which myopia progresses in individuals does not appear to be changing (Chandler et al., 2023; Khanal & Dhakal, 2024; see Box 3-1). Therefore, the focus of this chapter will be to identify what is known about overall prevalence and best practices to determine current prevalence more accurately in the United States, including surveillance and accountability.

BOX 3-1
Higher Prevalence of Myopia but Same Rate of Progression

Has the rate of myopia progression for school-aged children become faster as myopia has become more common? A comparison between late 20th century studies and more recent work suggests that the answer is no. Myopia may be more common, but the rate of progression has largely remained the same across the last 60 years, at least in the United States. The data come primarily from observational studies and clinical trial control groups. The previous 1989 report on myopia from the National Research Council Committee on Vision summarized the existing literature from the 1960s through the early 1980s. Myopia progression at that time was typically −0.50 diopters* (D) per year with a range of −0.30 to −0.60 D/year. A 2012 meta-analysis summarizing literature from 1990 to 2012 found similar values (Donovan et al., 2012). The 2012 study's estimate was that myopia progressed at an annual rate of −0.55 D/year (95% CI = −0.39 to −0.72 D/year) for children of European heritage who had a mean age of 9.3 years when progression was measured.

More recent clinical trial results show similar rates of progression for young myopic children. In studies of multifocal contact lenses, Chamberlain et al. (2019) and Walline et al. (2020) reported −0.45 D/year and −0.38 D/year average annual myopia progression, respectively, in their control groups not receiving that treatment. In randomized studies of the effectiveness of low-dose atropine for slowing myopia progression in children, Repka et al. (2024) and Zadnik et al. (2023) reported annual progression rates in control groups receiving placebo (i.e., children without atropine treatment) of −0.41 D/year and −0.43 D/year, respectively. As noted in Chapter 5, the age at onset of myopia in U.S. children generally ranges from 7 years to 16 years (Kleinstein et al., 2012). For about 50% of children with myopia, the condition stabilizes, meaning it is no longer increasing, by age 15, and in 75% of children with myopia by age 18 (COMET Group, 2013). Younger children have faster rates of myopia progression (Chua et al., 2016; Jones-Jordan et al., 2021) and data from China suggest that recent cohorts of children are becoming myopic at younger ages (Wang et al., 2021). These two factors combined could increase the overall rate of progression when averaged across ages. The rate of progression at a given age, however, appears to be stable over time.

*For an explanation of diopters, see Box 2-1 in Chapter 2.

MEASURING MYOPIA

Refractive error is usually measured as the spherical equivalent in units of diopters (D). Spherical equivalent refractive error takes account of the patient's spherical refractive error as well as any astigmatism. The threshold for classifying a patient as myopic varies from study to study; most studies use a threshold level of spherical equivalent refractive error of −0.50, −0.75, or −1.00 D. Other researchers take account of astigmatism by defining myopia in any "meridian" or in one specific meridian; that is, along any astigmatic axis or along one specific axis. For example, an eye could potentially be farsighted in one meridian but myopic in another meridian, due to the presence of astigmatism (see Figure 3-1 and Table 3-1).

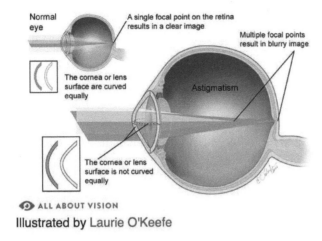

Illustrated by Laurie O'Keefe

FIGURE 3-1 Illustration of an eye with astigmatism and one with perfect optical balance.
NOTE: The larger image shows an eye with uneven optical power in the vertical and horizonal meridians, which produces multiple focal points on the retina and a blurry image. The smaller image shows a normal eye with perfect optical balance between meridians, which produces a single focal point on the retina in shown at the top for comparison.
SOURCE: Illustration by Laurie O'Keefe in Mangan, 2019. Image used with permission from AllAboutVision.com.

Another issue in measurement is whether the refractive measurements are made while the child's focusing system is temporarily paralyzed using eye drops that induce cycloplegia, which is a state of temporary paresis of the ciliary body muscles. Because a child's eye has a dynamic accommodative range in those muscles, changing focus from near to far distances with little effort, myopia may be overestimated without cycloplegia. With the focusing power made static using cycloplegic eye drops, a more predictable and reproducible measure of refractive error can be obtained. Empirical data comparing pre- and post-cycloplegic data show that teenage measurements are, on average, 0.26 D more myopic before cycloplegia. Adults have a less dynamic focusing range, and cyclopleged versus non-cyclopleged refractions are usually similar after approximately age 20 (Sanfillippo et al., 2014).

TABLE 3-1 Myopia as Studied

Study/Project	Definition of Myopia	Definition of Astigmatism	Definition of Aniso-Metropia
CLEERE (Collaborative Longitudinal Evaluation of Ethnicity and Refractive Error) Jones-Jordan et al., 2010	−0.75 D or more myopia in both meridians (by cycloplegic autorefraction)		
COMET (Correction of Myopia Evaluation Trial) Hyman et al., 2001	SER between −1.25 D and −4.50 D	Astigmatism < or = 1.50 D	Aniso < 1.00 D
IMI (International Myopia Institute) Flitcroft et al., 2019	SER of an eye is ≤ −0.50 D when ocular accommodation is relaxed		

BLINK (**Bifocal Lenses in Nearsighted Kids**) **Walline et al., 2020**	−0.75 D to −5.00 D of spherical component myopia	Astigmatism < 1.00 D	
MOSAIC (**Myopia Outcome Study of Atropine in Children**) **Loughman et al., 2024**	SER ≤ −0.50 D in both eyes		
MTS1 (**Myopia Treatment Study 1**) **Repka et al., 2023**	−1.00 D to −6.00 D SER	Astigmatism of 1.50 D or less in both eyes	Aniso < 1.00 D
CHAMPS (**Childhood Atropine for Myopia Progression**) **Zadnik et al., 2023**	−0.50 D to −6.00 D SER	No worse than −1.50 D astigmatism	
LAMP (**Low-concentration Atropine for Myopia Progression**) **Yam et al., 2019**	At least 1.0 D	Astigmatism of 2.5 D or less	
DOT (**Diffusion Optics Technology by SightGlass**) **Rappon et al., 2023**	SER between −0.75 and −4.50 D	Astigmatism greater than 1.25 D	No more than 1.50 D aniso
HALT (**Highly Aspherical Lenslet Technology by Essilor Stellest**) **Bao et al., 2022**	Cycloplegic SER between −0.75 D and −4.75 D	Astigmatism not exceeding 1.50 D	Aniso not exceeding 1.00 D based on SER

NOTE: Various large-scale randomized clinical trials have studied myopia using various quantitative definitions.

Some investigators simply ask participants (or their parents) if they are farsighted or nearsighted. Others evaluate the individual's most recent spectacle prescription. Still others use more objective means, such as an automated measure of myopia or a retinoscopy session with an eye care provider. Measurement error is reduced when objective measures are used. However, it may not be feasible at the population level to collect prevalence data using cycloplegic eye drops and an automated instrument. Screening data from uncyclopleged eyes and automated instruments are useful, but they might cause the rate of myopia to be over- or underestimated due to variable screening protocols within or outside of school systems. Diagnostic codes and their use can also be monitored, but not all eye care providers use the same codes, if they use any at all. Table 3-2 summarizes the strengths and weaknesses of different ways of measuring myopia in an individual and of estimating its prevalence at the population level. Table 3-3 presents options for reporting myopia in prevalence evaluations, and their feasibility at the population level and at the individual/local level.

The age at which myopia is measured may also affect prevalence rates. Data from the Collaborative Longitudinal Evaluation of Ethnicity and Refractive Error suggest that the average age of onset for myopia is 11 years old and ranges primarily from 7 to 16 years of age (Kleinstein et al., 2012). Therefore, if myopia is measured in the preschool years, the prevalence will be much smaller than it would be if it were measured in the late school-aged years. Some studies measure myopia in older generations and compare that to myopia prevalence in younger generations of the same population. If prevalence were increasing, one would expect to find more in younger generations. In fact, this is what was found, for example, in Singapore where one researcher measured the prevalence of myopia (worse than −0.50 D spherical equivalent) to be 81.6% in young adults (Koh et al., 2014) and another found myopia prevalence, using the same magnitude of myopia, to be 38.9% in adults over age 40 (Pan et al., 2013).

A small caveat on how myopia is measured is related to the natural aging of the human eye. Changes in the anterior part of the eye, including natural yellowing and hardening of the crystalline lens, are associated with aging, and these can lead to an increase in a person's nearsightedness without a change in the axial length. Similarly, natural changes in the power of the crystalline lens after age 50 years shift refractive error toward hyperopia, complicating comparisons between generations (Bomotti et al., 2018; Mutti & Zadnik, 2000).

TABLE 3-2 Methods for Detecting and Measuring Myopia

Ways to Measure Myopia	Pros	Cons	Feasible at the Population Level[a]	Feasible at the individual/ Local Level[b]
Distance visual acuity	Snellen or pediatric visual acuity charts are readily available.	The assumption that poor vision at distance indicates myopia may lead to over-estimation given that other refractive errors, amblyopia, and other conditions of the eye may result in poor distance vision.	Yes	Yes
Photorefraction	Takes fewer than 30 seconds to obtain measure in a cooperative child, including preschool-aged or younger children.	Instrument-based techniques may be cost-prohibitive; without cycloplegia, estimates of myopia may be inflated due to a child's strong accommodative system (Hu et al., 2015; Li et al., 2019)	Yes	Yes
Autorefraction	If used under cycloplegic conditions, this represents possibly one of the most accurate and objective	Instrument-based techniques may be cost-prohibitive. Without cycloplegia, estimates of myopia may be inflated due to	Possible, but an autorefractor is generally less portable than a photorefractor, which is often handheld;	Yes

	measures of refractive error.	strong accommodative system of child (Hu et al., 2015; Li et al., 2019).	Not readily feasible with cycloplegia but can be used for noncycloplegic estimates.	
Retinoscopy	Under cycloplegic conditions, this represents one of the most accurate and objective measures of refractive error.	Requires specially trained individuals, largely eye care professionals.	Not readily feasible under cycloplegic conditions. Possible under noncycloplegic conditions, but requires an expert, and the measure may be less consistent than under cycloplegic conditions.	Yes

[a]Population level: large-scale evaluations of prevalence including vision screenings in community/school/country.

[b]Individual/local level: smaller-scale, more in-depth evaluation, including comprehensive eye exams within a clinical office setting.

TABLE 3-3 Ways to Report Myopia When Evaluating Prevalence and Their Feasibility

Ways to Define Myopia	Feasible at the Population Level[a]	Feasible at the Individual/Local Level[b]
Magnitude in diopters	Yes	Yes
Magnitude in millimeters (length of the eyeball)	No	Yes
Self-report	Yes	Yes
Prescription evaluation	Yes	Yes
Lensometry (measuring prescription of spectacle lenses using an optical instrument)	No	Yes
Medicaid or other use of ICD-10 diagnostic codes[c]	No	Yes

[a]Population level: large-scale evaluations of prevalence including vision screenings in community/school/country.

[b]Individual/local level: smaller-scale, more in-depth evaluation, including comprehensive eye exams within a clinical office setting.

[c]ICD-10 codes are applicable diagnosis codes that providers and suppliers utilize when submitting medical claims to Medicare.

WORLDWIDE PREVALENCE

Myopia is one of the most prevalent eye disorders worldwide and is a major cause of visual impairment (Bourne et al., 2013; Resnikoff et al., 2008). The highest prevalence is observed in well-documented studies performed in countries in East and South-East Asia: 80–90% of children ages 17–18 from urban regions of Hong Kong, Singapore, China, Taiwan, and Japan are myopic (Morgan & Rose, 2005; Morgan et al., 2012) and evidence of steady increases in prevalence during the last 10 years (see, for example, Gwon & Lee, 2023 for longitudinal data from over 2 million Korean men reporting for mandatory physical exams at age 19). A comprehensive study of all 19-year-old males residing in urban Seoul, Korea, found an astonishing prevalence of over 96% (Jung et al., 2012).[1] In European countries, the overall prevalence of myopia is 24% across all age categories and 47% in young adults (Williams et al., 2015).

The rising prevalence in China was recently documented in a detailed analysis of 7.5 million Chinese children, which used data from 187 individual studies conducted in schools to calculate prevalence in five time periods from 1998 to 2015 (Wang et al., 2023b). There was a steady increase in the prevalence of myopia, especially in rural communities where the rate rose by 5% to 7% every 5 years, as compared to a slower but steady increase in urban communities (see Figure 3-2). Other studies from Asia found prevalence rates for high myopia already varying between 15% and 25% by the age of 10 (Matsumura & Hirai, 1999).

There data from China indicate a further increase in urban communities during the pandemic for children in Grades 1–9 (Wang et al., 2023a). In Hong Kong, where school closures were of longer duration than in mainland China, cross-sectional data from cyclopleged refraction indicates that the prevalence of myopia[2] in children 6–7 years old, which had been stable from 2015–2019, was higher during and after the lockdown (2020 and 2021; Zhang et al., 2023). At the same time, parental questionnaires indicated that the decrease in time outdoors and increased time on screens and doing near work that characterized the lockdown period did not completely reverse after it was lifted.

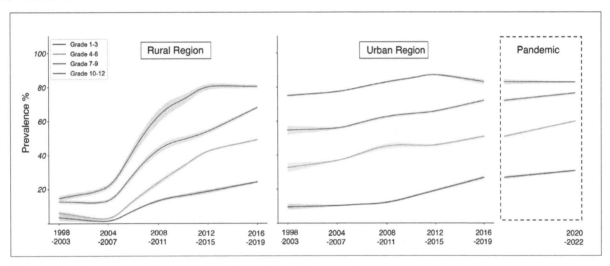

FIGURE 3-2 Prevalence of myopia in 7.5 million Chinese children in rural and urban regions by period of measurement.
NOTE: The left and middle panels show data from rural and urban regions, respectively; the right panel shows urban regions tested during the pandemic.
SOURCE: Reprinted from Wang et al., 2023b, under a Creative Commons Attribution-NonCommercial-No Derivatives 4.0 International License (https://creativecommons.org/licenses/by-nc-nd/4.0/).

While the largest increase in myopia has occurred in Asian populations, increases have also been observed in the United States and other countries worldwide (Sankaridurg et al., 2021; Vitale et al., 2009). It is estimated that by the year 2050, half of the world's population will be

---

[1]Worse than −0.50.

[2]−0.5D or worse.

myopic (3.6–6.1 billion), and almost 10% will be highly myopic and thus at greater risk for retinal issues and other comorbidities (Holden et al., 2016). The impact on those afflicted and on society is already significant, with reduction of or lost productivity and quality of life, as well as a high health care burden and costs (Sankaridurg et al., 2021).

Divergent Prevalence in Children by Age and Ethnicity

Several studies report on the prevalence of refractive error and myopia in children, generally finding lower prevalence in younger children and differences according to ethnicity (Goh et al., 2005; Kim et al., 2020; Logan et al., 2011; Matsumura & Hirai, 1999; Morgan et al., 2010; Vitale et al., 2009). For example, Czepita et al. (2008) studied myopia in Polish children from rural regions between the ages of 10 and 14. Among these children, all from the southeast part of Poland, they found a myopia prevalence rate of 6.3% at the age of 10, which increased to a prevalence of 9.7% at the age of 12. In another Polish study in a semirural population of children ages 6–18, the prevalence of myopia using the same methodology and cut-off was slightly higher: 11.0% in those age 10 and 14.4% in those age 12 (Czepita et al., 2008). Two studies in the United Kingdom of children of European descent, which looked at children ages 6 to 7 and ages 12 to 13, respectively, found a myopia prevalence of 2.8%–5.7% in the younger group and of 17.7%–18.6% in the older age group (Logan et al., 2011; O'Donoghue et al., 2010). All four of those studies used the same definition of myopia, namely at least −0.5D.

Ojaimi et al. (2005) studied schoolchildren ages 5 to 8 in Australia and found an overall myopia prevalence of 1.4%. They found a significant difference between children of European descent (0.79%) and those belonging to other racial groups (2.73%, $p < 0.001$). The Sydney Myopia Study (Ip et al., 2008), which examined children ages 11 to 14, determined an overall myopia prevalence of 11.9% but also found large differences in prevalence between children of European descent (4.6%) and those of East Asian descent (39.5%). In a representative sample of South Korean children aged 5–18 years old, prevalence of myopia was over 75% by age 13 (Kim et al., 2020). Comparatively, South Asian children also have relatively high prevalence rates from early childhood: 10.8% in those ages 6 to 7 and 36.8% in those ages 12 to 13 (Logan et al., 2011; see Goh et al., 2005 for similar data from Malaysia). These studies also used the same definition of myopia, namely at least −0.5D.

Lifestyle and Urbanization: Potential Causes of Divergent Prevalence

Although these ethnic differences are striking, they may reflect lifestyle differences among populations through which environmental factors may affect the onset and progression of myopia. These factors could include time spent outdoors, amount of near work, and educational exposure (see Chapter 5 on onset and progression). There is no genetic reason to expect major ethnic differences (Tedja et al., 2018). What these studies make clear is that the prevalence of myopia in most studies of children is non-trivial, regardless of ethnicity.

Data from studies in China suggest that prevalence is increasing faster in rural than in urban communities there (Wang et al., 2023b), although myopia manifested at an earlier age in the urban communities. This pattern raises concern that as more rural communities begin to urbanize, especially in developing countries, the prevalence of myopia globally will likely increase. Current data from Africa show this pattern already: the prevalence of myopia approximately doubled between 2000 and 2010 (reaching 2.9%) and again between 2011 and 2020 (reaching 5.6%), perhaps because of increased access to schooling (Kobia-Acquah et al.,

2022). These rates remain low by worldwide standards, but they raise concern that prevalence may increase dramatically with further development and urbanization across Africa.

While a heat map comparing prevalence levels across countries has not yet been developed, even informal comparisons are difficult to interpret. They are hampered by the varied methods of detection (manual retinoscopy versus multiple instruments, cycloplegia versus not), varied policies on population screening, and varied methods for measurement (Carlton et al., 2008; Goh et al., 2005; Multi-Ethnic Pediatric Eye Diseases Study, 2010; Pan et al., 2009; Taylor et al., 2010; Villarreal et al., 2003).

A rare exception to the difficulties in making direct comparisons concerns the inspection of data from Sydney, Australia, alongside that from Belfast, Northern Ireland. The first set of data are from a study of Australian children who were predominantly 6 years old at the time of cycloplegic autorefraction and among whom 1.4% had myopia[3] (Robaei et al., 2005). With the same definition and method of refractive-error assessment, the study in Northern Ireland reported that 2.8% of 661 children aged 6 to 7 had myopia. In older children, ages 12 to 13, 17.7% had myopia in the Belfast study (O'Donoghue et al., 2010). The observed differences might be caused by the slightly older cohort in Ireland and the possibility of differences in ethnic composition between the two populations, but they also might arise instead, or in addition, from behavioral differences that vary with culture.

PREVALENCE OF MYOPIA IN THE UNITED STATES

As stated earlier, the current prevalence of myopia in the United States is largely an estimate. Without formal policies on myopia surveillance and accountability, it is difficult to find rigorous, large-scale and (or) population-based estimates of childhood myopia prevalence in the country.

The best evidence of the prevalence of myopia in U.S. adults likely stems from the work of Susan Vitale and the studies she directed using the National Health and Nutrition Evaluation Survey (NHANES; Vitale et al., 2008). NHANES is an ongoing study of population characteristics in a nationally representative sample of the United States population that for many years included measures of refractive errors, including myopia.

Adult Population-Based Prevalence

NHANES: National Data

For the period 1999–2004 (Vitale et al., 2008), the prevalence of myopia in adults aged 20 and older was 33.1% (see Table 3-4). Individuals aged 60 and older were less likely to have myopia than younger participants, hinting at increasing prevalence in more recent generations since axial myopia is usually a lifelong condition. Again, inter-generational comparisons can be confounded by hyperopic shifts with age. Myopia was more common in non-Hispanic White people (35.2%) than in non-Hispanic Black people (28.6%) or Mexican American people (25.1%).

NHANES data have also been compared between the periods 1971–1975 and 1999–2004 (Vitale et al., 2009). For individuals aged 12–54, average prevalence increased from 25% in 1971–1975 to 41.6% in 1999–2004. It should be noted that for Americans of European descent

---

[3]Defined as worse than −0.50D.

myopia increased 1.63-fold; for African Americans it increased 2.59-fold. Perhaps of most concern, for high myopia (worse than or equal to –7.90 D myopia), there was an 8-fold increase in prevalence.

Rochester, Minnesota

The prevalence of myopia in adults has also been reported for the period between 1966 and 2019 in Olmsted County, which encompasses the Mayo Clinic in Rochester, Minnesota (Tailor et al., 2024). For adults there older than age 18, 57.1% had myopia in the 2010s. This represents a 68% increase from the 33.9% prevalence recorded in the 1960s. By the 2010s, the prevalence of myopia had increased to 53.3% in White people and to 41% in Black people. Of note, high myopia, defined as –6.00 D of myopia or more, had nearly tripled, from 2.8% in the 1960s to 8.3% in the 2010s. It should also be noted that this study is not representative of the United States, as nearly every participant in the 1960s was White, and in 2010, 85% of participants were White as well. Nevertheless, the Olmstead County study does represent a comprehensive look at the prevalence of myopia at the (county) population level and illustrates the increasing prevalence in the area. More population-based studies in more diverse areas of the United States will be required to obtain a more representative picture.

Pediatric Population-Based Prevalence

In 2013, a population-based study of refractive error and other eye conditions known as the Multi-Ethnic Pediatric Eye Disease Study (MEPEDS) was conducted in Los Angeles, California, in children ages 6 to 72 months. It found that the prevalence of myopia in the preschool years ranged from 1.2% to 6.6%, depending on ethnicity (see Table 3-4; MEPEDS, 2010; Wen et al., 2013).

An earlier study, known as the Baltimore Pediatric Eye Disease Study (BPEDS), was conducted in Baltimore, Maryland, with the same core definitions and age groups as MEPEDS. When MEPEDS and BPEDS participant data are combined, the total prevalence of myopia in preschool children comes out to 3.8%, with prevalence ranging from 1.0% to 5.8% depending on ethnicity and age (see Table 3-4; Borchert et al., 2011).

Medicaid Claims for Children

Crude prevalence data are also available from Medicaid claims between 2016 and 2019. In 2016, of 27,667,800 children (0 to 17 years old) with claims data, 6.75% of children were diagnosed with myopia (Vision & Eye Health Surveillance Systems, 2016). In 2019, of 34,094,900 children with claims, prevalence rose to 7.24% (Vision & Eye Health Surveillance Systems, 2019).

TABLE 3-4 Studies of U.S. Prevalence of Myopia

Study	Prevalence (period of measurement)	Myopia definition and measurement technique	Age (n)
NHANES 2008 (Vitale et al., 2008)	33.1% (1999–2004)	> –1.00 D SER myopia; non-cycloplegic autorefraction	> 20 years (12,010)
NHANES 2009	25.0% (1971–1972)	lensometry, pinhole visual acuity, and presenting visual acuity (for	12–54 years (4,436 in 1971–

(Vitale et al., 2009)	41.6% (1999–2004)	presenting visual acuity of at least 20/40) or retinoscopy (for presenting visual acuity of 20/50 or worse).	1972 and 8,339 in 1999–2004)
Olmsted County, MN (Tailor et al., 2024)	33.9% (1960s) 57.1% (2010s)	> −0.50 D SER myopia; refraction or lensometry	>18 years (81,706)
Los Angeles, CA (MEPEDS, 2010; Wen et al., 2013)	1.2% in White Americans 3.7% in Hispanic Americans 3.98% in Asian Americans 6.6% in African American Americans (2003–2011)	> −1.00 D SER myopia; cycloplegic examination	6–72 months (1,501 non-Hispanic White Americans; 3,030 Hispanic Americans, 1,507 Asian; 2,994 African Americans)
Los Angeles, CA, and Baltimore, MD (combined) (Borchert et al., 2011)	3.8% (all) 1.0% in White Americans, 3.3% in Hispanic Americans, 5.8% in African Americans (2003–2007)		(Combined: 9,970)
Medicaid Claims	6.75% (2016) 7.24% (2019)	Medicaid International Classification of Diseases diagnosis	0–17 years (27,667,800 in 2016; 34,094,900 in 2019)

SOURCE: Committee generated.

LESSONS FROM THREE REGIONS: THE INUIT, AUSTRALIA, AND ISRAEL

Lessons from the Inuit

Historically, population studies of Arctic communities found low rates of myopia (Rozema et al., 2021). After 1950, though, reports emerged of increasing prevalence in younger members of the community in studies from Canada, Alaska, and Greenland. A recent review shows this pattern by plotting the prevalence as a function of age and the decade of measurement (Figure 3-3; Rozema et al., 2021). It includes five studies from Alaska, one from Canada, and two from Greenland, with data collected from 1950 to 2010. From 1950 to 1980, there is higher prevalence of myopia for those ages 10 to 30 years than for older members of the community, suggesting that prevalence is increasing. For the intervals 1980–1990 and 1990–2010, the prevalence remains high at ages 10 to 30 but the peak shifts to older ages, as would be expected from the cumulative effect of a factor that began to affect children's eye growth around 1950. Results are similar in studies using a higher cut-off for myopia (e.g., Morgan et al., 1975).

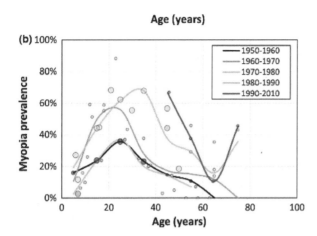

FIGURE 3-3 Myopia prevalence in northern native communities 1950–2010, by age.
NOTES: The prevalence of myopia of −0.25 D or worse in studies of northern native communities plotted as a function of age. Each dot represents an individual data point, with its size scaled to the size of the sample. The color coding represents the decade when the measurements were taken.
SOURCE: Reprinted from Rozema et al., 2021, with permission from John Wiley & Sons, Inc. Copyright © 1999–2024 John Wiley & Sons, Inc or related companies. All rights reserved, including rights for text and data mining and training of artificial intelligence technologies or similar technologies.

Two concerns emerge from the data depicted in Figure 3-3. First, there is a surprising uptick at the end for those ages 75 to 80 from a much lower prevalence at age 65. The uptick is based on studies with very small sample sizes (e.g., 11 participants ages 70−90; 7 participants ages 80+), while the remainder of the graphs are based on larger cohorts. The uptick may also be due to concomitant age-related changes to the human lens called nuclear sclerosis, which can cause a myopic shift in older adults (Lee et al., 1999). Second, one study was omitted, as the authors wrote that the "Myopia percentage makes no sense" (see also Rozema et al., 2021). This omitted study covered 138 Inuit individuals who lived on Canada's Belcher Island,[4] most of whom were under age 50 (Woodruff & Samer, 1976). Only 6.9% of the eyes were myopic,[5] mostly in those in the age range of 10−20 years, and only 23% had any negative refractive error at all. One possible reason for the low incidence suggested by the authors is the relatively little western contact of this community, except for a period of iron ore mining in the 1950s.

Collectively, these studies show an initially low incidence of myopia in northern native populations and a recent increase in prevalence in many, but not all of these communities (see comment on Belcher Island, above). The most likely cause of the increased prevalence is increased early childhood school attendance, with which it correlates almost perfectly (Rozema et al., 2021). The correlation is often explained by the increase in near work that happens with schooling, but it is important to remember that there is a corresponding decrease in time outdoors. The importance of the latter is also signaled by the way myopia correlates with latitude, that is, with the angle and amount of sunlight in winter and summer. However, latitude cannot explain the increasing prevalence over time in any given locale.

---

[4]Measurements were taken of 77% of the population by a vision team from the University of Waterloo's School of Optometry.
[5]Myopia worse than −1.0D.

Lessons from Australia

Australians are known as a people who enjoy spending significant time at beaches and, perhaps as a result, who have a higher risk of developing skin cancer (Mackey, 2023). Prevalence figures suggest lower rates of myopia there than in other countries of similar economic development. As early as 2000, the prevalence of myopia[6] in adults older than 40 years was noted to be lower in Australia than in western Europe or the United States: the estimated prevalences for these three regions as of 2000 were 16.4%, 26.6%, and 25.4%, respectively (Kempen et al., 2004). Figure 3-4 shows that the prevalence of myopia[7] across four large-scale population studies of Australian adults aged 40 and older ranged from 13.6% to 23.9%—all significantly lower than rates for the comparison group used by the authors from the U.K. Biobank study of adults ages 40 to 69 (27.8%). In one of the Australian studies, prevalence was lower in those with a history of skin cancer (and presumably more sun exposure) at 11.9% than in those with no such history, at 21.6% (Franchina et al., 2014). For high myopia,[8] all four Australian samples had a significantly lower prevalence than the U.K. sample (0.7–2.7% versus 6.1%).[9] Inspection of Figure 3-4 hints at increasing prevalence over decades because it is higher at ages 49–54 than at ages 65–70. This might reflect lifestyle changes, such as increasing education, or hyperopic shifts in the aging eye (Lee et al.,1999).

Although the low prevalence in Australians is notable, comparisons to the U.K. Biobank data might not be appropriate because of likely differences in social class and education (which are higher in the U.K. sample; Cumberland et al., 2015). A more appropriate comparison might be the data from the Gutenberg Health Study. With similar cutoffs,[10] the prevalence in the German adults ages 35–74 was 35% and the prevalence of high myopia was 3.5% (Wolfram et al., 2014). Although the definition of myopia and age range do not match those in the Australian studies exactly, the German prevalence figures are higher than any of those from Australia.

Studies of Australian adolescents also indicate a relatively low incidence of myopia by worldwide standards, especially when the analysis is restricted to those of European ancestry. For example, one comparison of Sydney, Australia, and Northern Island found a prevalence of <10% at age 12 years (2 samples) and of 17.7% at age 17 years (1 sample) in Sydney schools, both of which were lower than the prevalence in comparable samples in Northern Ireland (French et al., 2012, 2013). A longitudinal study of children born in a Perth, Western Australia hospital in 1989–1991 found that 25.8% of those tested at age 20 years had myopia and 1.4% had high myopia[11] (Lee et al., 2022). Myopia was more likely if they were currently studying, if they were non-White, if the concentration of serum 25(OH)D was lower at ages 17 or 20, suggesting less exposure to sunlight, and if there was more parental myopia (Lingham et al., 2021). By age 28 years, the prevalence had increased to 33.2%; the incidence of high myopia

---

[6]Myopia of at least −1.0 D.

[7]Myopia of at least −0.5 D.

[8]High myopia of −5.0 D or worse.

[9]The study also included data from a much smaller sample of 1,098 parents of children born 26 years earlier at a Perth hospital, with 22% of eligible mothers and 16% of eligible fathers participating; this study is omitted from the summary given here because the smaller number of participants may not be a representative sample, since they were parents who were willing to participate for 26 years.

[10]Myopia worse than –0.50D (rather than –0.05D or worse in the Australian study) and high myopia equal to –6D or worse (rather than –5.00 D or worse in the Australian study).

[11]Myopia of –0.5D or worse; high myopia of –6.0D or worse; n = 1328; longitudinal study, n = 801.

had not changed (1.5% vs. 1.4% at age 20). Importantly, the longitudinal data showed that the onset of myopia can occur between age 20 and 28 years: of the 516 participants without myopia at age 20 years, 72 (14%) had developed it by age 28 years. Multivariate analyses indicated that the increase of myopia between age 20 and 28 years was related to female gender, East Asian (as opposed to White) ethnicity, less sun exposure, parental myopia, and reporting more time working on a computer either at both ages or increasing to high usage over this period of time (Lee et al., 2023). The reported amount of TV time (including gaming) and reported amount of screen time (smartphones and tablets) were unrelated to the myopia results (Lee et al., 2022).

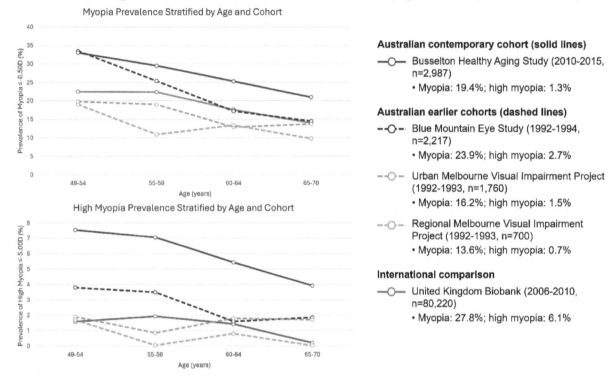

FIGURE 3-4 (A) Myopia prevalence stratified by age and cohort. (B) High myopia prevalence stratified by age and cohort.
NOTES: The prevalence of myopia (top panel; −0.50 D or worse) and of high myopia (bottom panel; −5.00 D or worse) in adults 40–70 years old in Australia and, for comparison, the United Kingdom. Shown are data collected in 1992–1994 in Australia: The Blue Mountain Eye Study assessment in two postal codes of urban Sydney and the Melbourne urban and regional assessments conducted in randomly selected areas of metropolitan Melbourne and regional Victoria. Also shown are data from an Australian study conducted in 2010–2015 in Busselton, a regional town in Western Australia (brown line, n = 5,907). For comparison, data are plotted from the United Kingdom Biobank study (purple line on the top; n= 80,220).
SOURCE: Adapted from Mackey et al., 2021, with permission from John Wiley & Sons, Inc. © 1999–2024 John Wiley & Sons, Inc, or related companies. All rights reserved, including rights for text and data mining and training of artificial intelligence technologies or similar technologies.

Lessons from Israel

Prevalence data from Israel are valuable because virtually the entire population of 17-year-olds is screened for mandatory military service, including males and females, except for married or pregnant women, mothers, Arabs and some other minority groups, and until 2013, the ultra-Orthodox. From 1971 and 1994 the prevalence of myopia[12] increased from 20.4% to 26.2%, with a higher prevalence in females than males at all time points (see Figure 3-5), possibly because they were more likely to have higher education (Shapira et al., 2019). Those of non-Jewish origin also had lower prevalence.

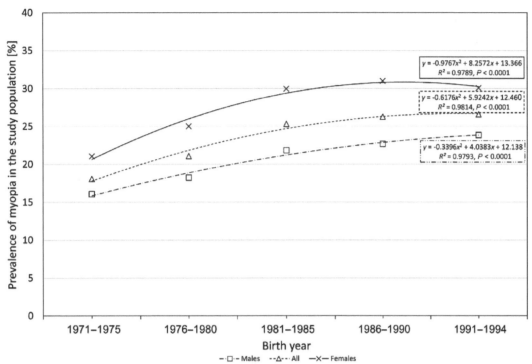

FIGURE 3-5 The prevalence of myopia of −0.5D or more in Israeli army recruits from 1971 to 1994. NOTES: The triangles are the overall data; the squares are the data from males; the x's, from females. Refractive error was measured in 104,689 young adults, excluding only the ultra-Orthodox, some ethnic minorities, multiparous females, and married females. Over this time, the prevalence of myopia increased, with a similar pattern for high myopia (6 D and higher), which increased from 1.54% to 1.75%. SOURCE: Reprinted from Shapira et al., 2019, with permission from Elsevier.

Data accumulated from 1990 through 2002 on 919,929 recruits in Israel show a continuation of this trend: an overall increase in prevalence from 20.3% in 1990 to 28.3% in 2002, with prevalence again higher in females, those with more years of higher education, and those of Jewish origin. Part of the increasing prevalence could be explained by an increase in higher education among male recruits and the increased pursuit of higher education among females (Dayan et al., 2005).

Particularly interesting are data for the 22,823 male recruits in 2013, a year when mandatory service included the ultra-Orthodox. The goal was to assess the entire male Jewish population of Israel at ages 17–18.[13] The prevalence of myopia was 37.8% overall, with large differences depending on where the recruit had studied or was studying (see Table 3-5). For those from the Orthodox educational system, where males study in single-sex classrooms and are

---

[12]Myopia of −0.5D or worse.

[13]The sample excluded recruits born abroad, of a different age, non-Jewish, those who had had surgical refractive correction, and all female recruits (because religious female recruits are not subject to military service).

expected to do 2–3 additional hours weekly of intensive study of religious texts, the prevalence was significantly higher than for those with secular schooling. It was higher yet for those from the ultra-Orthodox educational system, who begin formal school with an emphasis on reading religious texts in fine print from the age of three and who are expected to study up to 16 hours/day as they progress in school (Bez et al., 2019).

Similar differences are evident in the prevalence of high myopia. The differences remained significant after adjustment for age, country of origin, socioeconomic status, years of education, and body-mass index. With secular recruits as a reference, the odds ratio for having myopia in the ultra-Orthodox was 9.3:1. Note that the data suggest an influence of near work (and the consequent lack of time outside) from an early age in a population that also experiences very little screen time (Bez et al., 2019).

TABLE 3-5 The Prevalence of Refractive Error in Israeli Male Army Recruits in 2013 as a Function of the Educational System

Schooling	Refractive Error Worse than or Equal to −0.50D	Refractive Error Worse than or Equal to −6.00D
Secular	29.7%	2%
Orthodox	50.3%	7.1%
Ultra-Orthodox	82.2%	27.6%

SOURCE: Committee generated from data in Bez et al., 2019.

Lessons from the Inuit, Australia, and Israel

The relatively low prevalence among the Inuit and Australians suggests important lessons. For the Inuit, western contact and schooling appear to have led to an increase in myopia. However, the data for Australia, while also showing increasing prevalence, suggest that exposure to sunlight is prophylactic and may offset the effects of schooling. The data from Israel are especially valuable because of the use of large representative samples collected using the same methods over extended periods of time. They demonstrate convincingly that prevalence is increasing. Within the Israeli samples, education seems to be a factor, as those with more years of education were more likely to be nearsighted, as were those for whom near work was more intense and started at younger ages (the ultra-Orthodox). In Chapter 5, we evaluate evidence on the impact of near work and sunlight on the development of myopia, including the mechanisms by which they might have an impact. That evidence is clear for the benefit of sunlight but not for any independent effect of near work.

Trends in Myopia Prevalence

Although the National Academies 1989 myopia report (National Research Council, 1989) suggested no increase in prevalence at that time, it appears that myopia prevalence is now increasing in the United States and around the world (Mackey et al., 2021; Rozema et al., 2021; Shapira et al., 2019; Vitale et al., 2009). Of special concern is that high myopia, which creates a greater risk for retinal detachment, glaucoma, and myopic macular degeneration, appears to be increasing rapidly. Large-scale studies have not been funded recently in the United States, making it difficult to ascertain how the United States fits in with worldwide trends. Comparisons are difficult because of impactful methodological differences in how myopia is defined and measured. Estimates would be improved with formal policies on surveillance and accountability, including stipulations on how to measure refractive error and how to define myopia, as well as similar procedures for taking and reporting measurements in different jurisdictions.

INFLUENCES OF SEX AND ETHNICITY ON PREVALENCE

Some prevalence data suggests higher rates in females and in certain ethnic groups. Those data should be interpreted with caution, as they may be influenced by differences in lifestyle, education, access to care, and a variety of other confounders. Moreover, there is no known genetic explanation that would lead one to expect sex or ethnic differences (see Chapter 5).

CONCLUSIONS

In recent years, there has been growing concern over the escalating prevalence of myopia on a global scale, including within the United States. The increases appear related to increased near work, as exemplified by the data from studies of the Inuit, urbanized Chinese, and ultra-Orthodox Jewish scholars. However, the Australian counter-example suggests a protective effect of time outdoors, which may decrease as the amount of near work or schooling increases. Factors such as extensive indoor reading in childhood (in the data from Israel) and extra time in the sunlight (data from Australia) very likely affect prevalence. In Chapter 5, we consider the direct evidence on the relationship between the protective effect of time outdoors and increased near work.

Despite the clear worldwide trends, comprehensive and up-to-date data in the United States remain scarce. This scarcity can be attributed to various factors, including discrepancies in the definition, measurement techniques, and age of assessment across different states and studies. Moreover, the lack of recent funding for large-scale surveillance studies with representative populations further exacerbates this data deficit. Concurrently, as lifestyle patterns evolve, particularly in developing regions, there is a foreseeable surge in myopia rates worldwide, one that will likely have significant economic implications. Contextualizing U.S. data within this broader international landscape not only facilitates comparative analysis but also allows for the generation of innovative hypotheses concerning the etiology of myopia and treatment development.

Conclusion 3-1: The prevalence of myopia appears to be increasing worldwide, including in the United States. However, very little recent data exist for the United States, and even when data are available, measuring trends is difficult. This is partly because the definition, magnitude, measurement technique, and age of assessment vary across states and across studies. The needed large-scale surveillance studies with representative populations have not been funded in recent years.

Conclusion 3-2: Predictable changes in lifestyle factors in the developing world, such as spending less time outdoors and more time at school and in near work, are likely to lead to an increase in worldwide myopia with an associated economic burden. Placing U.S. data in the context of worldwide trends will allow for comparisons to formulate novel hypotheses about etiology and/or treatment development.

RECOMMENDATIONS

Recommendation 3-1: The Centers for Disease Control and Prevention and state health departments should collect consistent, harmonized data on the prevalence of myopia in the United States, prioritizing longitudinal surveillance on refractive error prevalence in children using standardized procedures. A central repository should be created so that consistent data can be uploaded into a central database using insight from existing repositories (e.g., National Alzheimer's Coordinating Center or the National Cancer Institute's Surveillance, Epidemiology, and End Results Program) to advance our understanding of this disease.

   a. **For such population statistics, the data should comprise objective measures at various ages, collected longitudinally from an early age and by repeated cross-sectional measurements using consistent methodology.**
   b. **The data should include the entire distribution of refractive errors, not just the mean and the age of onset. Otherwise, a shift in part of the distribution (e.g., high myopia) or age of onset (e.g., starting before Grade 1) that would suggest the need for different policy/practice responses could be obscured. This will also prevent biased conclusions from comparisons of studies using different values as the cut-off separating myopic from not-myopic.**
   c. **The repository should involve collaboration between government agencies, research institutions, healthcare providers, and advocacy organizations to ensure comprehensive data collection and dissemination.**

Recommendation 3-2: The Centers for Disease Control and Prevention should coordinate with the World Health Organization so that both organizations are using consistent, harmonized definitions and monitoring methods. Data subsequently collected should then consistently follow these methods so that future worldwide comparisons can be used to identify the influence of economic development, lifestyle, and ethnicity on the prevalence of refractive error.

REFERENCES

Bao, J., Yang, A., Huang, Y., Li, X., Pan, Y., Ding, C., Lim, E. W., Zheng, J., Spiegel, D. P., Drobe, B., Lu, F., & Chen, H. (2022). One-year myopia control efficacy of spectacle lenses with aspherical lenslets. *The British Journal of Ophthalmology, 106*(8), 1171–1176. https://doi.org/10.1136/bjophthalmol-2020-318367

Bez, D., Megreli, J., Bez, M., Avramovich, E., Barak, A., & Levine, H. (2019). Association between type of educational system and prevalence and severity of myopia among male adolescents in Israel. *JAMA Ophthalmology, 137*(8), 887. https://doi.org/10.1001/jamaophthalmol.2019.1415

Bomotti, S., Lau, B., Klein, B. E. K., Lee, K. E., Klein, R., Duggal, P., & Klein, A. P. (2018). Refraction and change in refraction over a 20-year period in the Beaver Dam Eye Study. *Investigative Ophthalmology & Visual Science, 59*(11), 4518–4524. https://doi.org/10.1167/iovs.18-23914

Borchert, M. S., Varma, R., Cotter, S. A., Tarczy-Hornoch, K., McKean-Cowdin, R., Lin, J. H., Wen, G., Azen, S. P., Torres, M., Tielsch, J. M., Friedman, D. S., Repka, M. X., Katz, J., Ibironke, J., Giordano, L., & Multi-Ethnic Pediatric Eye Disease Study and the Baltimore Pediatric Eye Disease Study Groups. (2011). Risk factors for hyperopia and myopia in preschool children: The multi-ethnic pediatric eye disease and Baltimore pediatric eye disease studies. *Ophthalmology, 118*(10), 1966–1973. https://doi.org/10.1016/j.ophtha.2011.06.030

Bourne, R. R., Stevens, G. A., White, R. A., Smith, J. L., Flaxman, S. R., Price, H., Jonas, J. B., Keeffe, J., Leasher, J., Naidoo, K., Pesudovs, K., Resnikoff, S., & Taylor, H. R. (2013). Causes of vision loss worldwide, 1990–2010: A systematic analysis. *Lancet Global Health, 1*, e339–e349. https://doi.org/10.1016/S2214-109X(13)70113-X

Carlton, J., Kamon, J., Czoski-Murray, C., Smith, K. J., & Marr, J. (2008). The clinical effectiveness and cost-effectiveness of screening programmes for amblyopia and strabismus in children up to the age of 4–5 years: A systematic review and economic evaluation. *Health Technology Assessment, 12*(25). https://doi.org/10.3310/hta12250

Chamberlain, P., Peixoto-de-Matos, S. C., Logan, N. S., Ngo, C., Jones, D., & Young, G. (2019). A 3-year randomized clinical trial of MiSight lenses for myopia control. *Optometry and Vision Science, 96*(8), 556–567. https://doi.org/10.1097/OPX.0000000000001410

Chandler, S., Sinnott, L., Mutti, D., Zadnik, K., Jordan, L., Fong, T., & Hemmati, H. (2023). *The CHAMP and CLEERE studies demonstrate similar rates of myopia progression over time* [Conference abstract]. Academy 2023: Annual Meeting of the American Academy of Optometry. New Orleans, LA, United States. https://aaopt.org/past-meeting-abstract-archives/?SortBy=&ArticleType=&ArticleYear=&Title=&Abstract=&Authors=&Affiliation=&PROGRAMNUMBER=230015

Chua, S. Y., Sabanayagam, C., Cheung, Y. B., Chia, A., Valenzuela, R. K., Tan, D., Wong, T. Y., Cheng, C. Y., & Saw, S. M. (2016). Age of onset of myopia predicts risk of high myopia in later childhood in myopic Singapore children. *Ophthalmic & Physiological Optics: The Journal of the British College of Ophthalmic Opticians (Optometrists), 36*(4), 388–394. https://doi.org/10.1111/opo.12305

COMET Group. (2013). Myopia stabilization and associated factors among participants in the Correction of Myopia Evaluation Trial (COMET). *Investigative Ophthalmology & Visual Science, 54*(13), 7871–7884. https://doi.org/10.1167/iovs.13-12403

Cumberland, P. M., Bao, Y., Hysi, P. G., Foster, P. J., Hammond, C. J., Rahi, J. S., & UK Biobank Eye and Vision Consortium. (2015). Frequency and distribution of refractive error in adult life: Methodology and findings of the UK Biobank Study. *PLOS ONE, 10*(10), e0139780. https://doi.org/10.1371/journal.pone.0139780

Czepita, D., Mojsa, A., & Zejmo, M. (2008). Prevalence of myopia and hyperopia among urban and rural schoolchildren in Poland. *Annales Academiae Medicae Stetinensis, 54*(1), 17–21. https://pubmed.ncbi.nlm.nih.gov/19127805/

Dayan, Y. B., Levin, A., Morad, Y., Grotto, I., Ben-David, R., Goldberg, A., Onn, E., Avni, I., Levi, Y., & Benyamini, O. G. (2005). The changing prevalence of myopia in young adults: A 13-year series of population-based prevalence surveys. *Investigative Ophthalmology & Visual Science, 46*(8), 2760. https://doi.org/10.1167/iovs.04-0260

Donovan, L., Sankaridurg, P., Ho, A., Naduvilath, T., Smith, E. L., 3rd, & Holden, B. A. (2012). Myopia progression rates in urban children wearing single-vision spectacles. *Optometry and Vision Science: Official Publication of the American Academy of Optometry, 89*(1), 27–32. https://doi.org/10.1097/OPX.0b013e3182357f79

Flitcroft, D. I., He, M., Jonas, J. B., Jong, M., Naidoo, K., Ohno-Matsui, K., Rahi, J., Resnikoff, S., Vitale, S., & Yannuzzi, L. (2019). IMI—Defining and classifying myopia: A proposed set of standards for clinical and epidemiologic studies. *Investigative Ophthalmology & Visual Science, 60*(3), M20–M30. https://doi.org/10.1167/iovs.18-25957

Franchina, M., Yazar, S., Hunter, M., Gajdatsy, A., deSousa, J., Hewitt, A. W., & Mackey, D. A. (2014). Myopia and skin cancer are inversely correlated: Results of the Busselton Healthy Ageing Study. *Medical Journal of Australia, 200*(9), 521–522. https://doi.org/10.5694/mja14.00086

French, A. N., Morgan, I. G., Burlutsky, G., Mitchell, P., & Rose, K. A. (2013). Prevalence and 5- to 6-year incidence and progression of myopia and hyperopia in Australian schoolchildren. *Ophthalmology, 120*(7), 1482–1491. https://doi.org/10.1016/j.ophtha.2012.12.018

French, A. N., O'Donoghue, L., Morgan, I. G., Saunders, K. J., Mitchell, P., & Rose, K. A. (2012). Comparison of refraction and ocular biometry in European Caucasian children living in Northern Ireland and Sydney, Australia. *Investigative Ophthalmology & Visual Science, 53*(7), 4021. https://doi.org/10.1167/iovs.12-9556

Goh, P. P., Abqariyah, Y., Pokharel, G. P., & Ellwein, L. B. (2005). Refractive error and visual impairment in school-age children in Gombak District, Malaysia. *Ophthalmology, 112*(4), 678–685. https://doi.org/10.1016/j.ophtha.2004.11.034

Gwon, S. H., & Lee, D. C. (2023). Factors associated with myopia in 19-year-old adult men in Korea between 2014 and 2020. *Scientific Reports, 13*(1), 11581. https://doi.org/10.1038/s41598-023-38569-w

Holden, B. A., Fricke, T. R., Wilson, D. A., Jong, M., Naidoo, K. S., Sankaridurg, P., Wong, T. Y., Naduvilath, T. J., & Resnikoff, S. (2016). Global prevalence of myopia and high myopia and temporal trends from 2000 through 2050. *Ophthalmology, 123*(5), 1036–1042. https://doi.org/10.1016/j.ophtha.2016.01.006

Hu, Y. Y., Wu, J. F., Lu, T. L., Wu, H., Sun, W., Wang, X. R., Bi, H. S., & Jonas, J. B. (2015). Effect of cycloplegia on the refractive status of children: The Shandong Children Eye Study. *PLOS ONE, 10*(2), e0117482. https://doi.org/10.1371/journal.pone.0117482

Hyman, L., Gwiazda, J., Marsh-Tootle, W. L., Norton, T. T., Hussein, M., & COMET Group. (2001). The Correction of Myopia Evaluation Trial (COMET): Design and general baseline characteristics. *Controlled Clinical Trials, 22*(5), 573–592. https://doi.org/10.1016/s0197-2456(01)00156-8

Ip, J. M., Huynh, S. C., Robaei, D., Kifley, A., Rose, K. A., Morgan, I. G., Wang, J. J., & Mitchell, P. (2008). Ethnic differences in refraction and ocular biometry in a population-based sample of 11–15-year-old Australian children. *Eye, 22*(5), 649–656. https://doi.org/10.1038/sj.eye.6702701

Jones-Jordan, L. A., Sinnott, L. T., Chu, R. H., Cotter, S. A., Kleinstein, R. N., Manny, R. E., Mutti, D. O., Twelker, J. D., Zadnik, K., & CLEERE Study Group. (2021). Myopia progression as a function of sex, age, and ethnicity. *Investigative Ophthalmology & Visual Science, 62*(10), 36. https://doi.org/10.1167/iovs.62.10.36

Jones-Jordan, L. A., Sinnott, L. T., Manny, R. E., Cotter, S. A., Kleinstein, R. N., Mutti, D. O., Twelker, J. D., Zadnik, K., & Collaborative Longitudinal Evaluation of Ethnicity and Refractive Error. (CLEERE) Study Group. (2010). Early childhood refractive error and parental history of myopia as predictors of myopia. *Investigative Ophthalmology & Visual Science, 51*(1), 115–121. https://doi.org/10.1167/iovs.08-3210

Jung, S. K., Lee, J. H., Kakizaki, H., & Jee, D. (2012). Prevalence of myopia and its association with body stature and educational level in 19-year-old male conscripts in Seoul, South Korea. *Investigative Ophthalmology & Visual Science, 53*(9), 5579–5583. https://doi.org/10.1167/iovs.12-10106

Kempen, J. H., Mitchell, P., Lee, K. E., Tielsch, J. M., Broman, A. T., Taylor, H. R., Ikram, M. K., Congdon, N. G., O'Colmain, B. J., & Eye Diseases Prevalence Research Group. (2004). The prevalence of refractive errors among adults in the United States, Western Europe, and Australia. *Archives of Ophthalmology, 122*(4), 495–505. https://doi.org/10.1001/archopht.122.4.495

Khanal, S., & Dhakal, R. (2024). Myopia progression trends from 1980 to 2020. *Investigative Ophthalmology & Visual Science, 65*(7), 173.

Kim, H., Seo, J. S., Yoo, W. S., Kim, G. N., Kim, R. B., Chae, J. E., Chung, I., Seo, S. W., & Kim, S. J. (2020). Factors associated with myopia in Korean children: Korea National Health and Nutrition Examination Survey 2016–2017 (KNHANES VII). *BMC Ophthalmology*, *20*(1), 31. https://doi.org/10.1186/s12886-020-1316-6

Kleinstein, R. N., Sinnott, L. T., Jones-Jordan, L. A., Sims, J., Zadnik, K., & Collaborative Longitudinal Evaluation of Ethnicity and Refractive Error (CLEERE) Study Group. (2012). New cases of myopia in children. *Archives of Ophthalmology*, *130*(10), 1274–1279. https://doi.org/10.1001/archophthalmol.2012.1449

Kobia-Acquah, E., Flitcroft, D. I., Akowuah, P. K., Lingham, G., & Loughman, J. (2022). Regional variations and temporal trends of childhood myopia prevalence in Africa: A systematic review and meta-analysis. *Ophthalmic and Physiological Optics*, *42*(6), 1232–1252. https://doi.org/10.1111/opo.13035

Koh, V., Yang, A., Saw, S. M., Chan, Y. H., Lin, S. T., Tan, M. M. H., Tey, F., Nah, G., & Ikram, M. K. (2014). Differences in prevalence of refractive errors in young Asian males in Singapore between 1996–1997 and 2009–2010. *Ophthalmic Epidemiology*, *21*(4), 247–255. https://doi.org/10.3109/09286586.2014.928824

Lee, K. E., Klein, B. E., & Klein, R. (1999). Changes in refractive error over a 5-year interval in the Beaver Dam Eye Study. *Investigative Ophthalmology & Visual Science*, *40*(8), 1645–1649. https://pubmed.ncbi.nlm.nih.gov/10393030/

Lee, S. S.-Y., Lingham, G., Sanfilippo, P. G., Hammond, C. J., Saw, S.-M., Guggenheim, J. A., Yazar, S., & Mackey, D. A. (2022). Incidence and progression of myopia in early adulthood. *JAMA Ophthalmology*, *140*(2), 162. https://doi.org/10.1001/jamaophthalmol.2021.5067

Lee, S. S.-Y., Lingham, G., Wang, C. A., Torres, S. D., Pennell, C. E., Hysi, P. G., Hammond, C. J., Gharahkhani, P., Clark, R., Guggenheim, J. A., & Mackey, D. A. (2023). Changes in refractive error during young adulthood: The effects of longitudinal screen time, ocular sun exposure, and genetic predisposition. *Investigative Ophthalmology & Visual Science*, *64*(14), 28. https://doi.org/10.1167/iovs.64.14.28

Lee, S. H., Tsai, P. C., Chiu, Y. C., Wang, J. H., & Chiu, C. J. (2024). Myopia progression after cessation of atropine in children: a systematic review and meta-analysis. *Frontiers in Pharmacology*, *15*, 1343698. https://doi.org/10.3389/fphar.2024.1343698

Li, T., Zhou, X., Zhu, J., Tang, X., & Gu, X. (2019). Effect of cycloplegia on the measurement of refractive error in Chinese children. *Clinical & Experimental Optometry*, *102*(2), 160–165. https://doi.org/10.1111/cxo.12829

Lingham, G., Mackey, D. A., Zhu, K., Lucas, R. M., Black, L. J., Oddy, W. H., Holt, P., Walsh, J. P., Sanfilippo, P. G., Chan She Ping-Delfos, W., & Yazar, S. (2021). Time spent outdoors through childhood and adolescence—assessed by 25-hydroxyvitamin D concentration—and risk of myopia at 20 years. *Acta Ophthalmologica*, *99*(6), 679–687. https://doi.org/10.1111/aos.14709

Lingham, G., Yazar, S., Lucas, R. M., Milne, E., Hewitt, A. W., Hammond, C. J., MacGregor, S., Rose, K. A., Chen, F. K., He, M., Guggenheim, J. A., Clarke, M. W., Saw, S., Williams, C., Coroneo, M. T., Straker, L., & Mackey, D. A. (2021). Time spent outdoors in childhood is associated with reduced risk of myopia as an adult. *Scientific Reports*, *11*(1). https://doi.org/10.1038/s41598-021-85825-y

Logan, N. S., Shah, P., Rudnicka, A. R., Gilmartin, B., & Owen, C. G. (2011). Childhood ethnic differences in ametropia and ocular biometry: the Aston Eye Study. *Ophthalmic & Physiological Optics: The Journal of the British College of Ophthalmic Opticians (Optometrists)*, *31*(5), 550–558. https://doi.org/10.1111/j.1475-1313.2011.00862.x

Loughman, J., Kobia-Acquah, E., Lingham, G., Butler, J., Loskutova, E., Mackey, D. A., Lee, S. S. Y., & Flitcroft, D. I. (2024). Myopia outcome study of atropine in children: Two-year result of daily 0.01% atropine in a European population. *Acta Ophthalmologica*, *102*(3), e245–e256. https://doi.org/10.1111/aos.15761

Mackey, D. (2023, December 5). Sunshine and nightshade to prevent myopia [Workshop presentation]. Workshop on the Rise in Myopia: Exploring Possible Contributors and Investigating Screening Practices, Policies, and Programs. National Academies of Sciences, Engineering, and Medicine, Washington, DC, United States. https://www.nationalacademies.org/event/41360_12-2023_workshop-on-the-rise-in-myopia-exploring-possible-contributors-and-investigating-screening-practices-policies-and-programs

Mackey, D. A., Franchina, M., Yazar, S., Hunter, M., Gajdatsy, A., deSousa, J., & Hewitt, A. W. (2014, April 30). Myopia and skin cancer are inversely correlated: Results of the Busselton Healthy Ageing Study. *Investigative Ophthalmology & Visual Science, 55*, 1274. https://iovs.arvojournals.org/article.aspx?articleid=2266491

Mackey, D. A., Lingham, G., Lee, S. S., Hunter, M., Wood, D., Hewitt, A. W., Mitchell, P., Taylor, H. R., Hammond, C. J., & Yazar, S. (2021). Change in the prevalence of myopia in Australian middle-aged adults across 20 years. *Clinical & Experimental Ophthalmology, 49*(9), 1039–1047. https://doi.org/10.1111/ceo.13980

Mangan, T. (2019, February 19). Astigmatism. *All About Vision*. https://www.allaboutvision.com/conditions/astigmatism.htm

Matsumura, H., & Hirai, H. (1999). Prevalence of myopia and refractive changes in students from 3 to 17 years of age. *Survey of Ophthalmology, 44*(Suppl 1), S109–S115. https://doi.org/10.1016/s0039-6257(99)00094-6

Morgan, I., & Rose, K. (2005). How genetic is school myopia? *Progress in Retinal and Eye Research, 24*(1), 1–38. https://doi.org/10.1016/j.preteyeres.2004.06.004

Morgan, I. G., Ohno-Matsui, K., & Saw, S.-M. (2012). Myopia. *The Lancet, 379*(9827), 1739–1748. https://doi.org/10.1016/S0140-6736(12)60272-4

Morgan, I. G., Rose, K. A., & Ellwein, L. B. (2010). Is emmetropia the natural endpoint for human refractive development? An analysis of population-based data from the refractive error study in children (RESC). *Acta Ophthalmologica, 88*(8), 877–884. https://doi.org/10.1111/j.1755-3768.2009.01800.x

Morgan, R. W., Speakman, J. S., & Grimshaw, S. E. (1975). Inuit myopia: An environmentally induced "epidemic"? *Canadian Medical Association Journal, 112*(5), 575–577. https://www.ncbi.nlm.nih.gov/pmc/articles/PMC1956268/

Multi-Ethnic Pediatric Eye Disease Study Group. (2010). Prevalence of myopia and hyperopia in 6- to 72-month-old African American and Hispanic children: The Multi-Ethnic Pediatric Eye Disease Study. *Ophthalmology, 117*(1), 140–147.e3. https://doi.org/10.1016/j.ophtha.2009.06.009

Mutti, D. O., & Zadnik, K. (2000). Age-related decreases in the prevalence of myopia: longitudinal change or cohort effect? *Investigative Ophthalmology & Visual Science, 41*(8), 2103–2107. https://pubmed.ncbi.nlm.nih.gov/10892850/

National Eye Institute. (2020). Projections for myopia (2010-2030-2050). Nearsightedness (myopia) tables. https://www.nei.nih.gov/learn-about-eye-health/eye-health-data-and-statistics/nearsightedness-myopia-data-and-statistics/nearsightedness-myopia-tables

National Research Council. (1989). *Myopia: Prevalence and progression*. National Academies Press. https://doi.org/10.17226/1420

O'Donoghue, L., McClelland, J. F., Logan, N. S., Rudnicka, A. R., Owen, C. G., & Saunders, K. J. (2010). Refractive error and visual impairment in school children in Northern Ireland. *The British Journal of Ophthalmology, 94*(9), 1155–1159. https://doi.org/10.1136/bjo.2009.176040

Ojaimi, E., Rose, K. A., Morgan, I. G., Smith, W., Martin, F. J., Kifley, A., Robaei, D., & Mitchell, P. (2005). Distribution of ocular biometric parameters and refraction in a population-based study of Australian children. *Investigative Ophthalmology & Visual Science, 46*(8), 2748–2754. https://doi.org/10.1167/iovs.04-1324

Pan, Y., Tarczy-Hornoch, K., Cotter, S. A., Wen, G., Borchert, M. S., Azen, S. P., Varma, R., & Multi-Ethnic Pediatric Eye Disease Study Group. (2009). Visual acuity norms in pre-school children: The Multi-Ethnic Pediatric Eye Disease Study. *Optometry and Vision Science: Official Publication of the American Academy of Optometry, 86*(6), 607–612. https://doi.org/10.1097/OPX.0b013e3181a76e55

Pan, C. W., Zheng, Y. F., Anuar, A. R., Chew, M., Gazzard, G., Aung, T., Chen, C.-Y., Wong, T. Y., & Saw, S.-M. (2013). Prevalence of refractive errors in a multiethnic Asian population: The Singapore Epidemiology of Eye Disease Study. *Investigative Ophthalmology & Visual Science, 54*(4), 2590–2598. https://doi.org/10.1167/iovs.13-11725

Rappon, J., Chung, C., Young, G., Hunt, C., Neitz, J., Neitz, M., & Chalberg, T. (2023). Control of myopia using diffusion optics spectacle lenses: 12-month results of a randomised controlled, efficacy and safety study (CYPRESS). *The British Journal of Ophthalmology, 107*(11), 1709–1715. https://doi.org/10.1136/bjo-2021-321005

Repka, M. X., Weise, K. K., Chandler, D. L., Wu, R., Melia, B. M., Manny, R. E., Kehler, L. A. F., Jordan, C. O., Raghuram, A., Summers, A. I., Lee, K. A., Petersen, D. B., Erzurum, S. A., Pang, Y., Lenhart, P. D., Ticho, B. H., Beck, R. W., Kraker, R. T., Holmes, J. M., Cotter, S. A., … Pediatric Eye Disease Investigator Group. (2023). Low-dose 0.01% atropine eye drops vs placebo for myopia control: A randomized clinical trial. *JAMA Ophthalmology, 141*(8), 756–765. https://doi.org/10.1001/jamaophthalmol.2023.2855

Resnikoff, S., Pascolini, D., Mariotti, S. P., & Pokharel, G. P. (2008). Global magnitude of visual impairment caused by uncorrected refractive errors in 2004. *Bulletin of the World Health Organization, 86*(1), 63–70. https://doi.org/10.2471/blt.07.041210

Robaei, D., Rose, K., Ojaimi, E., Kifley, A., Huynh, S., & Mitchell, P. (2005). Visual acuity and the causes of visual loss in a population-based sample of 6-year-old Australian children. *Ophthalmology, 112*(7), 1275–1282. https://doi.org/10.1016/j.ophtha.2005.01.052

Rozema, J. J., Boulet, C., Cohen, Y., Stell, W. K., Iribarren, L., van Rens, G. H. M. B., & Iribarren, R. (2021). Reappraisal of the historical myopia epidemic in native Arctic communities. *Ophthalmic and Physiological Optics, 41*(6), 1332–1345. https://doi.org/10.1111/opo.12879

Sanfilippo, P. G., Chu, B. S., Bigault, O., Kearns, L. S., Boon, M. Y., Young, T. L., Hammond, C. J., Hewitt, A. W., & Mackey, D. A. (2014). What is the appropriate age cut-off for cycloplegia in refraction. *Acta Ophthalmologica, 92*(6), e458–e462. https://doi.org/10.1111/aos.12388

Sankaridurg, P., Tahhan, N., Kandel, H., Naduvilath, T., Zou, H., Frick, K. D., Marmamula, S., Friedman, D. S., Lamoureux, E., Keeffe, J., Walline, J. J., Fricke, T. R., Kovai, V., & Resnikoff, S. (2021). IMI impact of myopia. *Investigative Ophthalmology & Visual Science, 62*(5), 2. https://doi.org/10.1167/iovs.62.5.2

Shapira, Y., Mimouni, M., Machluf, Y., Chaiter, Y., Saab, H., & Mezer, E. (2019). The increasing burden of myopia in Israel among young adults over a generation. *Ophthalmology, 126*(12), 1617–1626. https://doi.org/10.1016/j.ophtha.2019.06.025

Tailor, P. D., Xu, T. T., Tailor, S., Asheim, C., & Olsen, T. W. (2024). Trends in myopia and high myopia from 1966 to 2019 in Olmsted County, Minnesota. *American Journal of Ophthalmology, 259*, 35–44. https://doi.org/10.1016/j.ajo.2023.10.019

Taylor, H. R., Xie, J., Fox, S., Dunn, R. A., Arnold, A.-L., & Keeffe, J. E. (2010). The prevalence and causes of vision loss in Indigenous Australians: The National Indigenous Eye Health Survey. *Medical Journal of Australia, 192*(6), 312–318. https://doi.org/10.5694/j.1326-5377.2010.tb03529.x

Tedja, M. S., Wojciechowski, R., Hysi, P. G., Eriksson, N., Furlotte, N. A., Verhoeven, V. J. M., Iglesias, A. I., Meester-Smoor, M. A., Tompson, S. W., Fan, Q., Khawaja, A. P., Cheng, C. Y., Höhn, R., Yamashiro, K., Wenocur, A., Grazal, C., Haller, T., Metspalu, A., Wedenoja, J., Jonas, J. B., … Klaver, C. C. W. (2018). Genome-wide association meta-analysis highlights light-induced signaling as a driver for refractive error. *Nature Genetics, 50*(6), 834–848. https://doi.org/10.1038/s41588-018-0127-7

Villarreal, G. M., Ohlsson, J., Cavazos, H., Abrahamsson, M., & Mohamed, J. H. (2003). Prevalence of myopia among 12- to 13-year-old schoolchildren in northern Mexico. *Optometry and Vision Science: Official Publication of the American Academy of Optometry, 80*(5), 369–373. https://doi.org/10.1097/00006324-200305000-00011

Vision & Eye Health Surveillance System. (2016). Annual prevalence of diagnosed disorders of refection and accommodation, myopia, 2016 [Map]. Ceneters for Disease Control and Prevention. https://ddt-vehss.cdc.gov/LP?Level1=Vision+Problems+and+Blindness&Level2=Diagnosed+Vision+Disorders&Level3=Diagnosed+Refractive+Error&Level4=Diagnosed+Myopia&LocationId=&DataSourceId=MEDICARE&IndicatorId=QDXDC7~R7_1&ShowFootnotes=true&View=NationalMap&CompareViewYear=1&CompareId=&CompareId2=&YearId=YR7&ResponseId=R7_1&AgeId=AGE017&GenderId=GALL&RaceId=ALLRACE&RiskFactorId=RFALL&RiskFactorResponseId=RFTOT&DataValueTypeId=CRDPREV&MapClassifierId=quantile&MapClassifierCount=4&CountyFlag=N

___. (2019). Annual prevalence of diagnosed disorders of refection and accommodation, myopia, 2019 [Map]. Ceneters for Disease Control and Prevention. https://ddt-vehss.cdc.gov/LP?Level1=Vision+Problems+and+Blindness&Level2=Diagnosed+Vision+Disorders&Level3=Diagnosed+Refractive+Error&Level4=Diagnosed+Myopia&LocationId=&DataSourceId=MEDICARE&IndicatorId=QDXDC7~R7_1&ShowFootnotes=true&View=NationalMap&CompareViewYear=1&CompareId=&CompareId2=&YearId=YR11&ResponseId=R7_1&AgeId=AGE017&GenderId=GALL&RaceId=ALLRACE&RiskFactorId=RFALL&RiskFactorResponseId=RFTOT&DataValueTypeId=CRDPREV&MapClassifierId=quantile&MapClassifierCount=4&CountyFlag=N

Vitale, S., Ellwein, L., Cotch, M. F., Ferris, F. L., & Sperduto, R. (2008). Prevalence of refractive error in the United States, 1999-2004. *Archives of Ophthalmology, 126*(8), 1111–1119. https://doi.org/10.1001/archopht.126.8.1111

Vitale, S., Sperduto, R. D., & Ferris, F. L., III. (2009). Increased prevalence of myopia in the United States between 1971–1972 and 1999–2004. *Archives of Ophthalmology, 127*(12), 1632–1639. https://doi.org/10.1001/archophthalmol.2009.303

Walline, J. J., Walker, M. K., Mutti, D. O., Jones-Jordan, L. A., Sinnott, L. T., Giannoni, A. G., Bickle, K. M., Schulle, K. L., Nixon, A., Pierce, G. E., Berntsen, D. A., & BLINK Study Group. (2020). Effect of high add power, medium add power, or single-vision contact lenses on myopia progression in children: The BLINK randomized clinical trial. *JAMA, 324*(6), 571–580. https://doi.org/10.1001/jama.2020.10834

Wang, J., Han, Y., Musch, D. C., Li, Y., Wei, N., Qi, X., Ding, G., Li, X., Li, J., Song, L., Zhang, Y., Ning, Y., Zeng, X., Li, Y., Sun, L., Hua, N., Li, S., Jardines, S., & Qian, X. (2023a). Evaluation and follow-up of myopia prevalence among school-aged children subsequent to the COVID-19 home confinement in Feicheng, China. *JAMA Ophthalmology, 141*(4), 333–340. https://doi.org/10.1001/jamaophthalmol.2022.6506

Wang, J., Li, Y., Musch, D. C., Wei, N., Qi, X., Ding, G., Li, X., Li, J., Song, L., Zhang, Y., Ning, Y., Zeng, X., Hua, N., Li, S., & Qian, X. (2021). Progression of myopia in school-aged children after COVID-19 home confinement. *JAMA Ophthalmology, 139*(3), 293–300. https://doi.org/10.1001/jamaophthalmol.2020.6239

Wang, Y. X., Pan, Z., Wang, Z. Y., Li, Z., Huang, Y., Wang, J., Zhang, C., Li, F., Jonas, J. B., & Wong, T. Y. (2023b). 25-year trend in myopia prevalence in Chinese school children and adolescents: A nationwide analysis from 1998–2022. *Investigative Ophthalmology & Visual Science, 64*(8), 3821. https://iovs.arvojournals.org/article.aspx?articleid=2790769

Wen, G., Tarczy-Hornoch, K., McKean-Cowdin, R., Cotter, S. A., Borchert, M., Lin, J., Kim, J., Varma, R., & Multi-Ethnic Pediatric Eye Disease Study Group (2013). Prevalence of myopia, hyperopia, and astigmatism in non-Hispanic white and Asian children: Multi-ethnic pediatric eye disease study. *Ophthalmology, 120*(10), 2109–2116. https://doi.org/10.1016/j.ophtha.2013.06.039

Williams, K. M., Bertelsen, G., Cumberland, P., Wolfram, C., Verhoeven, V. J., Anastasopoulos, E., Buitendijk, G. H., Cougnard-Grégoire, A., Creuzot-Garcher, C., Erke, M. G., Hogg, R., Höhn, R., Hysi, P., Khawaja, A. P., Korobelnik, J. F., Ried, J., Vingerling, J. R., Bron, A., Dartigues, J. F., … European Eye Epidemiology Consortium. (2015). Increasing prevalence of myopia in Europe and the impact of education. *Ophthalmology, 122*(7), 1489–1497. https://doi.org/10.1016/j.ophtha.2015.03.018

Wolfram, C., Höhn, R., Kottler, U., Wild, P., Blettner, M., Bühren, J., Pfeiffer, N., & Mirshahi, A. (2014). Prevalence of refractive errors in the European adult population: The Gutenberg Health Study (GHS). *British Journal of Ophthalmology, 98*(7), 857–861. https://doi.org/10.1136/bjophthalmol-2013-304228

Woodruff, M. E., & Samek, M. J. (1976). The refractive status of Belcher Island Eskimos. *Canadian Journal of Public Health, 67*(4), 314–320. https://pubmed.ncbi.nlm.nih.gov/963652/

Yam, J. C., Jiang, Y., Tang, S. M., Law, A. K. P., Chan, J. J., Wong, E., Ko, S. T., Young, A. L., Tham, C. C., Chen, L. J., & Pang, C. P. (2019). Low-Concentration Atropine for Myopia Progression (LAMP) Study: A randomized, double-blinded, placebo-controlled trial of 0.05%, 0.025%, and 0.01% atropine eye drops in myopia control. *Ophthalmology, 126*(1), 113–124. https://doi.org/10.1016/j.ophtha.2018.05.029

Zadnik, K., Schulman, E., Flitcroft, I., Fogt, J. S., Blumenfeld, L. C., Fong, T. M., Lang, E., Hemmati, H. D., Chandler, S. P., & CHAMP Trial Group Investigators. (2023). Efficacy and safety of 0.01% and 0.02% atropine for the treatment of pediatric myopia progression over 3 years: A randomized clinical trial. *JAMA ophthalmology, 141*(10), 990–999. https://doi.org/10.1001/jamaophthalmol.2023.2097

Zhang, X. J., Zhang, Y., Kam, K. W., Tang, F., Li, Y., Ng, M. P. H., Young, A. L., Ip, P., Tham, C. C., Chen, L. J., Pang, C. P., & Yam, J. C. (2023). Prevalence of myopia in children before, during, and after COVID-19 restrictions in Hong Kong. *JAMA Network Open, 6*(3), e234080. https://doi.org/10.1001/jamanetworkopen.2023.4080

4
Assessment and Diagnostic Technologies

CURRENT STANDARD CLINICAL ASSESSMENTS AND DIAGNOSTIC TECHNOLOGIES

This chapter reviews the current assessments and diagnostic technologies used in screenings and clinical evaluations of myopia. The assessment and diagnostic measurements used in these evaluations shape researchers' understanding of myopia because they are the recorded, and therefore studied, characteristics of myopia.

Screening efforts are used to identify vision abnormalities, including refractive errors like myopia, in nonspecialist settings. These nonspecialist settings are usually settings where many target populations congregate (e.g., schools for children), public locales in the community at large (e.g., shopping centers), and primary or general medical clinics. Eye assessments in these settings include basic optotypes (e.g., presentation of letters at specified distances), autorefractor devices to directly measure an eye's refractive error, and photoscreeners. The original photoscreeners photographed the red reflex (red color within the eye's pupil during a flash photograph) from both eyes of a subject. Based on characteristics of the photographed red reflex, the image obtained could be used to identify refractive errors, obstructions in the visual axis (e.g., cataracts, tumors), and ocular misalignments associated with abnormal visual development.

Modern photoscreeners use infrared illumination and digital imaging, have autorefraction capabilities, and typically include some decision support (e.g., image quality assessment, screen pass/fail and need for referral). Modern photoscreeners include stand-alone devices such as the Spot and PlusoptiX and, more recently, smartphone-based variants such as the GoCheck Kids (Nallasamy et al., 2024). (For more details regarding vision screening including performance, accessibility, and barriers, see Chapter 8.)

Clinical History and Standard Eye Exam

Upon reaching the clinic, whether via screening or for an eye examination, the following describes the current assessments and diagnostic technologies someone with myopia would encounter in a clinical evaluation (Jacobs et al., 2022). As part of a comprehensive eye examination, the clinical assessment first includes obtaining the medical history. This includes (but is not limited to) recording the duration and progression of visual symptoms, past medical or surgical diagnoses, medication use, and family history. The duration and progression of visual symptoms provides information about the potential course of the myopia, with earlier onset and rapid progression increasing the likelihood of becoming highly myopic. Past medical or surgical diagnoses provide information about associated diseases or pathological forms of myopia. As an example of associated disease, primary congenital glaucoma can cause an increase in the size of the eye leading to axial myopia, due to globe wall distensibility with rapid expansion; as an example of myopia from prior other treatments, a scleral reinforcement buckle surgically placed to repair a retinal detachment can also increase the length of the eye, resulting in myopia. Medication use is also important, as some medications can cause myopia as a side effect (e.g., topiramate used for migraines or seizure control). A review of family history helps in identifying possible genetic or syndromic risks for myopia, given the strong heritability of myopia (Tedja et al., 2019).

Next, a physical examination is performed to assess the state of the eye. The physical examination includes measurements of visual acuity at distance (typically 20 ft or 6 m) both without and with correction. A refraction will be performed, which may consist of an auto-refractor measurement of the refractive state of the eye, an interactive subjective manifest refraction in which lenses are replaced (typically with a phoropter) based on the patient's perception of improvement or deterioration of vision, and/or a retinoscopy, in which the examiner replaces lenses based on assessing a streak of light reflected from the examined eye.

Children and young adults can dynamically adjust their lens power to focus on near objects by contracting the ciliary muscle, which changes the crystalline lens shape, a process called accommodation. For pediatric and young adult patients, pharmacologic cycloplegia (a temporary condition that paralyzes the eye's ciliary muscle, which controls accommodation) should be performed to determine the refractive state of the eye without the influence of accommodation.

Regarding accommodation, studies have noted accommodative lag differences in myopes compared to emmetropes (those with no refractive error). Specifically, there is an insufficiency of accommodation for near targets in myopes compared to emmetropes (Gwiazda et al., 1993). Accommodative lag is measured by having the individual look at targets varying from far to near distances, either physically or optically via lenses, and plotting the refraction measurements against the target distances. The slope of the accommodative response to the change in target distance is farther from 1:1 for myopes than it is for emmetropes. Typically, an autorefractor is used for these refraction measurements, and the target is placed along the line of sight. Performing this measurement requires specialized equipment, such as an open-field autorefractor (e.g., Grand Seiko WAM-5500), and a technician who must move the target either manually or by a motor and record the multiple measurements. Because accommodative lag has not been shown to predate the development of myopia (Mutti et al., 2006), the diagnostic value of this measurement appears to be limited compared to other, easier-to-obtain diagnostic measurements such as current refractive error (Zadnik et al., 2015). Accommodative measurements hence are not in widespread clinical use as an influence on myopia progression management.

After refraction, the remainder of the physical examination will include measurements of intraocular pressure, pupillary examination, an examination of the front of the eye, and a dilated exam of the back of the eye. Intraocular pressure is measured using tonometry. There are a variety of tonometer mechanisms and techniques, such as the air puff, thin filament rebound (which does not require anesthetic drops) and contact variants such as Goldmann tonometry (does require topical anesthesia). Increased intraocular pressure is a major risk factor for the development of glaucoma, which, as alluded to earlier, is associated with myopia.

The pupillary examination measures the response of the pupil to a light stimulus, both within the eye receiving the stimulus and in the other eye. The reflexive constrictive pupillary response to a light stimulus provides information on optic nerve and cortical visual pathway health. As detailed in the research diagnostics section later, the pupillary response may also provide information about specific neurons that can affect myopia development. The examination of the front of the eye is usually performed with a slit lamp biomicroscope, and the examination of the back of the eye is performed with direct or indirect ophthalmoscopy (a medical exam that allows a doctor to see the inside of the eye using a magnifying lens and light) after dilation with dilating drops.

These examination techniques provide magnified views of the anatomy of the eye, so that the practitioner can look for physical evidence that may be associated with or be a consequence of myopia.

Other diagnostic technologies are used to supplement this standard clinical assessment. They include fundus imaging, ocular biometry, optical coherence tomography (OCT), electroretinograms (ERGs), contrast sensitivity testing, and automated visual field testing.

Fundus Imaging

Fundus imaging provides a recorded, portable, and reviewable assessment of the posterior eye. Fundus imaging is typically performed with fundus photography or videography (Figure 4-1) or with scanning laser ophthalmoscopy. In fundus photography/videography—which is now mostly digital—one takes color images of the retina through a dilated pupil with approximately a 30° to 50° field of view through lenses specifically designed for imaging the posterior eye. Multiple images can be montaged together to provide a wider field of view. Fundus cameras range from purpose-specific models made by major ophthalmic device companies to add-ons for consumer cameras, including smartphone cameras.

Angiography, the mapping of blood vessels, is carried out to assess the retinal and deeper vasculature and can be obtained using injected dyes such as fluorescein and indocyanine green to provide contrast as the dyes circulate through the vasculature. Scanning laser ophthalmoscopy is another way to image the fundus and uses a confocal and scanning laser to obtain images. Depending on the laser wavelengths used, the retinal image obtained and reconstructed by this method may appear in pseudo-color. Modern commercial versions of this technique can have fields of view larger than regular fundus photography and can image through non-dilated pupils with proper alignment.

Overall, fundus imaging provides a recorded color view of the retina which should provide similar information to the clinical fundus examination to assess for posterior eye pathologies associated with myopia, including maculopathy, glaucoma, and retinal detachment.

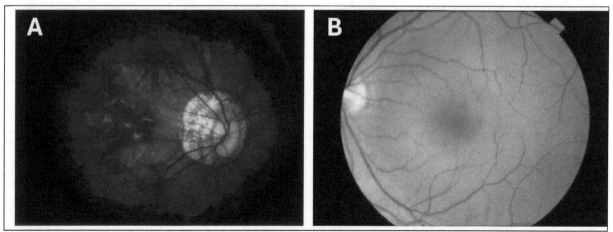

FIGURE 4-1 Fundus photograph images of (A) pathologic myopia and (B) normal fundus.
SOURCE: (A) American Academy of Ophthalmology, 2020; (B) National Eye Institute, 2020.

Ocular Biometry

Ocular biometry is used to measure the curvature of the optical elements within the eye and the length of the eye. The major application for ocular biometry devices is for cataract surgery, so most of the measurements from ocular biometry are those needed to calculate the optical power of intraocular lenses in the context of cataract surgery. These include curvature measurements of the cornea, which provide information about the power and astigmatism of the cornea, and central length measurements through the eye, such as central cornea thickness, anterior chamber depth, lens thickness, and axial length. Originally, the curvature and axial length information were captured using separate devices—a keratometer and ultrasound A-scan, respectively—but most modern ocular biometers combine those modalities into a single device. Modern ocular biometers include a keratometer and/or cross-sectional corneal imaging device such as OCT (see discussion below) or Scheimpflug photography to measure the corneal curvature. For the axial length measurements, optical interferometry is used either via partial coherence interferometry or OCT.

While many studies have investigated the relationships between myopia and these various ocular biometric measurements, the major measurement of concern for myopia is axial length (Jones et al., 2005; Mutti et al., 2007; Tideman et al., 2016; Wong et al., 2010). For fixed anterior segment optics, an axially longer eye results in the image being focused in front of the retina, a condition that defines myopia. Multiple studies have shown the relationship between increasing axial length, myopia, and pathologic myopia risk. Longitudinal axial length measurements are also used to assess the effects of myopia interventions and treatments aimed at slowing or stabilizing axial lengthening.

Optical Coherence Tomography

OCT is a micrometer-scale cross-sectional imaging technology that is a major advancement in clinical diagnostic information, particularly for retinal diseases (Figure 4-2). Current clinical OCT systems can image either the front of the eye (anterior segment OCT systems) or the back of the eye (retinal OCT systems), and their micrometer-scale cross-sectional imaging allows either corneal or retinal layers to be visualized in detail. In the context of myopia, retinal OCT is currently used to assess microstructural changes in the retina, particularly as they relate to myopic maculopathies.

More specifically, OCT imaging can show clinicians retinal layer thinning (associated with degeneration or glaucoma), disruptions in retinal layers (outer retinal degenerations), and accumulations of pathologic fluid (as might occur with neovascularization). A technique called OCT angiography is also available, making it possible to view microvasculature without the use of injected dyes as an alternative to standard (dye-based) angiography when examining vascular disruptions (Jia et al., 2015; Mariampillai, 2008) as might be seen in pathologic myopia (Wong et al., 2019; Zheng et al., 2022). OCT has also been used in research applications for morphometric and choroidal analysis (those research applications will be covered in a later section of this chapter).

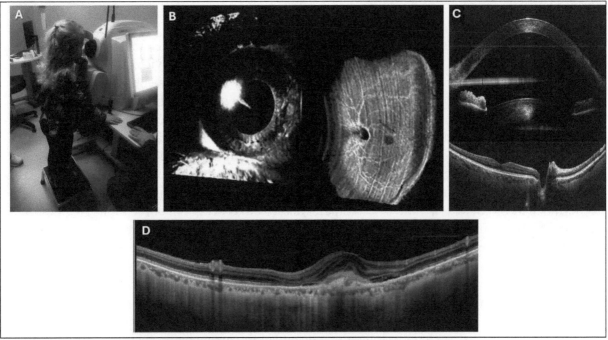

FIGURE 4-2 Examples of optical coherence tomography (OCT).
NOTES: (A) Though standard clinical OCT systems are not designed specifically for children, cooperative children can be imaged using them. (B) OCT is a three-dimensional imaging technique capable of imaging both the front and the back of the eye, both shown here, though standard clinical systems usually use only one image or the other. (C) The three-dimensional OCT volume is composed of two-dimensional slices termed B-scans as shown here. B-scans offer high-resolution cross-sectional views of ocular anatomy. They are typically viewed vertically as shown here. Anterior eye shown in top image and retina in bottom image. (D). An example of OCT to visualize pathologic myopia, specifically neovascularization (the "bump" just right of the middle of the image).
SOURCES: (A) Courtesy Katherine Weise, OD, University of Alabama at Birmingham; (B) and (C) reprinted with permission from McNabb et al., 2018; © Optica Publishing Group; (D) from Gupta et al., 2024.

Electroretinograms

ERGs are noninvasive clinical recordings of the electrical response of the retina in response to light (Ramkumar et al., 2024). Electrodes are placed on the anesthetized cornea or on the skin below the eye and record the electrical responses from the eye, similar to an electrocardiogram (EKG) for the heart or an electroencephalogram (EEG) for the brain. These responses are generally characterized as waveforms, and varying the visual stimulus allows different waveforms to be extracted. Aspects of these waveforms are thought to correspond largely or entirely to different cell types within the retina. More specifically, these electrical responses represent responses to light by the retinal photoreceptors and bipolar cells, with different parts of the waveform corresponding to those cell layers. Using different ambient conditions (dark/light) and light stimuli (full-field, multi-focal, pattern), different parts of the retinal circuitry and areas can be interrogated. The full-field ERG consists of two major waves: a negative a-wave generated by the photoreceptors and a positive b-wave generated by activity of the retinal ON bipolar cells. The ON and OFF neural pathways contain parallel retinal circuitry that signals when the retina responds to the onset or the offset of light stimuli, respectively

(Ichinose & Habib, 2022; Schiller, 1992; see Chapter 5, Stimulation of ON vs. OFF Visual Pathways). Certain inherited retinal diseases, like retinitis pigmentosa and congenital stationary night blindness, can result in development of myopia. Because the first of these two diseases causes photoreceptor loss and the second results in diminished or absent b-wave amplitudes, ERG can be used to assess the loss of photoreceptor or ON bipolar function (Frishman, 2013; Pardue & Peachey 2014). More directly related to myopia, there have been limited studies showing associations between myopia and changes in the nerve signals observed by ERG (Chan, 2022; Gupta et al., 2022; Poudel et al., 2024; Zahra, 2023). The underlying hypothesis is that local retinal signaling, such as through ON pathways, is involved in myopia development. The associations between ERG and myopia are thought to be related to changes in signaling, though the literature is not conclusive at this point, and ERG is not an ubiquitous myopia diagnostic for this purpose.

Contrast Sensitivity

Contrast sensitivity tests the ability of the eye to discriminate between differences in luminance or color. This is different from standard optotype testing such as the Snellen acuity test, which presents a high contrast black target on a white background. Contrast sensitivity can provide a better indication of subtle disturbances in visual function that high-contrast testing cannot provide. There are a variety of ways to carry out contrast sensitivity, ranging from specialized eye charts (e.g., Pelli-Robson contrast chart, Hamilton Veale chart) to machine-generated stimuli or gratings (e.g., ColorDome by Diagnosys, Functional Vision Analyzer by Stereo Optical; Liou & Chiu, 2001; Poudel et al., 2024). More recently, a computerized program displaying targets with combinations of spatial frequency and contrast combined with eye tracking was used to obtain contrast sensitivity testing in children and nonverbal individuals (Mooney et al., 2021). As discussed previously in the ERG section, myopia is associated with differences in ON-OFF retinal pathways, and given that ON pathways have higher contrast sensitivity, the disturbances in those pathways could be identified via contrast sensitivity testing. Clinically, contrast sensitivity is used in clinical trials of optical devices such as contact lenses, but its role as a myopia diagnostic tool is not widespread.

Visual Field Tests

Visual field tests are used clinically to systematically assess deficits in the patient's field of vision. Clinically, visual fields are currently obtained with automated perimeters using sophisticated algorithms to present lights of appropriate size and intensity at different locations in the patient's field of vision in a repeatable and reproducible fashion. The requirement for patient interaction nevertheless introduces a subjective component into the test. In the context of current myopia care, visual fields are used to assess vision loss related to the increased risk for glaucoma with myopia or directly from pathologic myopia changes.

Summary

A variety of assessments and diagnostic technologies are currently clinically available to identify and characterize the myopic eye. The mainstay of the current clinical assessment includes the history and physical—particularly a measurement of the refraction—and is supplemented by diagnostic technologies, particularly fundus imaging and ocular biometry.

Those assessments and diagnostic tests provide a snapshot of the myopic eye at the time of the exam. This in turn provides a baseline to track longitudinal trajectories and changes in refraction and axial length in response to therapies (see Box 4-1).

DIAGNOSTICS AND ASSESSMENTS IN CLINICAL RESEARCH

Additional diagnostic technologies have been used in clinical research to assess myopia. These are not currently used in standard clinical practice for myopia in the United States and are instead being developed and explored to better understand the myopic eye.

Ocular (Eye) Shape

Eye shape, also referred to as ocular shape, is known to be different in myopic eyes compared to non-myopic eyes. Measurements of eye shape are also important as physical data that can be used to create models of the eye, particularly when combined with refraction data. A variety of methods are used to measure eye shape, including neuroimaging (typically with magnetic resonance imaging [MRI]), ultrasound B-scans, multi-axis refraction and/or biometry, and OCT.

As described earlier, axial myopia results from an elongation of the eye's axial length. This is only a one-dimensional measurement, though, and researchers have examined the myopic eye in two and three dimensions (i.e., eye shape) to identify other differences in a myopic eye that has grown "too long" for the anterior segment optics. One could hypothesize that an axially elongating eye might produce a football-shaped eye (termed prolate) with the long axis in the anterior-posterior direction; an oblate eye would instead have the long axis in the lateral direction (Figure 4-3). The earliest studies used MRI and ultrasound to explore this and, in some cases, showed that myopic eyes were generally less oblate than non-myopic eyes (Atchison et al., 2005; Cheng et al., 1992).

A less oblate eye in myopia also dovetails well with the peripheral refraction concept of myopia, where in an aspheric posterior eye, peripheral hyperopic defocus can drive eye growth and elongation (Smith, 2011). Performing refractions on-axis and off-axis (central and peripheral) provides information about the position of the retinal image plane relative to the anterior segment optics (Mutti et al., 2000). Ocular biometry can similarly be performed on- and off-axis to provide a physical mapping and measurement of the shape of the posterior eye (Schmid, 2003; Verkicharla et al., 2015). Retinal OCT functions as an automated interferometric sweeping of the posterior eye and hence also provides a physical mapping and measurement of the shape of the posterior eye with better depth and sampling resolution. With the optical techniques, artifacts introduced by refraction and display rendering need to be removed to recover the actual morphometry. Additionally, the direct measurement from these optical techniques is optical path length, which requires assumed or nominal refractive indices to convert to physical distances. Once the artifacts have been removed, OCT recapitulates the findings of the MRI studies using a more readily available ophthalmic technology (Kuo et al., 2016).

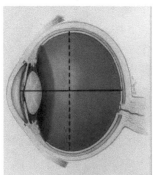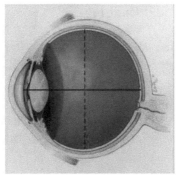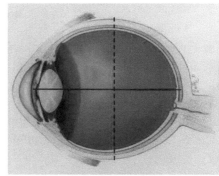

FIGURE 4-3 Illustrations of different eye shapes (exaggerated to illustrate the concept).
NOTE: The center image represents a nominally circular eye (or in three-dimensions, spherical). The left image represents an *oblate* eye shape where the equatorial axis (dashed line) is longer than the anterior-posterior axis (solid line, or axial length). The right image represents a *prolate* eye shape where the equatorial axis is shorter than the anterior-posterior axis (axial length). Again, these are exaggerated to illustrate the concept. In actuality, the differences in axes will usually require measurement rather than mere visual inspection, and few eyes will be at the extremes illustrated here.
SOURCE: Adapted from the eye illustration found at
https://medialibrary.nei.nih.gov/sites/default/files/media-images/NEI-medialibrary-2817499.png.

Figure 4-3 describes eye shape in global terms such as prolate, oblate, or spherical. However, global shape descriptors may not account for changes that only occur locally. As an example of a local shape change, a staphyloma is an outpouching of the eye due to a thinned sclera from extensive eye elongation in high myopia. More recently, using higher Tesla magnetic field MRI systems with more resolution, local differences have been shown in shape, particularly in pathologically myopic eyes (Moriyama et al., 2011). The MRIs showed the staphylomatous outpouchings as well as other localized disturbances even when a staphyloma was not identified on clinical exam by the fundus examination. Ultrasound is a more clinically accessible imaging technology in the eye care setting and can also be used to identify local changes such as staphylomas; despite its clinically accessibility, ultrasound has been used in few studies to assess these changes (Ito et al., 2022).

OCT represents resolution improved by an order of magnitude over both ultrasound and even the newer MRI systems used clinically, and in the context of eye shape OCT also shows local posterior eye shape changes in pathologically myopic eyes. OCT has been used to identify and report newly described conditions such as dome-shaped maculopathy (Gaucher et al., 2008), to create new cross-sectional anatomic definitions of staphylomas based on inflections in the profile of the posterior eye (Shinohara et al., 2017), and to enable methods to measure and describe local posterior eye shape variability (McNabb et al., 2021; Tan et al., 2021). The primary limitation of OCT relative to MRI and ultrasound is OCT's limited imaging range in width and depth, which is due to OCT light needing to reach the target tissue to form the image. Advances using contact techniques hold promise to increase light access to the extreme ocular periphery (Ni et al., 2023), and in myopic eyes with a thinned choroid OCT light is sometimes able to image the sclera of the posterior eye.

The morphology of the posterior eye differs in myopes from what it is in emmetropes, particularly with increasing degrees of myopia, in both global shape descriptors and local shape variability. While some of these morphologic changes can be qualitatively visualized from the image output of the diagnostic devices, quantitative measures have to date relied on research-specific software and image analysis that are not yet broadly available for general clinical use.

Choroidal Imaging

The choroid, situated between the retina and the sclera, is a vital layer of tissue in the eye responsible for supplying oxygen and nutrients to the retina, aiding in its health and function. It also regulates the amount of light entering the eye by absorbing excess stray light, thus preventing glare. Conversely, the sclera, the tough outer layer of the eye, encases and safeguards the eyeball while providing structural support to maintain its shape. Serving as an attachment site for the muscles controlling eye movement, the sclera ensures proper functionality and protection of the eye.

Measuring Choroidal Thickening and Thinning

Choroidal thickness is a compelling area to study in myopia because the choroid is adjacent to the sclera, which remodels in myopia. The vascular choroid can also thicken and thin on short time scales, resulting in anterior and posterior displacement of the retina relative to the anterior segment optics of the eye. The normal choroid in the macula is approximately 200 μm thick. The advent of optical interferometric imaging techniques with sufficient μm scale resolution have allowed the *in vivo* measurement of choroidal thickness; these techniques include one-dimensional optical biometers using partial-coherence interferometry and two- and three-dimensional OCT (Chiang et al., 2015; Read et al., 2010; Wang et al., 2016). These optical interferometric imaging techniques produce peaks at interface changes, such as between the vitreous and retinal surface, the retinal pigment epithelium at the outer retina-anterior choroidal interface, and the posterior interface between the choroid and the sclera.

The one-dimensional partial-coherence interferometric optical biometers do not automatically find the signal at the posterior choroidal boundary, so it is necessary to manually analyze and mark the waveform it generates to identify that interface and generate measures of choroidal thickness. Due to loss of light reflecting back to the detector in the case of deeper structures and/or noise in the measurements, the ability to identify the more posterior interfaces relies heavily on manual interpretation of the waveform. Similarly, two- and three-dimensional OCT both generate intensity peaks at interface changes, and due to the techniques' dimensional nature they produce histology-like cross-sectional images, which can be used to identify the anterior and posterior choroidal boundaries for thickness measurements (Figure 4-4).

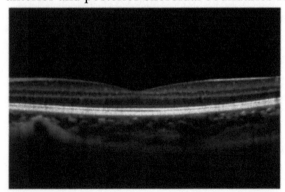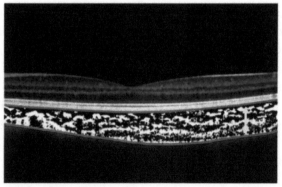

FIGURE 4-4 Optical coherence tomography (OCT) images of the choroid.
NOTE: The image on the left is an averaged B-scan, and the image on the right shows the anterior (blue) and posterior (red) boundaries labeled to then calculate a thickness value between the two boundaries.
SOURCE: Reprinted from Ostrin et al., 2023, under a Creative Commons Attribution-NonCommercial-No Derivatives 4.0 International License (https://creativecommons.org/licenses/by-nc-nd/4.0/).

The ability to identify choroidal boundaries is not typically provided in the software packaged with commercial OCT devices to date, so it requires manual, custom-automated, or semi-automated marking and labeling of the boundaries. Again, as an optical technique, OCT is subject to signal loss with tissue depth, a problem affected by such factors as the pigmentation of the imaged eye, the thickness of the choroid itself, and the characteristics and power of the light source of the particular OCT system.

Altogether, studies of human choroidal thickness have generally shown that myopes have a thinner choroid than non-myopes (Read et al., 2019). Measurements of short time-scale dynamic choroidal responses using partial-coherence interferometry and OCT have in some studies shown the expected changes, with transient thickening of the choroid in response to myopic defocus and thinning with hyperopic defocus (Chiang et al., 2015; Read et al., 2010). However, the scale of the changes has been on the order of the resolution of the imaging systems, and other studies have not detected the expected dynamic choroidal responses to defocus (Wang et al., 2016). Technical choices associated with choroidal image analysis, including those discussed earlier--such as manual vs. semi-automated vs. automated segmentation, masked vs. unmasked analysis, area vs. volume reporting--can contribute to the variability of current measurements. Additionally, other physiologic and logistical factors can confound measurements of choroidal thickness, such as time of day and previous fluid consumption (Ostrin et al., 2023).

Overall, though it is compelling and promising, dynamic choroidal imaging in humans remains an active area of study and development.

Measuring Choroidal Vasculature

In addition to choroidal thickness, the vasculature of the choroid itself can be studied. Dye-based angiographic techniques, such as indocyanine green angiography, have been used clinically for examination of the choroidal vasculature in myopia (e.g., Ohno-Matsui et al., 1996). OCT angiography is a more recent dye-free alternative that uses the motion of blood cells within the vessels as the contrast. OCT angiography has been used to image the choroidal vasculature and has shown flow deficits in pathologic myopia that are qualitatively visible on the *en face* projection, as noted earlier in the standard clinical assessments and diagnostics section.

Metrics have been developed to quantify vessel morphology, such as through measurements of length, branching, and density. However, it should be noted that technical constraints affect the information within a choroidal OCT angiography scan. These can include projection artifacts ("shadows" from more superficial vessels in the scan) and flow detection limits related to the OCT source and scan parameters (blood velocity above and below certain levels does not generate a signal; Corvi et al., 2021; Ferrara et al., 2016). Source image quality, noise, and motion artifacts also affect the derived measures. Resolving these artifacts is an active area of research in the effort to produce accurate depth-resolved angiograms (Wang et al., 2016).

The above-mentioned limits could affect the accuracy and reliability of indices and metrics describing choroidal vasculature morphology in OCT angiography. Nevertheless, setting those limits aside, most cross-sectional studies have generally reflected decreases in vessel density that appear to be consistent with the already noted decrease in choroidal thickness seen with higher myopia (Al-Sheikh et al., 2017; Devarajan et al., 2020; Liu et al., 2022; Wu et al., 2021; Xu et al., 2021), although other cross-sectional studies have not found differences in the vascular parameters (Chang et al., 2022; Scherm et al., 2019).

Scleral Imaging

Scleral imaging is an area of interest in studying myopia, given that elongation of the eye necessarily involves changes to the sclera, particularly the posterior sclera wall. Though ultrasound could be used to image the posterior sclera, there is sparse literature describing this. Optical techniques such as OCT are normally limited by signal loss through the retinal pigment epithelium and choroid, but the thinning of posterior eye layers with high myopia allows deeper OCT imaging and visualization of the full thickness of the posterior sclera (Imamura et al., 2011; Ohno-Matsui, 2012). Cross-sectional studies to date confirm the known clinical observations regarding thinning of posterior eye layers with higher myopia.

Newer directions include investigating *in vivo* differences in the collagenous organization within the posterior sclera and using the easier-to-access anterior sclera as a proxy for the posterior sclera. Recent attempts to investigate the collagenous organization within the posterior sclera in research participants have used polarization-sensitive OCT (Liu et al., 2023; Ohno-Matsui et al., 2024). Polarization-sensitive OCT can be used to detect scleral birefringence. Birefringence, or double refraction, occurs when a material is not uniformly organized at an atomic or molecular level which will cause light to travel differently through it depending on the polarization of the light and/or the direction light enters the material. In the case of the sclera, the bi-refringence is related to the organization and structure of the collagen within the sclera. Polarization sensitive OCT studies show cross-sectional differences in collagenous organization and structure within the sclera among myopes with and without pathologic features.

Turning to the anterior sclera, its anterior location makes it more clinically accessible and hence an area of interest in research. For instance, there are diagnostic tests for biomechanical properties, but they require direct access to the tissue. This makes them difficult to perform on the posterior sclera, but if there were a relationship between the anterior and posterior sclera properties, then measuring the anterior sclera could serve as a proxy for posterior sclera events. Study results to date using OCT to measure anterior scleral thickness have been mixed, with some studies showing a correlation between refractive errors and anterior scleral thickness (Dhakal et al., 2020; Vurgese et al., 2012; Zhou et al., 2023) and others not showing a correlation (Buckhurst et al., 2015; Pekel et al., 2015).

Pupillometry to Assess Rods, Cones, and Intrinsically Photosensitive Retinal Ganglion Cells (ipRGCs)

Retinal illumination triggers the pupillary light reflex (PLR), a reflexive constriction of the pupillary sphincter muscle. This response has long been exploited by clinicians to probe the integrity of the retina and optic nerve, the parasympathetic innervation of ocular structures (cranial nerve), and the brainstem regions where the two are linked. An example of a pupillometer used clinically is shown in Figure 4-5. The retinal circuitry that signals the pupillary light reflex overlaps heavily with those linked to effects of luminance on axial elongation of the eye. They carry a steady-state irradiance signal driven by the retinal ON channel.

In mice, selective ablation (removal or destruction of a body part or tissue or its function) of ipRGCs eliminates retinal input to the obligatory brainstem relay center and blocks the pupillary light reflex (Guler et al., 2008; Hatori et al., 2008; Hattar et al., 2006). In mouse models lacking rod and cone function, this reflex persists due to the intrinsic photosensitivity of the M1 subtype of ipRGCs. In wild-type mice, however, the pupillary light reflex reflects contributions from rods and cones as well as from melanopsin within, and this appears to be true in humans as well. The pupillary light reflex thus provides a practical way to assess the integrity of neuronal types and networks that encode luminance at the retinal level. These are ostensibly the same as networks implicated in dopaminergic mechanisms that suppress axial elongation during eye development, as discussed elsewhere in this report (see Chapter 6, Dopaminergic Amacrine Cells and ipRGCs—Irradiance-coding Cells and Circuits).

Methods are available for assessing the specific contributions of rod, cone, and melanopsin to the pupillary light reflex in clinical as well as research settings for animal and human subjects. These methods have been documented in a report from members of the International Pupil Colloquium establishing formal standards for various kinds of pupillometry (Kelbsch et al., 2019). For example, the shutoff of melanopsin phototransduction is slower than in rods and cones, so the post-illumination pupil response, measured well after the light is turned off, provides an index of melanopsin response with minimal rod or cone contribution.

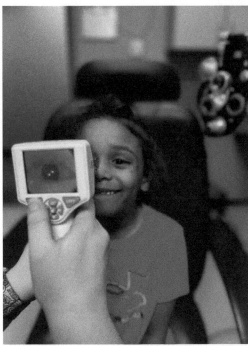

FIGURE 4-5 Example of a commercially available pupillometer being used clinically.
SOURCE: Courtesy of Katherine Weise, OD, University of Alabama at Birmingham.

Adaptive Optics

Adaptive optics is a technique used to improve the resolution of an imaging system by measuring and correcting for aberrations (optical imperfections or distortions) in the imaging path, typically by precise dynamic adjustment of deformable mirrors to compensate for the light distortions in the system. The technique was developed in astronomy to improve the imaging of celestial bodies by accounting for dynamic aberrations introduced by the earth's atmosphere. Adaptive optics was subsequently used in ophthalmology to correct for the aberrations introduced by the cornea and crystalline lens and obtain high resolution images of cells in the retina that would otherwise be blurred by the eye's optics in vivo. In addition, adaptive optics can be used to create visual stimuli on the retina that are limited only by diffraction due to the eye's pupil alone, or to create artificial optical conditions by superimposing new aberrations for vision simulation. Overall, adaptive optics has not only transformed the study of retinal structure and function in vivo in humans and animal models but provided new avenues for testing the impact of the eye's native and modified optics (via lenses, refractive surgery, intraocular lenses from cataract surgery, etc.) on visual function.

In the context of myopia, the adaptive optics scanning laser ophthalmoscope has revealed the structure of the foveal cone photoreceptor mosaic and how it varies with axial length (Dabir et al., 2015; Li et al., 2010 Wang et al., 2019). These findings have consequences for models of the expansion of the eye that determine its final shape and the factors that limit visual performance in myopia. Nevertheless, the effect of myopic retinal stretching on inner retinal anatomy and connectivity remains unknown. The use of OCT enhanced by adaptive optics and precise 3D image registration has shown the feasibility of imaging the topography of the ganglion cells in humans in vivo (Liu et al., 2017).

Aberrometry

Aberrometry—or measurement, analysis, and reporting of "optical imperfections" in an optical system—provides a holistic view of the optical quality of the eye and includes the sum of contributions from all the optical elements. This view, while not sufficient to pinpoint the specific optical quality of the crystalline lens or cornea, is very useful for describing the retinal image quality and refraction. Moreover, aberrometry accounts for changes in retinal shape that accompany axial elongation. Aberrometry has advantages over other methods for quantifying refractive error and optical quality in general in the context of myopia. For example, traditional autorefractor and retinoscopic measures of refraction often use smaller pupils compared to the wavefront sensor. The interaction between different aberrations significantly impacts the best image plane (Applegate et al., 2003). The higher-order aberrations are further exaggerated for larger pupils and peripheral eccentricities. Peripheral wavefront sensors are available that allow measuring aberrations across a wide visual field to characterize image quality (Jaeken & Artal, 2012; Jaeken et al., 2011; Pusti et al., 2023). Importantly, the measured aberrations can be converted to metrics of retinal image quality to assess how the image varies with factors such as accommodation and pupil size (Marsack et al., 2004). The application of aberrometry to evaluate the myopic eye is described in Chapter 6 (Eye Models).

Overall, aberrometry, in conjunction with morphometry of the cornea and crystalline lens, lays the foundation for an ideal eye model that would form the basis for testing new treatments and detailing the optics of the myopic eye. To this end, longitudinal studies of aberrometry and morphometry of the cornea and crystalline lens are needed, both early in childhood and prior to myopia onset, so that the causality and progression of the optical changes in normal and myopic eye growth can be investigated.

BOX 4-1
Diagnostic Technologies for Children

While the diagnostic technologies discussed in this chapter (specifically fundus photography, biometry, OCT, ERGs, contrast testing, visual fields, pupillometry, and aberrometry) are primarily used in adults and were not designed specifically for children, they can also be performed in children—especially school-aged and older depending on the degree of cooperation from the child and the patience of the person performing the test.

Some younger children may also be able to participate in the testing. Large-scale, randomized clinical trials of children with myopia often include several of the tests listed. However, there will be older children who will not have the attention or motivation to complete testing on a given day. In such cases, returning for retesting alone may be helpful to maximize attention and motivation and minimize apprehension.

To make diagnostic technology explicitly child-friendly, manufacturers should consider testing that:

- does not require direct contact with the eye: the further from the child, the better
- takes no more than a few seconds to minutes to obtain the measurement
- can be adjusted for varying sizes of children
- is portable or handheld so it can be applied in various settings
- avoids needing long instructions
- avoids using very bright lights
- has pictures for matching response or requested task
- has normative data for children if it is expected to differ from that of an adult.

Regarding the last bullet, some diagnostic devices will assist in interpretation of the measurement results by comparing them to normative databases of the measurement. If the measurement was not designed specifically for children, the normative database is typically based on adult measurements (e.g., OCT nerve fiber layer thicknesses for glaucoma). Hence, to be useful in children, normative databases for specific diagnostic measurements should also include data for children.

DIAGNOSTICS FOR ASSESSING THE ENVIRONMENT

The visual environment has been associated with the development of myopia in many studies. This includes associations with increased myopia and near work (Guo et al., 2016; Pärssinen & Kauppinen, 2019) and decreased myopia with more outdoor activity (He et al., 2015; Jones et al., 2007; Rose et al., 2008; Wu et al., 2020). Near work and outdoor time have predominantly been assessed using surveys and questionnaires or indirectly, such as by using educational attainment or occupation as a proxy for the amount of near work. To further study these environmental conditions, methods to objectively measure specific environmental variables have been developed. These include wearable light meters (because light is one of the principal aspects of the outdoors) and depth-sensing cameras to measure the distance of objects in the environment.

Wearable Light Meters

Wearable light meters are used to detect and record the wearer's environmental exposure to light. Reported wearable light meters to date have included dedicated, single-function light sensors worn as a pendant or affixed to clothing (Read et al., 2018), dedicated light sensors that can be attached to worn eyeglasses (Stampfi et al., 2023; Wen et al., 2021), and multi-function wristwatches with an incorporated light sensor (Read et al., 2015; Verkicharla et al. 2017; Ye et al., 2019). Depending on the configurations, the multi-function wristwatches could also measure other parameters (date/time, geographic position) that in turn could be used to obtain other associated data (e.g., weather) used to supplement the light measurement data. The light sensors on these wristwatches typically measure visible light intensity, though some have ultraviolet or near infrared measurement capabilities dependent on the included sensor. The published wristwatch studies have used either commercially available software and hardware (Philips Actiwatch 2), custom-developed software for a commercially available smartwatch (FitSight: custom app on a Sony SmartWatch), or custom-developed hardware and software (MuMu). As an aside, contemporary iOS and Android smartwatches do include light sensors in their suite of sensors. Though there have not yet been reports of their use in myopia studies, these in-built sensors appear to present an opportunity to obtain the desired light measurement from a relatively general-purpose device.

Depth-Sensing Cameras

Depth-sensing cameras are used for detecting the position of objects in the environment relative to the camera. A variety of techniques can be used for depth sensing, including structured illumination, by which a pattern is used to illuminate a scene and changes in the pattern are used to estimate the 3D position of elements in the scene; time-of-flight, which like radar or ultrasound uses the time it takes emitted energy to reflect from the scene back to the detector and is used to calculate the position of that element in the scene relative to the camera; and stereo cameras, where two or more cameras with a fixed relationship are used to image the scene and differences between the two imaged perspectives are used to calculate the position of objects in the scene.

In the study of myopia, wearable depth-sensing cameras can record the position of objects in the workspace of the wearer to provide direct measurements of the distance of objects during near work or outdoor activities. Consumer-grade (i.e., readily commercially attainable) depth-sensing cameras have only become available in the last decade, and the application of this technology in myopia is still new. Recent studies attaching these cameras to spectacle-like frames or helmets have demonstrated their potential use not only in relatively stationary indoor environments (García et al., 2017; Read et al., 2023) but even in dynamic, open outdoor environments (Banks, 2024). Alternatively, some current smartphones also have integrated depth-sensing cameras. Smartphone cameras designed and intended for face-scanning of the user can measure spatial relationships between the phone and its user. In the context of myopia, this information is used by on-device apps (e.g., Apple's Screen Distance) and has been used by researchers to objectively record viewing distance for children using smartphones (Richards et al., 2024).

Altogether, these increasingly accessible environment-sensing diagnostics and technologies are likely to constitute critical technologies for measuring and understanding the world that the myopic eye experiences, which this report refers to as the "visual diet."

OTHER ASSESSMENT AND DIAGNOSTIC TECHNOLOGIES

Artificial intelligence (including machine learning and deep learning) is a rapidly advancing area in general and specifically in ophthalmic research. While the concept of artificial intelligence is not new, within the last decade deep learning approaches such as convolutional neural networks have made rapid gains in tasks such as image classification that rival human performance (e.g., ImageNet challenge). The widespread use of diagnostic imaging in ophthalmology and optometry have benefited from these recent advances in artificial intelligence-based image classification. This research has progressed to the point that there are now U.S. Federal Drug Administration approved artificial intelligence–based diabetic retinopathy diagnostics for fundus photographs (U.S. Food & Drug Administration, 2018).

Artificial intelligence approaches are particularly suitable for complex entities with multi-parameter and/or nonlinear associations and typically depend on large, labeled datasets for training. Because myopia has complex genetic/hereditary and environmental underpinnings and exists in a field where diagnostic imaging is common, myopia seems particularly amenable to artificial intelligence approaches. Efforts to date in the myopia space have focused on diagnostic classification of images (e.g., presence of myopia, degree of myopia), identification of pathologic myopia features within images, prediction of targeted parameters (e.g., refractive errors, related parameters from other imaging modalities) from diagnostic imaging, and prediction of progression from biometric data, refraction data, or other recorded medical data (Du & Ohno-Matsui, 2022).

Artificial intelligence for myopia is still nascent and growing, and there is not yet broad usage or consensus as to its role in current clinical practice for myopia. Even for research, the ability to investigate associations, perform classifications, and create predictions is linked to the availability of the underlying data. Investigations are limited to recorded data; in other words, if one wants to predict the future axial-length elongation of an eye from refraction measurements, at some point a dataset with refraction and longitudinal axial-length data will need to be used for training. Clinical datasets will inherently be limited to the available diagnostic measurements. Also, the set of training data required for deep learning approaches is typically large, though if a similar model already exists, transfer learning approaches can be used that decrease the size of new training data.

Electronic health records hold the promise of large pools of medical data. However, because one clinician may qualitatively describe the same entity differently than another clinician or some data may simply not be recorded, the variability and consistency of the recording of granular data require an extensive investment in data preprocessing, cleaning, and harmonization before its use for applications such as artificial intelligence. There are current efforts underway to perform these tasks in the ophthalmic space, such as that of the Sight Outcomes Research Collaborative,[1] to pool ophthalmic data in electronic health records across multiple large academic medical centers. For both artificial intelligence and electronic health records, there can be limitations in representation and hence resultant bias. For instance, the underrepresentation of populations—whether they be underrepresented by ethnicity, by age, by lack of clinical usage, or by other characteristics—will be perpetuated in subsequent models or analyses whether in a training dataset for artificial intelligence or in an electronic health record

---

[1]For more information, see https://www.sourcecollaborative.org/about

dataset (Evans et al. 2022). The potential of artificial intelligence approaches to assist in myopia diagnostics has certainly been recognized, and the field is currently actively developing the data sources and defining the desired associations to realize that potential.

CONCLUSIONS

The landscape of myopia assessment and diagnosis remains marked by a notable absence of consensus regarding mandatory components within clinical examinations. While routine or comprehensive examination standards exist, specific guidelines for patients with myopia lack uniformity, leading to a spectrum of variability in clinical practices. This lack of standardization not only affects the consistency of clinical care but also hampers the availability of cohesive data types crucial for subsequent analyses, including population studies and advancements in artificial intelligence. Despite this challenge, the horizon is bright with the emergence of promising diagnostic biomarkers poised to revolutionize myopia diagnostics, management, and our understanding of the disease. However, their definitive role in both research and clinical care necessitates further exploration through rigorous clinical studies.

Furthermore, given that children represent the demographic most susceptible to myopia progression, there is a pressing need to develop assessment and diagnostic technologies tailored specifically for this vulnerable population. Such initiatives hold the potential to significantly enhance accessibility and efficacy of myopia management strategies targeted toward children, thus addressing a critical aspect of public health concern.

Conclusion 4-1: There is no consensus as to the mandatory assessment and diagnostic components of a clinical examination of the myopic patient aside from clinical standards for routine/comprehensive examinations in general. This lack of standardization creates variability in clinical care and affects the availability of data for downstream analyses such as for population studies and artificial intelligence efforts. When available and feasible, the following clinical tools may enhance the assessment of the myopic eye.

- *In addition to a dilated fundus exam, fundus imaging is valuable to assessing posterior eye pathologies associated with myopia, as it records color views of the retina.*
- *Optical coherence tomography provides high-resolution cross-sections for more detailed assessment of structural retinal changes.*
- *Devices that measure axial length allow for more detailed assessment of eye growth, which may help assess risk to eye health.*

Conclusion 4-2: There are promising diagnostic biomarkers (e.g., axial elongation, changes in choroidal thickness and ocular shape, optical aberrations) and technologies (electroretinograms based on the hypothesis that outer-retinal neuron signaling affects myopia development) that may be useful for myopia diagnostics, management, and understanding of the disease. Further work in clinical studies is needed to definitively establish their role in research and clinical care of myopia.

Conclusion 4-3: Children are most at risk of myopia progression, and designing assessment and diagnostic technologies for children enhances the description of their myopic eyes, which may allow for more precise treatment in this critical population.

RECOMMENDATIONS

Recommendation 4-1: Ophthalmologists and optometrists should always use cycloplegic eye drops in children to obtain a consistent retinoscopy/refractive error reading along with pupillary dilation for visualizing the health of the middle and back of the eye, particularly for younger patients who have large accommodative and pupil constriction ability. If possible and available, other objective structural measurements of the eye should be obtained, such as axial length and optical coherence tomography. Payors (e.g., health/vision insurances) should reimburse for these examinations and tests to ensure their performance longitudinally.

Recommendation 4-2: Researchers and developers of assessment and diagnostic technologies should design assessments and tests to better understand the myopic eye, its development, and its environment (the visual diet). In addition to identifying eyes that are already myopic, there is also a need to identify eyes at risk for myopia in childhood and to identify other key events (e.g., pre-pathologic myopia state in adulthood). Other diagnostic technologies to support these goals include, for example, biometric and functional measurements to develop individualized eye modeling, improved choroidal imaging, and methods to sense and measure the visual environment.

Recommendation 4-3: Professionals examining the eye and organizations representing them (such as the American Academy of Pediatrics, American Academy of Pediatric Ophthalmology and Strabismus, American Academy of Optometry, and American Academy of Ophthalmology), together with researchers and other stakeholders in the field of myopia, should discuss and develop consensus standards for the assessments and diagnostics they deem most important for population-level studies. Development of a consortium/network repository for myopia-related clinical data by international or national entities (e.g., International Myopia Institute, National Eye Institute) would further these efforts. This would benefit standardization not only for clinical care but also for research, particularly with artificial intelligence efforts.

Recommendation 4-4: Developers of assessment and diagnostic technologies should consider the ability to use the technology in multiple age groups and settings as major design criteria. This includes making the technology time-efficient and "child-friendly." To ensure the broadest adoption, such technologies should also be made as portable and cost-effective for the end user as is feasible.

REFERENCES

Al-Sheikh, M., Phasukkijwatana, N., Dolz-Marco, R., Rahimi, M., Iafe, N. A., Freund, K. B., Sadda, S. R., & Sarraf, D. (2017). Quantitative OCT angiography of the retinal microvasculature and the choriocapillaris in myopic eyes. *Investigative Ophthalmology & Visual Science, 58*(4), 2063–2069. https://doi.org/10.1167/iovs.16-21289

American Academy of Ophthalmology. (2020). Pathologic myopia with tilted disc and peripapillary atrophy of RPE and choroid [Image]. Eyewiki. https://eyewiki.org/File:AA0_13422.jpg

Applegate, R. A., Hilmantel, G., Thibos, L. N., & Hong, X. (2003). Interaction between aberrations to improve or reduce visual performance. *Journal of Cataract & Refractive Surgery, 29*(8), 1487–1495. http://dx.doi.org/10.1016/S0886-3350(03)00334-1

Atchison, D. A., Pritchard, N., Schmid, K. L., Scott, D. H., Jones, C. E., & Pope, J. M. (2005). Shape of the retinal surface in emmetropia and myopia. *Investigative Ophthalmology & Visual Science, 46*(8), 2698–2707. https://doi.org/10.1167/iovs.04-1506

Banks, M. (2023). *Depth statistics of indoor and outdoor light* [Workshop presentation]. Workshop on the Rise in Myopia: Exploring Possible Contributors and Investigating Screening Practices, Policies, and Programs. National Academies of Sciences, Engineering, and Medicine. Washington, DC, United States. https://www.nationalacademies.org/event/41360_12-2023_workshop-on-the-rise-in-myopia-exploring-possible-contributors-and-investigating-screening-practices-policies-and-programs

Buckhurst, H. D., Gilmartin, B., Cubbidge, R. P., & Logan, N. S. (2015). Measurement of scleral thickness in humans using anterior segment optical coherent tomography. *PLOS One, 10*(7), e0132902. https://doi.org/10.1371/journal.pone.0132902

Chan, H. H. L., Choi, K. Y., Ng, A. L. K., Choy, B. N. K., Chan, J. C. H., Chan, S. S. H., Li, S. Z. C., & Yu, W. Y. (2022). Efficacy of 0.01% atropine for myopia control in a randomized, placebo-controlled trial depends on baseline electroretinal response. *Scientific Reports, 12*(1), 11588. https://doi.org/10.1038/s41598-022-15686-6

Chang, X., Li, M., Lv, L., Yan, X., Liu, Y., Zhu, M., Wang, J., Wang, P., & Xiang, Y. (2022). Assessment of choroidal vascularity and choriocapillaris blood perfusion after accommodation in myopia, emmetropia, and hyperopia groups among children. *Frontiers in Physiology, 13*, 854240. https://doi.org/10.3389/fphys.2022.854240Cheng, H. M., Singh, O. S., Kwong, K. K., Xiong, J., Woods, B. T., & Brady, T. J. (1992). Shape of the myopic eye as seen with high-resolution magnetic resonance imaging. *Optometry and Vision Science, 69*(9), 698–701. https://doi.org/10.1097/00006324-199209000-00005

Chiang, S. T., Phillips, J. R., & Backhouse, S. (2015). Effect of retinal image defocus on the thickness of the human choroid. *Ophthalmic & Physiological Optics, 35*(4), 405–413. https://doi.org/10.1111/opo.12218

Corvi, F., Su, L., & Sadda, S. R. (2021). Evaluation of the inner choroid using OCT angiography. *Eye, 35*(1), 110–120. https://doi.org/10.1038%2Fs41433-020-01217-y

Dabir, S., Mangalesh, S., Schouten, J. S., Berendschot, T. T., Kurian, M. K., Kumar, A. K., Yadav, N. K., & Shetty, R. (2015). Axial length and cone density as assessed with adaptive optics in myopia. *Indian Journal of Ophthalmology, 63*(5), 423–426. https://doi.org/10.4103/0301-4738.159876

Devarajan, K., Sim, R., Chua, J., Wong, C. W., Matsumura, S., Htoon, H. M., Schmetterer, L., Saw, S. M., & Ang, M. (2020). Optical coherence tomography angiography for the assessment of choroidal vasculature in high myopia. *The British Journal of Ophthalmology, 104*(7), 917–923. https://doi.org/10.1136/bjophthalmol-2019-314769Dhakal, R., Vupparaboina, K. K., & Verkicharla, P. K. (2020). Anterior sclera undergoes thinning with increasing degree of myopia. *Investigative Ophthalmology & Visual Science, 61*(4), 6. https://doi.org/10.1167/iovs.61.4.6

Du, R., & Ohno-Matsui, K. (2022). Novel uses and challenges of artificial intelligence in diagnosing and managing eyes with high myopia and pathologic myopia. *Diagnostics (Basel), 12*(5), 1210. https://doi.org/10.3390%2Fdiagnostics12051210

Evans, N. G., Wenner, D. M., Cohen, I. G., Purves, D., Chiang, M. F., Ting, D. S. W., & Lee, A. Y. (2022). Emerging ethical considerations for the use of artificial intelligence in ophthalmology. *Ophthalmology Science*, 2(2), 100141. https://doi.org/10.1016/j.xops.2022.100141

Ferrara, D., Waheed, N. K., & Duker, J. S. (2016). Investigating the choriocapillaris and choroidal vasculature with new optical coherence tomography technologies. *Progress in Retinal and Eye Research*, 52, 130–155. https://doi.org/10.1016/j.preteyeres.2015.10.002

Frishman, L. J. (2013). Electrogenesis of the electroretinogram. In S. R. Sadda (Ed.), *Ryan's Retinal Imaging and Diagnostics* (pp. e178–e202). https://doi.org/10.1016/b978-0-323-26254-5.00007-7

García, M. G., Ohlendorf, A., Schaeffel, F., & Wahl, S. (2017). Dioptric defocus maps across the visual field for different indoor environments. *Biomedical Optics Express*, 9(1), 347–359. https://doi.org/10.1364/BOE.9.000347

Gaucher, D., Erginay, A., Lecleire-Collet, A., Haouchine, B., Puech, M., Cohen, S. Y., Massin, P., & Gaudric, A. (2008). Dome-shaped macula in eyes with myopic posterior staphyloma. *American Journal of Ophthalmology*, 145(5), 909–914. https://doi.org/10.1016/j.ajo.2008.01.012

Guo, L., Yang, J., Mai, J., Du, X., Guo, Y., Li, P., & Zhang, W. H. (2016). Prevalence and associated factors of myopia among primary and middle school-aged students: A school-based study in Guangzhou. *Eye*, 30(6), 796–804. https://doi.org/10.1038/eye.2016.39

Gupta, S. K., Chakraborty, R., & Verkicharla, P. K. (2022). Electroretinogram responses in myopia: A review. *Documenta Ophthalmologica*, 145, 77–95. https://doi.org/10.1007/s10633-021-09857-5

Gupta, Y., Weng, C. Y., & Lim, J. I. (2024). Myopic CNVM. *EyeWiki*. American Academy of Ophthalmology. https://eyewiki.org/Myopic_CNVM

Gwiazda, J., Thorn, F., Bauer, J., & Held, R. (1993). Myopic children show insufficient accommodative response to blur. *Investigative Ophthalmology & Visual Science*, 34(3), 690–694. https://pubmed.ncbi.nlm.nih.gov/8449687/

Hattar, S., Kumar, M., Park, A., Tong, P., Tung, J., Yau, K. W., & Berson, D. M. (2006). Central projections of melanopsin-expressing retinal ganglion cells in the mouse. *Journal of Comparative Neurology*, 497(3), 326–349. https://doi.org/10.1002/cne.20970

He, M., Xiang, F., Zeng, Y., Mai, J., Chen, Q., Zhang, J., Smith, W., Rose, K., & Morgan, I. G. (2015). Effect of time spent outdoors at school on the development of myopia among children in China: A randomized clinical trial. *JAMA*, 314(11), 1142–1148. https://doi.org/10.1001/jama.2015.10803

Ichinose, T., & Habib, S. (2022). ON and OFF Signaling Pathways in the Retina and the Visual System. *Frontiers in Ophthalmology*, 2, 989002. https://doi.org/10.3389/fopht.2022.989002

Imamura, Y., Iida, T., Maruko, I., Zweifel, S. A., & Spaide, R. F. (2011). Enhanced depth imaging optical coherence tomography of the sclera in dome-shaped macula. *American Journal of Ophthalmology*, 151(2), 297–302. https://doi.org/10.1016/j.ajo.2010.08.014

Ito, K., Lye, T. H., Dan, Y. S., Yu, J. D. G., Silverman, R. H., Mamou, J., & Hoang, Q. V. (2022). Automated classification and detection of staphyloma with ultrasound images in pathologic myopia eyes. *Ultrasound in Medicine & Biology*, 48(12), 2430–2441. https://doi.org/10.1016/j.ultrasmedbio.2022.06.010

Jacobs, D. S., Afshari, N. A., Bishop, R. J., Keenan, J. D., Lee, J. K., Shen, T. T., & Vitale, S. (2022). *Refractive errors Preferred Practice Pattern guideline 2022*. American Academy of Ophthalmology. https://www.aao.org/education/preferred-practice-pattern/refractive-errors-ppp-2022

Jaeken, B., & Artal, P. (2012). Optical quality of emmetropic and myopic eyes in the periphery measured with high-angular resolution. *Investigative Ophthalmology & Visual Science*, 53(7), 3405–3413. https://doi.org/10.1167/iovs.11-8993

Jaeken, B., Lundström, L., & Artal, P. (2011). Fast scanning peripheral wave-front sensor for the human eye. *Optics Express*, 19(8), 73–82. https://doi.org/10.1364/oe.19.007903

Jia, Y., Bailey, S. T., Hwang, T. S., McClintic, S. M., Gao, S. S., Pennesi, M. E., Flaxel, C. J., Lauer, A. K., Wilson, D. J., Hornegger, J., Fujimoto, J. G., & Huang, D. (2015). Quantitative optical coherence tomography angiography of vascular abnormalities in the living human eye. *Proceedings of the National Academy of Sciences of the United States of America, 112*(18), E2395–E2402. https://doi.org/10.1073/pnas.1500185112

Jones, L. A., Mitchell, G. L., Mutti, D. O., Hayes, J. R., Moeschberger, M. L., & Zadnik, K. (2005). Comparison of ocular component growth curves among refractive error groups in children. *Investigative Ophthalmology & Visual Science, 46*(7), 2317–2327. https://doi.org/10.1167/iovs.04-0945

Jones, L. A., Sinnott, L. T., Mutti, D. O., Mitchell, G. L., Moeschberger, M. L., & Zadnik, K. (2007). Parental history of myopia, sports and outdoor activities, and future myopia. *Investigative Ophthalmology & Visual Science, 48*(8), 3524–3532. https://doi.org/10.1167/iovs.06-1118

Kelbsch, C., Strasser, T., Chen, Y., Feigl, B., Gamlin, P. D., Kardon, R., Peters, T., Roecklein, K. A., Steinhauer, S. R., Szabadi, E., Zele, A. J., Wilhelm, H., & Wilhelm, B. J. (2019). Standards in Pupillography. *Frontiers in Neurology, 10*, 129. https://doi.org/10.3389/fneur.2019.00129

Kuo, A. N., Verkicharla, P. K., McNabb, R. P., Cheung, C. Y., Hilal, S., Farsiu, S., Chen, C., Wong, T. Y., Ikram, M. K., Cheng, C. Y., Young, T. L., Saw, S. M., & Izatt, J. A. (2016). Posterior eye shape measurement with retinal OCT compared to MRI. *Investigative Ophthalmology & Visual Science, 57*(9), OCT196–OCT203. https://doi.org/10.1167/iovs.15-18886

Li, K. Y., Tiruveedhula, P., & Roorda, A. (2010). Intersubject variability of foveal cone photoreceptor density in relation to eye length. *Investigative Ophthalmology & Visual Science, 51*(12), 6858–6867. https://doi.org/10.1167/iovs.10-5499

Liou, S. W., & Chiu, C. J. (2001). Myopia and contrast sensitivity function. *Current Eye Research, 22*(2), 81–84. https://doi.org/10.1076/ceyr.22.2.81.5530

Liu, L., Zhu, C., Yuan, Y., Hu, X., Chen, C., Zhu, H., & Ke, B. (2022). Three-dimensional choroidal vascularity index in high myopia using swept-source optical coherence tomography. *Current Eye Research, 47*(3), 484–492. https://doi.org/10.1080/02713683.2021.2006236

Liu, X., Jiang, L., Ke, M., Sigal, I. A., Chua, J., Hoang, Q. V., Chia, A. W., Najjar, R. P., Tan, B., Cheong, J., Bellemo, V., Chong, R. S., Girard, M. J. A., Ang, M., Liu, M., Garhöfer, G., Barathi, V. A., Saw, S. M., Villiger, M., & Schmetterer, L. (2023). Posterior scleral birefringence measured by triple-input polarization-sensitive imaging as a biomarker of myopia progression. *Nature Biomedical Engineering, 7*(8), 986–1000. https://doi.org/10.1038/s41551-023-01062-w

Liu, Z., Kurokawa, K., Zhang, F., Lee, J. J., & Miller, D. T. (2017). Imaging and quantifying ganglion cells and other transparent neurons in the living human retina. *Proceedings of the National Academy of Sciences of the United States of America, 114*(48), 12803–12808. https://doi.org/10.1073/pnas.1711734114

Mariampillai, A., Standish, B. A., Moriyama, E. H., Khurana, M., Munce, N. R., Leung, M. K., Jiang, J., Cable, A., Wilson, B. C., Vitkin, I. A., & Yang, V. X. (2008). Speckle variance detection of microvasculature using swept-source optical coherence tomography. *Optics Letters, 33*(13), 1530–1532. https://doi.org/10.1364/ol.33.001530

Marsack, J. D., Thibos, L. N., & Applegate, R. A. (2004). Metrics of optical quality derived from wave aberrations predict visual performance. *Journal of Vision, 4*(4). https://doi.org/10.1167/4.4.8

McNabb, R. P., Polans, J., Keller, B., Jackson-Atogi, M., James, C. L., Vann, R. R., Izatt, J. A., & Kuo, A. N. (2018). Wide-field whole eye OCT system with demonstration of quantitative retinal curvature estimation. *Biomedical Optics Express, 10*(1), 338–355. https://doi.org/10.1364/BOE.10.000338

McNabb, R. P., Liu, A. S., Gospe, S. M., 3rd, El-Dairi, M., Meekins, L. C., James, C., Vann, R. R., Izatt, J. A., & Kuo, A. N. (2021). Quantitative topographic curvature maps of the posterior eye utilizing optical coherence tomography. *Retina, 41*(4), 804–811. https://doi.org/10.1097/IAE.0000000000002897

Mooney, S. W. J., Alam, N. M., & Prusky, G. T. (2021). Tracking-based interactive assessment of saccades, pursuits, visual field, and contrast sensitivity in children with brain injury. *Frontiers in Human Neuroscience, 15*, 737409. https://doi.org/10.3389/fnhum.2021.737409

Moriyama, M., Ohno-Matsui, K., Hayashi, K., Shimada, N., Yoshida, T., Tokoro, T., & Morita, I. (2011). Topographic analyses of shape of eyes with pathologic myopia by high-resolution three-dimensional magnetic resonance imaging. *Ophthalmology, 118*(8), 1626–1637. https://doi.org/10.1016/j.ophtha.2011.01.032

Mutti, D. O., Hayes, J. R., Mitchell, G. L., Jones, L. A., Moeschberger, M. L., Cotter, S. A., Kleinstein, R. N., Manny, R. E., Twelker, J. D., Zadnik, K., & CLEERE Study Group. (2007). Refractive error, axial length, and relative peripheral refractive error before and after the onset of myopia. *Investigative Ophthalmology & Visual Science, 48*(6), 2510–2519. https://doi.org/10.1167/iovs.06-0562

Mutti, D. O., Mitchell, G. L., Hayes, J. R., Jones, L. A., Moeschberger, M. L., Cotter, S. A., Kleinstein, R. N., Manny, R. E., Twelker, J. D., Zadnik, K., & CLEERE Study Group. (2006). Accommodative lag before and after the onset of myopia. *Investigative Ophthalmology & Visual Science, 47*(3), 837–846. https://doi.org/10.1167/iovs.05-0888

Mutti, D. O., Sholtz, R. I., Friedman, N. E., & Zadnik, K. (2000). Peripheral refraction and ocular shape in children. *Investigative Ophthalmology & Visual Science, 41*(5), 1022–1030. https://pubmed.ncbi.nlm.nih.gov/10752937/

Nallasamy, S., Silbert, D. I., & Chang, L. (2024). EyeWiki: Photoscreening. *EyeWiki*. American Academy of Ophthalmology. https://eyewiki.aao.org/Photoscreening

National Eye Institute. (n.d.). Illustrations of different eye shapes [Image]. https://medialibrary.nei.nih.gov/media/3551

___. (2020). Normal retina: Fundus photograph-normal retina [Image]. https://medialibrary.nei.nih.gov/media/3825

Ni, S., Nguyen, T. P., Ng, R., Woodward, M., Ostmo, S., Jia, Y., Chiang, M. F., Huang, D., Skalet, A. H., Campbell, J. P., & Jian, Y. (2023). Panretinal optical coherence tomography. *IEEE Transactions on Medical Imaging, 42*(11), 3219–3228. https://doi.org/10.1109/TMI.2023.3278269

Ohno-Matsui, K., Akiba, M., Moriyama, M., Shimada, N., Ishibashi, T., Tokoro, T., & Spaide, R. F. (2012). Acquired optic nerve and peripapillary pits in pathologic myopia. *Ophthalmology, 119*(8), 1685–1692. https://doi.org/10.1016/j.ophtha.2012.01.047

Ohno-Matsui, K., Igarashi-Yokoi, T., Azuma, T., Sugisawa, K., Xiong, J., Takahashi, T., Uramoto, K., Kamoi, K., Okamoto, M., Banerjee, S., & Yamanari, M. (2024). Polarization-sensitive OCT imaging of scleral abnormalities in eyes with high myopia and dome-shaped macula. *JAMA Ophthalmology, 142*(4), 310–319. https://doi.org/10.1001/jamaophthalmol.2024.0002

Ohno-Matsui, K., & Tokoro, T. (1996). The progression of lacquer cracks in pathologic myopia. *Retina, 16*(1), 29–37. https://doi.org/10.1097/00006982-199616010-00006

Ostrin, L. A., Harb, E., Nickla, D. L., Read, S. A., Alonso-Caneiro, D., Schroedl, F., Kaser-Eichberger, A., Zhou, X., & Wildsoet, C. F. (2023). IMI—The dynamic choroid: New insights, challenges, and potential significance for human myopia. *Investigative Ophthalmology & Visual Science, 64*(6), 4. https://doi.org/10.1167/iovs.64.6.4

Pardue, M. T., & Peachey, N. S. (2014). Mouse b-wave mutants. *Documenta Ophthalmologica. Advances in Ophthalmology, 128*(2), 77–89. https://doi.org/10.1007/s10633-013-9424-8

Park, H., Tan, C. C., Faulkner, A., Jabbar, S. B., Schmid, G., Abey, J., Iuvone, P. M., & Pardue, M. T. (2013). Retinal degeneration increases susceptibility to myopia in mice. *Molecular Vision, 19*, 2068–2079. https://www.ncbi.nlm.nih.gov/pmc/articles/PMC3786452/

Pärssinen, O., & Kauppinen, M. (2019). Risk factors for high myopia: A 22-year follow-up study from childhood to adulthood. *Acta Ophthalmologica, 97*(5), 510–518. https://doi.org/10.1111/aos.13964

Pekel, G., Yağcı, R., Acer, S., Ongun, G. T., Çetin, E. N., & Simavlı, H. (2015). Comparison of corneal layers and anterior sclera in emmetropic and myopic eyes. *Cornea, 34*(7), 786–790. https://doi.org/10.1097/ICO.0000000000000422

Poudel, S., Jin, J., Rahimi-Nasrabadi, H., Dellostritto, S., Dul, M. W., Viswanathan, S., & Alonso, J. M. (2024). Contrast sensitivity of ON and OFF human retinal pathways in myopia. *The Journal of Neuroscience, 44*(3), e1487232023. https://doi.org/10.1523/jneurosci.1487-23.2023

Pusti, D., Kendrick, C. D., Wu, Y., Ji, Q., Jung, H. W., & Yoon, G. (2023). Widefield wavefront sensor for multidirectional peripheral retinal scanning. *Biomedical Optics Express, 14*(9), 4190–4204. https://doi.org/10.1364%2FBOE.491412

Ramkumar, H. L., Epley, D., Shah, V. A., Kumar, U. R., Tripathy, K., Prakalapakorn, S. G., Hyde, R. A., Lim, J. I., Griffiths, D., Karth, P. A., & Rodriguez, S. (2024). Electroretinogram. *EyeWiki*. American Academy of Ophthalmology. https://eyewiki.aao.org/Electroretinogram

Read, S. A., Collins, M. J., & Sander, B. P. (2010). Human optical axial length and defocus. *Investigative Ophthalmology & Visual Science, 51*(12), 6262–6269. https://doi.org/10.1167/iovs.10-5457

Read, S. A., Collins, M. J., & Vincent, S. J. (2015). Light exposure and eye growth in childhood. *Investigative Ophthalmology & Visual Science, 56*(11), 6779–6787. https://doi.org/10.1167/iovs.14-15978

Read, S. A., Fuss, J. A., Vincent, S. J., Collins, M. J., & Alonso-Caneiro, D. (2019). Choroidal changes in human myopia: Insights from optical coherence tomography imaging. *Clinical & Experimental Optometry, 102*(3), 270–285. https://doi.org/10.1111/cxo.12862

Read, S. A., Vincent, S. J., Tan, C. S., Ngo, C., Collins, M. J., & Saw, S. M. (2018). Patterns of daily outdoor light exposure in Australian and Singaporean children. *Translational Vision Science & Technology, 7*(3), 8. https://doi.org/10.1167/tvst.7.3.8

Richards, J., Jakulski, M., Rickert, M., & Kollbaum, P. (2024). Digital device viewing behavior in children. *Ophthalmic and Physiological Optics, 44*(3), 546–553. https://doi.org/10.1111/opo.13288

Rose, K. A., Morgan, I. G., Ip, J., Kifley, A., Huynh, S., Smith, W., & Mitchell, P. (2008). Outdoor activity reduces the prevalence of myopia in children. *Ophthalmology, 115*(8), 1279–1285. https://doi.org/10.1016/j.ophtha.2007.12.019

Scherm, P., Pettenkofer, M., Maier, M., Lohmann, C. P., & Feucht, N. (2019). Choriocapillary blood flow in myopic subjects measured with OCT angiography. *Ophthalmic Surgery, Lasers & Imaging Retina, 50*(5), e133–e139. https://doi.org/10.3928/23258160-20190503-13

Schiller, P. H. (1992). The ON and OFF channels of the visual system. *Trends in Neurosciences, 15*(3), 86–92. https://doi.org/10.1016/0166-2236(92)90017-3

Schmid, G. F. (2003). Axial and peripheral eye length measured with optical low coherence reflectometry. *Journal of Biomedical Optics, 8*(4), 655–662. https://doi.org/10.1117/1.1606461

Shinohara, K., Shimada, N., Moriyama, M., Yoshida, T., Jonas, J. B., Yoshimura, N., & Ohno-Matsui, K. (2017). Posterior staphylomas in pathologic myopia imaged by widefield optical coherence tomography. *Investigative Ophthalmology & Visual Science, 58*(9), 3750–3758. https://doi.org/10.1167/iovs.17-22319

Smith, E. L. III. (2011). Prentice Award Lecture 2010: A case for peripheral optical treatment strategies for myopia. *Optometry and Vision Science, 88*(9), 1029–1044. https://doi.org/10.1097%2FOPX.0b013e3182279cfa

Stampfli, J. R., Schrader, B., di Battista, C., Häfliger, R., Schälli, O., Wichmann, G., Zumbühl, C., Blattner, P., Cajochen, C., Lazar, R., & Spitschan, M. (2023). The light-dosimeter: A new device to help advance research on the non-visual responses to light. *Lighting Research & Technology, 55*(4-5), 474–486. https://doi.org/10.1177/14771535221147140

Tan, B., McNabb, R. P., Zheng, F., Sim, Y. C., Yao, X., Chua, J., Ang, M., Hoang, Q. V., Kuo, A. N., & Schmetterer, L. (2021). Ultrawide field, distortion-corrected ocular shape estimation with MHz optical coherence tomography (OCT). *Biomedical Optics Express, 12*(9), 5770–5781. https://doi.org/10.1364/BOE.428430

Tideman, J. W., Snabel, M. C., Tedja, M. S., van Rijn, G. A., Wong, K. T., Kuijpers, R. W., Vingerling, J. R., Hofman, A., Buitendijk, G. H., Keunen, J. E., Boon, C. J., Geerards, A. J., Luyten, G. P., Verhoeven, V. J., & Klaver, C. C. (2016). Association of axial length with risk of uncorrectable visual impairment for Europeans with myopia. *JAMA Ophthalmology*, *134*(12), 1355–1363. https://doi.org/10.1001/jamaophthalmol.2016.4009

U.S. Food & Drug Administration. (2018, April 11). *FDA permits marketing of artificial intelligence-based device to detect certain diabetes-related eye problems* [Press release]. https://www.fda.gov/news-events/press-announcements/fda-permits-marketing-artificial-intelligence-based-device-detect-certain-diabetes-related-eye

Verkicharla, P. K., Ramamurthy, D., Nguyen, Q. D., Zhang, X., Pu, S. H., Malhotra, R., Ostbye, T., Lamoureux, E. L., & Saw, S. M. (2017). Development of the FitSight Fitness Tracker to increase time outdoors to prevent myopia. *Translational Vision Science & Technology*, *6*(3), 20. https://doi.org/10.1167/tvst.6.3.20

Verkicharla, P. K., Suheimat, M., Pope, J. M., Sepehrband, F., Mathur, A., Schmid, K. L., & Atchison, D. A. (2015). Validation of a partial coherence interferometry method for estimating retinal shape. *Biomedical Optics Express*, *6*(9), 3235–3247. https://doi.org/10.1364%2FBOE.6.003235

Vurgese, S., Panda-Jonas, S., & Jonas, J. B. (2012). Scleral thickness in human eyes. *PLOS One*, *7*(1), e29692. https://doi.org/10.1371/journal.pone.0029692

Wang, Y., Bensaid, N., Tiruveedhula, P., Ma, J., Ravikumar, S., & Roorda, A. (2019). Human foveal cone photoreceptor topography and its dependence on eye length. *eLife*, *8*, e47148. https://doi.org/10.7554/eLife.47148

Wang, D., Chun, R. K., Liu, M., Lee, R. P., Sun, Y., Zhang, T., Lam, C., Liu, Q., & To, C. H. (2016). Optical defocus rapidly changes choroidal thickness in schoolchildren. *PloS One*, *11*(8), e0161535. https://doi.org/10.1371/journal.pone.0161535

Wen, L., Cheng, Q., Cao, Y., Li, X., Pan, L., Li, L., Zhu, H., Mogran, I., Lan, W., & Yang, Z. (2021). The Clouclip, a wearable device for measuring near-work and outdoor time: Validation and comparison of objective measures with questionnaire estimates. *Acta Ophthalmologica*, *99*(7), e1222–e1235. https://doi.org/10.1111/aos.14785

Wolffsohn, J. S., Flitcroft, D. I., Gifford, K. L., Jong, M., Jones, L., Klaver, C. C. W., Logan, N. S., Naidoo, K., Resnikoff, S., Sankaridurg, P., Smith, E. L., 3rd, Troilo, D., & Wildsoet, C. F. (2019). IMI—Myopia control reports overview and introduction. *Investigative Ophthalmology & Visual Science*, *60*(3), M1–M19. https://doi.org/10.1167/iovs.18-25980

Wong, H. B., Machin, D., Tan, S. B., Wong, T. Y., & Saw, S. M. (2010). Ocular component growth curves among Singaporean children with different refractive error status. *Investigative Ophthalmology & Visual Science*, *51*(3), 1341–1347. https://doi.org/10.1167/iovs.09-3431

Wong, C. W., Teo, Y. C. K., Tsai, S. T. A., Ting, S. W. D., Yeo, Y. S. I., Wong, W. K. D., Lee, S. Y., Wong, T. Y., & Cheung, C. M. G. (2019). Characterization of the choroidal vasculature in myopic maculopathy with optical coherence tomographic angiography. *Retina*, *39*(9), 1742–1750. https://doi.org/10.1097/iae.0000000000002233

Wu, P. C., Chen, C. T., Chang, L. C., Niu, Y. Z., Chen, M. L., Liao, L. L., Rose, K., & Morgan, I. G. (2020). Increased time outdoors is followed by reversal of the long-term trend to reduced visual acuity in Taiwan primary school students. *Ophthalmology*, *127*(11), 1462–1469. https://doi.org/10.1016/j.ophtha.2020.01.054

Wu, H., Xie, Z., Wang, P., Liu, M., Wang, Y., Zhu, J., Chen, X., Xu, Z., Mao, X., & Zhou, X. (2021). Differences in retinal and choroidal vasculature and perfusion related to axial length in pediatric anisomyopes. *Investigative Ophthalmology & Visual Science*, *62*(9), 40. https://doi.org/10.1167/iovs.62.9.40

Xu, A., Sun, G., Duan, C., Chen, Z., & Chen, C. (2021). Quantitative assessment of three-dimensional choroidal vascularity and choriocapillaris flow signal voids in myopic patients using SS-OCTA. *Diagnostics*, *11*(11), 1948. https://doi.org/10.3390/diagnostics11111948

Ye, B., Liu, K., Cao, S., Sankaridurg, P., Li, W., Luan, M., Zhang, B., Zhu, J., Zou, H., Xu, X., & He, X. (2019). Discrimination of indoor versus outdoor environmental state with machine learning algorithms in myopia observational studies. *Journal of Translational Medicine, 17*(1), 314. https://doi.org/10.1186/s12967-019-2057-2

Zadnik, K., Sinnott, L. T., Cotter, S. A., Jones-Jordan, L. A., Kleinstein, R. N., Manny, R. E., Twelker, J. D., Mutti, D. O., & Collaborative Longitudinal Evaluation of Ethnicity and Refractive Error (CLEERE) Study Group (2015). Prediction of juvenile-onset myopia. *JAMA Ophthalmology, 133*(6), 683–689. https://doi.org/10.1001/jamaophthalmol.2015.0471

Zahra, S., Murphy, M. J., Crewther, S. G., & Riddell, N. (2023). Flash electroretinography as a measure of retinal function in myopia and hyperopia: A systematic review. *Vision, 7*(1), 15. https://doi.org/10.3390%2Fvision7010015

Zheng, F., Chua, J., Ke, M., Tan, B., Yu, M., Hu, Q., Cheung, C. M. G., Ang, M., Lee, S. Y., Wong, T. Y., SNEC Retina Group, Schmetterer, L., Wong, C. W., & Hoang, Q. V. (2022). Quantitative OCT angiography of the retinal microvasculature and choriocapillaris in highly myopic eyes with myopic macular degeneration. *The British Journal of Ophthalmology, 106*(5), 681–688. https://doi.org/10.1136/bjophthalmol-2020-317632

Zhou, J., He, H., Yang, Q., Wang, J.-Y., You, Z.-P., & Liu, L.-L. (2023). Comparison of anterior sclera thickness in emmetropes and myopes. *BMC Ophthalmology, 23*(1), 67. https://doi.org/10.1186/s12886-023-02775-x

5

Onset and Progression of Myopia

This chapter covers genetic and environmental factors that may contribute to the onset and progression of myopia. Evidence is presented on how myopia development may be influenced by genetic factors, visual behaviors such as near work or use of electronic devices, and the visual environment while indoors versus outdoors. Here the committee defines "myopia onset" as the first occurrence of a refractive error that meets the formal definition of myopia, usually a spherical or spherical equivalent refractive error between –0.5 and –1.0 D.[1] While most of this chapter focuses on human studies and randomized clinical trials, results from animal studies are also included as evidence for, or against, the effects of particular risk factors. The committee had the opportunity to develop recommendations from a holistic, societal perspective to address what is controllable about environmental risks for myopia, management of the condition, and improving equity in access to diagnosis and treatment of myopia.

During the past decade, insufficient time spent outdoors has emerged as a major factor for increasing the risk of myopia onset. The risk of myopia caused by insufficient time outdoors is amenable to study in randomized controlled trials, which have yielded convincing evidence for its role in myopia onset and, potentially, myopia progression. Researchers have also explored the possible roles of education and near-work, including the use of electronic devices such as smartphones. These investigations have relied predominantly on cross-sectional and longitudinal epidemiology study designs, which require strong assumptions for causal inference. Existing research suggests that genetics does not explain the surge in myopia prevalence over recent decades. Nevertheless, genetics research has provided insight into causal biological mechanisms and helped to explain differences between individuals in their susceptibility to environmental risk factors. Much of the change in myopia incidence is likely attributable to changes in exposure to lifestyle-related risk factors, the potential interaction of lifestyle and genetic risk factors, and the ways that parents and society manage children's experiences. See Box 5-1 for an explanation of the correlation between earlier-onset myopia and higher amounts of myopia.

---

[1] As a reminder, refractive error covers the spectrum from farsightedness (hyperopia) to nearsightedness (myopia), measured in units called diopters (D).

BOX 5-1
Earlier Onset of Myopia Typically Means Higher Amounts of Myopia

The speed with which the eye elongates is highest at younger ages. Axial elongation shows an early exponential phase of rapid elongation in infancy, followed by a slower "quadratic" phase in early childhood, until stability is reached, on average during the teenage years (Gordon et al., 1985; Larsen, 1971; Mutti et al., 2018). In the myopic eye, the optics of the eye cannot compensate for the axial elongation, so the vast majority of eye growth translates into progressively worse myopic refractive error. Elongation is also faster in myopic eyes than in non-myopic eyes (Mutti et al., 2007; Rozema et al., 2019), adding to the more rapid rate of myopic progression in younger eyes. The net result is that children whose onset of myopia occurs at a young age are more likely to develop a higher amount of eventual myopia than children with onset at older ages. In cohorts from the United States, a three-to-five-year earlier onset results in −2.00 D or more additional myopia in later childhood (The COMET Group, 2013; Jones-Jordan et al., 2021). Singaporean children whose myopia started at age 5 years developed nearly −4.00 D more myopia than children whose onset was at age 9 years. Younger age of onset was associated with nearly a threefold increase in the odds of becoming highly myopic (OR = 2.86; 95% CI: 2.39 to 3.43; Chua et al., 2016). Long-term longitudinal results from China show that 53.9% of children with onset at 7–8 years of age become highly myopic (as or more myopic than −6.00 D) compared to only 1.3% whose onset is at age 12 years or older (Hu et al., 2020).

GENETIC FACTORS ASSOCIATED WITH MYOPIA

The role of genetics in the etiology of refractive errors has been of long-standing interest, and its importance has been demonstrated by twin, family, and gene-level association and linkage analysis studies (Baird et al., 2020; Tedja et al., 2019). Modern lifestyles in high- and middle-income countries expose the majority of the population to risk factors for myopia (He et al., 2015; Mountjoy et al., 2018). Thus, an often-misinterpreted consequence of this ubiquitous exposure to lifestyle risk factors is that genetic differences explain much of the variation in refractive error between individuals, despite genetics not being the primary 'driver' of myopia development. In general, genetic differences between individuals confer upon each person a relatively high or low level of susceptibility to myopia when they are exposed to environmental risk factors, rather than acting in a purely deterministic manner (Pozarickij et al., 2019).

Genes Associated with Myopia and Refractive Error Development

The variance in a trait explained by genetic differences between individuals is termed heritability. The heritability of refractive error varies from population to population but is typically within the range of 30–80% (Sanfilippo et al., 2010). Genome-wide association studies (GWAS) have been extremely successful in identifying specific genetic variants associated with susceptibility to myopia (Tedja et al., 2019). A powerful approach has been to meta-analyze multiple datasets (mostly population-based) through collaborative consortia such as CREAM (the Consortium for Refractive Error and Myopia). In the most recent GWAS meta-analysis, which assessed a total of more than half a million participants, 449 genomic regions harboring refractive error-associated genetic variants were identified (Hysi et al., 2020). GWAS findings have been very highly reproducible both within and across European ancestry and Asian ancestry study samples. African ancestry GWAS samples have been underrepresented to date.

Current evidence suggests that most genetic risk variants associated with myopia are shared between European and Asian ancestry groups and have similar effect sizes, which despite differences in allele frequencies between ancestry groups argues against genetics as an explanation for the widely differing prevalence levels observed between these geographic regions (Tedja et al., 2018). More research on mechanisms is needed to better understand how genetic variants affect refractive error development.

A current gap in knowledge is the mechanism by which the hundreds of known refractive error-associated variants confer susceptibility to myopia. (See Box 5-2 for information about mechanisms regulating normal and myopic eye growth.) Existing research to address this question has taken advantage of the genetic tractability of mouse and zebrafish models (Koli et al., 2021; Mazade et al., 2024; Quint et al., 2023; van der Sande et al., 2022). However, the difficulty of detecting subtle phenotypic effects in mice and zebrafish is a limitation, since most genetic variants discovered in GWAS analyses have only small effects. In addition, most GWAS variants are in *non-coding regions* of the genome, suggesting their effects are mediated *not* by the elimination of the protein product of a gene, but rather by altering a nearby gene's level of expression or the timing and context of its expression. Completely knocking out a gene in a mouse or zebrafish is arguably a poor model for studying this type of genetic variant, even if such models can provide insight into the key biological pathways.

The term 'monogenic' refers to a genetic disorder caused by a mutation in a single gene. Monogenic disorders often affect several members of a family, due to the segregation of the mutation through the pedigree. The causative mutation often varies from one family to another, and a mutation in a different gene can give rise to the same disease. Mutations in approximately 20 different genes have been identified as the cause of non-syndromic, monogenic high myopia (Cai et al., 2019). High myopia is more likely to be monogenic in origin if it has an onset prior to the age of 7 years. For instance, in a study of 298 individuals with early-onset high myopia, rare mutations in nine genes in nine individuals (3% of the cohort) were identified with high probability as being the cause of the high myopia (Jiang et al., 2015). Mutations that give rise to monogenic high myopia usually have a direct, adverse functional impact and thus may offer insight into the etiology of myopia in the general population; alternatively, they may simply identify genes and proteins that need to be functional for the eye and visual system to develop normally (see Box 5-2).

BOX 5-2
Are the Mechanisms Regulating Normal Eye Growth and Myopic Eye Growth the Same?

Like general growth parameters for the body (height, weight), there are intrinsic signals such as the insulin growth factor-1 hormone system that control the development of eye size. There appear to be separate signals that modulate eye growth, targeting an optimal refractive state of the eye (i.e., emmetropization) as well as passive, non-visually-targeted eye growth. Emmetropization represents coordinated growth where the eye's focal length tends to match its physical length. Myopic eye growth occurs when the eye's physical elongation either exceeds the capacity of the crystalline lens to maintain coordinated, proportional growth or the eye's elongation becomes decoupled and independent of compensatory optical changes. As illustrated in Figure 5-1 below, comparison of the growth curves for body height, the eye's axial length, and refractive error in humans and many other species indicates that normal emmetropization reaches a plateau while growth in body length or the eye's axial length continues to increase (Mazade et al., 2024).

In chicks, genetic variants that regulate normal eye size are distinct from the variants that confer susceptibility to visually driven changes in eye growth (Chen et al., 2011). There is also evidence in humans that commonly occurring genetic variants controlling normal eye size are distinct from those involved in myopic eye growth (Plotnikov, 2021). Rare mutations also provide insight into this question. Myopia can occur due to a mutation that has an effect in one specific ocular structure: For instance, a defect in a protein needed to convert light energy into a neuronal signal, inter-retinoid binding protein (IRBP), causes excessive axial length and myopia from birth (Markand et al., 2016). However, there is no evidence currently that IRBP plays a role in emmetropization or common myopia, nor that IRBP mutations influence body weight or stature. Thus, while there is some evidence that normal eye growth and myopic eye growth may have separate mechanisms, more studies are needed to determine the causal mechanisms of both to be conclusive.

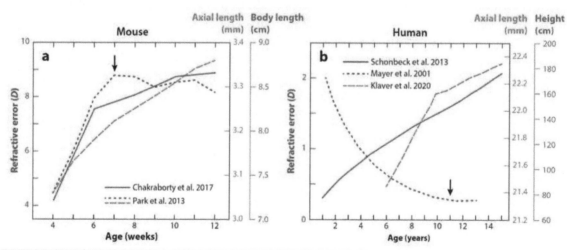

FIGURE 5-1 Growth curves for height, axial length, and refractive error in mice and humans. NOTE: Refractive development plateaus before ocular and body development. Refractive error (red) compared to ocular (green) and body growth (blue) in young mice (A) and children (B). Arrows indicate the age when refractive error reaches a steady state.
SOURCE: Mazade et al., 2024.

A current gap in knowledge is the contribution of rare genetic variants to refractive error in the general population and to the burden of high myopia. Past studies have had limited statistical power to identify rare variants associated with high myopia (Guggenheim et al., 2022a; Su et al., 2023). Addressing this issue will require the assembly of very large cohorts of high myopia cases and controls, subjected to whole-genome sequencing.

Syndromic Myopia

A disease 'syndrome' refers to a cluster of clinical features that tend to co-occur; disease syndromes often have a monogenic origin. Myopia and high myopia are frequent features of monogenic disease syndromes (Flitcroft et al., 2023; Wildsoet, 1998). For example, characteristic clinical features of Stickler syndrome are high myopia and hearing loss (Richards et al., 2010). Each monogenic disease syndrome is generally rare, yet in aggregate syndromic myopia accounts for a significant proportion of cases. This is most evident for early-onset high myopia, where up to 40% of cases may be monogenic/syndromic in origin (Logan et al., 2004). A recent study by the Myopia Associated Genetics and Intervention Consortium examined 75 candidate genes in a sample of 6,215 school-aged children with high myopia (Yu et al., 2023). Putative disease-causing mutations were identified in 15% of the cohort. Preliminary research suggests there exists an above-chance level of overlap between genes that cause syndromic myopia and those implicated in 'common' myopia (Flitcroft et al., 2018).

Myopia is very often a feature of certain inherited retinal dystrophies, including congenital stationary night blindness and subtypes of retinitis pigmentosa (Hendriks et al., 2017). The mutations that cause these syndromes have been shown to cause myopia or increased myopia susceptibility in mouse models (Mazade et al., 2024) and also have roles in ON-bipolar cell signaling, one of two main pathways in the retina that process visual information from photoreceptors to retinal ganglion cells (Hendriks et al., 2017). How these mutations lead to myopia is an area of active investigation (Zeitz et al., 2023). Apart from a genetic cause, early-onset myopia can also occur as a result of prematurity, especially in infants with retinopathy of prematurity (Mao et al., 2019).

The *OPN1LW* and *OPN1MW* genes encoding the cone opsin photopigments, most responsive to long-wavelength red light (L-opsin) and middle-wavelength green light (M-opsin), are located together on the X-chromosome; the high level of sequence similarity between these opsin genes predisposes them to mutations. A rare combination of sequence variants in the *OPN1LW* gene can cause Bornholm Eye Disease (BED), a disease syndrome with the clinical features of high myopia, color vision deficiency, reduced visual acuity, and reduced cone responses on electroretinography (ERG; McClements et al., 2013). A notable finding in BED is a reduction in the amount of opsin photopigment in affected L-cones, often associated with a molecular defect known as exon-skipping. This results in the retinal cone mosaic of patients with BED containing a mixture of normal M-cones and viable but poorly responsive L-cones. It has been hypothesized that this mixture of normal M-cones and abnormal L-cones promotes eye growth and myopia via spurious activation of ON- and OFF-bipolar cells when viewing low-contrast images (Neitz et al., 2022). While still speculative, this hypothesis has been extended by suggesting a role for commonly occurring L-opsin gene variants with mild effects, and the ratio of L vs. M-cones, in predisposing individuals to low myopia (Neitz et al., 2022). The hypothesis has also been suggested to relate to the mechanism of spectacle lenses designed to slow myopia progression by subtly lowering retinal contrast (marketed as SightGlass Vision DOT® lenses)

(Rappon et al., 2023). This topic is discussed further in the section on Reduction in Contrast vs. Peripheral Myopic Blur as Mechanisms of Spectacle Treatments, in Chapter 7.

Gene–Environment Interactions

If the hypothesis is correct that genetic factors determine susceptibility to myopia while environmental risk factors trigger myopia development and progression (Tedja et al., 2019), then the majority of the hundreds of known refractive-error-associated genetic variants probably exert their effects through gene–environment interactions. Attempts to identify specific genetic variants with gene–environment interaction effects on refractive error in humans are generally in agreement with this hypothesis, yet these studies have been far less fruitful than GWAS analyses aiming to detect direct genetic effects (Clark et al., 2022; Pozarickii et al., 2019; see Box 5-3 on GWAS). The reasons for this lack of success and the poor record of replication for gene–environment interaction studies are twofold. First, biobank-scale genetic studies rarely measure myopia-related risk factors, such as time spent outdoors during childhood, which limits the available sample size for gene–environment interaction studies. Second, the statistical power to identify gene–environment interaction effects is necessarily lower than for detecting direct genetic effects. To date, only a handful of genetic variants with replicated gene–environment interaction effects have been discovered; in all cases, the variants interact with education level, such that the risk allele is associated with a greater shift in refractive error toward myopia as the level of education increases (Baird et al., 2020; Clark et al., 2022).

Gene–environment interactions have also been investigated with animal studies, particularly in mice, in which both genes and environment can be manipulated. Some of these experiments have revealed that the genetic defect alone was not sufficient to generate a myopic phenotype. However, combining myopigenic stimuli with the genetic defect demonstrated increased susceptibility for myopia. For instance, mice with mutations in the ON-pathway (*nyx*) (Pardue et al. 2008) or causing retinal degenerations (*Pde6b^{rd1}* and *Pde6b^{rd10}*; Park et al., 2013) had normal hyperopic refractions throughout the juvenile ocular development period, yet these mice also showed increased susceptibility to experimental myopia using form deprivation (Mazade et al., 2024). Alternatively, a knock-out model of *Aplp2*, a gene associated with glycinergic amacrine cells that have an inhibitory role in the retina, resulted in hyperopia and reduced susceptibility to form-deprivation myopia (Tkatchenko et al., 2015). These animal studies support the hypothesis that the visual environment interacts with genetic factors to determine whether myopia develops and to what extent.

BOX 5-3
Genome-Wide Association Studies (GWAS)

The human genome is about 3 billion 'letters' (DNA nucleotides or molecular base pairs) long. The genome sequence is not identical in any two individuals (except for identical twins, prior to mutations that arise over the twins' lifetimes). Differences in sequence between individuals are called either mutations, variants, or polymorphisms, depending on the context. Some genetic variants occur rarely while others occur commonly. For example, 50% of people in a sample may have an 'A' nucleotide at a particular position in the genome and 50% may have a 'C' nucleotide in that same position.

A GWAS is a systematic method for identifying genetic variants associated with a trait or disease. The method was developed for studying commonly occurring diseases and for traits that do not cluster strongly in families; for rare diseases that do cluster in families, in-depth genetic evaluation of the individual families works better. Participants in a GWAS for a disease are selected based on their status as a disease case or as controls. Participants in a GWAS of a trait are typically chosen as a representative sample of the full population. To perform a GWAS, each and every common genetic variant in the human genome is tested, in turn, for an association with the disease status or trait. This step-by-step approach gives each genetic variant an equal chance of being discovered as a disease-associated risk factor; hence a GWAS is sometimes referred to as being 'hypothesis free'. There are several million common genetic variants in the human genome, so a GWAS entails performing this many separate statistical tests.

To account for all this statistical testing, which is prone to false positive discoveries, geneticists have established a p-value threshold of $P < 5 \times 10^{-8}$ for declaring genome-wide significant association. To have a realistic chance of reaching such a stringent p-value threshold, GWAS sample sizes need to be very large. To make matters worse, genetic predisposition for most common diseases and traits tends to be spread widely across thousands of genetic variants scattered throughout the genome (a so-called 'polygenic' genetic architecture). Thus, most genetic variants have a tiny impact on disease risk. This means that GWAS sample sizes of hundreds of thousands or even millions of participants are needed (see Figure 5-2).

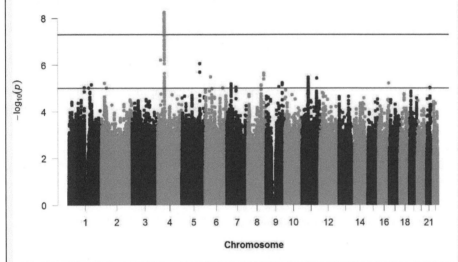

FIGURE 5-2 Manhattan plot from a Genome-Wide Association Studies (GWAS) analysis. NOTE: The results of a GWAS are presented graphically as a 'Manhattan plot' displaying the level of statistical association of each genetic variant, plotted according to its location in the genome. "Skyscrapers" in the plot indicate genomic regions with multiple strongly associated genetic variants. Further research through statistical 'fine mapping' or functional studies is needed to pinpoint the precise genetic variant(s) in each skyscraper region that have a causal impact on disease risk or trait level.
SOURCE: Committee generated.

Polygenic Scores (PGS) and Polygenic Risk Scores (PGRS)

A GWAS for refractive error yields a series of regression coefficients quantifying the shift in refractive error toward myopia or hyperopia associated with carrying one or two copies of the non-reference allele for thousands or millions of genotyped or imputed genetic variants from across the human genome. A polygenic score reverses the logic of a GWAS analysis. First, the shift in refractive error toward myopia or hyperopia is identified at each locus, corresponding to the GWAS regression coefficient multiplied by the number of copies of the non-reference allele. This is done for each of the thousands or millions of genetic variants carried by an individual person. The resulting values are summed to produce a single value quantifying their genetically predicted refractive error (Sugrue & Desikan, 2019). Initial PGS studies took account of just the top GWAS variants with the strongest association to refractive error (Hysi et al., 2020; Tedja et al., 2018), while later studies demonstrated improved accuracy by incorporating up to a million genetic variants (Clark et al., 2023b; Kassam et al., 2022).

The accuracy of a PGS is quantified as the 'incremental R-squared' in an independent test sample. That is, accuracy is measured as the variance in refractive error explained by the PGS over and above that explained by demographic characteristics such as age and sex. Current PGS for refractive error have an incremental R-squared of approximately 20% (Clark et al., 2023b). To put this level of prediction accuracy in context, the main known environmental risk factor for myopia, time spent outdoors (quantified objectively using a spectacle-mounted light level sensor), explained only 3% of the variance in refractive error in a (non-independent) test sample (Li et al., 2020). (However, see Figure 5-3 for a discussion of why the predictive accuracy of environmental risk factors may be underestimated compared to genetic factors.)

Whereas PGS predicts the level of a quantitative trait, PGRS identify individuals who are at high risk of developing a specific disorder (Sugrue & Desikan, 2019). PGRS for high myopia can predict the condition with an area under the receiver operating characteristics curve of approximately 80% in independent samples (Clark et al., 2023b; Hysi et al., 2020). This level of prediction accuracy approaches that required for use in the clinic. Compared to existing methods of predicting high myopia development, PGRS have the unique advantage of being able to be implemented in young children before the gradual transition from hyperopia to myopia starts to occur. This makes them well-suited to identifying 'pre-myopic' children who would benefit from prophylactic treatment interventions such as atropine eye drops (Yam et al., 2023) and increased time outdoors. Importantly, current PGRS for high myopia perform far better in individuals of European ancestry compared to those of non-European ancestry (Clark et al., 2023b; Kassam et al., 2022). Thus, a current research priority is to narrow the performance gap of polygenic scores across ancestry groups (Kachuri et al., 2024).

PGS and PGRS of sufficient predictive power have the potential to improve the assessment of myopia interventions in two different ways. First, because by definition they account for relevant genetic variation within a population, PGS can serve as regressors that reduce standard errors and thus allow for the better discernment of treatment effects, particularly in the context of gene–environment interactions (e.g. Barcellos et al. 2018). Second, using PGS or PGRS to select participants in clinical trials can potentially improve their efficiency through a combination of "prognostic enrichment" (effectively increasing the event rate by selecting people at higher risk for the disease) and by "predictive enrichment" (effectively increasing the treatment's effect size).

For example, in a retrospective analysis of trials of statins for cardiovascular disease, Fahed et al. (2022, p. 2) showed that:

> a trial that enrolled only those participants in the top quintile of the polygenic score might have required only 2360 participants—a greater than 90% reduction from the 27,564 studied—and demonstrated a 31% relative risk reduction as compared to the 20% observed in the overall trial population.

While collecting such data might be prohibitive for any given clinical trial and would require careful ethical oversight, in an official statement the American Heart Association has pointed out the value of a single concerted national effort to conduct broad genetic profiling of a large population, combined with detailed health information, to aid in the treatment and diagnosis of cardiovascular disease (O'Sullivan et al., 2022). Such a project would also have real benefits for better understanding gene–environment interactions in myopia.

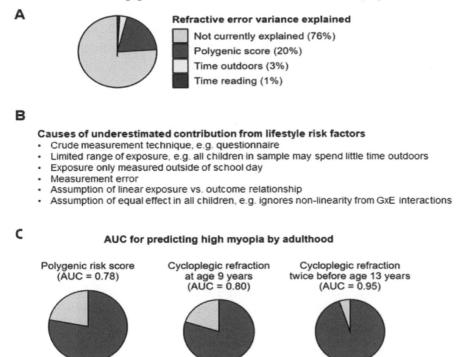

FIGURE 5-3 Predicting refractive error and high myopia: Reasons why predictive accuracy of lifestyle risk factors may have been underestimated.
NOTES: (A) Variance in refractive error predicted or explained by a polygenic score in individuals of European ancestry (Clark et al., 2023b) or time outdoors measured with a Clouclip sensor (Li et al., 2020) or near work ascertained using a parent-completed questionnaire (Guggenheim et al., 2015). (B) Some of the reasons why the role of lifestyle risk factors may have been underestimated in longitudinal epidemiology studies of myopia. (C) Predictive accuracy in identifying children who will become highly myopic by adulthood. Performance of a polygenic score in individuals of European ancestry (Clark et al., 2023b) compared with cycloplegic autorefraction (Chen et al., 2019). AUC = Area under the curve for a receiver-operating characteristics curve; GxE = Gene–environment interaction.
SOURCE: Committee generated, based on data from the sources cited in the note above.

Genetic Contribution to Myopic Maculopathy and Retinal Detachment

Aside from its value in helping to identify children at an increased risk of developing high myopia when they get older, genetic profiling might also be useful in patients with existing high myopia to identify those at greatest risk of myopic maculopathy or retinal detachment—although whether such a risk assessment is possible remains a current gap in knowledge. If it is possible, this knowledge would be valuable in stratifying patients to receive more or less frequent routine clinical follow-up. Patients with high myopia due to Stickler syndrome are at a high risk of retinal detachment (Richards et al., 2010) and GWAS analyses of retinal detachment cases and controls have observed an overlap with myopia-predisposing loci, as well as unique genetic risk factors (Johnston et al., 2016).

Genetic predisposition to myopia, as quantified by a polygenic score, was found to be no better at predicting the risk of myopic maculopathy than knowledge of the degree of high myopia (Sugrue & Desikan, 2019). To date, GWAS analyses of cases with high myopia and myopic maculopathy vs. highly myopic controls free from maculopathy have utilized small sample sizes, which have limited power to identify risk loci (Hosoda et al., 2018; Wong et al., 2019). Future research to address this question will require the assembly of a very large cohort of patients with high myopia, who have been genotyped and assessed clinically for signs of myopic maculopathy or retinal detachment.

Epigenetics

Epigenetic effects are defined as changes in gene expression (or other phenotypes) that occur without a change to the underlying DNA sequence. The most well-studied epigenetic mechanisms involve DNA methylation and histone modification, which are dynamic processes operating in the cell nucleus. Research into the role of epigenetics in myopia development has been limited, with just two large-scale genome-wide epigenetic studies reported to date. One study of 3-year-old infants with myopia vs. non-myopic controls identified five specific genomic regions that had a reduced level of methylation. The other study reported a link between myopia and the paternal grandmother's smoking during pregnancy, which the authors argued implicated a trans-generational epigenetic mechanism (Seow et al., 2019; Williams et al., 2019b). Research investigating methylation levels in specific regions of the genome has also been carried out; for example, one recent study targeted regions harboring miRNA-encoding genes was associated with high myopia (Swierkowska et al., 2022).

Epigenetic studies may hold promise by providing insight into how lifestyle risk factors lead to myopia development. However, existing studies have been underpowered due to small sample sizes, lack of longitudinal measurement of methylation levels and refractive error, and potential bias from confounding factors. As an example of the potential for confounding, smoking is known to produce changes to the epigenome (Wiklund et al., 2019), so the negative association that also exists between smoking and education level would be expected to lead to differences in methylation status between myopia cases and controls.

Parental Myopia as an Indicator of Genetic Risk

Parental myopia is a well-established risk factor for myopia and, accordingly, has been included in some myopia prediction algorithms. Initial research suggests that parental myopia and a polygenic score for refractive error provide complementary predictive information, consistent with the premise that parents with myopia expose their children to a more myopigenic home environment (such as one where reading indoors is favored over playing or working outside) than non-myopic parents (Mojarrad et al., 2018). Simply counting whether a child has zero, one, or two parents with myopia ignores valuable information concerning the exact refractive error of parents; accordingly, the component of parental myopia corresponding to purely genetic effects (i.e., excluding the home environment component) has a theoretical upper limit of explaining about 5% of the variation in a child's refractive error (Guggenheim et al., 2017). This compares poorly with current polygenic scores, which already can explain approximately 20% of the variation in a child's refractive error and, in theory, have the potential to explain as much as 30% to 50% of the variation (Clark et al., 2023b).

It has recently been discovered that for some traits, genetic predisposition is not, for the most part, transmitted directly from parents to children via the germline, but instead is transmitted indirectly via the home environment that parents create for their children (a phenomenon termed 'genetic nurture'; Guggenheim et al., 2017). Most notably, about three-quarters of a child's genetic predisposition to educational attainment (heritability = 17%) is transmitted via genetic nurture, while one-quarter is transmitted directly via the germline. At present, the available evidence suggests that the transmission of genetic predisposition to refractive error occurs predominantly via direct transmission through the germline rather than via genetic nurture (Guggenheim et al., 2022).

ENVIRONMENTAL FACTORS

While genetic factors influence refractive development and the prevalence of myopia, genetic factors in a population do not change rapidly. Given the rapid increase in myopia prevalence which began some decades ago, environmental factors have been implicated as driving the "myopia boom" (Dolgin, 2015). This section highlights the potential influence on myopia of near work, visual environment, and behavior.

Near Work—Re-Examining a Classic Risk Factor for Myopia

Near work, meaning any activity requiring ocular accommodation for clear vision at a close working distance, has been considered a risk factor for myopia for centuries. Below, we detail the evidence for near work as a risk factor for the onset and progression of myopia and discuss the limitations of prior studies on the topic.

Near Work and Education

Research over several decades has documented a close link between education and myopia (Morgan & Rose, 2004). It has been noted for more than 150 years that the prevalence of myopia is higher among professionals and those engaged in "white collar" indoor jobs requiring more years of schooling compared to those whose livelihoods involve more time outdoors, such as manual laborers or workers in agriculture (Goldschmidt, 1968). Ware (1813) believed that the higher prevalence of myopia among officers in the military and among university students compared to rank-and-file enlisted men was due to the more intense near work environment associated with advanced study (Ware, 1813). Cohn, in his monograph *The Hygiene of the Eye in Schools* (1886), attributed the higher prevalence of myopia in urban gymnasia compared to that found in rural schools to the intensity of near work required for their more rigorous curriculums, along with close working distances and poor indoor illumination (Cohn, 1886).

In the 20th century, the classic Inuit studies by Young et al. (1969) documented increasing prevalence of myopia among school-aged children compared to their parents and grandparents, a shift attributed to the increased level of near work that accompanied the children's newly instituted compulsory schooling (Young et al., 1969; see Chapter 3 for more details). An intense near-work environment in school is still frequently cited as a risk factor for myopia. A classic example is the study of Orthodox rabbinical students conducted in Israel by Zylbermann et al. (1993). The study found that more than 80% of male Orthodox students were myopic compared to less than half that prevalence among their sisters, who were also attending Orthodox schools, and among males or females attending general schools. The near work demands for Orthodox males, mainly reading and writing, were as high as 16 hours per day, as compared to 2–3 hours per day for the other students (Zylbermann et al., 1993; see Chapter 3 for similar data collected in Israel).

Recent work comparing the prevalence of myopia in different countries and academic test scores from children residing in those countries, using data from the Program in Secondary Assessment (PISA) system created by the Organisation for Economic Co-operation and Development, has confirmed the relationship between education and myopia (Jong et al., 2023). In a statistical model, PISA scores could account for 31% to 64% of the variation in myopia between countries (albeit not addressing whether the relationship was causal in nature). Economic development and urbanization are frequently associated with a higher prevalence of myopia compared to populations living in rural areas within the same country (Ip et al., 2008). The prevalence of myopia typically increases as societies become more affluent; for example, central African countries are predicted to undergo sharp increases in myopia prevalence, from 9.8% currently to 27.9% by 2050 (Holden et al., 2016).

The level of education was associated with increased odds of being myopic, particularly in the presence of risk alleles for refractive error and myopia identified in the CREAM consortium (Verhoeven et al., 2013). A child's exposure to education is not readily amenable to investigation in randomized trials. Instead, the Mendelian randomization analysis method (Mountjoy et al., 2018) has been used to gauge the potential causal effect of education on myopia: this approach aims, in theory, to reduce the effect of potentially confounding variables, thereby isolating the effects of the environmental variable of interest. An analysis of U.K. Biobank participants showed that each year of additional education was associated with −0.27 D (95% CI: −0.37 to −0.17) less hyperopic/more myopic refractive error; the study had 80% power to detect an effect of time spent in education on refractive error ≥ 0.14 D/year (Mountjoy et al., 2018).

A second research method that has been used to examine the causal effect of education on myopia is regression discontinuity analysis. Plotnikov et al. (2020) took advantage of a 'natural experiment' in which a government policy raised the school-leaving age of U.K. children from 15 to 16 years. In those affected by the education reform, refractive error was shifted in the direction of myopia by −0.77 D (95% CI: −1.53 to −0.02 D). In China, the effect of education on myopia has recently been quantified in children using data gathered through nationwide screening programs. One more grade level of education in China was associated with an increase in the prevalence of myopia by a consistent increment compared to children of similar age but with one grade level less of education. This phenomenon was evident at least until the prevalence of myopia began to reach a plateau, in high school (He et al., 2021). A regression discontinuity study of 910,000 children ages 4–14 years living in Shanghai, China, estimated that an additional year of schooling at age 6 years caused a −0.19 D (95% CI: −0.09 to −0.30 D) shift toward myopia, while at age 14 years an additional year of schooling caused a shift of −0.67 D (95% CI: −0.21 to −1.14 D; He et al., 2021).

These independent sets of results from Mendelian randomization and regression discontinuity studies underscore the effect of increasing education on the risk of having a myopic refractive error, but they do not shed light on potential biological mechanisms. Less time outdoors because of more years spent in education may contribute to the link between education and myopia. For instance, when time outdoors was accounted for in a Mendelian randomization analysis of education level, the effect size of −0.27 D for each year of education was reduced by roughly 40% to −0.17 D per year (Clark et al., 2023a). Further research to determine the relative importance of *more* near work versus *less* time outdoors, or other factors, will be important in understanding the link between education and myopia.

Near Work and Myopia Onset vs. Progression

The role of near work in myopia has recently been reviewed by Huang et al. (2015), Gajjar & Ostrin (2022), and Dutheil et al. (2023). However, the role of near work remains contentious (Mutti & Zadnik, 2009), in large part due to the conflicts between cross-sectional and longitudinal studies and the methods used to quantify near work. Near work has traditionally been assessed through surveys of parents estimating the time their children spend in various activities. Having parents estimate children's time in an activity is simple to incorporate into a survey, but it lacks detail, averages activities into one estimate over perhaps a year's length of time, asks parents to make an estimate of activity time they have not witnessed in person, and is subject to recall bias. Despite these limitations, some trends have emerged from survey-based research. Working distance and prolonged periods of near work are recurring themes in recent studies that could be evaluated on an individual basis using electronic monitoring technology (Gaijar & Ostrin, 2022; Guo, 2016; Huang et al., 2019). Minimally invasive electronic monitoring technology now permits a child's working distance and the duration of periods of near work to be evaluated over hours or days (Bhandari et al., 2022; Li et al., 2020; Williams et al., 2019a; see Chapter 4). Working distance and the temporal dynamics of near work, along with more detailed assessments of children's visual experience in both indoor and outdoor environments, deserve more attention in future longitudinal research.

Notwithstanding the limitations of the methods used to quantify near work, associations between levels of near work and myopia have been reported less consistently in cross-sectional and longitudinal studies than associations between time outdoors and myopia. Cross-sectional studies often evaluate the association between near work and myopia in individuals who are already myopic unless they are undertaken at an early age. Prospective longitudinal studies ask whether increased near work in non-myopic children increases their risk of myopia onset. Here, some of the key findings from these studies are summarized. The CLEERE study (Zadnik et al., 2015) was a multi-ethnic longitudinal study in the United States that monitored refractive development in more than 4,000 children, represented at each baseline age from 6 to 11 years old, with up to 7 years follow-up until the 8th grade. It found that the odds ratio for incident myopia associated with a one-unit increase in 'diopter-hours' of near work was estimated to be precisely 1.00 (95% CI: $< \pm 0.01$). In the 3-year longitudinal SCORM study, which followed 994 children residing in Singapore ages 7–9 years at baseline, the relative risk of incident myopia was 1.01 (95% CI: 0.97–1.05) for each additional book read per week (Saw et al., 2006). A one-year longitudinal study of nearly 1,500 Chinese children in grades 1–4 found no association between time spent in near work and increased risk of onset.

In contrast to many negative results for near work and risk of myopia onset in school-aged children, near work exposures prior to school age or early in school may increase risk. In the Generation R study (Enthoven et al., 2020), a birth cohort study that monitored more than 5,000 children in The Netherlands, incident myopia at age 9 was modestly but significantly associated with computer use at age 3 years (OR = 1.005, 95% CI: 1.002–1.010) and computer use at age 6 years (OR = 1.009, 95% CI: 1.002–1.017). In the SAVES study (French et al., 2013), which followed approximately 2,000 Australian children for 5–6 years, younger children in the high tertile for near work had a greater risk of incident myopia (OR = 2.35. 95% CI: 1.30–4.27) while older children in the high tertile for near work had an increased risk that was not statistically significant (OR = 1.31, 95% CI: 0.83–2.06). In contrast, a recent longitudinal study of initially non-myopic Chinese high school aviation cadets found that spending more than 8 hours in class per day, frequent periods of continuous reading for over one hour, and a near working distance of less than 30 cm—but not reading for more than 4 hours per day—were all significantly associated with a higher incidence rate of myopia over 20 months of follow-up (Yao et al., 2019). This finding is consistent with animal models of myopia that show temporal nonlinearities in the effects of hyperopic defocus, while "total amount of near work" may be a relatively poor measure for exactly these reasons (Wallman & Winnower, 2004). Reports of the association between near work and the progression of existing myopia have been similarly mixed (Dutheil et al., 2023; Gajjar & Ostrin, 2022; Huang et al., 2015). Also discussed below, early exposures to near work may be more significant regarding future myopia progression. However, at later ages, the following studies suggest that once myopic progression begins, near work may have limited effect on progression.

Research by the COMET Group found that near work at baseline had no effect on the proportion of children whose myopia stabilized by age 15, although the amount of myopia at stabilization as a function of near work was not presented (The COMET Group, 2013). A remarkable 23-year follow-up of Finnish participants enrolled at an average age of 11 years found no association between myopia progression and near work assessed in childhood and again at the follow-up visits at either 24 or 35 years of age (Parssinen et al., 2014). A 1-year longitudinal study of nearly 5,000 Chinese children in grades 1–4 found no association between time spent in near work and either axial elongation or change in refractive error (You et al., 2016).

Two studies show an effect on myopia progression from near work. In one study, however, it was an effect of reading distance more than time spent reading, and the effect was small. This two-year longitudinal study of nearly 4,000 Taiwanese children 9–11 years of age examined the association between progression and two near-work behaviors: reading distance and whether near work was uninterrupted for 30 minutes. Refractive errors were compared between groups dichotomized for exhibiting the better visual hygiene for each behavior (reading distance ≥ 30 cm and uninterrupted near work ≤ 30 minutes). There was statistically significantly less myopia in the "protective" group throughout follow-up, although it is unclear if these differences existed at baseline or developed over the course of follow-up. Over the two years of follow-up, the close reading distance group progressed 0.15 D more and the uninterrupted group progressed 0.07 D more than the respective "protective" group children (Huang et al., 2020). These groups were not randomized, and it is unclear how many children were in each group. The other significant association was found in a longitudinal study of 1,279 children ages 5–15 years from India. The odds ratio for progressing in myopia by at least −0.25 D in one year associated with spending more than 42 hours of near work per week compared to spending less than 35 hours was 2.10 (95% CI = 1.24-3.56). Spending more than 7 hours per week using a computer or playing video games was also associated with showing myopia progression (n = 629) vs. having a stable myopic refractive error (n = 650). Time watching television was not significantly related to myopia progression (Saxena et al., 2017).

More detailed assessments of working distance and uninterrupted time in near work seem warranted, as well as longitudinal studies beginning at earlier ages.

A Case for Re-Examining the Theories for the Effects of Near Work on Myopia: Does Defocus Have a Consistent Effect in Driving Eye Growth?

Animal experimental models of myopia produced by lens defocus are often cited as the theoretical framework supporting near work as a major risk factor for myopia incidence. Accommodation in children for near work is typically less than the amount required by the dioptric demand, resulting in under-accommodation, or accommodative lag (Gwiazda et al., 1999; Mutti et al., 2006). The sign of this defocus is hyperopic, with the conjugate point of the near reading material or computer screen in focus behind the retina. The analogous condition in animal experiments is hyperopic defocus imposed by minus lenses, a stimulus that reliably accelerates the elongation of the eyes of young animals across a wide variety of species (Pardue et al., 2008; Schaeffel et al., 1988; Smith & Hung, 1999; Wallman, 1987). The hypothesized connection between animal models and childhood myopia is that prolonged time in near work in the presence of accommodative lag provides the same form of growth signal from hyperopic defocus, thereby increasing the risk of myopia onset.

Accelerated eye growth in response to hyperopic defocus is quite reliable in animals, but the results of interventions in humans that prevent hyperopic defocus during accommodation are disappointing in comparison. If near work and hyperopic defocus were as detrimental to the eye as assumed from animal models, bifocal spectacles would have solved the problem long ago. Clinical trials of segmented multifocal or progressive-addition lenses have failed to produce clinically meaningful results in slowing myopia (Berntsen et al., 2012; Fulk et al., 2012; Gwiazda et al., 2003). The current emphasis in optical treatments is to provide myopic defocus as a 'stop' signal in the retinal periphery to inhibit overall elongation while not interfering with visual acuity. These peripheral optical treatments take many forms: contact lenses, overnight orthokeratology, and specialty spectacles (see Chapter 7). The treatment benefit from this approach is greater than from bifocal spectacles, but there are important limitations, as elaborated in Chapter 6. The treatment benefit seems to have a ceiling, limited to 0.50 D to 0.75 D less progression of myopia in treated children compared to controls (Chamberlain et al., 2019; Lam et al., 2020; Walline et al., 2020).

More importantly, the greatest effect is seen early in most myopia control treatments, with diminishing additional treatment benefit in later years. In the BLINK study of multifocal contact lenses, for example, significant inhibition of axial elongation was observed only in the first two of its three years (Mutti et al., 2022). A Cochrane review of myopia treatments shows that this is typical for both optical and pharmaceutical approaches to myopia control (Walline et al., 2011). A child destined to have −6.00 D of myopia may instead become −5.25 D. While this is an improvement, no clinical data exist to support a claim that current myopia control could make the final refractive error of that child −3.00 D. The pattern of inhibition of ocular growth in the BLINK study was also inconsistent with prediction from animal models. Elongation was indeed inhibited at every peripheral point measured out to 30° in the retinal periphery, but the inhibition compared to controls was greatest at the fovea, not in three of the four quadrants of the periphery where myopic defocus was present.

Control of ocular growth by defocus was also inconsistent, with similar amounts of inhibition seen between the vertical and horizontal meridians of the eye despite the substantially greater peripheral myopic defocus vertically (Mutti et al., 2022). Accommodative lag is supposed to be a visual risk factor for myopia onset and progression, but longitudinal results show excess lag in myopes to be more a consequence of myopia rather than a cause (Mutti et al., 2006). Once lag increases after the onset of myopia, the degree of lag is unrelated to the rate of myopia progression (Berntsen et al., 2011). Hyperopic peripheral defocus is also unrelated to increased risk of onset (Mutti et al., 2011; Sng et al., 2011).

As with accommodative lag, once hyperopic peripheral defocus increases in myopia, studies in the United States, Singapore, the United Kingdom, and China show that the rate of progression is either unrelated or inconsistently related to the amount of relative peripheral hyperopia (Atchison et al., 2015; Mutti et al., 2022; Radhakrishnan et al., 2013; Sng et al., 2011). Animal results clearly point to local control of eye growth through defocus (Gawne et al., 2022; Leng et al., 2010), suggesting that treatments directed at controlling myopic progression through modification of peripheral defocus should be more effective than they currently appear to be. It is difficult to explain why animal experimental results do not translate more effectively when applied to children. Given that clinical interventions based on animal models only show incremental progress against myopia, animal models may not be the strongest foundation for building an argument for near work as a risk factor for myopia onset. At the same time, there is insufficient understanding of how treatments, and even natural near viewing (Labhishetty et al., 2021), affect retinal image quality and defocus under various viewing conditions—whether it is through accommodative effort or pupil size, for example (reviewed in Chapter 7). This gap in knowledge underscores the need to establish more detailed models of retinal image quality during the various visual experiences of childhood when hypothesized associations between environmental exposures and myopia are studied.

Accommodation and Emmetropization in Infancy

Induction of myopia in animal models clearly shows a sensitive period (McBrien & Norton, 1992). The responses to deprivation or defocus are greatest in young animals and diminish with age (Smith et al., 1999; Wallman & Adams, 1987). This age effect could be one reason why interventions that reduce hyperopic defocus in humans are only partially effective in slowing myopia progression: the treated children may be outside of this sensitive period. The effects of accommodation and near work may be overstated in childhood and underappreciated at earlier ages. Emmetropization, the reduction in both the absolute level of hyperopia and the variance in refractive error, is the major characteristic of infant refractive error development (Mutti et al., 2018). Hyperopia in infancy drives eye growth in a negative feedback loop to be self-correcting. The tuning mechanism by which the distribution of refractive error is transformed from a normal distribution at birth into its characteristic leptokurtic shape (far more children than by chance near the average than in a normal [bell-shaped] curve) after the first two years of life is widely considered to be driven by visual feedback. Most researchers working with animal models consider hyperopic defocus to be the operative visual signal.

This hypothesis deserves reconsideration. The accommodative response stimulated by early levels of hyperopia may represent a candidate visual signal for emmetropization. The assumption is that when a negative lens is placed over a neonate eye that the animal is experiencing hyperopic defocus. However, accommodation and the effective refractive state of the animal are rarely assessed. When accommodation was assessed in a key study in macaques, Smith and co-workers made an important statement in their discussion (Smith et al., 1999):

> animals that failed to compensate for large hyperopic errors did not overcome the imposed errors via accommodation. The eyes that failed to compensate for large negative lenses, both anisometropic and equal-powered binocular lenses, appeared

to exhibit no effort to accommodate for the imposed error. As a result, these eyes chronically experienced a high degree of hyperopic defocus. (p. 1428)

In other words, compensation for imposed hyperopia required a robust accommodative response.

Human infants can produce an adult level of accommodation at 3–4 months of age, which is the age at which the variance in neonatal refractive error begins to narrow (Banks, 1980; Gabriel & Mutti, 2009; Haynes et al., 1965; Mayer et al.; 1995, Mutti, 2007). The effects of defocus and accommodation can be untangled, because they represent equal and opposite sides of dioptric demand. Infants are either experiencing defocus or they are accommodating and experiencing less defocus. The necessary measurements for the analysis are distance refractive error and the accommodative state during a near task. Such an analysis was performed on the 262 infants in the Berkeley Infant Biometry Study. Cycloplegic refractive error was measured at 3 months and again at 9 months, a time period when the majority of emmetropization takes place. After accounting for the effects of underlying hyperopic refractive error, the poorest emmetropization was seen in infants with the greatest amount of hyperopic defocus, both at near and far test distances. More accurate accommodation at 3 months of age translated into more effective emmetropization by 9 months of age (Mutti et al., 2009). Horwood and Riddell found similar results, that non-emmetropizing hyperopic infants under 6 months of age showed high amounts of hyperopic defocus at distance because of poor accommodation, in contrast to the more accurate accommodation of emmetropizing infants (Horwood & Riddell, 2011). Effective accommodation was associated with emmetropization, not hyperopic defocus, in their sample.

Studies that employ spectacle correction of infant hyperopia are difficult to interpret. Spectacles would be predicted to inhibit emmetropization under both theories; correction reduces both hyperopic defocus and the accommodative demand. The key question is the effect of spectacle correction on accommodative response. Unfortunately, this measurement has not been made in these studies. The two major studies of correction of infant hyperopia had conflicting results. Ingram found inhibition of emmetropization after spectacle correction of non-strabismic highly hyperopic infants, while Atkinson found no significant differences between treated and control infants (Atkinson et al., 2000; Ingram et al., 2000).

In sum, accommodation may be an underappreciated potential driver of infant eye growth that deserves greater attention in studies of human emmetropization.

Near Work and Accommodation May Have a Greater Influence on Infant and Early Childhood Refractive Error than Later in Childhood

Accommodation could influence refractive error through the action of the ciliary muscle on ocular shape. An accelerated rate of axial elongation, a distortion in the shape of the eye toward a less oblate shape, and a cessation in the thinning, flattening, and power loss of the crystalline lens all characterize the onset of myopia (Mutti et al., 2007a, 2012). Proportional expansion of the eye axially and peripherally along with compensatory changes in the crystalline lens that have occurred from birth all cease with the onset of myopia. The increase in accommodative lag and in the AC/A ratio (the amount of convergence resulting from one diopter of accommodation) suggest that a possible source of interruption to the necessary changes in the crystalline lens is equatorial restriction from a thickened ciliary muscle (Mutti et al., 2006, 2017). If the ciliary muscle can influence the development of myopia in childhood, perhaps it can be a factor in emmetropization. If the distortion in ocular shape from ciliary muscle tension plays a negative role in childhood myopia by accelerating axial elongation, it could also be a positive influence in hyperopic infants.

Data supporting the role of accommodation in emmetropization and experimental myopia using animal models are mixed. Chicks, marmosets, and rhesus monkeys all have active accommodation and have been used to investigate the influence of accommodation on emmetropic or myopic eye growth (Chakraborty et al., 2020). Studies have blocked accommodation by lesioning the Edinger-Westphal nuclei, or by performing optic nerve or ciliary nerve section, and have then examined the response to lens-induced myopia (Schaeffel et al., 1990; Raviola & Wiesel, 1990). These studies reported that the response to myopigenic signals remained intact with the lack of accommodation. Additionally, the protective effects of atropine on experimental myopia were first thought to produce paralysis of the ciliary muscle and inhibition of accommodation through atropine's action as a nonspecific muscarinic antagonist (Chakraborty et al., 2020). However, later studies in chicks found that atropine did not affect the ciliary muscle in the chick, so atropine was likely not preventing myopia by inhibiting accommodation (McBrien et al., 1993).

Another point of dissonance with accommodation contributing to lens-induced myopia is that accommodation changes focus uniformly across the visual field, while regional stimulation of the retina with negative or positive defocus can produce local changes in eye growth (Diether & Schaeffel, 1997). Evidence supporting accommodation in modulating refractive eye growth includes studies showing that brief periods of normal vision during exposure to negative lenses can inhibit experimental myopia (Kee et al. 2007; Schmid & Wildsoet, 1996; Shaikh et al., 1999). Thus, eliminating defocus through accommodation could inhibit myopia development. Further supporting this possibility, accommodative performance before and after inducing experimental myopia in marmosets revealed that increased accommodative lag was present after lens-induced defocus and did not predict the amount of induced myopia (Troilo, 2007). Finally, blocking accommodation in chicks with ciliary nerve section resulted in myopia, suggesting that accommodation may play a role in evaluating the sign of defocus (Diether & Wildsoet, 2005). These conflicting results were summarized by Chakraborty et al. (2020), stating "a complex relationship exists between accommodation and emmetropization, involving multiple neural pathways, feedback loops, and interactions between temporal and spatial patterns of defocus." Given these various findings, accommodation as a visual signal for emmetropization deserves further study.

If accommodation might reduce hyperopia in a beneficial manner in infancy, how long is this sensitive period? If it extends into early childhood, what would the effect be of intense near work on the eye of a toddler? Gordon-Shaag et al. (2021) studied Israeli schoolchildren and found that the more myopic ultra-Orthodox children learned to read 1–2 years earlier (at an average of 4.3 ± 0.8 years of age) than the less myopic religious or secular students (see Chapter 3). Early computer use at age 3 was associated with later myopia at ages 6 and 9 in the Generation R study (Enthoven et al., 2020). The age at which children learn to read is not a variable typically included in studies of myopia, but it may be one that deserves more attention. The epidemiology of myopia emphasizes this point. The children of East Asia and of Scandinavia have widely different prevalences of myopia. Prevalence in Taiwan may be as high as 80%, while in Scandinavia it may be 16% or lower (Hagen et al., 2018; Lin et al., 2004). "Finnish children first learn the letter sounds at school when they are 7 years old" (Brandslet, 2023). Chinese children in preschool as young as 3 years old may begin to learn to read, and more than 80% of Chinese children attend preschool in a more intensive near work environment, one with an emphasis on learning to read at an early age (Jiang et al., 2021). In Scandinavia the emphasis in preschool is on play and social interaction, with a considerable amount of time spent outdoors each day regardless of the weather. The data from China suggest that starting school increases the prevalence of myopia relative to children of similar age who begin school one year later, an increase that carries through the elementary grades (Xu et al., 2021).

Summary for Near Work

Addressing near work in childhood is a challenge. Near work is an essential and inescapable part of the reading and learning necessary for productive citizenship. Changing the research emphasis to investigating the effects of near work performed earlier in childhood may be more productive in understanding the role it plays in the onset of myopia. Investigating the effects of early near work, accommodation, and the visual environment of children (including their visual diet in the educational setting) on later myopia development may be a novel and important new area in myopia research.

ELECTRONIC DEVICES

As children increasingly engage with electronic devices at younger ages and their screen time rises, it is imperative to fully understand the association between electronic device usage and ocular health (Liu et al., 2021). Electronic device use has been suggested as one of the environmental risk factors for myopia (Martínez-Albert et al., 2023). Recent studies have shown a significant increase in screen time at earlier first-exposure ages among young children (Byrne et al., 2021; Dumuid, 2020), and even more so during the COVID-19 pandemic (Wong et al., 2021).

For example, the percentages of kids from 8 to 18 years old who own smartphones steadily increased from 2015 to 2021; as of 2021, the 8- to 12-year-olds used screen media about 5.5 hours per day and the 13- to 18-year-olds used it about 8.5 hours per day (see Figure 5-4; Common Sense, 2021). Among households with children younger than age 8, smartphone ownership increased from 41% to 97% and tablet ownership increased from 8% to 75% from 2011 to 2020 (Laricchia, 2022). While the global rise in myopia prevalence predates the advent of smart devices, the recent surge in electronic device usage has been argued to further add to the already high rates of myopia (Dirani et al., 2019; Foreman et al., 2021; Lanca & Saw, 2020). Gaining an understanding of the effects of electronic device use on myopia is crucial for shaping public health policies, educational strategies, clinical practice guidelines, and parenting approaches.

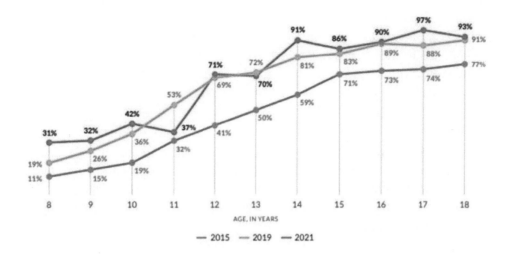

FIGURE 5-4 Smartphone ownership, by individual age, 2015–2021: Percent of 8- to 18-year-olds who have their own smartphone.
SOURCE: The Common Sense Census, 2021.

There have been mixed perspectives on the contribution of electronic devices to the increase in myopia (Lanca & Saw, 2020). For example, some vision researchers claim uniquely influential features of using electronic devices, such as different eye-movement patterns induced and light exposure while using them (e.g., Jian, 2022; Miranda et al., 2018), whereas others view electronic device usage as a case of near-vision work, with a byproduct of reduced time outdoors (e.g., Alvarez-Peregrina et al., 2020; Huang et al., 2015). While assessing its impact, it is important to understand the underlying mechanisms associated with electronic device usage.

The following sections will first distinguish among the different types of electronic devices primarily based on the viewing distance, and then discuss the potential mechanisms of any effect on myopia induction and production related to the physical features of the electronic devices and the behavioral consequences of screen use. The chapter then reviews current measures of screen use, related development of recent technologies, and potential influences of the COVID-19 pandemic on screen use and myopia.

Distinguishing Electronic Devices

When discussing electronic devices in the context of myopia, it is critical to distinguish between those with smaller screens (e.g., smartphones and tablets), which are typically viewed close to the observer (like a book) and therefore require active accommodation, versus those with larger screens (e.g., televisions) typically viewed at optically "far" distances. The nature of screen time and consumption in young children has largely changed in the last decade (Milkovich & Madigan, 2020). Recent studies have shown more time spent on near-viewing screens than is spent on far-viewing screens (Cyril Kurupp et al., 2022; Mohan et al., 2022; Wang et al., 2021; Zhang et al., 2021).

It is critical to note that viewing smaller, handheld devices is a type of near work, no different from reading a book in terms of the accommodative state of the eye. Increased near viewing screen time, sustained near work, and decreased time outdoors often go hand-in-hand (Alvarez-Peregrina et al., 2021; Aslan & Sahinoglu-Keskek, 2022; Lanca et al., 2022). An earlier study by Lee et al. (2013) compared the effects on myopia of reading, using a computer, and watching TV. This survey study of male military conscripts in Taiwan showed that time spent reading was a significant predictor of myopia, whereas time spent using a computer and watching TV were not. More reading time was associated with higher refractive error and computer use was related to axial length, but watching TV was not a significant predictor of either measure. These differences might be due to different accommodation and defocus patterns in these different conditions (Charman, 2011).

In a recent systematic review by Lanca and Saw (2020), studies involving TV screen time were intentionally excluded because they were not performed at near distance. In a 2022 study of 12,241 children in Asian countries from the Sunflower Myopia Asian Eye Epidemiology Consortium, digital screen time use was defined to include the use of TV, smartphone, tablet, and computer. After adjusting for other factors (e.g., parental myopia, outdoor time), screen time, including TV, was not associated with myopia. The authors acknowledge that the inclusion of TV could have changed the results, as TV is viewed at a greater distance than the other digital devices. Thus, when referring to electronic devices or screen time in relation to myopia, it is essential to define the types of devices studied and their typical viewing distances.

Optical Features of Electronic Devices

Electronic device use intrinsically differs from other types of near work in physical characteristics such as the light emitted by the screen—its chromatic content, luminance, and contrast—as well as features such as screen flicker (Loughman & Flitcroft, 2021; Thomson, 1998). These physical characteristics are potential candidates contributing to the effects of screen use on myopia. For example, the light emitted from screens has considerable energy at the blue end of the chromatic spectrum, and this has been of interest in relation to myopia development. Although the sun has much higher unweighted irradiance in blue light than other sources, screens of electronic devices produce high levels of blue light (de Gálvez et al., 2022), more so than other types of near work such as reading given the same level of ambient lighting.

Chang et al. showed that the light-emitting LE-eBooks used by their participants were more short-wavelength-enriched than printed books (see Figure 5-5) depending on the luminant. Other electronic devices show similar spectral peaks, except Kindle, which is not light-emitting (see Table 5-1; Chang et al., 2015). Gringras et al. (2015) measured light emissions of a tablet, e-reader, and smartphone. They also showed that the content displayed on the electronic devices affected the light emission's intensity, not necessarily its spectrum (see Figure 5-6). With the prolonged periods of screen use and the proximity of screens to our eyes in today's digital age, users may be exposed to significant amounts of blue light from electronic devices. However, the mechanisms by which blue light affects ocular health and myopia remain unclear (Cougnard-Gregoire et al., 2023; Iqbal et al., 2023). Future studies can focus on the effects of blue light, as well as various spectral profiles, to inform the design of screens and related products (e.g., light-filtering lenses).

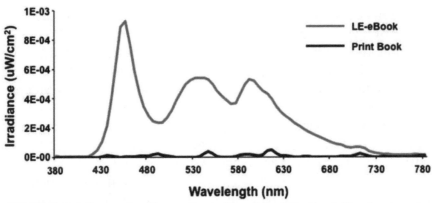

FIGURE 5-5 Spectral radiometric profile of the LE-eBook Device (gray) and incident light reflected by the printed book (black).

NOTE: The peak irradiance for the LE-eBook eReader is ~450 nm and for the reflected light is 612 nm.

SOURCE: Chang et al., 2015.

TABLE 5-1 Screen Size, Irradiance, and Peak Spectral Wavelength of Print Books and Electronic Reading Devices

Device	Size, in	Irradiance, W/m^2	Spectral peak, nm
Book*	NA	3.23×10^{-3}	612
iPad	9.7	1.03×10^{-1}	452
iPad2	9.7	8.91×10^{-2}	452
iPhone	3.5	2.50×10^{-2}	452
iPod Touch	3.5	2.05×10^{-2}	456
Kindle*	6	3.84×10^{-3}	612
Kindle Fire	7	4.31×10^{-2}	448
Nook Color	7	2.72×10^{-2}	448

A diagonal measurement was used for the screen size dimension. Light readings were taken while devices were at their maximum brightness setting, and all measurements were recorded from the same distance (38–40 cm) from the screen and in the same background conditions. NA, not applicable. *Neither the book nor the Kindle eReader emitted light; the irradiance measured was the ambient room light emitted by the ceiling fixtures and reflected by the printed book or the Kindle screen. The iPad, iPad2, iPhone, and iPod Touch are registered trademarks of Apple Inc. The Kindle and Kindle Fire are registered trademarks of Amazon.com, Inc. The Nook Color is a trademark of Barnes & Noble, Inc. Patent Pending.

SOURCE: Chang et al., 2015.

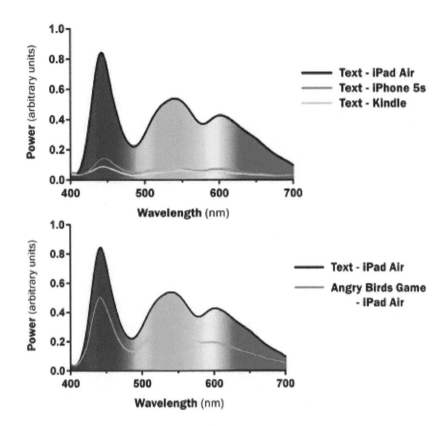

FIGURE 5-6 Spectral profile of text (A) comparing identical text on three devices and (B) compared to game (same device).
SOURCE: Gringras et al., 2015.

Contrast has been found to significantly influence retinal processing, potentially impacting the onset and progression of myopia. The act of reading a text with dark letters against a bright background primarily stimulates the retinal OFF pathway, resulting in thinner choroids, which is linked to the onset of myopia (Aleman et al., 2018). Conversely, reading text with bright letters on a dark background (i.e., inverted text contrast) produces the opposite effect. These effects have been shown with exposure to text on screens. Swiatczak & Schaeffel (2022) found that inverted text contrast also elicited axial eye shortening for myopic subjects after reading a large screen at a 2-meter distance for 45 minutes. This effect of text contrast was shown to be dependent on text size, only eliciting significant differences in axial length with large text (Swiatczak & Schaeffel, 2022). This effect of contrast polarity has been further shown to have different effects on retinal processing in myopic and emmetropic eyes (Wagner & Strasser, 2023).

These results may guide the designers of screens to consider screen contrast for the purpose of protection against myopia. However, it is important to note that the contrast ratio between the characters and the background also affect legibility and readability. Although white-on-black and black-on-white texts have the same contrast ratio, white-on-black text is more difficult to read than black-on-white text (Proctor & Van Zandt, 2018; Taylor, 1934).

Behaviors Associated with Screen Use

Besides the intrinsic characteristics of screens, screen use is associated with different behaviors that may affect the user's ocular health, even when performing the same tasks (e.g., reading on different platforms). Bao et al. (2015), working with 120 myopic children aged 6 to 13 years in China, compared their near-vision posture during various tasks: playing a video game on a handheld electronic device, reading on paper, and writing on paper. They found that, although all tasks were performed at a desk, the viewing distance was significantly closer when playing the video game (21.3 cm) than when reading (27.2 cm) and writing (24.9 cm), with head declination being greater when playing the video game (63.5°) than reading (37.1°) and writing (44.5°). Similarly, Read et al. (2023) conducted a controlled experiment to compare the effects of reading platform (smartphone vs. paper) and environment (indoor vs. outdoor) on gaze behaviors for adult myopes and emmetropes. They showed that a closer viewing distance was used for smartphone-based reading than for paper-based reading, and this difference was greater for myopes. The mean 20° peripheral scene relative defocus was also greater for smartphone-based reading, which was likely due to the closer viewing effect and smaller size of the smartphone. One study compared the print-based tasks of writing on paper and reading books with electronic tasks done on an iPad and a cellphone and found no difference between the print tasks and the electronic tasks (Bhandari & Ostrin, 2022). However, their writing task was set up on a desk, while the other tasks were handheld or on the participants' laps. Thus, further research is needed to understand the differences between using electronic devices and traditional media while performing similar tasks in the context of myopia onset and progression.

Children report that they are drawn indoors by interesting activities, including the use of electronic devices (Larson et al., 2019). Larson et al. (2019) surveyed 543 6th to 8th graders in rural South Carolina and reported that screen time and outdoor time were negatively correlated, and that the amount of screen time was higher than the outdoor time for almost all groups. On the contrary, a survey on 5,844 children ages 9–11 years from 12 countries showed that greater outdoor time spent outside of school hours was associated with higher screen time, with a possible reason being that those who spent more time outdoors were compensated with more screen time (LeBlanc et al., 2015). However, for children at a much earlier age, 2 years, screen time was shown to be negatively associated with outdoor play in 885 children in Japan (Sugiyama et al., 2023). Similarly, a study of 1,772 preschool children in urban and rural China showed that urban children spent more time playing outdoors and less time on screens (Wang et al., 2020). Thus, there seems to be at least a trend in which using electronic devices is associated with less time spent outdoors.

Children can use screens for extended periods of time before they are even able to read, at very early ages. Among 390 children who were ages 2–5 years old in Korea, 31.3% started using smartphones before 2 years of age and 23.4% used smartphones for over an hour on weekends (Chang et al., 2018). Hinkley et al. (2018) found that 575 children aged 2–5 years were reported to have an average of 2.1 hours of screen time per day. Radesky et al. (2020) found that about 15% of children between the ages of 3 and 5 used their mobile devices over 4 hours per day, among the 346 children they studied in Michigan, United States. Xu et al. (2016) study on over 500 children showed that one-year-old children in Sydney, Australia, had an average of 0.64 hours of screen time per day, with 26% having more than one hour per day. The mean screen time increased to 1.37 hours, 2.48 hours, and 2.25 hours for 2-year-olds, 3.5-year-olds, and 5-year-olds, respectively. Moreover, screen time during infancy at age one was found to be predictive of children's screen time from ages 2 to 5. These behavior patterns, shown in studies across different countries, are concerning given that rapid eye elongation occurs at young ages.

Measurements of Screen Use

To further the research on the potential impact of screen time on myopia in young children, it is essential to enhance the rigor of measures and reporting. The methodological consideration of how to measure screen time among children has received little attention until recently. Byrne et al. (2021) summarized measurements of screen time in children ages 0 to 6 years old. One finding is a notable increase in articles measuring screen time on mobile devices in addition to TV starting in 2015, which is an indication of increased interest in this topic. Among the 622 articles included in their review, the overwhelming majority (92.4%) of the studies used questionnaires, while the remaining used 24-hour diary logs. In addition, most reported duration of screentime rather than the frequency of screen viewing. Moreover, the majority of the studies did not report psychometric properties, such as the validity and reliability of the measures. It is also notable that device-based usage event monitoring was not used in any of the studies.

In an effort to ensure the psychometric soundness of the measures, Hutton and colleagues (Hutton et al., 2020) developed a composite parent-report measure of screen-based media use (ScreenQ) and provided a psychometric assessment of its validity and reliability. ScreenQ reflects four dimensions cited in current American Academy of Pediatrics recommendations: access to screens, frequency of use, media content, and caregiver-child co-viewing. This measure has been validated among 69 children ages 36 to 63 months old in the United States and among young Portuguese children (from 6 months to 9.9 years old) with strong psychometric properties, including internal consistency, reliability, and concurrent validity (Hutton et al., 2020; Monteiro et al., 2022).

Recent measures for assessing children's screen usage beyond parent-report surveys are also under development (Milkovich & Madigan, 2020; Radesky et al., 2020). Radesky et al. (2020) used a method called "mobile device sampling" to objectively measure mobile device use among children ages 3 to 5 years old. This method used data gathered by the device operating system (a monitoring app on Android devices and the battery feature on iOS devices) and found that only about 30% of the parents had subjective retrospective reports of children's device use that were deemed accurate, with 36% deemed to be underestimates and 35% deemed overestimates of their children's device usage. This device sampling method has a problem, however, in that it cannot accurately measure usage when individuals share devices (Milkovich & Madigan, 2020).

Recent Technologies

In addition to screentime measurement, which is enabled by emerging technologies, measuring screen distance has also become a feature incorporated into mobile devices. For example, the Screen Distance feature (see Figure 5-7 below) is available on iPhones and iPads starting with iOS 17 and iPadOS, as announced by Apple in 2023. This feature, using a TrueDepth camera, detects and alerts users when the mobile device is held closer than 12 inches from the user's eyes "for an extended period" (Apple, 2024). This feature is based on the assumption that "Viewing a device (or a book) too closely for an extended period of time can increase the risk of myopia for younger users and eye strain for users of all ages." In addition to this built-in feature in iOS, mobile applications (apps) are available to remind or force users to hold their mobile devices at appropriate distances (e.g., Samsung Safety Screen available since 2016, the EyesPro App by Parental Control Kroha available since 2020). Potentially, these apps and features could be used for measuring screen time and distance in research to obtain objective measures. Recent studies have also shown the potential of using smartphones as an optical sensing and analysis platform (e.g., as spectrometers), utilizing their advanced on-board sensors (Di Nonno & Ulber, 2021; Fratto et al., 2023). Research has also made it possible to detect when small children are using smart devices, such as through speech and facial features (Li et al., 2013; Qawaqneh et al., 2017), tap and swipe analysis (Li et al., 2018; Vatavu et al., 2015), as well as touch- and sensor-based approaches (Nguyen et al., 2019).

Other recent developments in technologies such as virtual reality (VR) and augmented reality (AR), utilizing head-mounted displays and head-up displays, have been used to convey virtual visual information to operators in applications such as aircraft (Gu et al., 2020), automobiles (Park & Im, 2020), and games (Munsamy et al., 2020). In VR/AR, eye convergence can be manipulated through rotation of the virtual cameras used to present information to the left and right eyes through automatic virtual convergence (State et al., 2001). The convergence distance can be fixed at a predetermined value, such as a few feet away or infinity (Sherstyuk & State, 2010). However, the accommodation distance is determined by the distance of the light rays, which has been measured to be around 3 to 7 meters (Itoh et al., 2021; Kramida, 2015). The mismatch between convergence distance and accommodation distance is called the vergence-accommodation conflict (see Figure 5-8), which is a major source of motion sickness caused by using VR (Itoh et al., 2021).

Recent efforts by both industry and the academy have developed several mitigation solutions to the vergence-accommodation conflict, with examples such as varifocal displays (Stevens et al., 2018), multifocal displays (Rolland et al., 2000), and retinal displays (Topliss et al., 2023). Apple's VisionPro, a mixed reality headset announced on June 5, 2023, utilizes a retinal display designed to tackle the accommodation-convergence conflict (Topliss et al., 2023). In the VisionPro's direct retinal projector system developed for the retinal display, light beams are projected to the eyes through scanning mirrors, rather than images being viewed on a screen or surface as in conventional VR/AR systems. However, this direct retinal projector system does not eliminate the vergence-accommodation conflict, although it is believed to "at least partially" (Topliss et al., 2023, p. 4) help eliminate the conflict.

VR/AR is regarded as having the potential to help prevent and manage myopia through accommodation training (Turnbull & Phillips, 2017; Zhao et al., 2018). However, the effects on ocular health of extended use of VR/AR and exposure to the artificial lights in VR/AR displays is under-researched (Jonnakuti & Frankfort, 2023). Despite remarkable advances in these technologies, they have a long way to go before they can ensure proper depth perception, visual comfort, positive user experience, and ocular health (Cebeci et al., 2024; Kramida, 2015).

To utilize the recent technologies for measuring, monitoring, and preventing myopia, a clearer understanding of the mechanisms that cause myopia is needed. Future research is needed to further the potential of electronic-device-based systems to objectively measure myopia and to monitor other environmental risk factors for myopia, as well as design advanced training and prevention techniques.

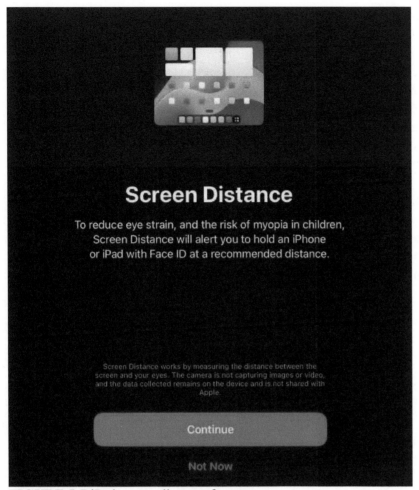

FIGURE 5-7 iPad screen distance feature.
SOURCE: Screenshot taken on committee member iPad.

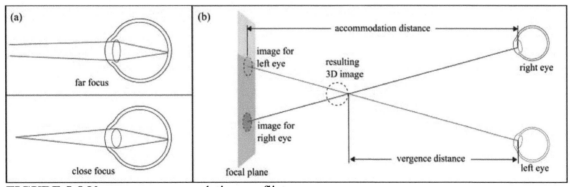

FIGURE 5-8 Vergence-accommodation conflict.
SOURCE: Kramida, 2015.

Impact of COVID-19

"Quarantine myopia" is a term used to describe myopia developed during the COVID-19 home quarantine (Aslan & Sahinoglu-Keskek, 2022). School-age kids (3 to 17 years old) in various countries had increased screen time due to online schooling requirements (Bergmann et al., 2022; see Table 5-2). Bergmann et al. (2022) found similar patterns during COVID-19 lockdown for younger children from ages 8 to 36 months, who had no online schooling requirements, in 12 countries. They found that longer durations of lockdown were associated with a more significant rise in screen time and that caregivers reported more screen time during the pandemic compared to before.

The latter outcome might be influenced by the age difference in the children studied, as they were older during the pandemic than before. Older children, in general, reported longer screen times compared to their younger counterparts (Bergmann et al., 2022). In China, Sun et al. (2020) found that nearly half of their 6,416 respondents reported increased internet use during COVID-19. Among students in grade schools, more than 50% of students used smartphones for online learning (Wang et al., 2021). Similarly, in India, Mohan et al. (2022) found that 96.7% of their study population, who were 6- to 18-year-olds, used smartphones for online learning during COVID-19. They also showed an association between rapid myopia progression and using smartphones for video games for more than one hour per day. Children had increased use of electronic devices in many countries during the COVID-19 pandemic.

TABLE 5-2 Previous Findings on Lockdown-Related Increases to Children's Screen Time

Country	Age	Screen time effect
Canada	5 to 11 years	95% of children not meeting guidelines for physical activity due to sedentary behaviour including screen time (Moore et al., 2020)
China	6 to 17 years	30 h more screen time per week (Xiang et al., 2020)
France	6 to 10 years	62% of children had increased screen time (Chambonniere et al., 2021)
Germany	4 to 17 years	One hour more screen time per day (Schmidt et al., 2020)
Italy	6 to 18 years	Almost 5 h more screen time per day in children with obesity (Pietrobelli et al., 2020)
Netherlands	6 to 14 years	Self-reported screen time increased by 59–62 min per day (ten Velde et al., 2021)
South Korea	age not reported	81% of children had increased screen time (Guan et al., 2020)
Spain	8 to 16 years	2 h more screen time per day (Medrano et al., 2020)
USA	< 18 years	'Dramatic' increase in screen time (Hartshorne et al., 2020)
Multi-country	3 to 7 years	50 min more screen time per day (Ribner et al., 2021)

SOURCE: Bergmann et al., 2022, under a Creative Commons Attribution-NonCommercial-No Derivatives 4.0 International License (https://creativecommons.org/licenses/by/4.0/).

Studies conducted and data collected during the pandemic may provide invaluable evidence for the impact of electronic devices on myopia. A systematic review (Cyril Kurupp et al., 2022) on the impact of the COVID-19 pandemic on myopia progression in children, which highlighted reduced outdoor time and increased electronic device use during home confinement, concluded that the heightened usage of electronic devices (e.g., mobile phones and tablets) among children during the pandemic had a significant impact on the progression of myopia. The review included 10 research papers published between 2019 and 2022, most of them focused on grade school children. However, it is worth noting that most of the studies reviewed by Cyril Kurupp et al. (2022) used questionnaires to study the risk factors of myopia progression, which lack objective measures.

In summary, the causal effect of electronic device usage on myopia is under-explored. The lack of consistency in definitions and measures of both electronic device use and myopia makes it challenging to reach an agreement on whether electronic device usage has a causal effect on myopia. Although recent developments in the technologies of mobile sensors, monitoring and alerting systems, and VR/AR are promising, more research is needed to allow for recommendations regarding the usage and design of electronic devices.

INDOOR VERSUS OUTDOOR VISION

The Nature of the Problem and Its Distal Causes

There are stark differences between the optical environment of the outdoors, where all visual systems evolved, and the *indoor* setting of the modern home or classroom, which includes a variety of viewing screen technologies. Several lines of evidence indicate that something, or more likely some *things*, about these differences are causing the worldwide increase in the prevalence and severity of myopia.

Initial studies of this problem were observational and correlational, but nevertheless strongly suggestive. These have been nicely reviewed elsewhere (e.g., Wallman & Winawer, 2004) and summarized in other parts of this report, and so will only be mentioned here. They include the fact that myopia increases with the level of education attained (Goldschmidt, 1968; Sperduto et al., 1983), that cultures in which people still lead outdoor lives have little myopia (Morgan & Rose, 2005), and that the introduction of compulsory education to the children of Native American & Inuit peoples led to dramatic increases in myopia within one generation (Bear, 1991).

More directly relevant to the indoor/outdoor issue, a seminal, large cross-sectional study of Australian school children (Rose et al., 2008) revealed that those who engaged in more near work and spent less time outdoors had, on average, significantly more myopia. And even after stratification for amount of near work and adjustment for other relevant factors, such as ethnicity and parental refractive errors, children who spent more time outdoors were less likely to be myopic. It should be noted, however, that the effect size was rather small, amounting to a difference in spherical equivalent refraction between the two groups of only about 0.3 D. Other observational studies have largely supported the original findings from Australia. For example, a prospective cohort study in Taiwan (Wu et al., 2020) revealed an impressive slowing, and then reversal, in myopia incidence following school-based interventions that promoted time outdoors.

From early observational studies, one of the most relevant analyses for present purposes was performed by Jones et al. (2007), using survey data from the Orinda Longitudinal Study of Myopia to predict which children subsequently became myopic. They performed a logistic regression analysis and identified two key predictive factors: time outdoors and parental myopia history, including a significant interaction between the two such that children at higher genetic risk benefitted more from time outdoors (Figure 5-9). Interestingly, once these two major risk factors were accounted for, the number of hours a child spent reading per week failed to provide significantly additional predictive power. This latter observation, however, could be confounded by the aforementioned "genetic nurture" if, for example, myopic parents encourage their children to read or otherwise provide an environment that is more supportive of reading (e.g., having lots of books around the house). Similar results were reported in another large longitudinal study of children in the United Kingdom (Shah et al., 2017). The salutary effects of time outdoors were apparent in children as young as age 3, and they remained sizeable (Hazard ratios of ~0.9 per SD of hours outdoors per day) after adjusting for sex, number of myopic parents, and time spent reading.

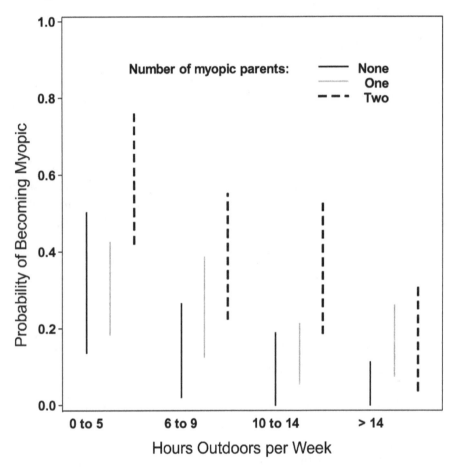

FIGURE 5-9 Width of the 95% CI associated with the probability of myopia among the levels of sports and outdoor activity per week stratified by number of myopic parents.
NOTE: The figure is from the Orinda Longitudinal Study of Myopia (Orinda, California). Greater outdoor/sports activity per week in 514 third-grade children reduced the probability of the onset of myopia by the eighth grade.
SOURCE: Adapted from Jones et al., 2007, Figure 4.

Subsequent randomized controlled trials (RCTs) have clearly demonstrated a causal benefit of increased time outdoors. But as with previous observational studies, the magnitude of the benefits has been modest. For example, a cluster-randomized (i.e., by school) intervention with 1st-graders in China (He et al., 2015) found that an additional 40 minutes a day of outdoor time produced a decrease in 3-year, cumulative rates of myopia (defined as spherical equivalent refraction of < -0.5 D) from 39.5% in the control group to 30.4% in the intervention group. Again, this is a small decrease (9 percentage point decrease; 95% CI of a 4 to 14% decrease), but it is a convincingly real effect. Likewise, a large cluster RCT in Taiwan (Wu et al., 2018) found small (but highly significant) beneficial effects of time outdoors after one year: a difference of 0.11 D for children who were non-myopic at baseline, but a larger difference of 0.23 D in children who were already myopic at the beginning of the study. When normalized for the respective pooled standard deviations (Cohen's d-prime), these amount to effect sizes of 0.18 (generally interpreted as a "small" effect) and 0.6 (a "moderate" effect), respectively. In agreement with this, a recent meta-analysis of five RCTs with a total of 3,014 participants found an overall beneficial effect size of 0.15 D (0.06 to 0.23) and a risk ratio for developing new myopia of 0.76 (0.67 to 0.87).

Taken together, these data overwhelmingly demonstrate that time outdoors matters, particularly when referring to reduction in the risk of myopia onset. Yet the magnitude of the beneficial effects with respect to myopia progression seem rather small. To put them in perspective, these data can be compared to other interventions, including optical interventions using spectacles or contact lenses and medical interventions with atropine eyedrops.

Caveats in Estimating Effect Size

There are several caveats to consider when considering the RCT-based effect-size estimates above. One is that all these studies were done in school-age children—the youngest being 6-year-olds—and mainly focused on the rate of myopia progression, rather than on a delay in onset. Delay in onset has been suggested by some studies (He et al., 2015; Jin et al. 2015; Jones et al., 2007; Wu et al. 2013) as the major beneficial effect of time outdoors. The RCT-based studies thus may be suffering from the same problem pointed out above concerning near work, namely not focusing on *early exposure* and on *prevention*. Second, the magnitude of the intended treatment may have been insufficient. Even though children in the treatment group were encouraged to spend more time outdoors, they were still, relatively speaking, spending most of their school day indoors. For example, in the RCT conducted by He et al. (2015), children in the treatment group received an additional 40 minutes of outdoor recess during school, but this is only about 8% of an 8-hour school day. The data shown in Figure 5-9 suggest that 2 hours per day or 14 hours per week provides the maximum effect (Jones et al., 2007).

Finally, over and above the problem of a low dose of outdoors in the treatment group, the actual differences in time outdoors between the treatment and the control groups may not have been as large as one would desire from a scientific perspective. In this regard, the trial reported in Wu et al. (2018) is worth a closer look, as children in both groups wore light meters, giving the investigators an objective measure of light exposure. The investigators reported the number of minutes per week that children spent in four different luminance categories: ≥ 1000 lux, ≥ 3000 lux, ≥ 5000 lux, and $\geq 10,000$ lux (Table 4, p. 1246), both at baseline and at the end of the study for both treatment (n = 267) and control (n = 426) groups. The values in Table 5-3 represent a rough integral of light exposure (lux-minutes/week), taken by multiplying the average number of minutes per week that each group spent in each of the four luminance categories and summing the resulting values.

Curiously, *both* groups rather dramatically increased their total light exposure: the treatment group increased by about 40%, as expected, but the control group's exposure also increased, by 32%. When Wu et al. (2018) used the raw values for each child—and they had large enough samples for considerable statistical power—they found no statistically significant difference in time spent in any of the four light-exposure categories, either at baseline or during the study, with unadjusted p-values ranging from 0.37 to 0.97 (median, 0.80). It was only when they combined objective data from the light meters with data from self-report diaries that they found a significant in-study difference, which amounted to about 70 minutes/week more time outdoors for the treatment group.

TABLE 5-3 Integral of Light Exposure.

	Control (lux-minutes/week)	**Treatment** (lux-minutes/week)
Baseline	1,111,720	1,092,290
Study	1,468,710	1,528,930

SOURCE: Wu et al., 2018.

What might have accounted for this puzzling result? As with all behavioral modifications, noncompliance in the treatment group appeared to be an issue (Wu et al., 2018). However, there also appeared to be some "self-treatment" in the control group (Table 5-3). Some of this latter effect may have been due to parallel initiatives launched by the Taiwanese government, "Sport & Health 150" and "Tien-Tien 120," both of which promoted time outdoors for school children.

In summary, virtually all studies on the effect of time outdoors—both observational and interventional—have found statistically significant, beneficial effects of small to moderate size. The most consistent benefit has been a delay in the onset of myopia, while slowing of progression in pre-existing myopes has been less frequently observed.

How Does Spending Time Outdoors Protect Against Myopia?

In addition to suggesting interventions for myopia prevention, the beneficial effects of time outdoors give us important clues as to the possible "sensed variables" (Figure 5-10) in the visual environment that are most directly relevant to emmetropization. These are variables that may serve as more convenient points of intervention than the modifications in education and behavior entailed by the "increased time outdoors" approach. To take a simple—and currently hypothetical—example: Insofar as differences in the brightness and color spectrum between the indoor and outdoor environments were found to be causal factors, easier-to-implement changes in classroom design (e.g. larger windows to admit more natural light or specific improvements in artificial lighting) might be effective interventions.

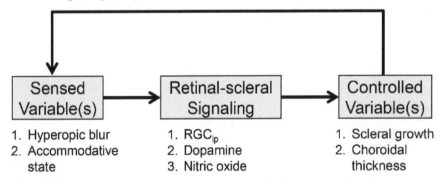

FIGURE 5-10 A simple control systems model of emmetropization.
NOTE: The items enumerated beneath each box are only examples for purposes of illustration and are not intended to be comprehensive lists.
SOURCE: Committee generated.

One problem is that such a list of the differences in the "visual diet" (Poudel et al., 2023) provided by indoor vs. outdoor experience is long, particularly when possible differences in oculomotor behavior are also considered. Further complicating the problem, there is likely to be redundancy at multiple levels of the emmetropization system, including which specific variables are sensed under different conditions. Moreover, the critical variables may interact with each other in nonlinear ways and may differ, subtly but importantly, in different species. Even so, differences in the visual environment are an important starting point, and the Committee believes that developing sophisticated models of how the environment, whether indoors or outdoors, influences early visual processing will be critical for advancing our understanding of emmetropization (see Chapter 6, Myopia Pathogenesis: From Retinal Image to Scleral Growth). This will require collecting large data sets of the visual environment experienced by observers under different conditions (e.g., Flitcroft, 2012), combined with good models of the eye's optics (Hastings et al., 2024) and movements (Rucci & Victor, 2018) to determine how the environment is spatio-temporally sampled. Ultimately, the environment's influence on photoreceptors and the ensuing retinal circuitry relevant to emmetropization will need to be considered. This effort calls for improvements in technology that will allow the longitudinal monitoring of the visual environment at a fine-grained level in children, during the critical period for emmetropization.

One other wrinkle is that the visual diet, regardless of *where* one is, depends largely on *what* one is doing. Because most extended periods of near work (e.g., reading) are performed indoors, this introduces correlations among several groups of potential sensed variables. To disambiguate these variables, it would help to find epidemiological circumstances that break these correlations. For example, are there groups of children who spend time indoors but do not engage in much near work? Or, vice versa, are there schools that make use of outdoor classrooms? Below we have focused on the major characteristics of the visual diet that have been investigated experimentally: luminance, chromaticity, dioptric environment, eye movements, and contrast (ON/OFF pathway stimulation).

Effects of Luminance

Because of the remarkable ability of our visual system to adapt to different levels of illumination (Rieke & Rudd, 2009), we are blissfully unaware of even rather large differences: the intensity of outdoor sunlight is roughly 100 times that of a well-lit room (Lanca et al., 2019). This has several consequences for retinal processing that may be relevant to emmetropization and myopigenesis.

There is very strong evidence from studies in animal models that high levels of illumination alone (i.e., absent other features of outdoor vision) are protective against the development of myopia. The ability of bright light to slow eye growth during both form deprivation and lens-induced myopia has been demonstrated in chickens, guinea pigs, rhesus monkeys, mice, and tree shrews (see reviews: Mazade et al., 2024; Muralidharan et al., 2022). It was found in chicks for both form-deprivation myopia (Ashby et al., 2009) and lens-induced myopia (Ashby & Schaeffel, 2010), and in monkeys for form-deprivation myopia (Smith et al., 2012). In the chick form-deprivation myopia model, continuous bright light was more effective than an equivalent amount of intermittent light (Backhouse et al., 2013), and the beneficial effect appeared to be mediated by retinal dopamine (Ashby & Schaeffel, 2010; Muralidharan et al., 2022).

However, it is important to point out that light intensity, *per se*, cannot be a signal for emmetropization, because it offers no possibility of a differential signal for myopic versus hyperopic defocus that could be used in a negative feedback loop to regulate eye growth. With respect to the benefits of high luminance (outdoors), there are two possibilities: First, high luminance might induce a general signal (e.g., dopamine) that slows eye growth, which would be beneficial in a situation of hyperopic defocus—the starting point for human children (Mazade et al., 2024)—but could be counterproductive under other circumstances. Indeed, Ashby & Schaeffel (2010), using the chick lens-induced myopia model, found that bright light decreased the rate of eye-length compensation for negative lenses and increased it for positive lenses. Alternatively, high luminance might improve the overall operation of emmetropization mechanisms.

The findings of Ashby & Schaeffel (2010) argue strongly for the first possibility. While luminance may not be a signal *per se*, it can have a huge effect on retinal circuits. Thus, if contrast were an important signal for eye growth, bright light vs. dim light would activate different retinal pathways that could provide different retinal signals for growth.

Because the pupil constricts in response to light, the eye's optics are improved in bright light: (a) there is better depth of focus, meaning that, other things being equal, an eye with a smaller pupil will experience less blur when viewing objects at different distances from the focal plane and (b) optical aberrations besides defocus and astigmatism are reduced. However, the pupil also constricts as part of the accommodation reflex during near work, so pupil size, *per se*, may not be a major luminance-related mechanism for the beneficial effects of time outdoors.

Effects of Chromaticity

The sunlight experienced on earth is subject to filtering by clouds and to the effects of Rayleigh scattering in the atmosphere, but under a wide variety of conditions it has roughly equal power at the wavelengths to which the human eye is sensitive (Figure 5-11). In other words, it is "broad spectrum" illumination. In addition, sunlight contains considerable power at wavelengths below 400 nm—so-called ultraviolet light—which are not experienced by the retina due to their absorption by the lens and cornea but affect the production of vitamin D by the skin. By contrast, the spectral composition of indoor lighting varies widely depending on the source (Figure 5-12).

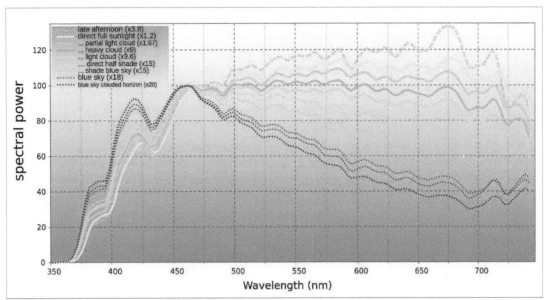

FIGURE 5-11 Spectral composition of sunlight at approximately sea level.
NOTE: Illumination by direct sunlight is compared with direct sunlight scattered by cloud cover and with indirect sunlight by varying degrees of cloud cover. The yellow line shows the power spectrum of direct sunlight under optimal conditions. To aid comparison, the other illumination conditions are scaled by the factor shown in the key, so they match at about 470 nm (blue light).
SOURCE: Wikimedia Commons, 2023.

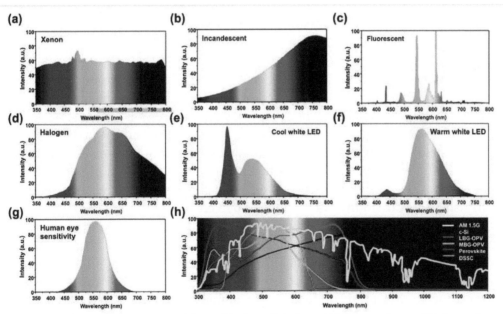

FIGURE 5-12 Spectral composition of indoor lighting. (A) Xenon lamp, (B) incandescent lamp, (C) fluorescent lamp, (D) halogen lamp, (E) cool white LED, (F) warm white LED, (G) human eye sensitivity spectrum, and (H) AM 1.5G spectrum overlaid with spectral response of various photovoltaic devices.
SOURCE: Kim et al., 2019.

The power of traditional incandescent lighting is heavily concentrated toward the red end of the spectrum, whereas fluorescent lighting tends to be bluer. Increasingly, LED-based lights can have their color spectra tailored from "cooler" (i.e., shorter wavelengths or "bluer") to "warmer" (longer/redder). Humans are normally unaware of these wavelength differences, due to extensive spatial-chromatic processing in the retina and beyond. This processing endows our visual systems with the ability to compute the *relative* reflectance of different surfaces (e.g., the color of paint, independent of the spectral composition of the lighting), largely eliminating the effect of the color spectrum of the light source on our perception of the color of things.

However, just because our visual systems can "discount the illuminant" for color perception, it does not follow that emmetropization has the same capacity or that it does not use chromatic signals that could be affected by the ambient color spectrum. For example, one proposed mechanism by which the retina detects the sign of defocus involves the use of longitudinal chromatic aberration: because shorter wavelengths are refracted by the eye's optics *more* than longer wavelengths, hyperopic defocus will result in relatively more retinal blur for longer wavelengths than for shorter; and vice versa for myopic defocus (Figure 5-13).

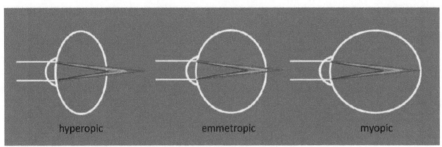

FIGURE 5-13 Effects of longitudinal chromatic aberration.
NOTE: Illustration depicting the multiple planes of focus in a hyperopic (left), emmetropic (middle), and myopic (right) eye. In each case, shorter wavelength light (blue) is focused more strongly than medium (green) or long (red) wavelength light.
SOURCE: Wallman & Winawer, 2004.

Thus, a comparison of retinal signals for channels that have different chromatic sensitivities could act as one of the sensed variables for emmetropization. The evidence in animal models is mixed: there is reported evidence that chickens and tree shrews, at least, make use of chromatic cues (Khanal et al. 2023; Muralidharan et al., 2021; Rucker & Wallman, 2009, 2012; Troilo et al., 2019), and also reports that chickens show *no* effect of chromatic stimulation (Rohrer et al., 1992; Schaeffel & Howland, 1991; Wildsoet et al., 1993). Insofar as spectra from artificial lighting alter the balance in activity between different chromatic channels, they could perturb such a mechanism. This possibility was examined by Gawne & Norton (2020), who performed simulations of the effects on emmetropization of different common sources of artificial lighting using a specific model of longitudinal chromatic aberrations (LCA), the so-called "opponent dual-detector spectral drive model." The results of their simulations suggested that these artificial sources were chromatically rich enough so as not to perturb emmetropization.

Numerous experiments have been conducted with animals raised under narrow-band illumination, with results varying according to the color of light and the species (see Table 5-4). The consensus from studies in chicks and Guinea pigs is that short-wavelength light promotes hyperopia and is protective against interventions that induce myopia; vice versa for longer-wavelength light (e.g., Foulds et al., 2013; Liu et al., 2011; Seidemann & Schaeffel, 2002; Wang et al., 2018; see Table 5-4 for other references). However, the relationship between wavelength and refractive effect appears to be reversed in rhesus monkeys and tree shrews, with long-wavelength light slowing eye growth (Gawne et al., 2017; Hung et al., 2018; Smith et al., 2015; Ward et al., 2018), and protecting against form deprivation myopia in rhesus monkeys (Hung et al., 2018; reviewed in Muralidharan et al., 2021). At present, the reasons for the apparent species-related differences are unclear. One important factor that has only recently been identified is the possible differential pre-retinal filtering of light by the cornea and lens. For example, a recent study (Grytz, 2023) found that the tree shrew lens absorbs considerably more violet light than does that of the mouse.

TABLE 5-4 Effect of Raising Different Animals Under Narrow-Band Illumination

Study	Animal	Light Color	Refractive Effect (Relative to White Light Group)
Seidemann & Schaeffel (2002)	Chick	Bue	Hyperopic
Foulds et. al (2013)	Chick	Blue (15% green)	Hyperopic
Wang et. al (2018)	Chick	Blue	Hyperopic
Wang et. al (2018)	Chick	Ultraviolet	Hyperopic
Seidemann & Schaeffel (2002)	Chick	Red	Myopic
Foulds et. al (2013)	Chick	Red (10% yellow-green)	Myopic
Wang et. al (2018)	Chick	Red	Myopic
Liu et. al (2011)	Guinea pig	Blue	Hyperopic
Jiang et. al (2014)	Guinea pig	Blue	Nil effect
Qian et. al (2013)	Guinea pig	Blue	Hyperopic
Zou et. al (2018)	Guinea pig	Blue	Hyperopic
Liu et. al (2011)	Guinea pig	Green	Myopic
Qian et. al (2013)	Guinea pig	Green	Myopic
Zou et. al (2018)	Guinea pig	Green	Myopic
Jiang et. al (2014)	Guinea pig	Red	Myopic
Gawne et. al (2018)	Tree shrew	Blue	Myopic
Gawne et. al (2018)	Tree shrew	Red	Hyperopic
Ward et. al (2018)	Tree shrew	Red	Hyperopic
Hung et. al (2018)	Rhesus monkey	Red	Hyperopic
Smith et. al (2015)	Rhesus monkey	Red	Hyperopic

SOURCE: Lingham et al., 2020, with permission from BMJ Publishing Group Ltd.

Another route by which the spectral composition of the illuminant might affect emmetropization involves intrinsically photosensitive retinal ganglion cells (ipRGC). In the primate retina, this mechanism begins with a population of giant ganglion cells that express melanopsin, a photopigment whose spectral sensitivity, though complex, is relatively blue-shifted (peak sensitivity at 482 nm), and that appear to roughly (log-)linearly encode retinal irradiance over at least 3–4 log units of intensity (Dacey et al., 2005). These ipRGCs provide excitatory input to dopaminergic amacrine cells (Roy & Field 2019), the principal source of retinal dopamine, which may be an important molecule in retinal-scleral signaling for emmetropization (see Chapter 6). Sunlight, by virtue of both its broader spectrum and greater intensity, clearly provides sufficient power to stimulate the ipRGC pathway, but certain forms of artificial lighting, such as incandescent lights and "warm" white LEDs, may provide a weaker stimulus. Direct evidence for such a possibility was recently obtained using mouse genetics to target melanopsin or ipRGCs (Chakraborty et al., 2022; Liu et al., 2022). In these studies, investigators eliminated or replaced *Opn4* which encodes melanopsin and found altered response to form deprivation or lens defocus myopia, respectively. Furthermore, investigators have found that other atypical opsins, Opn3 and Opn5, which are sensitive to blue or violet wavelengths and are also found in RGCs, might be involved in myopia development. Jiang et al. (2021) found that lens-induced myopia suppression by violet light depended on both the time of day when the treatment was administered and the presence of neuropsin (OPN5). Linne et al. (2023) found that a germline knock-out of Opn3 had more myopic refractions. Overall, this appears to be a promising and important direction for future research.

Effects of Dioptric Environment

The refractive power of the eye's optics—measured in diopters (D; see definition in Box 2-1)—required to render objects in focus on the retina is inversely related to the distance of the objects targeted. Hence objects at distances less than about 2 meters require positive refraction and, in the emmetropic eye, objects at distances greater than a few meters are essentially "far" (optically speaking, "at infinity"; see Figure 5-14). The term "dioptric environment" is used to denote the distribution of distances of visual surfaces from the observer across the entire visual field.

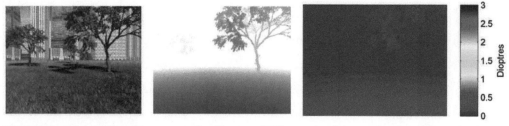

FIGURE 5-14 Refractive power (in diopters [D]) required to render far objects in focus.
SOURCE: Flitcroft, 2012.

The outdoor and indoor dioptric environments are radically different (Flitcroft 2012; Gibaldi & Banks, 2019; Marcos, 2024; Sprague et al., 2015; see Figure 5-15). Outdoors, under normal viewing conditions, virtually the entire optical environment is effectively at infinity, whereas indoors there is a much greater range of nearer objects. This dramatic difference could have major implications for the defocus experienced by the retina—particularly the peripheral retina, which for purely geometrical reasons exerts an outsized influence on retinal signals relevant to emmetropization.

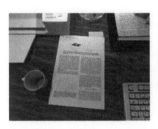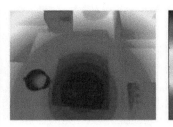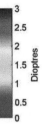

FIGURE 5-15 Refractive power (in diopters [D]) required to render near objects in focus. SOURCE: Flitcroft, 2012.

With respect to defocus, the animal literature seems to argue that the observer needs to experience nearly constant hyperopic defocus to produce a myopic eye. On the face of it, this would seem unlikely to ever occur in human children, although the indoor environment, with its greater representation of near surfaces, would potentially create greater amounts of hyperopic defocus than the outdoors. This depends, however, on the viewer's accommodative state. As illustrated by Flitcroft (2012; see panel B in Figure 5-16), a person reading a book in a school or office setting would experience a small amount of hyperopic defocus near the fovea (due to accommodative lag), but the majority of the retinal surface would be experiencing *myopic* defocus. Based on animal studies of lens-induced myopia, this myopic defocus should slow eye growth and thus be protective against myopia. If the point of regard shifts to a distant object— such as when a student looks at the teacher in the front of the room—then surfaces near the student (her desk and objects thereupon) produce *hyperopic* defocus, especially in the lower visual field (Flitcroft 2012; see panel A in Figure 5-16).

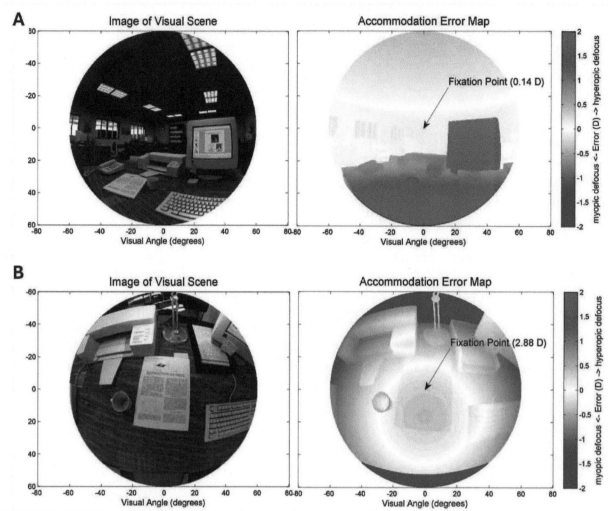

FIGURE 5-16 Dioptric error generated when viewing a near or distant visual scene.
SOURCE: Flitcroft, 2012.

Flitcroft's (2012) simulations provide a useful starting point, but they are limited by his use of computer-generated images and by their failure to consider the potential differences in retinal defocus patterns for different observers with differences in eye shape and optical aberrations (for more detail, see Chapter 6). To fully determine the retinal defocus experienced by real children in the indoor environment will require further research to supply (a) comprehensive data sets of the dioptric environments experienced by children during the critical period for emmetropization, (b) appropriate eye models to reveal actual patterns of defocus across the entire retina for differently shaped eyes, and (c) models of fixational eye movements (see below) to characterize the spatiotemporal contrast patterns experienced by the retina by different observers, in different environments, performing different visual tasks.

Effect of Eye Movements

The eyes of foveate animals are in constant motion. At the macroscopic level, primates make several saccades (eye movements between fixation points) every second as they seek to bring high-acuity foveae onto regions of interest in a scene. These relatively large eye movements have the effect of rapidly bringing visual stimuli into the receptive fields of retinal neurons, producing strong luminance contrast modulation. This is relevant, because experiments in chicks (Rucker et al., 2015) have shown that rapid changes in luminance contrast slow eye growth. Insofar as there are differences in saccade size and frequency in different environments, they could influence emmetropization.

There is precious little relevant data, but at least one study suggests that indoor-vs-outdoor differences in saccade frequency could contribute. Zhang & Vera-Diaz (2016) reported that "Subjects made significantly fewer fixation changes for all indoor tasks (Mean 22 ± 8 fixations), including walking indoors, compared to outdoor tasks (Mean 37 ± 13 fixations; $p < 0.01$), even for the same task (walking while using an iTouch [a kind of smart watch] indoors vs. outdoors, $p = 0.03$)." If this result generalizes, it will indicate that more frequent saccades, combined with higher luminance, could be one of the mechanisms by which time spent outdoors has a beneficial effect on delaying myopia onset.

Even when humans believe they are holding their eyes still during periods of fixation, their eyes are in perpetual motion due to so-called fixational eye movements (FEMs), consisting of drift, tremor, and microsaccades. These eye movements have a profound effect on the actual pattern of spatial contrast experienced by the retina and, as such, they are highly relevant to considerations of defocus during emmetropization (Rucci & Victor, 2018). FEMs interact with the spatial frequency distribution of natural images—which have a $1/f^2$ power spectrum (Simoncelli & Olshausen 2001)—to "whiten" the input to the retina. Interestingly, this effect of FEMs could serve to decrease the indoor-outdoor differences in spatial frequency content: The greater high-spatial frequency content of outdoor scenes compared with indoor (Flitcroft et al., 2019) would be low-pass-filtered by FEMs, tending to homogenize the spatial frequency distributions of indoor and outdoor environments. However, experts do not yet know whether there are indoor-outdoor differences in FEMs with respect to their spatial and temporal characteristics. As noted above, such data will be critical for a proper comparison of retinal blur in the two different environments.

Another aspect of myopia research for which FEMs are relevant is the interspecies comparisons implicit in the use of animal models of myopia (Troilo et al., 2019, Wallman & Winawer, 2004). Not much is known about miniature eye movements in other species, but what is known suggests that these movements are quite different in species that lack a fovea (Martinez-Conde & Macknik, 2008). This potentially muddies the interpretation of studies showing, for example, that high spatial frequency environments decrease the development of myopia in chicks (Hess et al. 2006; Tran et al., 2008). Until one knows the spatio-temporal properties of an animal's eye movements, it is difficult to translate spatial changes in the environment into changes in the optical diet experienced by the retina.

Stimulation of ON vs. OFF Visual Pathways

At the first retinal synapse, between photoreceptors and bipolar cells, visual signal processing is split between a positive-contrast sensing set of channels—the so-called "ON" pathway—and a negative-contrast sensing set of channels—the OFF pathway (Ichinose & Habib, 2022; Schiller, 1992). Because all mammalian photoreceptors hyperpolarize in response to light, the OFF pathway is produced by a sign-conserving, ionotropic glutamate receptor on the dendrites of OFF-bipolar cells, whereas the ON pathway uses a sign-inverting metabotropic glutamate receptor (mGluR6; Figure 5-17). To a first approximation, the two channels can be thought of as full-wave rectifier that converts both light increments and decrements to a positive signal. This process appears to be fundamental for vision, emerging from models that are built to encode natural scenes efficiently (Gjorgjieva et al., 2014; Karklin & Simoncelli 2011).

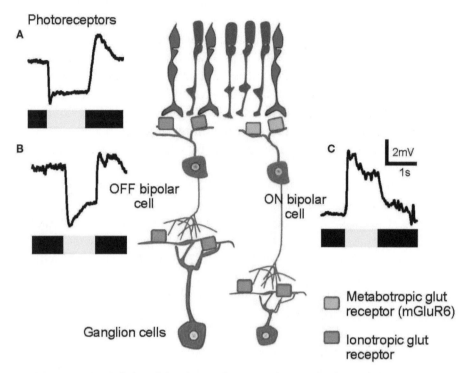

FIGURE 5-17 Origin of the ON and OFF pathways in the retina.
NOTES: (A) Photoreceptors hyperpolarize in response to light stimuli (yellow bars) and activate either OFF or ON bipolar cells through ionotroic or metabotropic glutamate receptors, respectively. (B) OFF bipolar cells hyperpolarize in response to light and decrease ganglion cells firing, signaling light decrements. (C) ON bipolar cells depolarize in response to light and increase ganglion cell firing, signaling light increments. mV=microvolt, s=second.
SOURCE: Reprinted from Ichinose & Habib, 2022, under a Creative Commons Attribution 4.0 International CC BY License (https://creativecommons.org/licenses/by/4.0).

However, there are also functional asymmetries between the ON and OFF pathways that are relevant for emmetropization and how it might be influenced by indoor-outdoor differences in the visual diet. The upshot is that a number of the features of the outdoor visual diet, such as higher luminance and higher spatial frequencies, favor the response properties of the ON pathway (Jansen et al. 2019; Luo-Li et al., 2018; Mazade et al. 2019). In addition, certain key players in the retinal-scleral signaling that regulates eye growth, including dopaminergic amacrine cells and ipRGCs, are driven mainly by inputs from the ON pathway (see Retinal Cells and Circuits Regulating Eye Growth in Chapter 6).

With respect to ON vs. OFF pathways, a *range* of luminance levels may also be important. The outdoor environment contains a broad luminance range (i.e., sunlight to shade), while the indoor environment has a narrow luminance range (i.e., uniform artificial lighting). When testing contrast sensitivity across broad versus narrow luminance ranges using the electroretinogram, ON pathways have a larger response than OFF and this difference increases with luminance range (Poudel et al., 2024). Supporting the benefit of exposure to both dim and bright luminance, exposure to dim ambient light that stimulates mostly rod photoreceptor and

ON pathways may also be protective for myopia in mice (Landis et al., 2021) and children (Landis et al., 2018).

A related issue is the amount of residual retinal motion—i.e., motion not compensated by vestibular reflexes—that is created by movements of the head and body as the observer moves about her environment. This residual motion is a powerful cue to visual stabilization reflexes, such as the optokinetic response, which are driven predominantly by ON pathways (Emran et al., 2007; Sugita et al., 2013; Wang et al. 2023). Insofar as children tend to move around more when they are outdoors (Khawaja et al., 2020), this would present a potentially additional benefit of the outdoor environment for driving ON pathways (Poudel et al., 2023).

These features have led some to propose that a relative under-stimulation of ON pathways during indoor vision may favor the onset and progression of myopia (Poudel et al., 2023). This idea is largely supported by both clinical and basic research findings, which indicate that genetic mutations that selectively degrade ON pathway function are myopigenic, and manipulations that increase ON pathway activation are protective (Crewther & Crewther, 2002; Aleman et al., 2018). For example, patients with congenital stationary night blindness (CSNB) are likely to develop high myopia (Zeitz et al., 2023). And mice with mutations affecting the ON pathway are more susceptible to experimentally induced myopia (Chakraborty et al., 2015; Mazade et al., 2015; Pardue et al., 2008). However, two other studies in which the pathways were manipulated pharmacologically (Crewther & Crewther, 2003; Smith et al., 1991) yielded contrary results, indicating a need for more research (see Chapter 6 for more detail).

Finally, it appears that myopia itself can lead to under-stimulation of retinal ON pathways. A recent study (Poudel et al., 2024) that measured retinal responses using both electroretinography (ERG) and the pupillary light response in human emmetropes and myopes found that as axial eye length increased, the ERG component corresponding to ON-pathway activation decreased. Moreover, luminance increases became less effective at driving pupillary constriction. This result raises the possibility of a pernicious, myopigenic positive feedback loop in which initial myopic changes—whether caused by under-stimulation of ON pathways by the indoor visual diet or other factors—themselves lead to progressively poorer activation of retinal ON circuitry, further diminishing the stop signal to eye growth.

One important caveat to the preceding discussion is that the ON and OFF pathways are each composed of multiple, parallel processing channels, only a subset of which are likely to be relevant to emmetropization and myopigenesis. Because the cleanest distinction between ON and OFF pathways exists at the first synapse, between photoreceptors and bipolar cells, all manipulations performed to date have affected all of the different processing channels that comprise the ON pathways. Given that ON/OFF functional differences may vary for different "pairs" of on-off pathways (Ravi et al., 2018), it will be critical for future studies to home in on the specific inputs that are relevant to myopigenesis. Insofar as particular downstream cell types, such as, for example, dopaminergic amacrine cells and ipRGCs, are implicated in providing signals critical for guiding eye growth, their inputs can be identified using both anatomical and physiological techniques and serve as targets for more specific manipulation.

Sleep Patterns

Human and animal studies have suggested a link between circadian rhythms and myopia (Chakraborty et al., 2018; Hussain et al., 2023). Therefore, it is plausible that a specific aspect of sleep quality also acts as a risk factor for myopia. Recent cross-sectional and longitudinal epidemiology studies have produced mixed results regarding the association between sleep duration or sleep quality and myopia (Liu et al., 2023). Of the associations identified to date, a shorter sleep duration is the trait that has been most consistently linked to myopia risk, reported in seven of 15 studies addressing this question (Liu et al., 2023). However, shorter sleep duration is also associated with education level, household income, and self-reported race/ethnicity (Whinnery et al., 2014), which means that observational epidemiology studies hold limited scope to address the role of sleep in myopia development, due to the likelihood of bias from residual confounding. Currently, Mendelian randomization cannot be applied to explore the role of sleep duration and myopia, since genetic variants robustly associated with sleep duration in children have yet to be identified; notably, genetic variants associated with sleep duration in adults are not associated with sleep duration in children (Marinelli et al., 2016).

CONCLUSIONS

The recent surge in myopia prevalence has sparked intense interest in discerning its underlying causes, with growing evidence pointing toward environmental rather than solely genetic factors. Shared genetic risk variants across populations with varying prevalence levels strongly suggest the dominant influence of environmental factors on myopia. Notably, inadequate outdoor time among recent generations emerges as a significant environmental variable, with compelling evidence indicating the protective effect of more outdoor time against myopia onset. Studies highlight increased luminance outdoors, likely modulating dopaminergic signaling, as a key factor in this protective effect.

However, further exploration of other environmental disparities between indoor and outdoor settings is warranted. While near work's role remains less consistently supported, it remains a crucial area for investigation. Disparities in light spectra also emerge as potential influencers of eye growth, although human studies are currently sparse. The "ON/OFF imbalance hypothesis" presents a compelling framework linking visual differences between indoor and outdoor environments to retinal pathways implicated in myopigenesis. Moreover, while the rise of electronic devices coincides with the myopia surge, conclusive evidence regarding their independent role remains elusive, necessitating focused research. However, their association with decreased outdoor time and increased near work underscores the need for nuanced investigation into their impact on myopia risk, especially considering their widespread use among children. Addressing these knowledge gaps is paramount to developing effective strategies for mitigating the myopia epidemic.

Conclusion 5-1: The recent, rapid increase in myopia prevalence over the past few decades, concomitant with heightened industrialization and mandatory primary education, suggests greater weight of environmental influences relative to genetics as causal for this increase. However, genetics contribute strongly to an individual's susceptibility to environmental risk factors for myopia.

Conclusion 5-2: The environmental variable with the highest level of evidence is the protective effect of time outdoors. The implication is that the prevalence of myopia is increasing, at least in part, because of inadequate time spent outdoors by recent generations of children. Of the features of the outdoor environment that may be beneficial in delaying the onset of myopia, the strongest evidence is for increased luminance, which likely works, at least in part, through dopaminergic signaling. Studies addressing other salient differences between the indoor and outdoor environments have yet to be tested widely in humans.

Conclusion 5-3: Evidence for the role of near work is less consistent than for time outdoors. The role of near work remains an important gap in knowledge.

Conclusion 5-4: Differences in the spectra of different light sources can clearly influence eye growth in animal models, but studies in humans are currently lacking.

Conclusion 5-5: The "ON/OFF imbalance hypothesis" potentially links many salient visual differences between the outdoor and indoor environments with retinal pathways that have been implicated in myopigenesis, including dopaminergic amacrine cells and intrinsically photosensitive retinal ganglion cells.

Conclusion 5-6: The beginning of the myopia boom preceded the introduction of mobile devices, such as smartphones. Limitations with existing studies make it difficult to determine if use of electronic devices increases the risk of myopia over and above the risk from other near-work activities. This is an important gap in knowledge. Electronic device use does encourage children to spend less time outdoors and more time engaged in near work at close distances for long periods of time and at ever younger ages.

RECOMMENDATIONS

Recommendation 5-1: The Centers for Disease Control should produce evidence-based guidelines, supported by Departments of Education and healthcare providers, promoting more time outdoors (at least one hour per day in school and up to 2 hours total) for children. Consideration should be given to:
- **Ensure that outdoor time is safe for the skin and eye by using sunscreen and other protection against short-wavelength exposure.**
- **Determine the relative importance of *more* near work versus *less* time outdoors, or other factors to better understand the link between education and myopia.**
- **Build comprehensive datasets concerning children's changing visual diet.**
- **Include children across the age range of 3 to 16 years.**

Recommendation 5-2: The National Institutes of Health and other funding agencies should solicit and fund research to investigate novel questions about the genetic and environmental mechanisms in myopia with special emphasis on the following:
- **Studies to identify specific features of the indoor and outdoor visual diet that cause or inhibit myopia development, including potential stimulation through ON and OFF pathways;**

- Longitudinal studies of environmental risk factors for myopia that incorporate technologies for capturing data on working distance, temporal properties of near activities, and spectral characteristics of indoor and outdoor activities;
- Experiments in animal models to better understand the mechanisms through which genetic and environmental influences lead to myopia;
- Studies to assess both genetic factors—including polygenic scores—and environmental factors to account for confounding and interactive effects, including better studies of the risk of retinal detachment (etc.) among those with high myopia, by using large cohorts of gene-profiled subjects;
- A single concerted national effort with careful ethical oversight to conduct broad genetic profiling of a large population, combined with detailed health information, that would allow the generation of polygenic scores for myopia (and a number of common diseases) with only small incremental costs;
- The effects of near work, including use of digital devices in preschool children as well as school-aged children, with special attention to the ages at which children are first exposed to these devices;
- The unique risks of developing high myopia, including studies of genetic contributions;
- Better models to understand defocusing across the whole retina as well as fixational eye movement and whether accommodation is a driver of infant eye growth; and
- Better measures of the effects of varying ages when children learn to read.

Recommendation 5-3: Industry partners have an important role in providing:
- Comprehensive quantification of the features of the visual diet of preschool and school-age children;
- Sensors that can be used by researchers to accurately monitor the visual diet of children;
- Research—perhaps in collaboration with academic scientists—on:
  - The visual consequences of the use of their electronic devices, especially in children at risk for the development of myopia;
  - Working distance and the temporal dynamics of near work, along with more detailed assessments of children's visual experience in both indoor and outdoor environments; and
  - Better comparisons of the differing effects of electronic devices vs. traditional media.

REFERENCES

Aleman, A. C., Wang, M., & Schaeffel, F. (2018). Reading and myopia: Contrast polarity matters. *Scientific Reports, 8*(1), 10840. https://doi.org/10.1038/s41598-018-28904-x

Alvarez-Peregrina, C., Martinez-Perez, C., Villa-Collar, C., Andreu-Vázquez, C., Ruiz-Pomeda, A., & Sánchez-Tena, M. Á. (2021). Impact of COVID-19 home confinement in children's refractive errors. *International Journal of Environmental Research and Public Health, 18*(10). https://doi.org/10.3390/ijerph18105347

Alvarez-Peregrina, C., Sánchez-Tena, M. Á., Martinez-Perez, C., & Villa-Collar, C. (2020). The relationship between screen and outdoor time with rates of myopia in Spanish children. *Frontiers in Public Health, 8*, 560378. https://doi.org/10.3389/fpubh.2020.560378

Apple. (2024, February 20). Protect vision health with screen distance—iPad. https://support.apple.com/guide/ipad/protect-vision-health-screen-distance-ipad977a93d1/ipados

Ashby, R. S., & Schaeffel, F. (2010). The effect of bright light on lens compensation in chicks. *Investigative Ophthalmology & Visual Science, 51*(10), 5247–5253. https://doi.org/10.1167/iovs.09-4689

Ashby, R., Ohlendorf, A., & Schaeffel, F. (2009). The effect of ambient illuminance on the development of deprivation myopia in chicks. *Investigative Ophthalmology & Visual Science, 50*(11), 5348–5354. https://doi.org/10.1167/iovs.09-3419

Aslan, F., & Sahinoglu-Keskek, N. (2022). The effect of home education on myopia progression in children during the COVID-19 pandemic. *Eye, 36*(7), 1427–1432. https://doi.org/10.1038/s41433-021-01655-2

Atchison, D. A., Li, S. M., Li, H., Li, S. Y., Liu, L. R., Kang, M. T., Meng, B., Sun, Y. Y., Zhan, S. Y., Mitchell, P., & Wang, N. (2015). Relative peripheral hyperopia does not predict development and progression of myopia in children. *Investigative Ophthalmology & Visual Science, 56*(10), 6162–6170. https://doi.org/10.1167/iovs.15-17200

Atkinson, J., Anker, S., Bobier, W., Braddick, O., Durden, K., Nardini, M., & Watson, P. (2000). Normal emmetropization in infants with spectacle correction for hyperopia. *Investigative Ophthalmology & Visual Science, 41*(12), 3726–3731.

Backhouse, S., Collins, A. V., & Phillips, J. R. (2013). Influence of periodic vs continuous daily bright light exposure on development of experimental myopia in the chick. *Ophthalmic & Physiological Optics: The Journal of the British College of Ophthalmic Opticians (Optometrists), 33*(5), 563–572. https://doi.org/10.1111/opo.12069

Baird, P. N., Saw, S. M., Lanca, C., Guggenheim, J. A., Smith Iii, E. L., Zhou, X., Matsui, K. O., Wu, P. C., Sankaridurg, P., Chia, A., Rosman, M., Lamoureux, E. L., Man, R., & He, M. (2020). Myopia. *Nature Reviews: Disease Primers, 6*(1), 99. https://doi.org/10.1038/s41572-020-00231-4

Banks, M. S. (1980). The development of visual accommodation during early infancy. *Child Development, 51*(2), 646–666. https://pubmed.ncbi.nlm.nih.gov/7418504/

Bao, J., Drobe, B., Wang, Y., Chen, K., Seow, E. J., & Lu, F. (2015). Influence of near tasks on posture in myopic Chinese schoolchildren. *Optometry and Vision Science, 92*(8), 908–915. https://doi.org/10.1097/OPX.0000000000000658

Barcellos, S. H., Carvalho, L. S., & Turley, P. (2018). Education can reduce health differences related to genetic risk of obesity. *Proceedings of the National Academy of Sciences, 115*(42). https://doi.org/10.1073/pnas.1802909115

Bear, J. C. (1991). Epidemiology and genetics of refractive anomalies. In T. D. Grosvenor & M. C. Flom (Eds.), *Refractive Anomalies: Research and Clinical Applications*. Butterworth-Heinemann.

Bergmann, C., Dimitrova, N., Alaslani, K., Almohammadi, A., Alroqi, H., Aussems, S., Barokova, M., Davies, C., Gonzalez-Gomez, N., Gibson, S. P., Havron, N., Horowitz-Kraus, T., Kanero, J., Kartushina, N., Keller, C., Mayor, J., Mundry, R., Shinskey, J., & Mani, N. (2022). Young children's screen time during the first COVID-19 lockdown in 12 countries. *Scientific Reports, 12*(1), 2015. https://doi.org/10.1038/s41598-022-05840-5

Berntsen, D. A., Sinnott, L. T., Mutti, D. O., & Zadnik, K. (2012). A randomized trial using progressive addition lenses to evaluate theories of myopia progression in children with a high lag of accommodation. *Investigative Ophthalmology & Visual Science, 53*(2), 640–649. https://doi.org/10.1167/iovs.11-7769

Brandslet, S. (2023, July 6). New teaching method can even out children's reading skills. *Norwegian SciTech News.* https://norwegianscitechnews.com/2023/07/new-teaching-method-can-even-out-childrens-reading-skills/

Berntsen, D. A., Sinnott, L. T., Mutti, D. O., Zadnik, K., & CLEERE Study Group (2011). Accommodative lag and juvenile-onset myopia progression in children wearing refractive correction. *Vision Research, 51*(9), 1039–1046. https://doi.org/10.1016/j.visres.2011.02.016

Bhandari, K. R., & Ostrin, L. A. (2022). Objective measures of viewing behaviour in children during near tasks. *Clinical & Experimental Optometry, 105*(7), 746–753. https://doi.org/10.1080/08164622.2021.1971049

Byrne, R., Terranova, C. O., & Trost, S. G. (2021). Measurement of screen time among young children aged 0–6 years: A systematic review. *Obesity Reviews, 22*(8), e13260. https://doi.org/10.1111/obr.13260

Cai, X.-B., Shen, S.-R., Chen, D.-F., Zhang, Q., & Jin, Z.-B. (2019). An overview of myopia genetics. *Experimental Eye Research, 188*, 107778. https://doi.org/10.1016/j.exer.2019.107778

Cebeci, B., Askin, M. B., Capin, T. K., & Celikcan, U. (2024). Gaze-directed and saliency-guided approaches of stereo camera control in interactive virtual reality. *Computers & Graphics, 118*(C), 23–32. https://doi.org/10.1016/j.cag.2023.10.012

Chakraborty, R., Landis, E. G., Mazade, R., Yang, V., Strickland, R., Hattar, S., Stone, R. A., Iuvone, P. M., & Pardue, M. T. (2022). Melanopsin modulates refractive development and myopia. *Experimental Eye Research, 214*, 108866. https://doi.org/10.1016/j.exer.2021.108866

Chakraborty, R., Ostrin, L. A., Benavente-Perez, A., & Verkicharla, P. K. (2020). Optical mechanisms regulating emmetropisation and refractive errors: Evidence from animal models. *Clinical & Experimental Optometry, 103*(1), 55–67. https://doi.org/10.1111/cxo.12991

Chakraborty, R., Ostrin, L. A., Nickla, D. L., Iuvone, P. M., Pardue, M. T., & Stone, R. A. (2018). Circadian rhythms, refractive development, and myopia. *Ophthalmic & Physiological Optics: The Journal of the British College of Ophthalmic Opticians (Optometrists), 38*(3), 217–245. https://doi.org/10.1111/opo.12453

Chakraborty, R., Park, H. N., Hanif, A. M., Sidhu, C. S., Iuvone, P. M., & Pardue, M. T. (2015). ON pathway mutations increase susceptibility to form-deprivation myopia. *Experimental Eye Research, 137*, 79–83. https://doi.org/10.1016/j.exer.2015.06.009

Chamberlain, P., Peixoto-de-Matos, S. C., Logan, N. S., Ngo, C., Jones, D., & Young, G. (2019). A 3-year randomized clinical trial of MiSight Lenses for myopia control. *Optometry and Vision Science: Official Publication of the American Academy of Optometry, 96*(8), 556–567. https://doi.org/10.1097/OPX.0000000000001410

Chambonniere, C., Lambert, C., Fearnbach, N., Tardieu, M., Fillon, A., Genin, P., Larras, B., Melsens, P., Bois, J., Pereira, B., Tremblay, A., Thivel, D., & Duclos, M. (2021). Effect of the COVID-19 lockdown on physical activity and sedentary behaviors in French children and adolescents: New results from the ONAPS national survey. *European Journal of Integrative Medicine, 43*, 101308. https://doi.org/10.1016/j.eujim.2021.101308

Chang, A. M., Aeschbach, D., Duffy, J. F., & Czeisler, C. A. (2015). Evening use of light-emitting eReaders negatively affects sleep, circadian timing, and next-morning alertness. *Proceedings of the National Academy of Sciences, 112*(4), 1232–1237. https://doi.org/10.1073/pnas.1418490112

Chang, H. Y., Park, E. J., Yoo, H. J., Lee, J. W., & Shin, Y. (2018). Electronic media exposure and use among toddlers. *Psychiatry Investigation, 15*(6), 568–573. https://doi.org/10.30773/pi.2017.11.30.2

Charman W. N. (2011). Keeping the world in focus: How might this be achieved? *Optometry Vision Science: Official Publication of the American Academy of Optometry, 88*(3), 373–376. https://doi.org/10.1097/OPX.0b013e31820b052b

Chen, Y., Han, X., Guo, X., Li, Y., Lee, J., & He, M. (2019). Contribution of genome-wide significant single nucleotide polymorphisms in myopia prediction: Findings from a 10-year cohort of Chinese twin children. *Ophthalmology, 126*(12), 1607–1614. https://doi.org/10.1016/j.ophtha.2019.06.026

Chen, Y. P., Prashar, A., Erichsen, J. T., To, C. H., Hocking, P. M., & Guggenheim, J. A. (2011). Heritability of ocular component dimensions in chickens: Genetic variants controlling susceptibility to experimentally induced myopia and pretreatment eye size are distinct. *Investigative Ophthalmology & Visual Science, 52*(7), 4012–4020. https://doi.org/10.1167/iovs.10-7045

Chua, S. Y., Sabanayagam, C., Cheung, Y. B., Chia, A., Valenzuela, R. K., Tan, D., Wong, T. Y., Cheng, C. Y., & Saw, S. M. (2016). Age of onset of myopia predicts risk of high myopia in later childhood in myopic Singapore children. *Ophthalmic & Physiological Optics: The Journal of the British College of Ophthalmic Opticians (Optometrists)*, *36*(4), 388–394. https://doi.org/10.1111/opo.12305

Clark, R., Kneepkens, S. C. M., Plotnikov, D., Shah, R. L., Huang, Y., Tideman, J. W. L., Klaver, C. C. W., Atan, D., Williams, C., Guggenheim, J. A., & U.K. Biobank Eye and Vision Consortium. (2023a). Time Spent Outdoors Partly Accounts for the Effect of Education on Myopia. *Investigative Ophthalmology & Visual Science*, *64*(14), 38. https://doi.org/10.1167/iovs.64.14.38

Clark, R., Lee, S. S., Du, R., Wang, Y., Kneepkens, S. C. M., Charng, J., Huang, Y., Hunter, M. L., Jiang, C., Tideman, J. W. L., Melles, R. B., Klaver, C. C. W., Mackey, D. A., Williams, C., Choquet, H., Ohno-Matsui, K., Guggenheim, J. A., CREAM Consortium, & U.K. Biobank Eye and Vision Consortium. (2023b). A new polygenic score for refractive error improves detection of children at risk of high myopia but not the prediction of those at risk of myopic macular degeneration. *EBioMedicine*, *91*, 104551. https://doi.org/10.1016/j.ebiom.2023.104551

Clark, R., Pozarickij, A., Hysi, P. G., Ohno-Matsui, K., Williams, C., Guggenheim, J. A., & U.K. Biobank Eye and Vision Consortium. (2022). Education interacts with genetic variants near GJD2, RBFOX1, LAMA2, KCNQ5 and LRRC4C to confer susceptibility to myopia. *PLoS Genetics*, *18*(11), e1010478. https://doi.org/10.1371/journal.pgen.1010478

Cohn, H. (1886). *The hygiene of the eye in schools*. Simpkin, Marshall and Co.

Common Sense. (2021). *The Common Sense Census: Media use by tweens and teens*. https://www.commonsensemedia.org/sites/default/files/research/report/8-18-census-integrated-report-final-web_0.pdf

Cougnard-Gregoire, A., Merle, B. M. J., Aslam, T., Seddon, J. M., Aknin, I., Klaver, C. C. W., Garhöfer, G., Layana, A. G., Minnella, A. M., Silva, R., & Delcourt, C. (2023). Blue light exposure: ocular hazards and prevention-a narrative review. *Ophthalmology and Therapy*, *12*(2), 755–788. https://doi.org/10.1007/s40123-023-00675-3

Crewther, D. P., & Crewther, S. G. (2002). Refractive compensation to optical defocus depends on the temporal profile of luminance modulation of the environment. *Neuroreport*, *13*(8), 1029–1032. https://doi.org/10.1097/00001756-200206120-00010

Cyril Kurupp, A. R., Raju, A., Luthra, G., Shahbaz, M., Almatooq, H., Foucambert, P., Esbrand, F. D., Zafar, S., Panthangi, V., & Khan, S. (2022). The impact of the COVID-19 pandemic on myopia progression in children: A systematic review. *Cureus*, *14*(8), e28444. https://doi.org/10.7759/cureus.28444

Dacey, D. M., Liao, H. W., Peterson, B. B., Robinson, F. R., Smith, V. C., Pokorny, J., Yau, K. W., & Gamlin, P. D. (2005). Melanopsin-expressing ganglion cells in primate retina signal colour and irradiance and project to the LGN. *Nature*, *433*(7027), 749–754. https://doi.org/10.1038/nature03387

de Gálvez, E. N., Aguilera, J., Solis, A., de Gálvez, M. V., de Andrés, J. R., Herrera-Ceballos, E., & Gago-Calderon, A. (2022). The potential role of UV and blue light from the sun, artificial lighting, and electronic devices in melanogenesis and oxidative stress. *Journal of Photochemistry and Photobiology B: Biology*, *228*, 112405. https://doi.org/10.1016/j.jphotobiol.2022.112405

Di Nonno, S., & Ulber, R. (2021). Smartphone-based optical analysis systems. *Analyst*, *146*(9), 2749–2768. https://pubs.rsc.org/en/content/articlelanding/2021/an/d1an00025j

Diether, S., & Schaeffel, F. (1997). Local changes in eye growth induced by imposed local refractive error despite active accommodation. *Vision Research*, *37*(6), 659–668. https://doi.org/10.1016/s0042-6989(96)00224-6

Diether, S., & Wildsoet, C. F. (2005). Stimulus requirements for the decoding of myopic and hyperopic defocus under single and competing defocus conditions in the chicken. *Investigative Ophthalmology & Visual Science*, *46*(7), 2242–2252. https://doi.org/10.1167/iovs.04-1200

Dirani, M., Crowston, J. G., & Wong, T. Y. (2019). From reading books to increased smart device screen time. *The British Journal of Ophthalmology*, *103*(1), 1–2. https://doi.org/10.1136/bjophthalmol-2018-313295

Dirani, M., Tong, L., Gazzard, G., Zhang, X., Chia, A., Young, T. L., Rose, K. A., Mitchell, P., & Saw, S. M. (2009). Outdoor activity and myopia in Singapore teenage children. *The British Journal of Ophthalmology, 93*(8), 997–1000. https://doi.org/10.1136/bjo.2008.150979

Dolgin, E. (2015). The myopia boom. *Nature, 519*(7543), 276–278. https://doi.org/10.1038/519276a

Dumuid, D. (2020). Screen time in early childhood. *The Lancet Child & Adolescent Health, 4*(3), 169–170. https://doi.org/10.1016/S2352-4642(20)30005-5

Emran, F., Rihel, J., Adolph, A. R., Wong, K. Y., Kraves, S., & Dowling, J. E. (2007). OFF ganglion cells cannot drive the optokinetic reflex in zebrafish. *Proceedings of the National Academy of Sciences, 104*(48), 19126–19131. https://doi.org/10.1073/pnas.0709337104

Enthoven, C. E., Tideman, J. W. L., Polling, J. R., Yang-Huang, J., Raat, H., & Klaver, C. C. W. (2020). The impact of computer use on myopia development in childhood: The Generation R Study. *Preventive Medicine, 132*, 105988. https://doi.org/10.1016/j.ypmed.2020.105988

Fahed, A. C., Philippakis, A. A., & Khera, A. V. (2022). The potential of polygenic scores to improve cost and efficiency of clinical trials. *Nature Communications, 13*(1), 2922. https://doi.org/10.1038/s41467-022-30675-z

Flitcroft, D. I. (2012). The complex interactions of retinal, optical and environmental factors in myopia aetiology. *Progress in Retinal and Eye Research, 31*(6), 622–660. https://doi.org/10.1016/j.preteyeres.2012.06.004

Flitcroft, I., Ainsworth, J., Chia, A., Cotter, S., Harb, E., Jin, Z. B., Klaver, C. C. W., Moore, A. T., Nischal, K. K., Ohno-Matsui, K., Paysse, E. A., Repka, M. X., Smirnova, I. Y., Snead, M., Verhoeven, V. J. M., & Verkicharla, P. K. (2023). IMI-management and investigation of high myopia in infants and young children. *Investigative Ophthalmology & Visual Science, 64*(6), 3. https://doi.org/10.1167/iovs.64.6.3

Flitcroft, D. I., Harb, E. N., & Wildsoet, C. F. (2020). The spatial frequency content of urban and indoor environments as a potential risk factor for myopia development. *Investigative Ophthalmology & Visual Science, 61*(42). https://doi.org/10.1167/iovs.61.11.42

Flitcroft, D. I., Loughman, J., Wildsoet, C. F., Williams, C., & Guggenheim, J. A. (2018). Novel myopia genes and pathways identified from syndromic forms of myopia. *Investigative Ophthalmology & Visual Science, 59*(1), 338–348. https://doi.org/10.1167/iovs.17-22173

Foreman, J., Salim, A. T., Praveen, A., Fonseka, D., Ting, D. S. W., Guang He, M., Bourne, R. R. A., Crowston, J., Wong, T. Y., & Dirani, M. (2021). Association between digital smart device use and myopia: A systematic review and meta-analysis. *The Lancet Digital Health, 3*(12), e806–e818. https://doi.org/10.1016/S2589-7500(21)00135-7

Foulds, W. S., Barathi, V. A., & Luu, C. D. (2013). Progressive myopia or hyperopia can be induced in chicks and reversed by manipulation of the chromaticity of ambient light. *Investigative Ophthalmology & Visual Science, 54*(13), 8004–8012. https://doi.org/10.1167/iovs.13-12476

Fratto, B. E., Culver, E. L., Davis, G., Deans, R., Goods, J. B., Hwang, S., Keller, N. K., Lawrence, J. A., 3rd, Petty, A. R., Swager, T. M., Walish, J. J., Zhu, Z., & Cox, J. R. (2023). Leveraging a smartphone to perform time-gated luminescence measurements. *PloS One, 18*(10), e0293740. https://doi.org/10.1371/journal.pone.0293740.

French, A. N., Morgan, I. G., Mitchell, P., & Rose, K. A. (2013). Risk factors for incident myopia in Australian schoolchildren: The Sydney Adolescent Vascular and Eye Study. *Ophthalmology, 120*(10), 2100–2108. https://doi.org/10.1016/j.ophtha.2013.02.035

Gabriel, G. M., & Mutti, D. O. (2009). Evaluation of infant accommodation using retinoscopy and photoretinoscopy. *Optometry and Vision Science, 86*(2), 208–215. https://doi.org/10.1097/opx.0b013e3181960652

Gajjar, S., & Ostrin, L. A. (2022). A systematic review of near work and myopia: Measurement, relationships, mechanisms and clinical corollaries. *Acta Ophthalmologica, 100*(4), 376–387. https://doi.org/10.1111/aos.15043

Gawne, T. J., & Norton, T. T. (2020). An opponent dual-detector spectral drive model of emmetropization. *Vision Research, 173*, 7–20. https://doi.org/10.1167%2Fjov.21.5.11

Gawne, T. J., She, Z., & Norton, T. T. (2022). Chromatically simulated myopic blur counteracts a myopiagenic environment. *Experimental Eye Research, 222*, 109187. https://doi.org/10.1016/j.exer.2022.109187

Gawne, T. J., Ward, A. H., & Norton, T. T. (2017). Long-wavelength (red) light produces hyperopia in juvenile and adolescent tree shrews. *Vision Research, 140*, 55–65. https://doi.org/10.1016/j.visres.2017.07.011

Gawne, T. J., Ward, A. H., & Norton, T. T. (2018). Juvenile tree shrews do not maintain emmetropia in narrow-band blue light. *Optometry and Vision Science: Official Publication of the American Academy of Optometry, 95*(10), 911–920. https://doi.org/10.1097/OPX.0000000000001283

Gibaldi, A., & Banks, M. (2019). Binocular eye movements are adapted to the natural environment. *Journal of Neuroscience, 39*(15), 2877–2888. https://doi.org/10.1523/JNEUROSCI.2591-18.2018

Gjorgjieva, J., Sompolinsky, H., & Meister, M. (2014). Benefits of pathway splitting in sensory coding. *The Journal of Neuroscience: The Official Journal of the Society for Neuroscience, 34*(36), 12127–12144. https://doi.org/10.1523/JNEUROSCI.1032-14.2014

Goldschmidt, E. (1968). *On the etiology of myopia: An epidemiological study*. Munksgaard.

Gordon, R. A., & Donzis, P. B. (1985). Refractive development of the human eye. *Archives of Ophthalmology, 103*(6), 785–789. https://doi.org/10.1001/archopht.1985.01050060045020

Gordon-Shaag, A., Shneor, E., Doron, R., Levine, J., & Ostrin, L. A. (2021). Environmental and behavioral factors with refractive error in Israeli boys. *Optometry and Vision Science, 98*(8), 959–970. https://doi.org/10.1097/opx.0000000000001755

Gringras, P., Middleton, B., Skene, D. J., & Revell, V. L. (2015). Bigger, brighter, bluer-better? Current light-emitting devices—Adverse sleep properties and preventative strategies. *Frontiers in Public Health, 3*, 233. https://doi.org/10.3389/fpubh.2015.00233

Grytz, R. (2023, December 5). Workshop on the rise in myopia: Exploring possible contributors and investigating screening practices, policies, and programs. National Academies of Sciences, Engineering, and Medicine. Washington, DC, United States. https://www.nationalacademies.org/event/41360_12-2023_workshop-on-the-rise-in-myopia-exploring-possible-contributors-and-investigating-screening-practices-policies-and-programs

Gu, C., Jia, A. B., Zhang, Y. M., & Zhang, S. X. (2022). Emerging electrochromic materials and devices for future displays. *Chemical Reviews, 122*(18), 14679–14721. https://doi.org/10.1021/acs.chemrev.1c01055

Gu, L., Cheng, D., Liu, Y., Ni, J., Yang, T., & Wang, Y. (2020). Design and fabrication of an off-axis four-mirror system for head-up displays. *Applied Optics, 59*(16), 4893. https://doi.org/10.1364/ao.392602

Guan, H., Okely, A. D., Aguilar-Farias, N., Del Pozo Cruz, B., Draper, C. E., El Hamdouchi, A., Florindo, A. A., Jáuregui, A., Katzmarzyk, P. T., Kontsevaya, A., Löf, M., Park, W., Reilly, J. J., Sharma, D., Tremblay, M. S., & Veldman, S. L. C. (2020). Promoting healthy movement behaviours among children during the COVID-19 pandemic. *The Lancet. Child & Adolescent Health, 4*(6), 416–418. https://doi.org/10.1016/S2352-4642(20)30131-0

Guggenheim, J. A., Clark, R., Cui, J., Terry, L., Patasova, K., Haarman, A. E. G., Musolf, A. M., Verhoeven, V. J. M., Klaver, C. C. W., Bailey-Wilson, J. E., Hysi, P. G., Williams, C., CREAM Consortium, & UK Biobank Eye Vision Consortium (2022a). Whole exome sequence analysis in 51 624 participants identifies novel genes and variants associated with refractive error and myopia. *Human Molecular Genetics, 31*(11), 1909–1919. https://doi.org/10.1093/hmg/ddac004

Guggenheim, J. A., Clark, R., Zayats, T., Williams, C., & UK Biobank Eye and Vision Consortium. (2022b). Assessing the contribution of genetic nurture to refractive error. *European Journal of Human Genetics, 30*(11), 1226–1232. https://doi.org/10.1038/s41431-022-01126-6

Guggenheim, J. A., Ghorbani Mojarrad, N., Williams, C., & Flitcroft, D. I. (2017). Genetic prediction of myopia: prospects and challenges. *Ophthalmic & Physiological Optics, 37*(5), 549–556. https://doi.org/10.1111/opo.12403

Guo, L., Yang, J., Mai, J., Du, X., Guo, Y., Li, P., Yue, Y., Tang, D., Lu, C., & Zhang, W. H. (2016). Prevalence and associated factors of myopia among primary and middle school-aged students: A school-based study in Guangzhou. *Eye*, *30*(6), 796–804. https://doi.org/10.1038/eye.2016.39

Gwiazda, J., Grice, K., & Thorn, F. (1999). Response AC/A ratios are elevated in myopic children. *Ophthalmic and Physiological Optics*, *19*(2), 173–179. https://doi.org/10.1046/j.1475-1313.1999.00437.x

Gwiazda, J., Hyman, L., Hussein, M., Everett, D., Norton, T. T., Kurtz, D., Leske, M. C., Manny, R., Marsh-Tootle, W., & Scheiman, M. (2003). A randomized clinical trial of progressive addition lenses versus single vision lenses on the progression of myopia in children. *Investigative Ophthalmology & Visual Science*, *44*(4), 1492. https://doi.org/10.1167/iovs.02-0816

Hagen, L. A., Gjelle, J. V. B., Arnegard, S., Pedersen, H. R., Gilson, S. J., & Baraas, R. C. (2018). Prevalence and possible factors of myopia in Norwegian adolescents. *Scientific Reports*, *8*(1), 13479. https://doi.org/10.1038/s41598-018-31790-y

Hartshorne, J. K., Huang, Y., Oppenheimer, K., Robbins, P. T., Molina, M. D. V., & Aulestia, P. M. L. P. (2020, September 17). Screen time as an index of family distress. *PsyArXiv*. https://doi.org/10.31234/osf.io/zqc4t

Hastings, G. D., Tiruveedhula, P., & Roorda, A. (2024). Wide-field optical eye models for emmetropic and myopic eyes. *Journal of Vision*, *24*(7), 9. https://doi.org/10.1167/jov.24.7.9

Haynes, H., White, B. L., & Held, R. (1965). Visual accommodation in human infants. *Science*, *148*(3668), 528–529. https://doi.org/10.1126/science.148.3669.528

He, M., Xiang, F., Zeng, Y., Mai, J., Chen, Q., Zhang, J., Smith, W., Rose, K., & Morgan, I. G. (2015). Effect of Time Spent Outdoors at School on the Development of Myopia Among Children in China: A Randomized Clinical Trial. *JAMA*, *314*(11), 1142–1148. https://doi.org/10.1001/jama.2015.10803

He, X., Sankaridurg, P., Xiong, S., Li, W., Naduvilath, T., Lin, S., Weng, R., Lv, M., Ma., Y., Lu, L., Wang, J., Zhao, R., Resnikoff, S., Zhu, J., Zou, H., & Xu, X. (2021). Prevalence of myopia and high myopia, and the association with education: Shanghai Child and Adolescent Large-scale Eye Study (SCALE): A cross-sectional study. *BMJ Open*, *11*(12), e048450. https://doi.org/10.1136%2Fbmjopen-2020-048450

Hendriks, M., Verhoeven, V. J. M., Buitendijk, G. H. S., Polling, J. R., Meester-Smoor, M. A., Hofman, A., RD5000 Consortium, Kamermans, M., Ingeborgh van den Born, L., & Klaver, C. C. W. (2017). Development of refractive errors—What can we learn from inherited retinal dystrophies? *American Journal of Ophthalmology*, *182*, 81–89. https://doi.org/10.1016/j.ajo.2017.07.008

Hess, R. F., Schmid, K. L., Dumoulin, S. O., Field, D. J., & Brinkworth, D. R. (2006). What image properties regulate eye growth?. *Current Biology*, *16*(7), 687–691. https://doi.org/10.1016/j.cub.2006.02.065

Hinkley, T., Brown, H., Carson, V., & Teychenne, M. (2018). Cross sectional associations of screen time and outdoor play with social skills in preschool children. *PLoS One*, *13*(4), e0193700. https://doi.org/10.1371/journal.pone.0193700

Holden, B. A., Fricke, T. R., Wilson, D. A., Jong, M., Naidoo, K. S., Sankaridurg, P., Wong, T. Y., Naduvilath, T. J., & Resnikoff, S. (2016). Global prevalence of myopia and high myopia and temporal trends from 2000 through 2050. *Ophthalmology*, *123*(5), 1036–1042. https://doi.org/10.1016/j.ophtha.2016.01.006

Horwood, A. M., & Riddell, P. M. (2011). Hypo-accommodation responses in hypermetropic infants and children. *The British Journal of Ophthalmology*, *95*(2), 231–237. https://doi.org/10.1136/bjo.2009.177378

Hosoda, Y., Yoshikawa, M., Miyake, M., Tabara, Y., Shimada, N., Zhao, W., Oishi, A., Nakanishi, H., Hata, M., Akagi, T., Ooto, S., Nagaoka, N., Fang, Y., Nagahama Study group, Ohno-Matsui, K., Cheng, C. Y., Saw, S. M., Yamada, R., Matsuda, F., Tsujikawa, A., … Yamashiro, K. (2018). CCDC102B confers risk of low vision and blindness in high myopia. *Nature Communications*, *9*(1), 1782. https://doi.org/10.1038/s41467-018-03649-3

Hu, Y., Ding, X., Guo, X., Chen, Y., Zhang, J., & He, M. (2020). Association of age at myopia onset with risk of high myopia in adulthood in a 12-Year follow-up of a Chinese cohort. *JAMA Ophthalmology*, *138*(11), 1129. https://doi.org/10.1001/jamaophthalmol.2020.3451

Huang, H., Chang, D. S., & Wu, P. (2015). The association between near work activities and myopia in children—A systematic review and meta-analysis. *PLoS One*, *10*(10), e0140419. https://doi.org/10.1371/journal.pone.0140419

Huang, P. C., Hsiao, Y. C., Tsai, C. Y., Tsai, D. C., Chen, C. W., Hsu, C. C., Huang, S. C., Lin, M. H., & Liou, Y. M. (2020). Protective behaviours of near work and time outdoors in myopia prevalence and progression in myopic children: A 2-year prospective population study. *The British Journal of Ophthalmology*, *104*(7), 956–961. https://doi.org/10.1136/bjophthalmol-2019-314101

Huang, P. C., Hsiao, Y. C., Tsai, C. Y., Tsai, D. C., Chen, C. W., Hsu, C. C., Huang, S. C., Lin, M. H., & Liou, Y. M. (2020). Protective behaviours of near work and time outdoors in myopia prevalence and progression in myopic children: A 2-year prospective population study. *The British Journal of Ophthalmology*, *104*(7), 956–961. https://doi.org/10.1136/bjophthalmol-2019-314101

Hung, L. F., Arumugam, B., She, Z., Ostrin, L., & Smith, E. L., 3rd (2018). Narrow-band, long-wavelength lighting promotes hyperopia and retards vision-induced myopia in infant rhesus monkeys. *Experimental Eye Research*, *176*, 147–160. https://doi.org/10.1016/j.exer.2018.07.004

Hussain, A., Gopalakrishnan, A., Scott, H., Seby, C., Tang, V., Ostrin, L., & Chakraborty, R. (2023). Associations between systemic melatonin and human myopia: A systematic review. *Ophthalmic & Physiological Optics: The Journal of the British College of Ophthalmic Opticians (Optometrists)*, *43*(6), 1478–1490. https://doi.org/10.1111/opo.13214

Hutton, J. S., Huang, G., Sahay, R. D., DeWitt, T., & Ittenbach, R. F. (2020). A novel, composite measure of screen-based media use in young children (ScreenQ) and associations with parenting practices and cognitive abilities. *Pediatric Research*, *87*(7), 1211–1218. https://doi.org/10.1038/s41390-020-0765-1

Hysi, P. G., Choquet, H., Khawaja, A. P., Wojciechowski, R., Tedja, M. S., Yin, J., Simcoe, M. J., Patasova, K., Mahroo, O. A., Thai, K. K., Cumberland, P. M., Melles, R. B., Verhoeven, V. J. M., Vitart, V., Segre, A., Stone, R. A., Wareham, N., Hewitt, A. W., Mackey, D. A., Klaver, C. C. W., … Hammond, C. J. (2020). Meta-analysis of 542,934 subjects of European ancestry identifies new genes and mechanisms predisposing to refractive error and myopia. *Nature Genetics*, *52*(4), 401–407. https://doi.org/10.1038/s41588-020-0599-0

Ichinose, T., & Habib, S. (2022). ON and OFF signaling pathways in the retina and the visual system. *Frontiers in Ophthalmology*, *2*, 989002. https://doi.org/10.3389/fopht.2022.989002

Ingram, R. M., Gill, L. E., & Lambert, T. W. (2000). Effect of spectacles on changes of spherical hypermetropia in infants who did, and did not, have strabismus. *The British Journal of Ophthalmology*, *84*(3), 324–326. https://doi.org/10.1136/bjo.84.3.324

Ip, J. M., Rose, K. A., Morgan, I. G., Burlutsky, G., & Mitchell, P. (2008). Myopia and the urban environment: findings in a sample of 12-year-old Australian school children. *Investigative Ophthalmology & Visual Science*, *49*(9), 3858–3863. https://doi.org/10.1167/iovs.07-1451

Iqbal, M., Elmassry, A., & Said, O. (2023). Letter to the editor regarding "blue light exposure: ocular hazards and prevention-a narrative review". *Ophthalmology and Therapy*, *12*(5), 2813–2816. https://doi.org/10.1007/s40123-023-00759-0

Itoh, Y., Langlotz, T., Sutton, J., & Plopski, A. (2021). Towards indistinguishable augmented reality: A survey on optical see-through head-mounted displays. *ACM Computing Surveys (CSUR)*, *54*(6), 1–36. https://doi.org/10.1145/3453157

Jansen, M., Jin, J., Li, X., Lashgari, R., Kremkow, J., Bereshpolova, Y., Swadlow, H. A., Zaidi, Q., & Alonso, J. M. (2019). Cortical balance between ON and OFF Visual responses is modulated by the spatial properties of the visual stimulus. *Cerebral Cortex*, *29*(1), 336–355. https://doi.org/10.1093/cercor/bhy221

Jian, Y. C. (2022). Reading in print versus digital media uses different cognitive strategies: Evidence from eye movements during science-text reading. *Reading and Writing*, *35*, 1549–1568. https://doi.org/10.1007/s11145-021-10246-2

Jiang, D., Li, J., Xiao, X., Li, S., Jia, X., Sun, W., Guo, X., & Zhang, Q. (2014). Detection of mutations in LRPAP1, CTSH, LEPREL1, ZNF644, SLC39A5, and SCO2 in 298 families with early-onset high myopia by exome sequencing. *Investigative Ophthalmology & Visual Science, 56*(1), 339–345. https://doi.org/10.1167/iovs.14-14850

Jiang, L., Zhang, S., Schaeffel, F., Xiong, S., Zheng, Y., Zhou, X., Lu, F., & Qu, J. (2014). Interactions of chromatic and lens-induced defocus during visual control of eye growth in guinea pigs (cavia porcellus). *Vision Research, 94*, 24–32. https://doi.org/10.1016/j.visres.2013.10.020

Jiang, Y., Zhang, B., Zhao, Y., & Zheng, C. (2021). China's preschool education toward 2035: Views of key policy experts. *ECNU Review of Education, 5*(2), 345–367. https://doi.org/10.1177/20965311211012705

Jin, J. X., Hua, W. J., Jiang, X., Wu, X. Y., Yang, J. W., Gao, G. P., Fang, Y., Pei, C. L., Wang, S., Zhang, J. Z., Tao, L. M., & Tao, F. B. (2015). Effect of outdoor activity on myopia onset and progression in school-aged children in northeast China: The Sujiatun Eye Care Study. *BMC Ophthalmology, 15*, 73. https://doi.org/10.1186/s12886-015-0052-9

Johnston, T., Chandra, A., & Hewitt, A. W. (2016). Current understanding of the genetic architecture of rhegmatogenous retinal detachment. *Ophthalmic Genetics, 37*(2), 1–9. https://doi.org/10.3109/13816810.2015.1033557

Jones, L. A., Sinnott, L. T., Mutti, D. O., Mitchell, G. L., Moeschberger, M. L., & Zadnik, K. (2007). Parental history of myopia, sports and outdoor activities, and future myopia. *Investigative Ophthalmology & Visual Science, 48*(8), 3524–3532. https://doi.org/10.1167/iovs.06-1118

Jones, L. A., Sinnott, L. T., Mutti, D. O., Mitchell, G. L., Moeschberger, M. L., & Zadnik, K. (2007). Parental history of myopia, sports and outdoor activities, and future myopia. *Investigative Ophthalmology & Visual Science, 48*(8), 3524–3532. https://doi.org/10.1167/iovs.06-1118

Jones-Jordan, L. A., Sinnott, L. T., Chu, R. H., Cotter, S. A., Kleinstein, R. N., Manny, R. E., Mutti, D. O., Twelker, J. D., Zadnik, K., & CLEERE Study Group. (2021). Myopia progression as a function of sex, age, and ethnicity. *Investigative Ophthalmology & Visual Science, 62*(10), 36. https://doi.org/10.1167/iovs.62.10.36

Jong, M., Naduvilath, T., Saw, J., Kim, K., & Flitcroft, D. I. (2023). Association between global myopia prevalence and international levels of education. *Optometry and Vision Science: Official Publication of the American Academy of Optometry, 100*(10), 702–707. https://doi.org/10.1097/OPX.0000000000002067

Jonnakuti, V. S., & Frankfort, B. J. (2024). Seeing beyond reality: Considering the impact of mainstream virtual reality adoption on ocular health and the evolving role of ophthalmologists. *Eye, 38*(8), 1401–1402. https://doi.org/10.1038/s41433-023-02892-3

Kachuri, L., Chatterjee, N., Hirbo, J., Schaid, D. J., Martin, I., Kullo, I. J., Kenny, E. E., Pasaniuc, B., Polygenic Risk Methods in Diverse Populations (PRIMED) Consortium Methods Working Group, Witte, J. S., & Ge, T. (2024). Principles and methods for transferring polygenic risk scores across global populations. *Nature Reviews: Genetics, 25*(1), 8–25. https://doi.org/10.1038/s41576-023-00637-2

Karklin, Y., & Simoncelli, E. P. (2011). Efficient coding of natural images with a population of noisy Linear-Nonlinear neurons. *Advances in Neural Information Processing Systems, 24*, 999–1007. https://pubmed.ncbi.nlm.nih.gov/26273180/

Kassam, I., Foo, L., Lanca, C., Xu, L., Hoang, Q. V., Cheng, C., Hysi, P., & Saw, S. (2022). The potential of current polygenic risk scores to predict high myopia and myopic macular degeneration in multiethnic Singapore adults. *Ophthalmology, 129*(8), 890–902. https://doi.org/10.1016/j.ophtha.2022.03.022

Kee, C. S., Hung, L. F., Qiao-Grider, Y., Ramamirtham, R., Winawer, J., Wallman, J., & Smith, E. L., 3rd (2007). Temporal constraints on experimental emmetropization in infant monkeys. *Investigative Ophthalmology & Visual Science, 48*(3), 957–962. https://doi.org/10.1167/iovs.06-0743

Khanal, S., Norton, T. T., & Gawne, T. J. (2023). Limited bandwidth short-wavelength light produces slowly-developing myopia in tree shrews similar to human juvenile-onset myopia. *Vision Research, 204*, 108161. https://doi.org/10.1016%2Fj.visres.2022.108161

Khawaja, I., Woodfield, L., Collins, P., Benkwitz, A., & Nevill, A. (2020). Tracking children's physical activity patterns across the school year: A mixed-methods longitudinal case study. *Children, 7*(10), 178. https://doi.org/10.3390/children7100178

Kim, S., Jahandar, M., Jeong, J. H., & Lim, D. C. (2019). Recent progress in solar cell technology for low-light indoor applications. *Current Alternative Energy, 3*(1), 3–17. https://doi.org/10.2174/1570180816666190112141857

Koli, S., Labelle-Dumais, C., Zhao, Y., Paylakhi, S., & Nair, K. S. (2021). Identification of MFRP and the secreted serine proteases PRSS56 and ADAMTS19 as part of a molecular network involved in ocular growth regulation. *PLoS Genetics, 17*(3), e1009458. https://doi.org/10.1371%2Fjournal.pgen.1009458

Kramida, G. (2015). Resolving the vergence-accommodation conflict in head-mounted displays. *IEEE Transactions on Visualization and Computer Graphics, 22*(7), 1912–1931. https://doi.org/10.1109/TVCG.2015.2473855

Labhishetty, V., Cholewiak, S. A., Roorda, A., & Banks, M. S. (2021). Lags and leads of accommodation in humans: Fact or fiction? *Journal of Vision, 21*(3), 21. https://doi.org/10.1167/jov.21.3.21.

Lam, C. S. Y., Tang, W. C., Tse, D. Y., Lee, R. P. K., Chun, R. K. M., Hasegawa, K., Qi, H., Hatanaka, T., & To, C. H. (2020). Defocus Incorporated Multiple Segments (DIMS) spectacle lenses slow myopia progression: A 2-year randomised clinical trial. *The British Journal of Ophthalmology, 104*(3), 363–368. https://doi.org/10.1136/bjophthalmol-2018-313739

Lanca, C., & Saw, S.-M. (2020). The association between digital screen time and myopia: A systematic review. *Ophthalmic and Physiological Optics, 40*(2), 216–229. https://doi.org/10.1111/opo.12657

Lanca, C., Teo, A., Vivagandan, A., Htoon, H., Najjar, R., Spiegel, D., & Pu, S. (2019). The effects of different outdoor environments, sunglasses and hats on light levels: Implications for myopia prevention. *Translational Vision Science & Technology, 8*(7). https://doi.org/10.1167/tvst.8.4.7

Lanca, C., Yam, J. C., Jiang, W. J., Tham, Y. C., Hassan Emamian, M., Tan, C. S., Guo, Y., Liu, H., Zhong, H., Zhu, D., Hu, Y. Y., Saxena, R., Hashemi, H., Chen, L. J., Wong, T. Y., Cheng, C. Y., Pang, C. P., Zhu, H., Pan, C. W., Liang, Y. B., … Asian Eye Epidemiology Consortium (2022). Near work, screen time, outdoor time and myopia in schoolchildren in the Sunflower Myopia AEEC Consortium. *Acta Ophthalmologica, 100*(3), 302–311. https://doi.org/10.1111/aos.14942

Landis, E. G., Park, H. N., Chrenek, M., He, L., Sidhu, C., Chakraborty, R., Strickland, R., Iuvone, P. M., & Pardue, M. T. (2021). Ambient light regulates retinal dopamine signaling and myopia susceptibility. *Investigative Ophthalmology & Visual Science, 62*(1), 28. https://doi.org/10.1167/iovs.62.1.28

Landis, E. G., Yang, V., Brown, D. M., Pardue, M. T., & Read, S. A. (2018). Dim light exposure and myopia in children. *Investigative Ophthalmology & Visual Science, 59*(12), 4804. https://doi.org/10.1167/iovs.18-24415

Laricchia, F. (2022, April 4). Mobile device access among children in households in the United States 2011 to 2020. *Statistica.* https://www.statista.com/statistics/1293211/mobile-devices-us-households-children/

Larsen, J. S. (1971). The sagittal growth of the eye. IV. Ultrasonic measurement of the axial length of the eye from birth to puberty. *Acta Ophthalmologica, 49*(6), 873–886. https://doi.org/10.1111/j.1755-3768.1971.tb05939.x

Larson, R. W., & Verma, S. (1999). How children and adolescents spend time across the world: Work, play, and developmental opportunities. *Psychological Bulletin, 125*(6), 701–736. https://doi.org/10.1037/0033-2909.125.6.701

LeBlanc, A. G., Katzmarzyk, P. T., Barreira, T. V., Broyles, S. T., Chaput, J. P., Church, T. S., Fogelholm, M., Harrington, D. M., Hu, G., Kuriyan, R., Kurpad, A., Lambert, E. V., Maher, C., Maia, J., Matsudo, V., Olds, T., Onywera, V., Sarmiento, O. L., Standage, M., Tudor-Locke, C., … ISCOLE Research Group. (2015). Correlates of total sedentary time and screen time in 9-11 year-old children around the world: The International Study of Childhood Obesity, lifestyle and the environment. *PLoS One, 10*, e0129622. https://doi.org/10.1371/journal.pone.0129622

Lee, Y.-Y., Lo, C.-T., Sheu, S.-J., & Lin, J. L. (2013). What factors are associated with myopia in young adults? A survey study in Taiwan military conscripts. *Investigative Ophthalmology & Visual Science, 54*(2), 1026–1033. https://doi.org/10.1167/iovs.12-10480

Leng, Y., Lan, W., Yu, K., Liu, B., Yang, Z., Li, Z., Zhong, X., Zhang, S., & Ge, J. (2010). Effects of confined space and near vision stimulation on refractive status and vitreous chamber depth in adolescent rhesus monkeys. *Science China. Life Sciences, 53*(12), 1433–1439. https://doi.org/10.1007/s11427-010-4099-9

Li, L., Wen, L., Lan, W., Zhu, H., & Yang, Z. (2020). A novel approach to quantify environmental risk factors of myopia: Combination of wearable devices and big data science. *Translational Vision Science & Technology, 9*(13), 1–8. https://doi.org/10.1167%2Ftvst.9.13.17

Li, M., Han, K. J., & Narayanan, S. (2013). Automatic speaker age and gender recognition using acoustic and prosodic level information fusion. *Computer Speech & Language, 27*(1), 151–167. https://doi.org/10.1016/j.csl.2012.01.008

Li, X., Malebary, S., Qu, X., Ji, X., Cheng, Y., & Xu, W. (2018). iCare: Automatic and user-friendly child identification on smartphone. *HotMobile '18: Proceedings of the Nineteenth International Workshop on Mobile Computing Systems and Applications*, 43–48. https://doi.org/10.1145/3177102.3177119

Lin, L. L., Shih, Y. F., Hsiao, C. K., & Chen, C. J. (2004). Prevalence of myopia in Taiwanese schoolchildren: 1983 to 2000. *Annals of the Academy of Medicine, 33*(1), 27–33. https://pubmed.ncbi.nlm.nih.gov/15008558/

Linne, C., Mon, K. Y., D'Souza, S., Jeong, H., Jiang, X., Brown, D. M., Zhang, K., Vemaraju, S., Tsubota, K., Kurihara, T., Pardue, M. T., & Lang, R. A. (2023). Encephalopsin (OPN3) is required for normal refractive development and the GO/GROW response to induced myopia. *Molecular Vision, 29*, 39–57. https://pubmed.ncbi.nlm.nih.gov/37287644/

Liu, J., Chen, Q., & Dang, J. (2021). Examining risk factors related to digital learning and social isolation: Youth visual acuity in COVID-19 pandemic. *Journal of Global Health, 11*, 05020. https://doi.org/10.7189/jogh.11.05020

Liu, A. L., Liu, Y. F., Wang, G., Shao, Y. Q., Yu, C. X., Yang, Z., Zhou, Z. R., Han, X., Gong, X., Qian, K. W., Wang, L. Q., Ma, Y. Y., Zhong, Y. M., Weng, S. J., & Yang, X. L. (2022). The role of ipRGCs in ocular growth and myopia development. *Science Advances, 8*(23), eabm9027. https://doi.org/10.1126/sciadv.abm9027

Liu, R., Qian, Y. F., He, J. C., Hu, M., Zhou, X. T., Dai, J. H., Qu, X. M., & Chu, R. Y. (2011). Effects of different monochromatic lights on refractive development and eye growth in guinea pigs. *Experimental Eye Research, 92*(6), 447–453. https://doi.org/10.1016/j.exer.2011.03.003

Liu, X. N., Naduvilath, T. J., & Sankaridurg, P. R. (2023). Myopia and sleep in children—A systematic review. *Sleep, 46*(11). https://doi.org/10.1093/sleep/zsad162

Logan, N. S., Gilmartin, B., Marr, J. E., Stevenson, M. R., & Ainsworth, J. R. (2004). Community-based study of the association of high myopia in children with ocular and systemic disease. *Optometry and Vision Science: Official Publication of the American Academy of Optometry, 81*(1), 11–13. https://doi.org/10.1097/00006324-200401000-00004

Loughman, J., & Flitcroft, D. I. (2021). Are digital devices a new risk factor for myopia? *The Lancet Digital Health, 3*(12), e756–e757. https://doi.org/10.1016/S2589-7500(21)00231-4

Luo-Li, G., Mazade, R., Zaidi, Q., Alonso, J. M., & Freeman, A. W. (2018). Motion changes response balance between ON and OFF visual pathways. *Communications Biology, 1*, 60. https://doi.org/10.1038/s42003-018-0066-y

Macros, S. (2024). [Optical and visual diet in myopia]. Commissioned Paper for the Committee on Focus on Myopia: Pathogenesis and Rising Incidence.

Mao, J., Lao, J., Liu, C., Wu, M., Yu, X., Shao, Y., Zhu, L., Chen, Y., & Shen, L. (2019). Factors that influence refractive changes in the first year of myopia development in premature infants. *Journal of Ophthalmology*, *2019*, 7683749. https://doi.org/10.1155/2019/7683749

Marinelli, M., Pappa, I., Bustamante, M., Bonilla, C., Suarez, A., Tiesler, C. M., Vilor-Tejedor, N., Zafarmand, M. H., Alvarez-Pedrerol, M., Andersson, S., Bakermans-Kranenburg, M. J., Estivill, X., Evans, D. M., Flexeder, C., Forns, J., Gonzalez, J. R., Guxens, M., Huss, A., van IJzendoorn, M. H., Jaddoe, V. W., … Sunyer, J. (2016). Heritability and genome-wide association analyses of sleep duration in children: The EAGLE Consortium. *Sleep*, *39*(10), 1859–1869. https://doi.org/10.5665/sleep.6170

Mark, H. H. (1971). Johannes Kepler on the eye and vision. *American Journal of Ophthalmology*, *72*, 869–878. https://doi.org/10.1016/0002-9394(71)91682-5

Markand, S., Baskin, N. L., Chakraborty, R., Landis, E., Wetzstein, S. A., Donaldson, K. J., Priyadarshani, P., Alderson, S. E., Sidhu, C. S., Boatright, J. H., Iuvone, P. M., Pardue, M. T., & Nickerson, J. M. (2016). IRBP deficiency permits precocious ocular development and myopia. *Molecular Vision*, *22*, 1291–1308.

Martínez-Albert, N., Bueno-Gimeno, I., & Gené-Sampedro, A. (2023). Risk factors for myopia: A review. *Journal of Clinical Medicine*, *12*(18), 6062. https://doi.org/10.3390/jcm12186062

Martinez-Conde, S., & Macknik, S. L. (2008). Fixational eye movements across vertebrates: Comparative dynamics, physiology, and perception. *Journal of Vision*, *8*(14), 28–28. https://doi.org/10.1167/8.14.28

Mayer, D. L., Beiser, A. S., Warner, A. F., Pratt, E. M., Raye, K. N., & Lang, J. M. (1995). Monocular acuity norms for the Teller Acuity Cards between ages one month and four years. *Investigative Ophthalmology & Visual Science*, *36*(4), 671–685. https://pubmed.ncbi.nlm.nih.gov/7890497/

Mazade, R., Jin, J., Pons, C., & Alonso, J. M. (2019). Functional specialization of ON and OFF cortical pathways for global-slow and local-fast vision. *Cell Reports*, *27*(10), 2881–2894.e5. https://doi.org/10.1016/j.celrep.2019.05.007

Mazade, R., Palumaa, T., & Pardue, M. T. (2024). Insights into myopia from mouse models. *Annual Reviews of Vision Science*, *10*. https://doi.org/10.1146/annurev-vision-102122-102059

McBrien, N. A., Moghaddam, H. O., & Reeder, A. P. (1993). Atropine reduces experimental myopia and eye enlargement via a nonaccommodative mechanism. *PubMed*, *34*(1), 205–215. https://pubmed.ncbi.nlm.nih.gov/8425826

McBrien, N. A., & Norton, T. T. (1992). The development of experimental myopia and ocular component dimensions in monocularly lid-sutured tree shrews (Tupaia belangeri). *Vision Research*, *32*(5), 843–852. https://doi.org/10.1016/0042-6989(92)90027-g

McClements, M., Davies, W. I., Michaelides, M., Young, T., Neitz, M., MacLaren, R. E., Moore, A. T., & Hunt, D. M. (2013). Variations in opsin coding sequences cause x-linked cone dysfunction syndrome with myopia and dichromacy. *Investigative Ophthalmology & Visual Science*, *54*(2), 1361–1369. https://doi.org/10.1167/iovs.12-11156

Medrano, M., Cadenas-Sanchez, C., Oses, M., Arenaza, L., Amasene, M., & Labayen, I. (2021). Changes in lifestyle behaviours during the COVID-19 confinement in Spanish children: A longitudinal analysis from the MUGI project. *Pediatric Obesity*, *16*(4), e12731. https://doi.org/10.1111/ijpo.12731

Milkovich, L. M., & Madigan, S. (2020). Using mobile device sampling to objectively measure screen use in clinical care. *Pediatrics*, *146*(1), e20201242. https://doi.org/10.1542/peds.2020-1242

Miranda, A. M., Nunes-Pereira, E. J., Baskaran, K., & Macedo, A. F. (2018). Eye movements, convergence distance and pupil-size when reading from smartphone, computer, print and tablet. *Scandinavian Journal of Optometry and Visual Science*, *11*(1), 1–5. https://doi.org/10.5384/SJOVS.vol11i1p1

Mohan, A., Sen, P., Peeush, P., Shah, C., & Jain, E. (2022). Impact of online classes and home confinement on myopia progression in children during COVID-19 pandemic: Digital eye strain among kids (DESK) study 4. *Indian Journal of Ophthalmology, 70*(1), 241. https://doi.org/10.4103/ijo.IJO_1721_21

Mojarrad, N. G., Williams, C., & Guggenheim, J. A. (2018). A genetic risk score and number of myopic parents independently predict myopia. *Ophthalmic & Physiological Optics: The Journal of the British College of Ophthalmic Opticians (Optometrists), 38*(5), 492–502. https://doi.org/10.1111/opo.12579

Monteiro, R., Fernandes, S., Hutton, J. S., Huang, G., Ittenbach, R. F., & Rocha, N. B. (2022). Psychometric properties of the SCREENQ for measuring digital media use in Portuguese young children. *Acta Paediatrica, 111*(10), 1950–1955. https://doi.org/10.1111/apa.16439

Moore, S. A., Faulkner, G., Rhodes, R. E., Brussoni, M., Chulak-Bozzer, T., Ferguson, L. J., Mitra, R., O'Reilly, N., Spence, J. C., Vanderloo, L. M., & Tremblay, M. S. (2020). Impact of the COVID-19 virus outbreak on movement and play behaviours of Canadian children and youth: A national survey. *The International Journal of Behavioral Nutrition and Physical Activity, 17*(1), 85. https://doi.org/10.1186/s12966-020-00987-8

Morgan, I., & Rose, K. (2005). How genetic is school myopia? *Progress in Retinal and Eye Research, 24*(1), 1–38. https://doi.org/10.1016/j.preteyeres.2004.06.004

Mountjoy, E., Davies, N. M., Plotnikov, D., Smith, G. D., Rodriguez, S., Williams, C. E., Guggenheim, J. A., & Atan, D. (2018). Education and myopia: assessing the direction of causality by mendelian randomisation. *BMJ (Clinical Research Ed.), 361*, k2022. https://doi.org/10.1136/bmj.k2022

Munsamy, A. J., Paruk, H., Gopichunder, B., Luggya, A., Majola, T., & Khulu, S. (2020). The effect of gaming on accommodative and vergence facilities after exposure to virtual reality head-mounted display. *Journal of Optometry, 13*(3), 163–170. https://doi.org/10.1016/j.optom.2020.02.004

Muralidharan, A. R., Lança, C., Biswas, S., Barathi, V. A., Wan Yu Shermaine, L., Seang-Mei, S., Milea, D., & Najjar, R. P. (2021). Light and myopia: From epidemiological studies to neurobiological mechanisms. *Therapeutic Advances in Ophthalmology, 13*, 25158414211059246. https://doi.org/10.1177/25158414211059246

Muralidharan, A., Low, S., Chong Lee, Y., Barathi, V., Saw, S., & Milea, D. (2022). Recovery from dorm-deprivation myopia in chicks is dependent upon the fullness and correlated color temperature of the light spectrum. *Investigative Ophthalmology & Visual Science, 60*(61). https://doi.org/10.1167/iovs.63.2.16

Mutti, D. O. (2007). To emmetropize or not to emmetropize? The question for hyperopic development. *Optometry and Vision Science, 84*(2), 97–102. https://doi.org/10.1097/opx.0b013e318031b079

Mutti, D. O., Hayes, J. R., Mitchell, G. L., Jones, L. A., Moeschberger, M. L., Cotter, S. A., Kleinstein, R. N., Manny, R. E., Twelker, J. D., Zadnik, K., & CLEERE Study Group. (2007). Refractive error, axial length, and relative peripheral refractive error before and after the onset of myopia. *Investigative Ophthalmology & Visual Science, 48*(6), 2510–2519. https://doi.org/10.1167/iovs.06-0562

Mutti, D. O., Mitchell, G. L., Hayes, J. R., Jones, L. A., Moeschberger, M. L., Cotter, S. A., Kleinstein, R. N., Manny, R. E., Twelker, J. D., Zadnik, K., & CLEERE Study Group. (2006). Accommodative lag before and after the onset of myopia. *Investigative Ophthalmology & Visual Science, 47*, 837–846. https://doi.org/10.1167/iovs.05-0888

Mutti, D. O., Mitchell, G. L., Jones, L. A., Friedman, N. E., Frane, S. L., Lin, W. K., Moeschberger, M. L., & Zadnik, K. (2009). Accommodation, acuity, and their relationship to emmetropization in infants. *Optometry and Vision Science: Official Publication of the American Academy of Optometry, 86*(6), 666–676. https://doi.org/10.1097/OPX.0b013e3181a6174f

Mutti, D. O., Mitchell, G. L., Jones-Jordan, L. A., Cotter, S. A., Kleinstein, R. N., Manny, R. E., Twelker, J. D., Zadnik, K., & CLEERE Study Group. (2017). The response AC/A ratio before and after the onset of myopia. *Investigative Ophthalmology & Visual Science, 58*(3), 1594–1602. https://doi.org/10.1167/iovs.16-19093

Mutti, D. O., Mitchell, G. L., Sinnott, L. T., Jones-Jordan, L. A., Moeschberger, M. L., Cotter, S. A., Kleinstein, R. N., Manny, R. E., Twelker, J. D., Zadnik, K., & CLEERE Study Group (2012). Corneal and crystalline lens dimensions before and after myopia onset. *Optometry and Vision Science: Official Publication of the American Academy of Optometry, 89*(3), 251–262. https://doi.org/10.1097/OPX.0b013e3182418213

Mutti, D. O., Sinnott, L. T., Berntsen, D. A., Jones-Jordan, L. A., Orr, D. J., & Walline, J. J. (2022). The effect of multifocal soft contact lens wear on axial and peripheral eye elongation in the BLINK study. *Investigative Ophthalmology & Visual Science, 63*(10), 17. https://doi.org/10.1167/iovs.63.10.17

Mutti, D. O., Sinnott, L. T., Lynn Mitchell, G., Jordan, L. A., Friedman, N. E., Frane, S. L., & Lin, W. K. (2018). Ocular component development during infancy and early childhood. *Optometry and Vision Science: Official Publication of the American Academy of Optometry, 95*(11), 976–985. https://doi.org/10.1097/OPX.0000000000001296

Neitz, M., Wagner-Schuman, M., Rowlan, J. S., Kuchenbecker, J. A., & Neitz, J. (2022). Insight from OPN1LW gene haplotypes into the cause and prevention of myopia. *Genes, 13*(6), 942. https://doi.org/10.3390/genes13060942

Nguyen, T., Roy, A., & Memon, N. (2019). Kid on the phone! Toward automatic detection of children on mobile devices. *Computers & Security, 84*, 334–348. https://doi.org/10.48550/arXiv.1808.01680

O'Sullivan, J. W., Raghavan, S., Marquez-Luna, C., Luzum, J. A., Damrauer, S. M., Ashley, E. A., O'Donnell, C. J., Willer, C. J., & Natarajan, P. (2022). Polygenic risk scores for cardiovascular disease: a scientific statement from the American Heart Association. *Circulation, 146*(8). https://doi.org/10.1161/cir.0000000000001077

Pardue, M. T., Faulkner, A. E., Fernandes, A., Yin, H., Schaeffel, F., Williams, R. W., Pozdeyev, N., & Iuvone, P. M. (2008). High susceptibility to experimental myopia in a mouse model with a retinal ON pathway defect. *Investigative Ophthalmology & Visual Science, 49*(2), 706. https://doi.org/10.1167/iovs.07-0643

Park, H., Tan, C. C., Faulkner, A., Jabbar, S. B., Schmid, G., Abey, J., Iuvone, P. M., & Pardue, M. T. (2013). Retinal degeneration increases susceptibility to myopia in mice. *Molecular Vision, 19*, 2068–2079.

Park, K., & Im, Y. (2020). Ergonomic guidelines of head-up display user interface during semi-automated driving. *Electronics, 9*(4), 611. https://doi.org/10.3390/electronics9040611

Pärssinen, O., Kauppinen, M., & Viljanen, A. (2014). The progression of myopia from its onset at age 8-12 to adulthood and the influence of heredity and external factors on myopic progression: A 23-year follow-up study. *Acta Ophthalmologica, 92*(8), 730–739. https://doi.org/10.1111/aos.12387

Pietrobelli, A., Pecoraro, L., Ferruzzi, A., Heo, M., Faith, M., Zoller, T., Antoniazzi, F., Piacentini, G., Fearnbach, S. N., & Heymsfield, S. B. (2020). Effects of COVID-19 lockdown on lifestyle behaviors in children with obesity living in Verona, Italy: A longitudinal study. *Obesity, 28*(8), 1382–1385. https://doi.org/10.1002/oby.22861

Plotnikov, D., Cui, J., Clark, R., Wedenoja, J., Pärssinen, O., Tideman, J. W. L., Jonas, J. B., Wang, Y., Rudan, I., Young, T. L., Mackey, D. A., Terry, L., Williams, C., Guggenheim, J. A., & UK Biobank Eye and Vision Consortium and the CREAM Consortium. (2021). Genetic variants associated with human eye size are distinct from those conferring susceptibility to myopia. *Investigative Ophthalmology & Visual Science, 62*(13), 24. https://doi.org/10.1167/iovs.62.13.24

Plotnikov, D., Williams, C., Atan, D., Davies, N. M., Ghorbani Mojarrad, N., Guggenheim, J. A., & UK Biobank Eye and Vision Consortium. (2020). Effect of education on myopia: Evidence from the United Kingdom ROSLA 1972 reform. *Investigative Ophthalmology & Visual Science, 61*(11), 7. https://doi.org/10.1167/iovs.61.11.7

Poudel, S., Jin, J., Rahimi-Nasrabadi, H., Dellostritto, S., Dul, M. W., & Viswanathan, S., & Alonso, J.-M. (2024). Contrast sensitivity of ON and OFF human retinal pathways in myopia. *The Journal of Neuroscience: The Official Journal of the Society for Neuroscience, 44*(3), e1487232023. https://doi.org/10.1523/JNEUROSCI.1487-23.2023

Poudel, S., Rahimi-Nasrabadi, H., Jin, J., Najafian, S., & Alonso, J. M. (2023). Differences in visual stimulation between reading and walking and implications for myopia development. *Journal of Vision, 23*(4), 3. https://doi.org/10.1167/jov.23.4.3

Pozarickij, A., Williams, C., Hysi, P. G., Guggenheim, J. A., & U.K. Biobank Eye and Vision Consortium (2019). Quantile regression analysis reveals widespread evidence for gene-environment or gene-gene interactions in myopia development. *Communications Biology, 2*, 167. https://doi.org/10.1038/s42003-019-0387-5

Proctor, R. W., & Van Zandt, T. (2018). *Human factors in simple and complex systems.* CRC Press.

Qawaqneh, Z., Mallouh, A. A., & Barkana, B. D. (2017). Age and gender classification from speech and face images by jointly fine-tuned deep neural networks. *Expert Systems with Applications, 85*(C), 76–86. https://doi.org/10.1016/j.eswa.2017.05.037

Qian, Y. F., Dai, J. H., Liu, R., Chen, M. J., Zhou, X. T., & Chu, R. Y. (2013). Effects of the chromatic defocus caused by interchange of two monochromatic lights on refraction and ocular dimension in guinea pigs. *PloS One, 8*(5), e63229. https://doi.org/10.1371/journal.pone.0063229

Quint, W. H., Tadema, K. C. D., Kokke, N. C. C. J., Meester-Smoor, M. A., Miller, A. C., Willemsen, R., Klaver, C. C. W., & Iglesias, A. I. (2023). Post-GWAS screening of candidate genes for refractive error in mutant zebrafish models. *Scientific Reports, 13*(1), https://doi.org/10.1038/s41598-023-28944-y

Radesky, J. S., Weeks, H. M., Ball, R., Schaller, A., Yeo, S., Durnez, J., Tamayo-Rios, M., Epstein, M., Kirkorian, H., Coyne, S., & Barr, R. (2020). Young children's use of smartphones and tablets. *Pediatrics, 146*(1), e20193518. https://doi.org/10.1542/peds.2019-3518

Radhakrishnan, H., Allen, P. M., Calver, R. I., Theagarayan, B., Price, H., Rae, S., Sailoganathan, A., & O'Leary, D. J. (2013). Peripheral refractive changes associated with myopia progression. *Investigative Ophthalmology & Visual Science, 54*(2), 1573–1581. https://doi.org/10.1167/iovs.12-10278

Rappon, J., Chung, C., Young, G., Hunt, C., Neitz, J., Neitz, M., & Chalberg, T. (2023). Control of myopia using diffusion optics spectacle lenses: 12-month results of a randomised controlled, efficacy and safety study (CYPRESS). *The British Journal of Ophthalmology, 107*(11), 1709–1715. https://doi.org/10.1136/bjo-2021-321005

Ravi, S., Ahn, D., Greschner, M., Chichilnisky, E. J., & Field, G. D. (2018). Pathway-Specific Asymmetries between ON and OFF Visual Signals. *Journal of Neuroscience, 38*(45), 9728–9740. https://doi.org/10.1523/jneurosci.2008-18.2018

Raviola, E., & Wiesel, T. N. (1990). Neural control of eye growth and experimental myopia in primates. *Ciba Foundation Symposium, 155*, 22–44. https://doi.org/10.1002/9780470514023.ch3

Read, S. A., Alonso-Caneiro, D., Hoseini-Yazdi, H., Lin, Y. K., Pham, T. T. M., Sy, R. I., Tran, A., Xu, Y., Zainudin, R., Jaiprakash, A. T., Tran, H., & Collins, M. J. (2023). Objective measures of gaze behaviors and the visual environment during near-work tasks in young adult myopes and emmetropes. *Translational Vision Science & Technology, 12*(11), 18. https://doi.org/10.1167/tvst.12.11.18

Ribner, A. D., Coulanges, L., Friedman, S., Libertus, M. E., & I-FAM-Covid Consortium. (2021). Screen time in the coronavirus 2019 era: International trends of increasing use among 3- to 7-year-old children. *The Journal of Pediatrics, 239*, 59–66.e1. https://doi.org/10.1016/j.jpeds.2021.08.068

Richards, A. J., McNinch, A., Martin, H., Oakhill, K., Rai, H., Waller, S., Treacy, B., Whittaker, J., Meredith, S., Poulson, A., & Snead, M. P. (2010). Stickler syndrome and the vitreous phenotype: Mutations in COL2A1 and COL11A1. *Human Mutation, 31*(6), E1461–E1471. https://doi.org/10.1002/humu.21257

Rieke, F., & Rudd, M. E. (2009). The challenges natural images pose for visual adaptation. *Neuron, 64*(5), 605–616. https://doi.org/10.1016/j.neuron.2009.11.028

Rohrer, B., Schaeffel, F., & Zrenner, E. (1992). Longitudinal chromatic aberration and emmetropization: Results from the chicken eye. *The Journal of Physiology, 449*, 363–376. https://doi.org/10.1113/jphysiol.1992.sp019090

Rolland, J. P., Krueger, M. W., & Goon, A. (2000). Multifocal planes head-mounted displays. *Applied Optics, 39*(19), 3209–3215. https://doi.org/10.1364/AO.39.003209

Rose, K. A., Morgan, I. G., Ip, J., Kifley, A., Huynh, S., Smith, W., & Mitchell, P. (2008). Outdoor activity reduces the prevalence of myopia in children. *Ophthalmology, 115*(8), 1279–1285. https://doi.org/10.1016/j.ophtha.2007.12.019

Roy, S., & Field, G. D. (2019). Dopaminergic modulation of retinal processing from starlight to sunlight. *Journal of Pharmacological Sciences, 140*(1), 86–93. https://doi.org/10.1016/j.jphs.2019.03.006

Rozema, J., Dankert, S., Iribarren, R., Lanca, C., & Saw, S. M. (2019). Axial growth and lens power loss at myopia onset in Singaporean children. *Investigative Ophthalmology & Visual Science, 60*(8), 3091–3099. https://doi.org/10.1167/iovs.18-26247

Rucci, M., & Victor, J. D. (2018). Perspective: Can eye movements contribute to emmetropization? *Journal of Vision, 18*(7), 10. https://doi.org/10.1167/18.7.10

Rucker, F., Britton, S., Spatcher, M., & Hanowsky, S. (2015). Blue light protects against temporal frequency sensitive refractive changes. *Investigative Ophthalmology & Visual Science, 56*(10), 6121–6131. https://doi.org/10.1167/iovs.15-17238

Rucker, F. J., & Wallman, J. (2009). Chick eyes compensate for chromatic simulations of hyperopic and myopic defocus: Evidence that the eye uses longitudinal chromatic aberration to guide eye-growth. *Vision Research, 49*, 1775–83. https://doi.org/10.1016/j.visres.2009.04.014

Rucker F. J., & Wallman, J. (2012). Chicks use changes in luminance and chromatic contrast as indicators of the sign of defocus. *Journal of Vision, 12*(6), 23. https://doi.org/10.1167%2F12.6.23

Samsung. (2016, April 20). Samsung launches breakthrough application that protects your eyes. *Samsung Newsroom.* https://news.samsung.com/global/samsung-launches-breakthrough-application-that-protects-your-eyes

Sanfilippo, P. G., Hewitt, A. W., Hammond, C. J., & Mackey, D. A. (2010). The heritability of ocular traits. *Survey of Ophthalmology, 55*(6), 561–583. https://doi.org/10.1016/j.survophthal.2010.07.003

Saw, S. M., Shankar, A., Tan, S. B., Taylor, H., Tan, D. T., Stone, R. A., & Wong, T. Y. (2006). A cohort study of incident myopia in Singaporean children. *Investigative Ophthalmology & Visual Science, 47*(5), 1839–1844. https://doi.org/10.1167/iovs.05-1081

Saxena, R., Vashist, P., Tandon, R., Pandey, R. M., Bhardawaj, A., Gupta, V., & Menon, V. (2017). Incidence and progression of myopia and associated factors in urban school children in Delhi: The North India Myopia Study (NIM Study). *PloS One, 12*(12), e0189774. https://doi.org/10.1371/journal.pone.0189774

Schaeffel, F., & Feldkaemper, M. (2015). Animal models in myopia research. *Clinical & Experimental Optometry, 98*(6), 507–517. https://doi.org/10.1111/cxo.12312Schiller, P. (1992) The ON and OFF channels of the visual system, *Trends in Neurosciences, 15*(3), 86–92. https://doi.org/10.1016/0166-2236(92)90017-3

Schaeffel, F., Glasser, A., & Howland, H. C. (1988). Accommodation, refractive error and eye growth in chickens. *Vision Research, 28*(5), 639–657. https://doi.org/10.1016/0042-6989(88)90113-7

Schaeffel, F., & Howland, H. C. (1991). Properties of the feedback loops controlling eye growth and refractive state in the chicken. *Vision Research, 31*(4), 717–734. https://doi.org/10.1016/0042-6989(91)90011-s

Schaeffel, F., Troilo, D., Wallman, J., & Howland, H. C. (1990). Developing eyes that lack accommodation grow to compensate for imposed defocus. *Visual Neuroscience, 4*(02), 177–183. https://doi.org/10.1017/s0952523800002327

Schmidt, S. C. E., Anedda, B., Burchartz, A., Eichsteller, A., Kolb, S., Nigg, C., Niessner, C., Oriwol, D., Worth, A., & Woll, A. (2020). Physical activity and screen time of children and adolescents before and during the COVID-19 lockdown in Germany: A natural experiment. *Scientific Reports, 10*(1), 21780. https://doi.org/10.1038/s41598-020-78438-4

Schmid, K. L., & Wildsoet, C. F. (1996). Effects on the compensatory responses to positive and negative lenses of intermittent lens wear and ciliary nerve section in chicks. *Vision Research, 36*(7), 1023–1036. https://doi.org/10.1016/0042-6989(95)00191-3

Segala, F. G., Bruno, A., Martin, J. T., Aung, M. T., Wade, A. R., & Baker, D. H. (2023) Different rules for binocular combination of luminance flicker in cortical and subcortical pathways. *eLife, 12*. https://doi.org/10.7554/eLife.87048.2

Seidemann, A., & Schaeffel, F. (2002). Effects of longitudinal chromatic aberration on accommodation and emmetropization. *Vision Research, 42*(21), 2409–2417. https://doi.org/10.1016/s0042-6989(02)00262-6

Seow, T., & Fleming, S. M. (2019). Perceptual sensitivity is modulated by what others can see. *Attention Perception & Psychophysics, 81*(6), 1979–1990. https://doi.org/10.3758/s13414-019-01724-5

Shaikh, A. W., Siegwart, J. T., & Norton, T. T. (1999). Effect of interrupted lens wear on compensation for a minus lens in tree shrews. *Optometry and Vision Science, 76*(5), 308–315. https://doi.org/10.1097/00006324-199905000-00019

Shah, R. L., Huang, Y., Guggenheim, J. A., & Williams, C. (2017). Time outdoors at specific ages during early childhood and the risk of incident myopia. *Investigative Ophthalmology & Visual Science, 58*(2), 1158–1166. https://doi.org/10.1167%2Fiovs.16-20894

Sherstyuk, A., & State, A. (2010). Dynamic eye convergence for head-mounted displays. *VRST '10: Proceedings of the 17th ACM Symposium on Virtual Reality Software and Technology*, 43–46. https://doi.org/10.1145/1889863.1889869

Simoncelli, E. P., & Olshausen, B. A. (2001). Natural image statistics and neural representation. *Annual Review of Neuroscience, 24*, 1193–1216. https://doi.org/10.1146/annurev.neuro.24.1.1193

Smith, E. L., 3rd, Bradley, D. V., Fernandes, A., & Boothe, R. G. (1999). Form deprivation myopia in adolescent monkeys. *Optometry and Vision Science: Official Publication of the American Academy of Optometry, 76*(6), 428–432. https://doi.org/10.1097/00006324-199906000-00023

Smith, E. L., 3rd, & Hung, L. F. (1999). The role of optical defocus in regulating refractive development in infant monkeys. *Vision Research, 39*(8), 1415–1435. https://doi.org/10.1016/s0042-6989(98)00229-6

Smith, E. L., 3rd, Hung, L. F., Arumugam, B., Holden, B. A., Neitz, M., & Neitz, J. (2015). Effects of long-wavelength lighting on refractive development in infant rhesus monkeys. *Investigative Ophthalmology & Visual Science, 56*(11), 6490–6500. https://doi.org/10.1167/iovs.15-17025

Smith, E. L., 3rd, Hung, L. F., & Huang, J. (2012). Protective effects of high ambient lighting on the development of form-deprivation myopia in rhesus monkeys. *Investigative Ophthalmology & Visual Science, 53*(1), 421–428. https://doi.org/10.1167/iovs.11-8652

Sng, C. C., Lin, X. Y., Gazzard, G., Chang, B., Dirani, M., Lim, L., Selvaraj, P., Ian, K., Drobe, B., Wong, T. Y., & Saw, S. M. (2011). Change in peripheral refraction over time in Singapore Chinese children. *Investigative Ophthalmology & Visual Science, 52*(11), 7880–7887. https://doi.org/10.1167/iovs.11-7290

Sperduto, R. D., Seigel, D., Roberts, J., & Rowland, M. (1983). Prevalence of myopia in the United States. *Archives of Ophthalmology, 101*(3), 405–407. https://doi.org/10.1001/archopht.1983.01040010405011

Sprague, W. W., Cooper, E. A., Tošić, I., & Banks, M. S. (2015). Stereopsis is adaptive for the natural environment. *Science Advances, 1*(4), e1400254. https://doi.org/10.1126/sciadv.1400254

State, A., Ackerman, J., Hirota, G., Lee, J., & Fuchs, H. (2001). Dynamic virtual convergence for video see-through head-mounted displays: Maintaining maximum stereo overlap throughout a close-range workspace. *ISAR '01: Proceedings of the International Symposium on Augmented Reality*, 137–146. http://dx.doi.org/10.1109/ISAR.2001.970523

Stevens, R. E., Rhodes, D. P., Hasnain, A., & Laffont, P. Y. (2018). Varifocal technologies providing prescription and visual acuity correction mitigation in head-mounted displays using Alvarez lenses. *Proceedings of the SPIE, 10676*. https://doi.org/10.1117/12.2318397

Su, J., Yuan, J., Xu, L., Xing, S., Sun, M., Yao, Y., Ma, Y., Chen, F., Jiang, L., Li, K., Yu, X., Xue, Z., Zhang, Y., Fan, D., Zhang, J., Liu, H., Liu, X., Zhang, G., Wang, H., Zhou, M., … Qu, J. (2023). Sequencing of 19,219 exomes identifies a low-frequency variant in FKBP5 promoter predisposing to high myopia in a Han Chinese population. *Cell Reports*, *42*(5), 112510. https://doi.org/10.1016/j.celrep.2023.112510

Sugita, Y., Miura, K., Araki, F., Furukawa, T., & Kawano, K. (2013). Contributions of retinal direction-selective ganglion cells to optokinetic responses in mice. *European Journal of Neuroscience*, *38*(6), 2823–2831. https://doi.org/10.1111/ejn.12284

Sugiyama, M., Tsuchiya, K. J., Okubo, Y., Rahman, M. S., Uchiyama, S., Harada, T., Iwabuchi, T., Okumura, A., Nakayasu, C., Amma, Y., Suzuki, H., Takahashi, N., Kinsella-Kammerer, B., Nomura, Y., Itoh, H., & Nishimura, T. (2023). Outdoor play as a mitigating factor in the association between screen time for young children and neurodevelopmental outcomes. *JAMA Pediatrics*, *177*(3), 303–310. https://doi.org/10.1001/jamapediatrics.2022.5356

Sugrue, L. P., & Desikan, R. S. (2019). What are polygenic scores and why are they important? *JAMA*, *321*(18), 1820–1821. https://doi.org/10.1001/jama.2019.3893

Sun, Y., Li, Y., Bao, Y., Meng, S., Sun, Y., Schumann, G., Kosten, T., Strang, J., Lu, L., & Shi, J. (2020). Brief report: Increased addictive internet and substance use behavior during the COVID-19 pandemic in China. *The American Journal on Addictions*, *29*(4), 268–270. https://doi.org/10.1111/ajad.13066

Swiatczak, B., & Schaeffel, F. (2022). Transient eye shortening during reading text with inverted contrast: effects of refractive error and letter size. *Translational Vision Science & Technology*, *11*(4), 17. https://doi.org/10.1167/tvst.11.4.17

Swierkowska, J., Vishweswaraiah, S., Mrugacz, M., Radhakrishna, U., & Gajecka, M. (2022). Differential methylation of microRNA encoding genes may contribute to high myopia. *Frontiers in Genetics*, *13*, 1089784. https://doi.org/10.3389/fgene.2022.1089784

Taylor, C. D. (1934). The relative legibility of black and white print. *Journal of Educational Psychology*, *25*(8), 561–578. https://doi.org/10.1037/h0074746

Tedja, M. S., Haarman, A. E. G., Meester-Smoor, M. A., Kaprio, J., Mackey, D. A., Guggenheim, J. A., Hammond, C. J., Verhoeven, V. J. M., Klaver, C. C. W., & CREAM Consortium (2019). IMI - Myopia genetics report. *Investigative Ophthalmology & Visual Science*, *60*(3), M89–M105. https://doi.org/10.1167/iovs.18-25965.

Tedja, M. S., Wojciechowski, R., Hysi, P. G., Eriksson, N., Furlotte, N. A., Verhoeven, V. J. M., Iglesias, A. I., Meester-Smoor, M. A., Tompson, S. W., Fan, Q., Khawaja, A. P., Cheng, C. Y., Höhn, R., Yamashiro, K., Wenocur, A., Grazal, C., Haller, T., Metspalu, A., Wedenoja, J., Jonas, J. B., … Klaver, C. C. W. (2018). Genome-wide association meta-analysis highlights light-induced signaling as a driver for refractive error. *Nature Genetics*, *50*(6), 834–848. https://doi.org/10.1038/s41588-018-0127-7

ten Velde, G., Lubrecht, J., Arayess, L., van Loo, C., Hesselink, M., Reijnders, D., & Vreugdenhil, A. (2021). Physical activity behaviour and screen time in Dutch children during the COVID-19 pandemic: Pre-, during- and post-school closures. *Pediatric Obesity*, *16*(9), e12779. https://doi.org/10.1111/ijpo.12779

The COMET Group. (2013). Myopia stabilization and associated factors among participants in the Correction of Myopia Evaluation Trial (COMET). *Investigative Ophthalmology & Visual Science*, *54*, 7871–7884. https://doi.org/10.1167/iovs.13-12403

Thomson, W. (1998). Eye problems and visual display terminals—The facts and the fallacies. *Ophthalmic and Physiological Optics*, *18*(2), 111–119. https://doi.org/10.1016/S0275-5408(97)00067-7

Tkatchenko, A. V., Tkatchenko, T. V., Guggenheim, J. A., Verhoeven, V. J., Hysi, P. G., Wojciechowski, R., Singh, P. K., Kumar, A., Thinakaran, G., Consortium for Refractive Error and Myopia (CREAM), & Williams, C. (2015). APLP2 regulates refractive error and myopia development in mice and humans. *PLoS Genetics*, *11*(8), e1005432. https://doi.org/10.1371/journal.pgen.1005432

Topliss, R. J., Gelsinger-Austin, P. J., Gregory, T. M., Tsai, R. H., & Shpunt, A. (2023). *Display device including foveal and peripheral projectors* (U.S. Patent No. 11714284). U.S. Patent and Trademark Office. https://patents.justia.com/patent/11714284

Tran, N., Chiu, S., Tian, Y., & Wildsoet, C. F. (2008). The significance of retinal image contrast and spatial frequency composition for eye growth modulation in young chicks. *Vision Research, 48*(15), 1655–1662. https://doi.org/10.1016/j.visres.2008.03.022

Troilo, D. (2007). Experimental studies of emmetropization in the Chick. *Novartis Foundation Symposium*, 89–114. https://doi.org/10.1002/9780470514023.ch6

Troilo, D., Smith, E. L., 3rd, Nickla, D. L., Ashby, R., Tkatchenko, A. V., Ostrin, L. A., Gawne, T. J., Pardue, M. T., Summers, J. A., Kee, C. S., Schroedl, F., Wahl, S., & Jones, L. (2019). IMI—Report on experimental models of emmetropization and myopia. *Investigative Ophthalmology & Visual Science, 60*(3), M31–M88. https://doi.org/10.1167/iovs.18-25967

Turnbull, P. R. K., & Phillips, J. R. (2017). Ocular effects of virtual reality headset wear in young adults. *Scientific Reports, 7*, 16172. https://doi.org/10.1038/s41598-017-16320-6

van der Sande, E., Haarman, A. E. G., Quint, W. H., Tadema, K. C. D., Meester-Smoor, M. A., Kamermans, M., De Zeeuw, C. I., Klaver, C. C. W., Winkelman, B. H. J., & Iglesias, A. I. (2022). The Role of GJD2(Cx36) in refractive error development. *Investigative Ophthalmology & Visual Science, 63*(3), 5. https://doi.org/10.1167/iovs.63.3.5

Vatavu, R. D., Anthony, L., & Brown, Q. (2015). Child or adult? Inferring smartphone users' age group from touch measurements alone. *Proceedings of the Human-Computer Interaction*, 1–9.

Verhoeven, V. J., Buitendijk, G. H., Consortium for Refractive Error and Myopia (CREAM), Rivadeneira, F., Uitterlinden, A. G., Vingerling, J. R., Hofman, A., & Klaver, C. C. (2013). Education influences the role of genetics in myopia. *European Journal of Epidemiology, 28*(12), 973–980. https://doi.org/10.1007/s10654-013-9856-1

Wagner, S., & Strasser, T. (2023). Impact of text contrast polarity on the retinal activity in myopes and emmetropes using modified pattern ERG. *Scientific Reports, 13*(1), 11101. https://doi.org/10.1038/s41598-023-38192-9

Walline, J. J., Lindsley, K. B., Vedula, S. S., Cotter, S. A., Mutti, D. O., Ng, S. M., & Twelker, J. D. (2020). Interventions to slow progression of myopia in children. *The Cochrane Database of Systematic Reviews, 1*(1), CD004916. https://doi.org/10.1002/14651858.CD004916.pub4

Wallman, J., & Adams, J. I. (1987). Developmental aspects of experimental myopia in chicks: Susceptibility, recovery and relation to emmetropization. *Vision Research, 27*, 1139–1163. https://doi.org/10.1016/0042-6989(87)90027-7

Wallman, J., Gottlieb, M. D., Rajaram, V., & Fugate-Wentzek, L. A. (1987). Local retinal regions control local eye growth and myopia. *Science, 237*(4810), 73–77. https://doi.org/10.1126/science.3603011

Wallman, J., & Winawer, J. (2004). Homeostasis of eye growth and the question of myopia. *Neuron, 43*(4), 447–468. https://doi.org/10.1016/j.neuron.2004.08.008

Wang, A. Y. M., Kulkarni, M. M., McLaughlin, A. J., Gayet, J., Smith, B. E., Hauptschein, M., McHugh, C. F., Yao, Y. Y., & Puthussery, T. (2023). An ON-type direction-selective ganglion cell in primate retina. *Nature, 623*(7986), 381–386. https://doi.org/10.1038/s41586-023-06659-4

Wang, J., Li, Y., Musch, D. C., Wei, N., Qi, X., Ding, G., Li, X., Li, J., Song, L., Zhang, Y., Ning, Y., Zeng, X., Hua, N., Li, S., & Qian, X. (2021). Progression of myopia in school-aged children after COVID-19 home confinement. *JAMA Ophthalmology, 139*(3), 293–300. https://doi.org/10.1001/jamaophthalmol.2020.6239

Wang, M., Schaeffel, F., Jiang, B., & Feldkaemper, M. (2018). Effects of light of different spectral composition on refractive development and retinal dopamine in chicks. *Investigative Ophthalmology & Visual Science, 59*(11), 4413–4424. https://doi.org/10.1167/iovs.18-23880

Wang, Q., Ma, J., Maehashi, A., & Kim, H. (2020). The associations between outdoor playtime, screen-viewing time, and environmental factors in Chinese young children: The "Eat, Be Active and Sleep Well" study. *International Journal of Environmental Research and Public Health, 17*(13), 4867. https://doi.org/10.3390/ijerph17134867

Wang, W., Zhu, L., Zheng, S., Ji, Y., Xiang, Y., Lv, B., Xiong, L., Li, Z., Yi, S., Huang, H., Zhang, L., Liu, F., Wan, W., & Hu, K. (2021). Survey on the progression of myopia in children and adolescents in Chongqing during COVID-19 pandemic. *Frontiers in Public Health, 9*, 646770. https://doi.org/10.3389/fpubh.2021.646770

Ward, A. H., Norton, T. T., Huisingh, C. E., & Gawne, T. J. (2018). The hyperopic effect of narrow-band long-wavelength light in tree shrews increases non-linearly with duration. *Vision Research, 146-147*, 9–17. https://doi.org/10.1016/j.visres.2018.03.006

Ware, J. (1813). Observations relative to the near and distant sight of different persons. *Philosophical Transactions of the Royal Society of London, 103*, 31–50. https://doi.org/10.1098/rstl.1813.0007

Whinnery, J., Jackson, N., Rattanaumpawan, P., & Grandner, M. A. (2014). Short and long sleep duration associated with race/ethnicity, sociodemographics, and socioeconomic position. *Sleep, 37*(3), 601–611. https://doi.org/10.5665/sleep.3508

Wikimedia Commons (2023). Spectrum of sunlight. https://commons.wikimedia.org/wiki/File:Spectrum_of_Sunlight_en.svg

Wiklund, P., Karhunen, V., Richmond, R. C., Parmar, P., Rodriguez, A., De Silva, M., Wielscher, M., Rezwan, F. I., Richardson, T. G., Veijola, J., Herzig, K. H., Holloway, J. W., Relton, C. L., Sebert, S., & Järvelin, M. R. (2019). DNA methylation links prenatal smoking exposure to later life health outcomes in offspring. *Clinical Epigenetics, 11*(1), 97. https://doi.org/10.1186/s13148-019-0683-4

Wildsoet, C. F. (1998). Structural correlates of myopia. In M. Rosenfield & B. Gilmartin (Eds.), *Myopia and nearwork* (pp. 31–57). Butterworth-Heinemann.

Wildsoet, C. F., Howland, H. C., Falconer, S., & Dick, K. (1993). Chromatic aberration and accommodation: their role in emmetropization in the chick. *Vision Research, 33*(12), 1593–1603. https://doi.org/10.1016/0042-6989(93)90026-s

Williams, R., Bakshi, S., Ostrin, E. J., & Ostrin, L. A. (2019a). Continuous objective assessment of near work. *Scientific Reports, 9*(1). https://doi.org/10.1038/s41598-019-43408-y

Williams, C., Suderman, M., Guggenheim, J. A., Ellis, G., Gregory, S., Iles-Caven, Y., Northstone, K., Golding, J., & Pembrey, M. (2019b). Grandmothers' smoking in pregnancy is associated with a reduced prevalence of early-onset myopia. *Scientific Reports, 9*(1). https://doi.org/10.1038/s41598-019-51678-9

Wong, C. W., Tsai, A., Jonas, J. B., Ohno-Matsui, K., Chen, J., Ang, M., & Ting, D. S. W. (2021). Digital screen time during the COVID-19 pandemic: Risk for a further myopia boom? *American Journal of Ophthalmology, 223*, 333–337. https://doi.org/10.1016/j.ajo.2020.07.034

Wong, Y. L., Hysi, P., Cheung, G., Tedja, M., Hoang, Q. V., Tompson, S. W. J., Whisenhunt, K. N., Verhoeven, V. J. M., Zhao, W., Hess, M., Wong, C. W., Kifley, A., Hosoda, Y., Haarman, A. E. G., Hopf, S., Laspas, P., Sensaki, S., Sim, X., Miyake, M., Tsujikawa, A., … Consortium of Refractive Error, Myopia (CREAM) (2019). Correction: Genetic variants linked to myopic macular degeneration in persons with high myopia: CREAM consortium. *PloS One, 14*(10), e0223942. https://doi.org/10.1371/journal.pone.0223942

Wu, P. C., Chen, C. T., Lin, K. K., Sun, C. C., Kuo, C. N., Huang, H. M., Poon, Y. C., Yang, M. L., Chen, C. Y., Huang, J. C., Wu, P. C., Yang, I. H., Yu, H. J., Fang, P. C., Tsai, C. L., Chiou, S. T., & Yang, Y. H. (2018). Myopia prevention and outdoor light intensity in a school-based cluster randomized trial. *Ophthalmology, 125*(8), 1239–1250. https://doi.org/10.1016/j.ophtha.2017.12.011

Wu, P., Chen, C., Chang, L., Niu, Y., Chen, M., Liao, L., Rose, K., & Morgan, I. G. (2020). Increased time outdoors is followed by reversal of the long-term trend to reduced visual acuity in Taiwan primary school students. *Ophthalmology, 127*(11), 1462–1469. https://doi.org/10.1016/j.ophtha.2020.01.054

Wu, P. C., Tsai, C. L., Wu, H. L., Yang, Y. H., & Kuo, H. K. (2013). Outdoor activity during class recess reduces myopia onset and progression in school children. *Ophthalmology, 120*(5), 1080–1085. https://doi.org/10.1016/j.ophtha.2012.11.009

Xiang, M., Zhang, Z., & Kuwahara, K. (2020). Impact of COVID-19 pandemic on children and adolescents' lifestyle behavior larger than expected. *Progress in Cardiovascular Diseases*, *63*(4), 531–532. https://doi.org/10.1016/j.pcad.2020.04.013

Xu, H., Wen, L. M., Hardy, L. L. & Rissel, C. (2016). A 5-year longitudinal analysis of modifiable predictors for outdoor play and screen-time of 2- to 5-year-olds. *International Journal of Behavioral Nutrition and Physical Activity*, *13*, 96. https://doi.org/10.1186/s12966-016-0422-6

Xu, L., Ma, Y., Yuan, J., Zhang, Y., Wang, H., Zhang, G., Tu, C., Lu, X., Li, J., Xiong, Y. & Chen, F. (2021). COVID-19 quarantine reveals that behavioral changes have an effect on myopia progression. *Ophthalmology*, *128*(11), 1652–1654. https://doi.org/10.1016/j.ophtha.2021.04.001

Yam, J. C., Zhang, X. J., Zhang, Y., Yip, B. H. K., Tang, F., Wong, E. S., Bui, C. H. T., Kam, K. W., Ng, M. P. H., Ko, S. T., Yip, W. W. K., Young, A. L., Tham, C. C., Chen, L. J., & Pang, C. P. (2023). Effect of low-concentration atropine eyedrops vs placebo on myopia incidence in children: The LAMP2 randomized clinical trial. *JAMA*, *329*(6), 472–481. https://doi.org/10.1001/jama.2022.24162

Yao, L., Qi, L. S., Wang, X. F., Tian, Q., Yang, Q. H., Wu, T. Y., Chang, Y. M., & Zou, Z. K. (2019). Refractive change and incidence of myopia among a group of highly selected senior high school students in China: A prospective study in an aviation cadet prerecruitment class. *Investigative Ophthalmology & Visual Science*, *60*(5), 1344–1352. https://doi.org/10.1167/iovs.17-23506

You, X., Wang, L., Tan, H., He, X., Qu, X., Shi, H., Zhu, J., & Zou, H. (2016). Near work related behaviors associated with myopic shifts among primary school students in the Jiading district of Shanghai: A school-based one-year cohort study. *PloS One*, *11*(5), e0154671. https://doi.org/10.1371/journal.pone.0154671

Young, F. A., Leary, G. A., Baldwin, W. R., West, D. C., Box, R. A., Harris, E., & Johnson, C. (1969). The transmission of refractive errors within eskimo families. *American Journal of Optometry and Archives of American Academy of Optometry*, *46*(9), 676–685. https://doi.org/10.1097/00006324-196909000-00005

Yu, X., Yuan, J., Chen, Z. J., Li, K., Yao, Y., Xing, S., Xue, Z., Zhang, Y., Peng, H., An, G., Yu, X., Qu, J., Su, J., & Myopia Associated Genetics and Intervention Consortiums (2023). Whole-exome sequencing among school-aged children with high myopia. *JAMA Network Open*, *6*(12), e2345821. https://doi.org/10.1001/jamanetworkopen.2023.45821

Zadnik, K., Sinnott, L. T., Cotter, S. A., Jones-Jordan, L. A., Kleinstein, R. N., Manny, R. E., Twelker, J. D., Mutti, D. O., & Collaborative Longitudinal Evaluation of Ethnicity and Refractive Error (CLEERE) Study Group (2015). Prediction of juvenile-onset myopia. *JAMA Ophthalmology*, *133*(6), 683–689. https://doi.org/10.1001/jamaophthalmol.2015.0471

Zeitz, C., Roger, J. E., Audo, I., Michiels, C., Sánchez-Farías, N., Varin, J., Frederiksen, H., Wilmet, B., Callebert, J., Gimenez, M. L., Bouzidi, N., Blond, F., Guilllonneau, X., Fouquet, S., Léveillard, T., Smirnov, V., Vincent, A., Héon, E., Sahel, J. A., Kloeckener-Gruissem, B., Picaud, S. (2023). Shedding light on myopia by studying complete congenital stationary night blindness. *Progress in Retinal and Eye Research*, *93*, 101155. https://doi.org/10.1016/j.preteyeres.2022.101155

Zhang, A. & Vera-Diaz, F. (2016). Indoor and outdoor eye movements in myopia. *Investigative Ophthalmology & Visual Science*, *57*(12), 198–198. https://iovs.arvojournals.org/article.aspx?articleid=2559022

Zhang, X., Cheung, S. S. L., Chan, H.-N., Zhang, Y., Wang, Y. M., Yip, B. H., Kam, K. W., Yu, M., Cheng, C.-Y., Young, A. L., Kwan, M. Y. W., Ip, P., Chong, K. K.-L., Tham, C. C., Chen, L. J., Pang, C.-P., & Yam, J. C. S. (2021). Myopia incidence and lifestyle changes among school children during the COVID-19 pandemic: A population-based prospective study. *British Journal of Ophthalmology*, *106*(12), 1772–1778. https://doi.org/10.1136/bjophthalmol-2021-319307

Zhao, F., Chen, L., Ma, H., & Zhang, W. (2018). Virtual reality: A possible approach to myopia prevention and control? *Medical Hypotheses*, *121*, 1–3. https://doi.org/10.1016/j.mehy.2018.09.021

Zou, L., Zhu, X., Liu, R., Ma, F., Yu, M., Liu, H., & Dai, J. (2018). Effect of altered retinal cones/opsins on refractive development under monochromatic lights in guinea pigs. *Journal of Ophthalmology*, *2018*, 9197631. https://doi.org/10.1155/2018/9197631

Zylbermann, R., Landau, D., & Berson, D. (1993). The influence of study habits on myopia in Jewish teenagers. *Journal of Pediatric Ophthalmology and Strabismus, 30*(5), 319–322. https://doi.org/10.3928/0191-3913-19930901-12

6

Myopia Pathogenesis: From Retinal Image to Scleral Growth

This chapter considers how the diverse tissues of the eye interact with the visual environment in ways that could regulate refractive eye growth. First, the committee reviews how animal models have been used to study both emmetropization[1] and myopia. Then, the chapter covers how optical structures (cornea and crystalline lens) contribute to the retinal image; what evidence there is for retinal mechanisms of eye growth; the involvement of the retina, retinal pigment epithelium (RPE), choroid, and sclera; key signaling molecules in retino-scleral signaling (dopamine, retinoic acid, nitric oxide); and finally, the role of circadian rhythms.

KEY FINDINGS FROM ANIMAL MODELS OF EMMETROPIZATION AND MYOPIA

Animal models are instrumental in exploring the mechanisms of both healthy and diseased processes in the human body. The myopia field has used several different animal models to investigate environmental, cellular, and genetic factors that influence refractive eye growth. There is remarkable similarity in the response to experimental myopia across a diverse range of species, from fish to nonhuman primates, suggesting the presence of evolutionary conserved pathways for refractive eye growth. Regarding animal models that have been shown to respond to experimental myopia, Figure 6-1 shows that fish evolved the earliest, followed by birds, rodents, and nonhuman primates. This figure supports the theory that functional vision is important for survival and thus, it seems plausible that a fundamental pathway(s) could have evolved to carefully modulate the growth of the eye to match its optical power; thus, providing in-focus vision for survival. At the same time, it is feasible that differences have evolved across species. The myopia literature has many examples of species differences with respect to experimental myopia (see reviews in Bullimore, 2024; Chakraborty et al., 2020; Troilo et al., 2019). In this report, the committee focused on similarities among experimental myopia studies to find clues about the fundamentally conserved mechanisms that may underlie myopia across many species, including humans. At this time, there is not enough evidence to indicate whether some of the differences between species, like the response to monochromatic stimuli (see Table 5-4), reveal important modifications to myopia mechanisms or are due to artifacts or other experimental factors that have not yet been identified. From an evolutionary perspective, some animal models are closer to humans and may be more similar in mechanisms (see Figure 6-1). However, as with research on other physiological systems, different animal models are expected to provide essential insights into causal mechanisms of myopia at different levels (tissue, cells, genes, optics) that are needed to advance our understanding of emmetropia and myopia.

---

[1] As a reminder, emmetropization is the natural (ideal) development in the young eye that responds to the visual environment by steadily reshaping the ocular globe so that axial length allows image focus to land squarely on the retina.

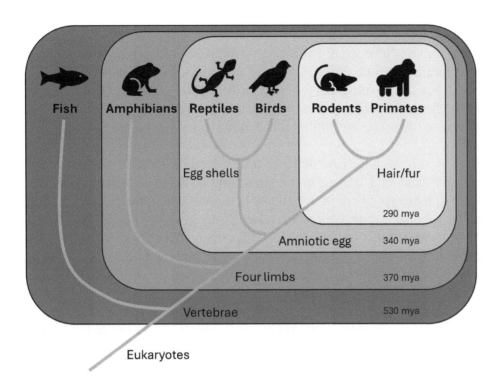

FIGURE 6-1 Plot of the evolutionary emergence of vertebrate animals on earth.
NOTE: MYA = million years ago.
SOURCE: Cornell, 2016.

Animal models have provided evidence that visually driven eye growth during development is an active process that can be disrupted (reviewed in Troilo et al., 2019; Wallman & Winawer, 2004). The first experiments to disrupt the normal growth of the eye to reach an emmetropic state used "form deprivation"—an experimental manipulation in which form vision is disrupted either by suturing the eyelid shut or by placing a diffuser lens in front of the eye—and showed that the eye became more myopic (reviewed in Gollender et al., 1979; Hodos & Kuenzel 1984; McKanna & Casagrande, 1978; Raviola & Wiesel, 1985; Sherman et al., 1977; Smith et al., 1980; Troilo et al., 2019; Wallman et al., 1978; Wiesel & Raviola, 1977; Yinon et al., 1980, 1983). Importantly, these studies in animals appear to model clinical conditions in which children with obstructed vision (due to congenital cataracts, corneal opacity, congenital optic neuropathy, etc.) or with low vision develop myopia (Bullimore, 2024; Rabin et al., 1981; Zadnik & Mutti, 1995), although myopia does not always develop in these cases (see Fledelius et al., 2014).

Additionally, removing the form-deprivation manipulation (referred to as "recovery") would reverse the myopia as the eye recovered back to emmetropia (Wallman & Adams, 1987). Further studies revealed that this regulation of refractive eye growth could be fine-tuned, as demonstrated by lens-induced myopia (reviewed in Troilo et al., 2019). Remarkably, chicks could quickly compensate for plus or minus lenses to the exact diopter to place the focal point back on the retina (Irving et al., 1991; Schaeffel et al., 1988, 1990).

As noted above, the ability to undergo emmetropization and respond to form deprivation or lens-induced myopia is conserved across a large range of species, including fish (Shen et al., 2005), chickens (Gottlieb et al., 1987; Irving et al., 1991; Schaeffel et al., 1990), mice (Barathi et al., 2008; Schaeffel et al., 2004), guinea pigs (Howlett & McFadden 2006; Lu et al., 2006), tree shrews (Siegwart & Norton, 1998), and nonhuman primates (Raviola & Wiesel, 1990; Smith et al., 1987; Troilo & Judge, 1993; von Noorden & Crawford, 1978). Considering the wide range of ocular features across these species—which differ in ocular anatomy, accommodative abilities, whether foveal or afoveal, degree of eye movement, binocularity, retinal circuitry, etc.—these results suggest a common fundamental pathway that exists across all species that controls refractive eye growth and can be disrupted by similar visual stimuli (see review by Troilo et al., 2019).

Additionally, these experiments have revealed a critical period for emmetropization and the response to form deprivation and lens defocus in mammals and chickens, which starts after eye opening and diminishes with age (see Bullimore, 2024). In contrast, fish, which grow continuously throughout life, are also responsive to experimental myopia beyond juvenile ages (Shen et al., 2005). These data suggest that myopia is most effectively induced in the actively growing eyes of juvenile animals. However, several studies have demonstrated that myopia can also be induced in adult chickens (Harman et al., 1999; Papastergiou et al., 1998; Saltarelli et al., 2004) and monkeys (Troilo et al., 2000b).

Researchers have employed animal models to investigate the origin of the refractive eye growth signals. Studies using partial occluders to deliver myopigenic stimuli to limited quadrants of the eye (Smith et al., 2009; Wallman et al., 1987), surgical methods to sever the optic nerve (Raviola & Wiesel, 1985; Troilo et al., 1987), or pharmacological inhibitors to block retinal ganglion cell activation of higher order visual circuits (Norton et al., 1994) have demonstrated that local retinal signals can control eye growth.

Animal models have also been instrumental in providing insights into the influence of ambient visual stimuli. Numerous animal models have shown that bright light is protective for experimental myopia, supporting the epidemiological findings in children (Muralidharan et al., 2021; Troilo et al., 2019). In addition, the use of animal models has revealed that dopamine levels are increased after bright light exposure (Cameron et al., 2009; French et al., 2013; Landis et al., 2021) and that blocking dopamine receptors blocks the beneficial effects of bright light in chicks (Ashby & Schaeffel, 2010), suggesting a potential mechanism of action. In the context of circadian rhythms, animal models have shown diurnal rhythms associated with refractive error, axial length and choroidal thickness (Campbell et al., 2012; Nickla et al., 1998; Nickla et al., 2017; Stone et al., 2024; Weiss & Schaeffel, 1993). In addition, deletion of melanopsin or clock genes have shown a modulatory effect on refractive development (Chakraborty et al., 2021; Stone et al., 2019). Spectral factors modulating refractive eye growth have also been extensively examined in animal models (reviewed in Gawne & Norton, 2020; Strickland et al., 2020; Troilo et al., 2019; Yoon et al., 2021).

The signaling pathways that modulate visually driven eye growth have remained elusive. The current understanding is that a signaling pathway is initiated with visual stimuli in the retina. Signaling molecule(s) then trigger other targets in the RPE and choroid or traverse these layers to ultimately induce scleral remodeling and ocular elongation. Each of these structures is covered below to consider how the structure and function of the retina, RPE, choroid, and sclera could align with a role in the signaling cascade for refractive eye growth. Additionally, identifying the components of the signaling pathway would provide potential pharmacological targets for novel myopia treatments. Many different signaling molecules have been implicated in the retina, including dopamine, nitric oxide, retinoic acid, and melanopsin (reviewed in Brown et al., 2022), which are discussed below.

OPTICAL MECHANISMS OF MYOPIA

Open and Closed-loop Control of Eye Growth

Broadly, an external stimulus can evoke an open or closed loop response from a biological system. The reflex of moving one's hand away from a hot object is an open loop response whereby the input (temperature) directly drives the response or output of the system (moving hand away). In contrast, the ability of the body to regulate its body temperature continuously over time in the face of changing external environmental conditions or internal physiology works in a closed-loop manner. The body can maintain temperature homeostasis because it has this ability to continuously drive itself toward a stable equilibrium in a closed loop. To implement a closed loop, the system consists of *sensors* that continuously measure the variable(s) of interest, *actuators* that effect a change in the system's response, and a *comparator* or control system that compares the output of the system against the input sensed variable(s) and finely tunes the actuator's response based on the differential, in case the output is offset from a set point.

Myopia is a case where the closed-loop homeostasis in the length and shape of the eye goes astray. Following the closed-loop control system model, the sensed variable of interest is the refractive error, while the actuators correspond to the changes in eye anatomy—eye length, choroid thickness, scleral growth and remodeling, properties of the cornea and crystalline lens—which all serve to alter the effective refractive state of the eye. The comparator or control loop's task is to deduce information about the eye's refractive state based on the retinal image and visual processing and instruct the actuators accordingly, to minimize the resultant refractive error. For this system to function appropriately during normal emmetropization requires an intricate closed-loop machinery that can precisely measure and continually adjust the refractive state of the eye.

These mechanisms by which the closed-loop system measures and fine-tunes the refractive state remain incompletely understood, but they undoubtedly utilize key retinal image features such as defocus (i.e., location of the optimal image plane in front of or behind the retina), higher-order optical blur (shape, size, and orientation), and contrast (spatial, spectral, and temporal). On the other hand, luminance is an aspect of the retinal image physically unrelated to the refractive state of the eye which cannot provide a differential feedback signal; thus, it cannot actively contribute to closed-loop emmetropization. Rather, the effect of luminance on myopic eye growth operates through an open loop (see also Chapter 5, under Effects of Luminance). In comparison to the closed-loop system tuning the refractive state, much is known about the retinal mechanisms that encode luminance and the molecular pathways by which this signal offers a protective effect for myopia.

The Role of the Eye's Optics in Emmetropization

The eye's optics—primarily the cornea and the crystalline lens—constitute the focusing elements of the eye, akin to the objective of a microscope. Rarely in any other part of the body are the rules of physics so elegantly applicable to biology as in the eye's optical elements. The similarities with a conventional optical lens, from the point of view of both its virtues *and* its limitations, have piqued the curiosity of astronomers, vision scientists, and physicists such as Helmholtz and Newton. Peering through telescopes and using an indirect ophthalmoscope to inspect a person's fundus led Helmholtz to the speculation that the eye is ridden with optical aberrations that are far more complex than those found in a traditional optical lens.

Many decades later, the application of sophisticated technologies to accurately measure the optical imperfections confirmed Helmholtz's prediction. Not only was it shown that the eye's optics are afflicted with aberrations beyond those that can be simply corrected with a spherocylindrical lens, but it was found that those aberrations vary with several factors—pupil size, wavelength, visual field, and eye shape. That the ensuing visual system can support a rich experience of the external world in a healthy eye, despite these fluid imperfections, is credit to the sophisticated and adaptable neural processing that takes place in the retina and the brain.

A recent review of published literature on ocular component development highlights the interplay between expansion of the globe and optical changes from the cornea and crystalline lens that together are both necessary to produce and then maintain emmetropia (Figure 6-2). The axial anterior-posterior length of the eye may increase by 5 mm between birth and maturity at age 20 years. Substantial amounts of myopia would be the result were it not for coordinated optical changes in other parts of the eye. Surface flattening of the refractive components and loss of optical power must occur during elongation to maintain balance between the eye's focal length and its physical length. These power losses come from flattening of the cornea early in infancy and then primarily from flattening, thinning, and power loss of the crystalline lens in childhood. This coordination between global expansion and optical compensation from the crystalline lens is due in large part to their anatomical connection by way of the ciliary body and zonules. The crystalline lens is continually adding new fibers throughout life, but its thinning from infancy through childhood indicates that it is being stretched into a thinner, flatter shape until the majority of global expansion is complete by age 10 years. At that point, the crystalline lens displays the net thickening seen throughout adulthood. Evidence from animal models suggests that the vitreous chamber depth drives the main compensation for changes in optical power in refractive development (Smith & Hung, 2000; Smith et al., 2013).

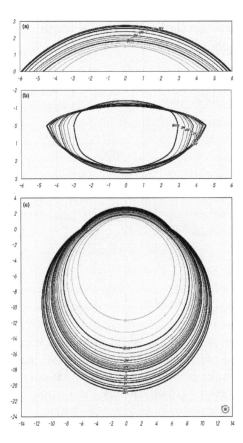

FIGURE 6-2 (A) Changes in the cornea, (B) lens, and (C) ocular globe with normal eye growth. SOURCE: Reprinted from Rozema, 2023, under a Creative Commons CC BY-NC 4.0 Attribution Non-Commercial International License (https://creativecommons.org/licenses/by-nc/4.0).

Ocular Component Characteristics Before, During, and After Myopia Onset

The criterion for the refractive error that defines myopia varies. The diagnosis may be made when myopic refractive error begins to affect distance visual acuity, for example at −0.50 diopters (D) spherical equivalent. Another definition might include the time when acceleration of axial elongation begins, several years before the appearance of negative diopters of refractive error. This process of elongation is depicted in Figure 6-3A, showing axial length at annual visits 5 years before onset (negative visit numbers), at myopia onset during visit 0 (refractive error reaching −0.75 D in all prescription meridians), and then during myopia progression following onset (positive visit numbers; Mutti et al., 2007).

The CLEERE study found that the axial lengths of age-, sex-, and ethnicity-matched children who remained emmetropic (open circles) were no different on average from the axial lengths of those who went on to become myopic (filled squares) 4–5 years before myopia onset. Axial elongation became significantly faster in children who eventually became myopic at visit 3, three years before myopia onset, and then during every subsequent year (Mutti et al., 2007). Axial elongation reached its maximum rate in the year of onset. Accelerated axial elongation in pre-myopic and myopic children compared to emmetropic children can also be seen in data from the Singapore Cohort Study of the Risk Factors for Myopia (SCORM) study 2–3 years before the age of myopia onset (more myopic than −0.50 D), where onset is marked in Figure 6-3B by a different colored dot for each age group (Rozema et al., 2019). Interestingly, both the SCORM and the CLEERE studies found that myopic diopters appeared when the average axial length reached roughly 23.8 mm, this despite being conducted in Singapore and the United States, respectively (Mutti et al., 2007; Rozema et al., 2019).

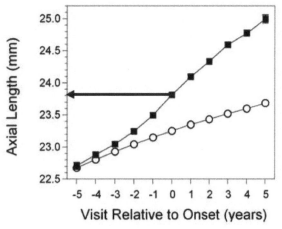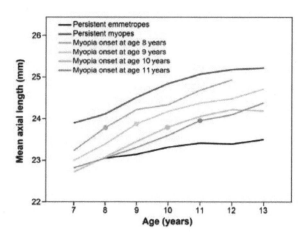

FIGURE 6-3 Axial elongation, relative to myopia onset and by age of onset.
NOTES: (A) Axial lengths from Collaborative Longitudinal Evaluation of Ethnicity and Refractive Error (CLEERE) before myopia onset (negative visit numbers), in the year of onset (visit 0), and after myopia onset (positive visit numbers). Data from children who remained always-emmetropic are shown as open circles, while data from those who eventually became myopic are shown as filled squares. Pre-myopic axial lengths −5 and −4 years before the onset of myopia are similar between the two groups, but acceleration occurred in the children who went on to develop myopia starting −3 years before myopia onset. The arrow indicates that the average axial length at onset was 23.8 mm. (B) Mean spherical equivalent refraction and axial length data in right eyes from the Singapore Cohort Study of the Risk Factors for Myopia (SCORM) according to age and split by ages of onset. The dots represent the value of axial length at the first myopic visit. The average axial length at onset was roughly 23.8 mm regardless of age at onset.
SOURCES: Mutti et al., 2007; Rozema et al., 2019.

The onset of myopia appears to be a discrete event. Accelerated axial elongation may occur for several years while distance acuity remains good. However, the onset of significant negative diopters of myopic refractive error typically takes place within one year. The shape of this relationship between refractive error and axial length is depicted in Figure 6-4A (Tideman et al., 2018) using data from the Generation R study (Dutch children measured at 6 and 9 years old; n = 6,934) and the Rotterdam Study III (Dutch adults 57 years old; n = 2957). The relationship is linear for moderate to low amounts of hyperopia, then flattens across a narrow range of axial lengths while emmetropia is maintained, then becomes linear again when refractive error becomes myopic (Tideman et al., 2018). This inflection point is something of a "cliff" for myopia onset. Onset is the time when axial elongation is rapid (Figures 6-4A and 6-4B) and when the crystalline lens no longer loses power in amounts adequate to compensate for axial elongation (Figure 6-4B; Mutti et al., 2007, 2012). Crystalline lens power changes are equal between children who remain emmetropic and those who become myopic prior to onset (visits −5 to −1). During the year of myopia onset (visit 0) and in each subsequent year (visits 1 to 5), myopic negative diopters of refractive error appear, because the crystalline lens no longer loses enough power to compensate for axial elongation (significant deficits in power loss are marked with asterisks in Figure 6-4B; Mutti et al., 2012).

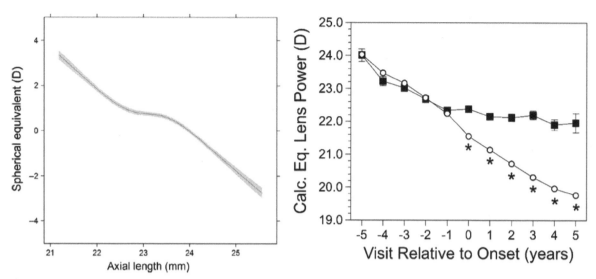

FIGURE 6-4 Onset of myopia is a discrete event.

NOTES: (A) Association between spherical equivalent and axial length at 9 years of age from the Generation R study and the Rotterdam Study III. The mean and 95% CI were adjusted for age, gender and height. Note the inflection points on the curve on either side of low levels of hyperopia, perhaps the first inflection indicating the start of acceleration of elongation and the second the point of failure of crystalline lens optical compensation. (B) Calculated lens equivalent powers from (CLEERE) before myopia onset (negative visit numbers), in the year of onset (visit 0), and after myopia onset (positive visit numbers). Always emmetropic data are shown as open circles and those who eventually became myopic are shown as filled squares. Asterisks mark significant differences (inadequate losses of lens power) between became-myopic and emmetropic children occurring at myopia onset and every year following onset.

SOURCES: (A) Reprinted from Tideman et al., 2018, under a Creative Commons CC BY 4.0 Attribution International License (https://creativecommons.org/licenses/by/4.0/); (B) Reprinted with permission from Mutti et al., 2012.

Importance of Optical Contributions to the Retinal Image

This section addresses the optical contributions to the retinal image and their implications for myopic eye growth. Many reviews have covered the research done in this area, and the purpose here is not to provide an exhaustive summary of them but to consider the key findings and open questions in this area.

The properties of the retinal image are fundamentally governed by the optics of the eye. The facets of this retinal image that provide the primary cues for normal emmetropization are currently unknown. While a lot of research has been dedicated to deciphering the critical properties of the retinal image that govern eye growth—blur, contrast, chromatic aberration, peripheral defocus among them—there remains a lack of consensus concerning what are the most potent cue(s). As the gatekeeper of the retinal image, the eye's optics have a critical role to play in shaping the cues that ultimately govern eye growth.

Specific to the properties of the retinal image, accumulating evidence suggests a potent role for time outdoors in delaying the onset of myopia progression as well as slowing eye growth once myopiogenesis is under way, though its underlying mechanisms remain unknown (see Chapter 5, Onset and Progression of Myopia). The role of light intensity outdoors is hypothesized to play a key role, and other factors—such as spectrum, chromaticity, as well as the spatial frequency and dioptric structure—may also play a role. The optics of the anterior eye encode these features of the visual environment, the so-called "visual diet," into the retinal image. Consequently, the ocular optics inform what critical feature(s) of the visual diet are most critical for eye length regulation.

A major unresolved question is whether the myopic axial elongation is a cause or consequence of the myopic eye's optics. There are both major changes in the myopic eye's optics (reviewed below) *and* large inter-subject variability. It remains unknown whether the changes in eye optics create an impairment in myopia early on to detect blur precisely to regulate eye length, leading to an open-loop eye elongation similar to the effect of form deprivation (Troilo et al., 2019). The converse possibility is that myopic eye growth is caused by the failure of another mechanism besides the optics, and that the changes in the eye's optics are all but a result of the changes the eye undergoes in its shape and anatomy as a result of normal eye growth.

Many optical treatments exist for slowing myopic eye growth (reviewed in Chapter 7), yet the mechanisms of their action remain inadequately characterized. This is a critical unknown that perhaps partly accounts for their variable efficacy. For any optical correction to work effectively and to devise new and better strategies for treatment requires understanding the interplay between the optics of the corrective device and the eye's own optics, and how the combined optical system (correction + native eye) interacts with the visual environment. Specifically, what is the interplay between the properties of the combined retinal image constructed by the eye's native and growing shape and its optics, coupled with the correction change, on the one hand, and retinal eccentricity, light wavelength, dioptric distance (near vs. far), accommodative demand, and spatial frequency content of the visual environment, on the other? Ultimately, individualized and average eye models are required to test-drive the treatments in order to deduce this interplay and devise the best corrective strategies.

Thus, to understand the mechanisms of both tightly regulated *and* uncontrolled eye growth, be equipped to suggest preventative strategies (time outdoors, for example), and devise new treatments, it is important to understand the optical factors that govern the retinal image.

AN IMPROVED FRAMEWORK FOR STUDYING THE ROLE OF THE RETINAL IMAGE IN REGULATING EYE GROWTH

*In the context of understanding eye growth a single sphero-cylindrical definition of foveal refraction is insufficient. Instead refractive error must be considered across the curved surface of the retina. This carries the consequence that local retinal image defocus can only be determined once the **3D structure of the viewed scene, off axis performance of the eye and eye shape** has been accurately defined. This, in turn, introduces an under-appreciated level of complexity and interaction between **the environment, ocular optics and eye shape** that needs to be considered when planning and interpreting the results of clinical trials on myopia prevention.* (Flitcroft, 2012, p. 622).

This text from Flitcroft indicates the need for a fresh framework to treat the retinal image in the context of the development of refractive error. Prior literature has emphasized the "foveocentric" framework—one in which defocus and the retinal image are defined at the fovea using paraxial optics, ocular shape is defined by axial length, and the spatial structure of the visual world is not relevant. While this framework has led to important findings as they relate to factors in the retinal image that drive visual acuity and accommodation, it is inadequate to describe properties of refractive error and image quality across the retina, and thus falls short in providing information on potential cues for emmetropization. Key results in animal models also indicate that the fovea isn't necessary for inducing myopia (Bullimore, 2024; Smith et al., 2005, 2009). With continued advancements in technologies to detail the visual environment (e.g., stereo scene cameras), the eye's optics (e.g., wavefront sensors, autorefractors), and the eye's shape (e.g., wide-field OCT), a more complete picture is beginning to emerge of the complex interaction between the three factors.

The need for such a framework arises based on the observation that the key mechanisms involving emmetropization involve the retinal periphery and the spatial structure of the visual stimulus (indoors vs. outdoors, for example). A paraxial, spherically symmetric, on-axis treatment of image formation cannot account for these observations. Furthermore, experimental evidence shows that local manipulations in the retinal image, based on an asymmetrically blurred visual field for example, can create similarly localized eye growth (Diether et al., 1997; Smith et al., 2009, 2010; Wallman et al., 1987). To make such deductions from the local defocus with the precision required for emmetropization requires having information about the dioptric and spatio-chromatic-temporal structure of the environment, the image-forming characteristics of the eye's optics, and the detection of the retinal image.

A Triangle of Interacting Factors

Figure 6-5 represents these interacting factors as a triangle, as opposed to a linear transformation, with the intention of denoting the strict interdependency between *any* two of them. That is, holding any two of the factors constant but allowing the third to vary can substantially alter the characteristics of the retinal image (Figure 6-4). For example, given the visual environment and image formation/detection specific to an individual's eye, the accommodative state, pupil size, and chromatic aberration all attributed to that eye's optics can drastically change the retinal image and hence the cues that are available to sense the focus error. A similar case can be made for the differences in the spatio-chromatic-temporal structure and dioptric content of the visual scene that reaches the retina. Holding the eye's optics and image formation machinery fixed, reading indoors versus riding a bike outdoors will result in very different retinal image distribution. Table 6-1, reproduced from Flitcroft (2012), lists the key differences between the foveocentric view and this retinocentric view of refraction.

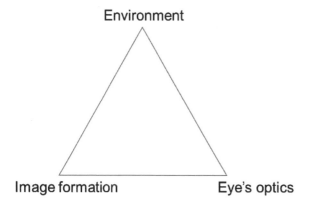

FIGURE 6-5 A framework for studying the role of the retinal image in regulating abnormal eye growth. NOTE: The three facets—features of the environment, the eye's optics and the factors relevant for early visual encoding that lead to retinal image formation—interact together to govern the visual diet. SOURCE: Committee generated.

TABLE 6-1 Differences Between the Foveocentric and Retinocentric Views of Refraction

Foveocentric view	Retinocentric view
An eye has a single refraction	An eye has a graded, complex pattern of refractions across the retinal surface
Refraction and retinal image blur are defined at a single point (the fovea)	Refraction and retinal image blur are defined across a 3-dimensional curved plane (the retina)
Spatial structure of the visual environment irrelevant	Spatial structure of the environment contributes to the defocus of the image at each point in the retinal image
Ocular shape unimportant apart from axial length	Three dimensional ocular shape is fundamentally important
Paraxial optics provides an adequate description of the eye's optics	Wide-angle ray tracing needed to fully define the eye's optics
Near work with a bifocal add is optically equivalent to far work	Near work with a bifocal add is not optically equivalent to far work
Relevant for visual acuity and accommodation	Relevant for understanding optical regulation of eye growth

SOURCE: Flitcroft, 2012, p. 654.

The following details the key characteristics of the three governing factors relevant to myopia in this retinocentric framework.

Environment

Chapter 5 (Onset and Progression) addresses the various factors in the environment pertinent to the onset and progression of myopia. Technologies that effectively quantify these environmental factors in children are rare and an important area of research and development where future resources may be devoted. Briefly, the environmental factors are light intensity, chromatic and spatial frequency spectra, dioptric variation, and temporal dynamics (due to eye, head, and body motion). These physical attributes are substantially different based on a person's location (indoors vs. outdoors, earth's latitude, etc.), their activity (doing near work vs. riding a bike), and time of day (dawn vs. dusk). The unknowns in this area concern characterizing the visual environment specific to children both prior to myopia onset *and* longitudinally, as children engage in their everyday activities.

Eye's Optics

The optical properties of the cornea and crystalline lens govern how light is channeled to the retina. Their shape (curvature, asphericity), refractive index distribution, effective optical zone diameter, and optical performance on- and off-axis, as well as their relative placement in space within the anterior chamber of the eye are all important parameters that together dictate the light distribution on the retina. Relevant in the context of axial elongation is how these parameters change longitudinally, especially in early childhood, with accommodation and with varying pupil diameters.

Image Formation

The early visual encoding of the retinal image involves sampling in space, time, and spectrum according to the shape of the eye, spatial and spectral topography of the photoreceptor mosaic, light adaptation in cone and rod phototransduction, and eye movements. Together these factors provide the signals from the external world that are available for detecting blur for regulating eye growth.

Computational Models of Retinal Image Formation and Visual Encoding

The framework described above allows any sequence of three-dimensional hyperspectral visual scenes (x, y, z, t, λ) to be transformed into the spatial (x, y, z), spectral (λ), and temporal (t) variations in the retinal image. These facets of the retinal image form the basis of downstream retinal circuits dedicated to signaling luminance, contrast, color, and form. The same facets of the image are critical as cues for eye growth. Naturally, computational models linking the environment, the eye's optics, and image formation would be instrumental in understanding mechanisms of normal eye growth, myopia pathogenesis, and treatments.

Eye Models

Many eye models exist in the literature that are based on anatomical parameters derived from biometry and imaging (reviewed in Atchison & Thibos, 2016). However, the classical eye models fall short in many ways. Most eye models are based on paraxial optics and are functional only for small fields of view (± 5 degrees), similar in spirit to the above noted foveocentric view. Thus, they do not fully reproduce the image quality and aberrations across the visual field relevant for myopia. In addition, they are based on population averages and cannot easily be generalized across variations in refractive error, accommodative state, or chromatic dispersion due to variations in ocular components, age, and eye shape.

Aberrometry provides a comprehensive account of the eye's optics (see Chapter 4) and can, in principle, account for inter-individual variations and the complex interactions between retinal shape, ocular surfaces, refractive index, and accommodation. It has long been appreciated that ray tracing through classical eye models falls short in precisely estimating the measured wavefront from aberrometry. Wide-angle eye models that best mimic the ocular anatomy and aberrations across a wide visual field are needed. While examples of such models exist (Polans et al., 2015), larger datasets of imaging and aberrometry will allow for better generalization of these models so they can be applied across the population and include the varying optical conditions relevant for myopia. Individualized eye models based on a retinocentric view are essential to further understand the mechanisms underlying the onset and progression of myopia, in particular how the visual environment interacts with the eye's optics, and to customize treatments specific to each eye.

Early Visual Encoding

Early visual encoding refers to the initial formation of an image on the retina by the eye's optics, the transduction of that image into electrical signals by the photoreceptors, and the subsequent transformations of the encoded image by retinal circuitry. The Image Systems and Engineering Toolbox for Biology (ISETBio; see Figure 6-6) is an example of a computational modelling platform for early vision that allows one to incorporate aspects of the environment/visual diet, the eye's optics, and image formation properties and yields cone photoreceptor signal outputs in response to any 3D hyperspectral visual scene (x, y, z, t, λ; Wandell et al., 2022; Zhang et al., 2022). It has found application in predicting spatial contrast sensitivity and color perception, among other visual tasks. Importantly, the ISETBio model allows probing the system at intermediate stages to quantify losses and encoding at various steps—for example, the physiological optics, the cone photoreceptor lattice, eye movements—and visualize the intermediate product of each processing unit. Refinements to existing parameters and later stages of retinal processing can be (and already are being) continually added into the software as more data from experiments become available. This is mentioned here to highlight an example of an existing framework for determining the retinal image from a visual scene after initial visual encoding and subject to the optical manipulations of the eye's optics. Moreover, it is constructed with the flexibility of taking as input personalized visual scenes, eye parameters, cone mosaics, eye movements and imposed treatments, and provides an avenue to ask mechanistic questions about the signals that the eye uses to sense blur and its sign.

Ocular Optics

The longitudinal changes in the focusing elements of the eye are shown in Figure 6-2. With respect to the corneal curvature, no specific trend—steep or flat—is characteristic of myopes or axial elongation, but rather curvature is associated with eye size (Guggenheim et al., 2013). Further, longer axial lengths and flatter corneas can confound the degree of myopia, so both parameters need to be measured simultaneously. Llorente et al. (2004) observed that the steeper myopic corneas had a higher negative asphericity (flatter in the periphery than the center), and the combined effect of curvature and asphericity led to an overall lower corneal spherical aberration in myopes.

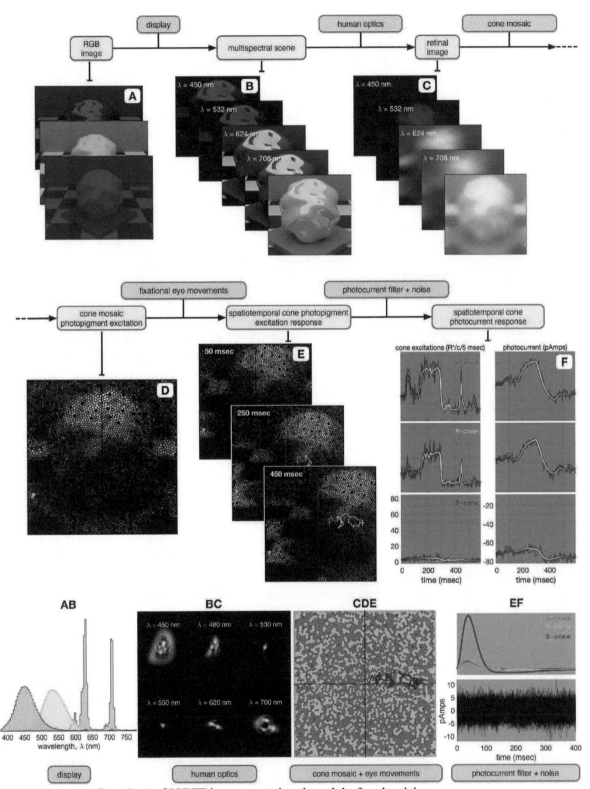

FIGURE 6-6 A flowchart of ISETBio computational model of early vision.
SOURCE: Reprinted from Cottaris et al., 2020, under a Creative Commons CC BY-NC-ND 4.0 License (https://creativecommons.org/licenses/by-nc-nd/4.0).

People with high myopia have been found to have a significantly thinner crystalline lens than emmetropes, specifically by a mean 0.046 mm. A decrease in −0.12 mm per mm of axial length (Muralidharan et al., 2019; Zhang et al., 2023) and an overall lower lens power of −1.2 D per mm of axial length is observed in the crystalline lens in myopic adults. Although this morphology is known, it remains unknown whether the gradient index properties of the crystalline lens are different in myopes, if at all. Differences in gradient index between emmetropes and myopes are important to consider in developing accurate eye models. Pupil size differences in myopes are also inconclusive—with studies indicating no differences (Orr et al., 2015) or else larger pupil size in myopes (Cakmak et al., 2010; Charman & Radhakrishnan, 2009; Guillon et al., 2016; Poudel et al., 2024).

With respect to aberrations besides spherical and cylindrical, in myopes one consistently observes one lower magnitude of primary-4th-order spherical aberration, consistent with a prolate shaped eye, its axial length longer than its width and height (Carkeet et al., 2002; Collins et al., 1995; Llorente et al., 2004). Chromatic aberrations do not seem to be affected by refractive error (Wildsoet et al., 1993), but in infants a larger amount of longitudinal chromatic aberration (LCA) is noted on account of the higher optical focusing power (Wang et al., 2018). In the periphery, myopes experience a positive refraction (image plane behind the retina) compared to emmetropes for whom the periphery is myopic (image plane in front of the retina; reviewed in Romashchenko et al., 2020). Besides the relatively less oblate shape in myopes compared to non-myopes, no other differences between eye shape are noted between refractive groups. These differences in eye shape have consequences for aberrations, including refraction and astigmatism. Changes in peripheral refraction may be more a consequence rather than a cause of myopia, given that peripheral refraction at baseline did not predict an onset of myopia in the future (Mutti et al., 2011; Sng et al., 2011). However, it is not clear to what degree these changes in peripheral shape contribute to myopia's progression, owing to the visual system's inability to detect blur and regulate eye growth.

Both young and adult myopes consistently show increased accommodative lag, and the accommodative response function decreases as myopia progresses (Abbott et al., 1998; Gwiazda et al., 1993; McBrien et al., 1986). This established observation is the basis of the near work hypothesis for myopia onset and progression discussed in detail in Chapter 5. Myopes showed different structural changes in response to an accommodative effort. A larger change in lens shape per diopter of change in accommodative focus is needed in myopes (Gwiazda et al., 1999; Mutti et al., 2017), accompanied with smaller reductions in ciliary muscle thickness but larger muscle movements (Bolz et al., 2007; Wagner et al., 2019; Wang et al., 2022).

The impact of accommodation on peripheral refraction deserves more study, since peripheral refraction is affected not only by eye shape but also by the peripheral focusing properties of the crystalline lens, such as its field curvature. Results are mixed on this issue. Whatham et al. (2009) showed hyperopic shifts in the near periphery with accommodation but the farther periphery either remained the same or demonstrated a myopic shift. A hyperopic shift is also noted by Walker & Mutti (2002). On the other hand, Davies & Mallen (2009), and Calver et al. (2007) found no associations due to accommodation between peripheral refractions (and their sign) and the refractive status. Overall, this large variability may be attributed to methodological differences as well as to the other lower and higher order aberrations, such as coma and astigmatism, which are large in magnitude and highly variable in the periphery and impact the best focus of the retinal image quality.

Photoreceptors: Retinal Density and Ratios

A few models have been proposed for the shape of eye growth that would predict different impacts of the linear and angular cone density in myopes in the foveal center (see Figure 3 in Strang et al., 1998). The model of global expansion suggests a proportional stretching of the retina with increasing eye length, such that the number of cones in each square millimeter area of the retina will decrease with increasing axial length, but the angular density will remain constant. The equatorial stretching model posits a simple posterior movement of the retina without expansion, such that the linear density remains the same, while the angular density increases with axial length. The over-development model suggests that the photoreceptors continue to migrate toward the fovea with eye elongation, leading to an increase in linear density and a still steeper increasing angular density with axial length. In marmosets, an increased linear cone density was observed with lens-induced eye growth (Troilo, 1998), and the overdevelopment model is inspired by this observation. Increasing linear cone spacing is also reported in chicks with eye growth that is unaccompanied by significant changes in angular cone density (Kisilak et al., 2012). An increased angular density would indicate better visual acuity in myopes compared to emmetropes.

Both histology and, more recently, *in vivo* adaptive optics imaging (see Chapter 4) have revealed the structure of the human photoreceptor mosaic (Curcio et al., 1990; Wang et al., 2019; Wells-Gray et al., 2016). Cone density peaks at the foveal center and decreases with eccentricity (Provis et al., 2013). The fovea is defined as the region of the highest cone density, ~1 mm in diameter, and with an absence of S-cones and rods. Rods begin to appear at ~1–2° from the foveal center, reaching high densities rivaling that of the cones at ~20° eccentricity. Rods outnumber cones by 10- to 20-fold between 10° and 30° eccentricity. Figure 6-7 shows the rod:cone ratio as a function of retinal eccentricity, imaged with an adaptive optics scanning laser ophthalmoscope (AOSLO), reproduced from Wells-Gray et al. (2016).

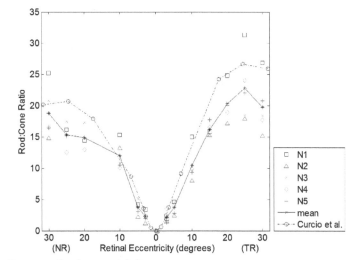

FIGURE 6-7 Rod:cone ratio vs. retinal eccentricity.
NOTE: Solid line is the mean of 5 subjects (N1–N5), and the OT dashed line is obtained from histology for comparison. NR = nasal retina; TR = temporal retina.
SOURCE: Wells-Gray et al., 2016.

Using a state-of-the-art adaptive optics scanning laser ophthalmoscope, Wang et al. (2019) revealed the structure of the foveal cone mosaic in emmetropes and myopes and found that, in general, shorter eyes have higher peak cone densities in linear units while longer eyes have lower linear peak cone density. Similar studies of rod topography in myopes are lacking. A lower linear cone density was also observed with an adaptive optics imaging study undertaken in children (ages 5.8 to 15.8 years) at eccentricities of 0.2 mm from the foveal center (Mirhajianmoghadam et al., 2020). These findings would be consistent with the global expansion model, in that longer eyes undergo an expansion at the fovea. However, when Wang et al. (2019) plotted the angular density in the fovea vs. axial length, they found an increasing trend.

Taken together, it becomes apparent that a combination of global expansion and equatorial stretching are needed to explain the foveal cone density in myopes, and that the foveal expansion does not occur in proportion to the length of the eye. The higher angular density in myopes would lead to a higher cone sampling density and predict better visual acuity when best corrected. However, this does not seem to be the case. Myopes routinely tend to have poorer acuity compared to emmetropes, even when the effect of the eye's optics is bypassed with the use of interference fringes (Atchison et al., 2006; Coletta & Watson, 2006) or with adaptive optics (Rossi et al., 2007). Prior to the adaptive optics imaging of the foveal cone mosaic by Wang et al. (2019), this would be attributed to the retinal stretching leading to reduced foveal cone density, but the reasons for these deficits must be post-receptoral. For example, it has been suggested that abnormal eye growth can lead to a loss of ganglion cells (Atchison et al., 2006). More work is needed to detail the inner retinal anatomy and wiring connectivity in myopia and assess whether the poorer visual performance is a cause or consequence of myopia.

Photoreceptors: Wavelength Sensitivity

The retinas of Old World primates, including humans, contain three different types of cones whose photopigments differ slightly in their sensitivity to different wavelengths of light. Each photopigment consists of a chromophore, 11-cis retinal, which is the same in all mammalian cones and undergoes photoisomerization when it absorbs a photon. This chromophore is covalently bound to an "opsin," a protein found in the visual system that "tunes" the spectral sensitivity of the photopigment. Each cone expresses only one of the three opsin genes, producing three unique types of cones that are relatively more sensitive to either short- (i.e., bluer), medium- or long- (i.e., redder) wavelength light, referred to as S-, M-, and L-cones for short. The signals from the three cone classes form the basis for color vision (among other visual capacities), and mutations in the opsin genes result in well-known inherited deficits in color vision, popularly but incorrectly referred to as "color blindness."

The distribution of cones varies across the retina, being most dense at the fovea and dropping off steeply with distance from the fovea (i.e., with eccentricity). In comparison with the cone mosaic's spatial topography, its spectral composition is relatively uncharacterized by its eccentricity, apart from the layout of the S-cones. This is because of the close similarity in the protein structure of L- and M-cones precluding their separation via histochemical markers. Nevertheless, S-cones are typically absent in the foveal center, peaking in their density at ~1–2° from the fovea and increasing in their proportions to reach ~10% of all cones by 10° (Curcio et al., 1991). Adaptive optics imaging has made it possible to detail the cone spectral types in humans (Roorda & Williams, 1999), yet the cone spectral type variation vs. eccentricity, especially in the foveal center, remains unknown. mRNA analysis of donor eyes has revealed that the retina becomes increasingly L-cone dominated in the far periphery (Neitz et al., 2006). Within individuals, variations in L:M cone ratios have been observed.

Related to this, an association has been suggested between the L:M cone ratio, cone opsin gene polymorphisms, and myopia. In a study conducted in a Norwegian population with a relatively low prevalence of myopia, it was suggested that the L:M cone ratio, combined with milder versions of L opsin gene polymorphisms, has a role to play in myopia (Hagen et al., 2019). High L:M cone ratios seemed protective in females, leading to lower degree of myopia in the Norwegian cohort, while lower L:M ratios, close to 1:1, were observed in East Asians (without concomitant measures of refractive error; Kuchenbecker et al., 2014) as compared to a 2:1 ratio observed in people of European ancestry (Carroll et al., 2002).

Cross-sectional studies reported conflicting results on the relationship between myopia and color vision deficiency (CVD). In Chinese high school students, ages 15–18 years (Qian et al., 2009), and in Iranian primary school students, ages 7–12 years (Ostadimoghaddam et al., 2014), a lower prevalence of myopia was noted in students with red-green CVD compared to color-normal individuals. However, no relationship was observed between red-green CVD and refractive error among Iranian children ages 7 to 12 years (Rajavi et al., 2015). A recent 5-year longitudinal study in China found lower cumulative incidence and change in spherical equivalent refraction in people with CVD: 35.4% (17/48) vs. 56.7% (1017/1794), and −1.81 D vs. −2.41 D respectively between CVD and the color-normal group (Gan et al., 2022). One limitation was the highly unbalanced number of children in both groups. The causal link between cone spectral composition, CVD, and myopia remains an open question. It has been suggested that chromatic cues, including transverse chromatic aberration and LCA, play a role in eye length regulation, and that there might be differences in the mechanisms by which these cues are encoded and utilized as cues in CVD, for example differences in cone contrast and their impact on accommodation.

While the recent myopia boom cannot naturally be attributed to the genetic differences inherent to people with CVD, these studies suggest a potential protective effect for myopigenic environmental factors in CVD via previously unknown mechanisms. LCA provides an important cue for accommodation and has been implicated in emmetropization using a model that compares the outputs of S-cones vs. LM-cone signals (Gawne & Norton, 2020). Thresholds for detecting S-cone increments and decrements of 3 cycles per degree grating patterns are shown to be worse in myopes; however, whether this reduced S-cone sensitivity constitutes one of the underlying causes for the impaired accommodative system in myopes is unknown. Again, as in the case of increased accommodative lag, longitudinal studies starting at an early age are required to establish whether the decrease in S-cone sensitivity in myopes is a cause or consequence of abnormal eye growth.

Retinal Periphery

Seminal work done in rhesus monkeys has implicated the essential role of the retinal periphery in both emmetropization and myopia pathogenesis, motivating treatments that focus on manipulating the quality of the peripheral retinal image (Smith et al., 2005, 2009). Few observations are of note, however. Peripheral form deprivation and lens-induced refractive error disrupted normal emmetropization and led to foveal myopia despite clear central vision (Smith et al., 2009). Foveal ablation of the central 5–6° did not impact the normal emmetropization of animals reared with unrestricted vision, nor the recovery of the animals from form deprivation myopia once the diffusers were removed, suggesting that the periphery beyond the central 5- to 6-degree region is sufficient for emmetropization (Huang et al., 2011; Smith et al., 2007). Taken together, these studies lead to the conclusion that the retinal periphery alone can regulate visually guided emmetropization, while the fovea and perifovea are not essential. The dominant role of the periphery in this may be attributed to its proportionally larger retinal area in comparison to the fovea, which occupies only a small fraction of the retina (Wallman & Winawer, 2004).

An alternative interpretation of these experiments is that cone photoreceptor circuits may not be the prominent retinal circuit guiding refractive eye growth. This hypothesis is further supported by studies in transgenic mouse models in which the rod or cone photoreceptor pathways were dysfunctional due to genetic mutations; the loss of rod function resulted in the eye not responding to experimentally induced myopia (Park et al., 2014) while the loss of cone function increased myopia susceptibility (Chakraborty et al., 2019). Hyperopic peripheral defocus as a risk factor and myopic peripheral defocus as treatments have their origins in these findings. However, such treatments have had limited success (as elaborated in Chapter 7).

Furthermore, studies on associations with near work, an activity purported to create peripheral hyperopic defocus, have led to inconsistent associations with myopia onset and progression. As indicated in Chapter 5, the negative impact of near work may be most potent during early age.

Role of the Non-foveal Retina in Accommodation

Near work is recognized as a risk factor for myopia (see Chapter 5). Given the importance of the retinal periphery in eye growth, it is worth considering if or whether the non-foveal retinal image makes a contribution to accommodative effort. There is evidence that even in the absence of a foveal stimulus, accommodative stimulation at 5–15° eccentricity creates a refractive change (Hartwig et al., 2011). An accommodative effort was observed when subjects fixated a foveal stimulus with no accommodative drive, while the retina was stimulated up to 30° with an accommodative demand (Gu & Legge, 1987). Patients with loss of foveal function due to juvenile macular degeneration also show a refractive change in response to an accommodative stimulus (White & Wick, 1995). In sum, the non-foveal retina can drive accommodation in the absence of a foveal near target.

Outside of these laboratory experiments, except in the case of diseases like macular degeneration, the fovea and the periphery are always stimulated together. To test how this real-life scenario affects peripheral contributions to accommodation, annular stimuli were used wherein the accommodative demand in the different parts of the fovea and periphery could be independently manipulated (Labhishetty et al., 2019). It was demonstrated that stimulating the retina in the perifovea with an annulus whose inner diameter was 8 degrees reaching up to 14 degrees eccentricity led to an accommodative effort, even though the fovea and parafovea were stimulated with the reverse accommodative demand.

Thus, peripheral hyperopia can drive an accommodative effort even when the foveal image is focused. This has consequences for how the accommodation system functions in the flatter vs. steeper dioptric environment found outdoors vs. indoors, respectively. In a flatter dioptric environment, accommodative demand is low and fairly uniform across the retina, exerting a proportionally lower impact on the periphery, compared to a steeper dioptric environment that has wider variability in accommodative stimuli (in diopters) and across the visual field. This larger variability indoors—both in dioptric distance and in its distribution across the retina—may lead to a conflict between the fovea and periphery, resulting in an ambiguous response of the accommodative system, in contrast to the outdoor environment where such a conflict is comparatively lower.

Peripheral Retinal Image Quality

The visual periphery has been the focus of many studies on aberrometry, including deducing the peripheral retinal shape and refraction from the experimental data (reviewed in Romashchenko et al., 2020). As stated earlier, myopes have peripheral hyperopia compared to emmetropes, for whom the periphery is myopic. Relative peripheral hyperopia seems to be a consequence rather than cause of myopic eye growth (Atchison et al., 2015; Mutti et al., 2011). That is, relative peripheral refraction depends on the magnitude of myopia, although these differences between the degree of myopia begin to appear only at 20° eccentric or greater. Relative refraction, or defocus, as a measure of the best image plane relative to the retina is challenging to determine precisely in the periphery. Image quality in the peripheral retina is affected by large magnitudes of coma, astigmatism, and other aberrations. Together, these expand the depth of focus significantly, and interactions between different aberrations lead to a shift in the defocus (compared to the relative refraction) where image quality is most optimal.

In contrast, aberrometry-derived metrics of retinal image quality, like modulation transfer function, better characterize images in the retinal periphery (Marsack et al., 2004). With distance foveal refraction, myopes have worse modulation transfer functions (poorer retinal image quality) along the horizontal visual field (calculated from aberrometry) than emmetropes do. This is the case from the fovea up until 20 degrees, after which the modulation transfer functions become similar between the two groups. These observations come from an analysis performed on wavefront aberration data of the horizontal visual field collected from 2,492 eyes (60% emmetropes, 20% each myopes and hyperopes) in Europe, Australia, and North America (Romashchenko et al., 2020). The same dataset was used to estimate the shape and orientation of blur (point-spread function) in the periphery in different refractive groups (Figure 6-8) (Zheleznyak, 2023). The blur study showed that along the horizontal nasal visual field from 0 to 30 degrees, the myopic retina experiences vertically elongated blur (circumferential or tangential), while emmetropic and hyperopic retinas experience horizontal or radially elongated blur when the fovea is refracted for distance vision. This radial to tangential anisotropy in blur orientation is attributed to the interaction of peripheral optics and retinal shape. It is known that in the periphery, the visual system has greater sensitivity for radially oriented targets compared to tangential ones. This preference is consistent with the peripheral optical blur orientation and resultant retinal images experienced habitually, given that even after optical corrections, the same bias holds in orientation preference, with some differences observed between refractive error groups (Leung et al., 2021; Zheleznyak et al., 2016).

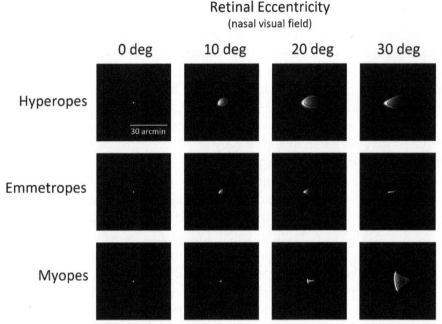

Retinal Eccentricity
(nasal visual field)

FIGURE 6-8 Shape and orientation of blur in the periphery in different refractive groups.
NOTE: Optical blur, shown as the point-spread function, for different refractive groups as a function of eccentricity. Pupil size was 4mm for the simulation, and monochromatic light was used.
SOURCE: Zheleznyak, 2023.

When published values of eccentricity-dependent chromatic aberrations—longitudinal and transverse—were incorporated, the retinal image (as estimated by the modulation transfer function) in the myopic peripheral retina was optimal for short wavelengths, while longer wavelengths were more optimal for hyperopes (Figure 6-9; Zheleznyak et al., 2024). This is denoted by the size of the point-spread function in the periphery; at wavelengths of 405 nm the point-spread function is relatively smaller in the myopes than at wavelengths of 695 nm, while the hyperopes show the opposite trend. Emmetropes and hyperopes exhibited more tangential blur at greater eccentricities (20° and 30°) for all wavelengths, while the blur shape for myopes depended on wavelength and eccentricity; at 30°, wavelengths greater than 505 nm (bluish-green) had a more vertical orientation bias. This optical blur anisotropy in the periphery, including the effects due to chromatic aberration, is suggested by the study as a potential cue for emmetropization that could be sensed by orientation-selective mechanisms in the retina.

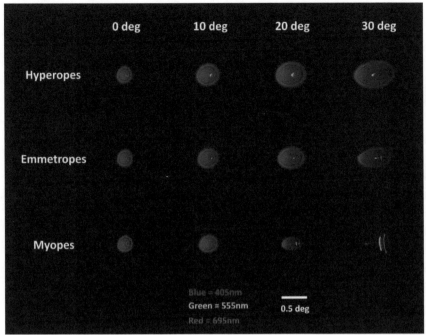

FIGURE 6-9 Polychromatic point-spread functions in the nasal visual field in different refractive groups.
NOTE: The three colors, red, green and blue, represent the blur on the retina created by 405 nm, 555 nm, and 695 nm wavelength light, respectively, considering the effects of monochromatic and chromatic aberrations as a function of eccentricity.
SOURCE: Reprinted from Zheleznyak et al., 2024, under a Creative Commons CC BY-NC-ND 4.0 License (https://creativecommons.org/licenses/by-nc-nd/4.0).

Summary

This section covered the characteristics of ocular optics and image formation that together determine the facets of the retinal image that may be pertinent as cues for emmetropization. These facets all vary in specific ways with defocus, eye shape, and retinal eccentricity. Deducing the direction of eye growth, therefore, is a problem of finding the most potent image facet(s) amenable to be detected by retinal cells and circuits to initiate the retinal-scleral signaling cascade (see next section). Here is listed a summary of these retinal image properties:

- Wavelength-dependent defocus or chromatic aberration: longitudinal and transverse
- Optical blur: shape, size, and orientation
- Contrast: spatial, spectral, and temporal contrast.

RETINAL CELLS AND CIRCUITS REGULATING EYE GROWTH

Earlier sections of this report implicate at least three sorts of retinal signals that could link specific features of the visual environment to dysregulation of eye growth in myopia. These are luminance (irradiance or light intensity), defocus or blur, and wavelength (color). This section surveys what is known about the specific retinal neurons and synaptic circuits that encode these stimulus features and their possible involvement in myopia pathogenesis.

The Retina's Central Role in Myopia Pathogenesis

The neural retina appears to be the key link between the properties of retinal images and the regulation of eye growth at the sclera. The retina has been shown to encode critical image features that have been linked to eye-growth regulation (including luminance, wavelength, and spatial contrast). Blurred or defocused images continue to affect eye growth even when the optic nerve is crushed, severing the link between eye and brain (McFadden & Wildsoet, 2020; Norton et al., 1994; Troilo & Wallman, 1991; Troilo et al., 1987; Wildsoet, 2003; Wildsoet & Pettigrew, 1988; Wildsoet & Wallman, 1995). Thus, post-retinal processing is not required for retinal images to affect eye growth. Though the brain and integrative visual behaviors may play some role, as discussed later, there is broad consensus that the retina is both necessary and sufficient as the neural link between retinal images and eye growth.

Diverse lines of evidence explored in this section reinforce the prevailing view that the retina is essential for encoding retinal image features that affect eye growth. For example, mutations in diverse genes disrupting retinal phototransduction or synaptic signaling in mice result in myopia or in the perturbation of dopamine levels (e.g., Nob [*nyx gene*], as reported in Pardue et al., 2008); mGluR6 (Grm6 gene), reported in Chakraborty et al., 2015; and Lrit3 and GPR179, reported in Zeitz et al., 2023; see review by Mazade et al., 2024). Retinal degenerative diseases are frequently associated with high myopia (Hendriks et al., 2017; Park et al., 2013; see Chapter 5 for additional information about genetics). Both dopamine and melanopsin have been implicated in myopigenesis, as discussed below, and their ocular expression is largely limited to the neural retina.

Retinal Cells and Circuits Encoding Light Intensity

The epidemiological and experimental animal studies considered in Chapter 5 suggest that environmental light intensity affects the propensity to develop myopia. Retinal irradiance or photon flux is thus among the best-established dimensions of the retinal image implicated in refractive development. This is significant because most retinal neurons are poorly suited for encoding luminance. The retina has evolved adaptation mechanisms that filter out responses to continuous background illumination in order to enhance spatio-temporal contrast. Due to lateral inhibition (Hartline & Ratliff, 1958; Kuffler 1953) and other mechanisms, most retinal neurons are unreliable reporters of environmental illumination (Barlow & Levick, 1969).

However, there is a specialized retinal network that does encode steady-state light intensity (Figure 6-10, panel A). This system was first probed as early as the 1960s (Barlow & Levick, 1969), but has been studied particularly intensively since the discovery of the intrinsically photosensitive retinal ganglion cells (ipRGCs; Aranda & Schmidt, 2020; Do et al., 2019). ipRGCs are unique among retinal ganglion cells (RGCs) in their capacity to respond directly to light, much like rod and cone photoreceptors, using melanopsin as their photopigment. The ipRGCs are also highly unusual among RGCs in their capacity to signal how much total visible light is in the environment. They encode light intensity stably over many hours and distribute this nerve signal to diverse brain regions. Their outputs to the brain drive constriction of the pupil, phase shifts of circadian rhythms, and reductions in melatonin levels in the bloodstream (Aranda & Schmidt, 2020; Do, 2019), among many other functions.

The 'luminance network' also includes the dopaminergic amacrine cells (DACs; Figure 6-10A). DACs, like ipRGCs, encode light intensity. Brighter ambient light triggers more DAC nerve-impulse spiking (Raviola, 2002; Zhang et al., 2008, 2017). This also increases dopamine release, which may act as a retino-scleral stop signal in refractive development (Norton & Siegwart, 2013; Schaeffel & Feldkaemper, 2013).

Both DAC and ipRGC signals are driven by light through a specialized component of the ON pathway (Figure 6-10A), that appears optimized for luminance coding and is highly conserved among mammals, including humans. This network encompasses a remarkable number of the retinal components implicated in eye-growth regulation in mammals, including dopamine, the ON pathway, and melanopsin. It also establishes a conceptual bridge to a much broader and burgeoning field of academic, clinical, design, and policy work informed by the effects of light on health. Examples in this field include sleep and circadian health, lighting and architectural design, human factors and shift work, and phototherapy for depression (Lucas et al., 2014). It is becoming increasingly clear that inadequate (or ill-timed) activation of this retinal luminance network, a hazard of contemporary lifestyles in urbanized environments, threatens physical and mental well-being in diverse ways.

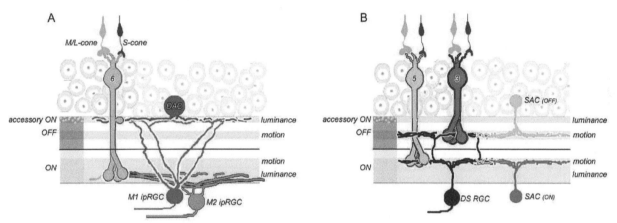

FIGURE 6-10 Distinct retinal neurons and synaptic circuits encoding luminance and image motion. NOTES: (A) Elements of the luminance network. Key synaptic connections are confined to the two gray 'luminance' sublayers, both driven by the ON pathway. The bottom (innermost) sublayer is the conventional ON sublayer. It is supplied with excitatory input from the main axon terminal field of certain types of ON bipolar cells. For simplicity, only a single type ("6") is shown here, in reference to mouse bipolar Type 6 and its probable primate equivalent, DB6. The upper luminance stratum—the "accessory ON sublayer"—lies (surprisingly) at the top margin of the inner plexiform layer (IPL), within a part of the OFF sublayer. There, descending ON bipolar axons that also supply the lower luminance band make *en passant* synapses in the accessory ON sublayer on their way by. Targets of this accessory ON channel drive include the dopaminergic amacrine cell (DAC; red) and some intrinsically photosensitive retinal ganglion cells (ipRGCs), including the M1 type (blue). Like all ipRGCs, M1 cells can respond directly to light through melanopsin phototransduction. Some DACs receive glutamatergic input from intra-retinal axons of M1 cells (not shown). The M2 ipRGC type (lavender), like most ipRGCs other than M1s, receives its synaptic input in the conventional ON sublayer. This network encodes environmental luminance much more faithfully than other retinal networks do. (B) Elements of the visual motion network. Key synaptic connections are largely confined to the two pink "motion" sublayers. The lower one sits in the middle of the ON sublayer and receives input from a set of ON bipolar cells (yellow; "5") distinct from those serving the luminance network. The upper 'motion' stratum is served by the OFF pathway, with input from axon terminals of OFF bipolar cells (purple; "3"). Starburst amacrine cells (SACs; green, with ON and OFF varieties) make their synaptic connections mainly within these two bands. Direction-selective retinal ganglion cells ("DS RGCs"; burgundy) are bistratified, with dendrites in both bands. They receive input from ON and OFF bipolar cells there, but also from the SACs. GABA inhibition from SACs to DS RGCs exhibits a highly ordered spatial asymmetry that tunes DS RGCs to

specific directions of image motion. These signals are used by the brain in diverse ways, including to detect image slip and thereby trigger image-stabilizing reflexes.
SOURCE: Committee generated.

Dopamine as a Stop Signal for Refractive Eye Growth

A growing body of work indicates that dopamine signaling in the retina is necessary for emmetropization and that the release of dopamine by DACs is protective for myopia development (Feldkaemper & Schaeffel, 2013; Mazade et al., 2024; Stone et al. 1989; Zhou et al. 2017). Experiments from multiple vertebrate species suggest that decreased retinal concentrations of dopamine are associated with increased ocular growth and myopia development, while increased retinal dopamine concentrations are associated with a slowing of ocular growth (Feldkaemper & Schaeffel, 2013). This is based on high-performance liquid chromatography results of retinal or vitreal dopaminergic amacrine (DA) and/or DOPAC (DA metabolite) that show reduced levels in response to form deprivation in primates (Iuvone et al., 1989), chickens (McBrien et al., 2001; Papastergiou et al., 1998; Stone et al., 1989), and guinea pigs (Dong et al., 2011), and negative lens defocus in chickens (Guo et al., 1995; Ohngemach et al., 1997). Moreover, it is well-established that retinal dopamine synthesis is stimulated by light, and a number of studies have shown that outdoor activity and/or bright light inhibits myopia, potentially through dopamine-mediated mechanisms (Ashby & Schaeffel, 2010; Chen et al., 2017; Cohen et al., 2012; Feldkaemper et al., 1999; Landis et al., 2021).

If dopamine levels and/or signaling are decreased during myopic eye growth, then increasing DA levels or DA receptor activity would be predicted to prevent myopia. This prediction is supported by experiments in which dopamine or dopamine agonists have shown protective effects on myopia development (Ashby et al., 2007; Brown et al., 2022; Dong et al., 2011; Iuvone et al., 1991; McCarthy et al., 2007; Rohrer et al., 1993; Schmid & Wildsoet, 2004; Stone et al., 1989; Yan et al., 2015). Additionally, dopamine antagonists (Wu et al., 2016) or mice genetically manipulated to eliminate tyrosine hydroxylase, a dopamine precursor (Bergen et al., 2016) have shown increased myopia susceptibility when dopamine levels are low. Together these studies suggest that DA receptor activation is needed for normal refractive eye growth under challenging/abnormal visual conditions (form deprivation or lens defocus) and that increasing DA levels in the eye can prevent myopic growth signals.

However, the role of dopamine in the control of postnatal ocular growth is likely complicated, as not all experiments to activate or inhibit dopamine signaling have similar results. For instance, treatment with the dopamine receptor antagonist 6-hydroxydopamine and the catecholamine depleting agent, reserpine, prevented (rather than facilitated) development of form-deprivation myopia in chickens by reducing axial eye growth (Schaeffel et al., 1995). Interestingly, dopamine agonists are not as effective for lens-induced myopia across multiple species (Ashby et al., 2007; Dong et al., 2011; Iuvone et al., 1991; McCarthy et al., 2007; Rohrer et al., 1993; Schmid & Wildsoet, 2004; Stone et al., 1989; Yan et al., 2015). Additionally, dopamine does not seem to affect eye growth under normal conditions, but only under myopigenic conditions as in the case of form-deprivation and lens-induced myopia (Dong et al., 2011; Junfeng et al., 2010; Landis et al., 2020; Rohrer et al., 1993; Yan et al., 2015). These findings suggest that modulation of visually driven eye growth is not simply due to the level of retinal dopamine.

Dopaminergic Amacrine Cells and ipRGCs—Irradiance-coding Cells and Circuits

DA cells are a type of retinal interneuron found in all vertebrate retinas. These widefield polyaxonal spiking amacrine cells are the sole source of dopamine within the eye (Witkovsky, 2004). Ample evidence from animal studies supports a role for dopamine as a retino-scleral signal in emmetropization (see review from Brown et al., 2022; Figure 6-10A). Mice lacking dopamine through tyrosine hydroxylase knockout (Bergen et al., 2016) or toxin administration (Wu et al., 2016) develop myopia. Both form-deprivation myopia and lens-induced myopia lower dopamine and DOPAC levels in most species tested (Dong et al., 2011; Guo et al., 1995; Iuvone et al., 1989; Ohngemach et al., 1997; Papastergiou et al., 1998; Stone et al., 1989; Sun et al., 2018). Dopamine receptor agonists or the dopamine precursor, L-DOPA, prevent form-deprivation myopia and to a smaller extent lens-induced myopia (Gao et al., 2006; Junfeng et al., 2010; Landis et al., 2020; Mao et al., 2016; Mao & Liu, 2017). The protective effect of high luminance on chick lens-induced myopia was abolished by a dopamine antagonist (spiperone; Ashby & Schaeffel, 2010). It is noteworthy that in some studies, manipulations of dopamine signaling only appear to affect axial elongation when visual input is disrupted (Landis et al., 2020; Mao et al., 2010).

Taken together, the evidence strongly backs the conclusion that dopamine acts as a 'stop' signal for axial elongation (Feldkaemper & Schaeffel, 2013) with roles in diverse myopia models. Dopamine is thus a key neural regulator of growth, though probably not the only one.

How does dopamine put the brakes on eye growth? DA diffuses throughout the retina, and although it may not actually reach the sclera, it does affect choroidal thickness (Mathis et al., 2023), which in turn is altered in many myopia models. This seems to be an indirect effect, since the choroid doesn't express DA receptors. The RPE may be the link between DACs and the choroid; RPE cells do express DA receptors (Dearry et al., 1990; Gallemore & Steinberg, 1990; Mathis et al., 2023).

Overall, the findings suggest that DA signaling is important for regulation of eye growth, but that its role is complex and best understood in the context of visually driven myopia and a broad retinal and ocular network of cellular intercommunication (see the section on the role of RPE below; Brown et al., 2022; Feldkaemper & Schaeffel, 2013; Mazade, Palumaa, & Pardue, 2024; Zhou et al., 2017). These findings implicate DACs in mechanisms of myopia pathogenesis, but these amacrine cells also play important roles in intrinsic circadian regulation of ocular tissues. Circadian mechanisms in turn have been suggested as playing some role in emmetropization (Chakraborty et al., 2018; Stone et al., 2020), so DACl may be implicated in this context as well. DACs are also key players during light adaptation and in regulating intercellular gap-junctional coupling among retinal cells (Goel & Mangel, 2021; McMahon & Dowling, 2023; Witkovsky, 2004).

DACs are ON-type retinal neurons: they respond to light increments by depolarizing and increasing their spike rate. There are many varieties of ON-type amacrine and ganglion cells, but DACs are unusual among them in having very sustained responses to steady illumination. Their firing rate is proportional to light intensity, so they can be said to encode luminance (Zhang et al., 2008). Increased spiking in DACs results in increased release of dopamine from their varicosities. This released dopamine acts in paracrine fashion at sites widely distributed within the retina, serving as the main signal for the transition of retinal circuitry from scotopic (dim light stimuli that activate only rod photoreceptors) to photopic (bright light stimuli that activate mainly cone and ipRGCs photoreceptors) vision (Jackson et al., 2012; see review in Bloomfield

& Volgyi, 2009). Paracrine signaling suits dopamine well for affecting other layers of the ocular globe, perhaps very far from the site of release (Popova, 1995).

The ON cone bipolar drive to DACs is unusual. Bipolar inputs to DACs, as to all RGCs and amacrine cells, are made in the *inner plexiform layer* (*IPL*), a synaptic layer in the inner retina interconnecting bipolar, amacrine and ganglion cells (Figure 6-10). OFF bipolar cells make their outputs in the outer (sclerad) part of the IPL (the "OFF sublayer") and ON bipolar cells do so in the inner (vitread) part of the IPL (the "ON sublayer"). Surprisingly, though both DACs and M1 ipRGCs are ON cells, their dendrites are found in the outermost margin of the IPL, abutting the cells of the inner nuclear layer, in what should be the OFF sublayer. The resolution of this paradox is that these two ON cell types get their excitatory ribbon synaptic input from *en passant* synapses from the axonal shafts of ON cone bipolar cells passing through the OFF sublayer on their way to the ON sublayer of the IPL (Dumitrescu et al., 2009; Hoshi et al., 2009). This thin isolated extra layer of ON-channel output has been called the 'accessory ON sublamina.'

The *en passant* output synapses of ON cone bipolar cells have a highly unusual ultrastructure, with multiple synaptic ribbons and only a single postsynaptic partner, unlike the dyad synapses found elsewhere in the IPL. These specializations may optimize the circuit's ability to stably encode irradiance. Segregation of this part of the ON channel in this way almost certainly means that this bipolar input is subject to a very different sort of pre- and post-synaptic amacrine-cell inhibition. This may help to explain why M1 cells have among the weakest receptive-field surrounds of any RGCs (Zhao et al., 2017). Bipolar drive to the DAC/ipRGC system comes from a subset of ON cone bipolar types. These appear to be reliable encoders of retinal irradiance (Sabbah et al.). They are also among those receiving the strongest input from the primary rod system (Demb & Singer 2012). This may relate to the outsized role of rods in driving dopamine release (Cameron et al., 2009; Pérez-Fernández et al., 2019; Zhou et al., 2017).

DACs contribute significantly to light-adaptation mechanisms in the retina. Dopamine levels are high in the presence of light, but they are also higher during the biological day regardless of lighting due to autonomous intraretinal circadian rhythmicity (see review in Ko, 2020). Retinal melatonin exhibits the inverse relationship to light exposure and circadian phase (Ko, 2020). Dopamine is a master regulator of retinal sensitivity, helping to shift the retina into a light-adapted state optimized for daylight conditions by influencing many specific neuronal types and their intercommunications with each other. The capacity of the DAC to link light intensity to diverse actions and physiological effects and to do so at remote locations through paracrine signaling seems nicely matched to the requirements of retino-scleral signaling for refractive eye growth. Nevertheless, mechanistic details have not been identified at this point.

One way dopamine affects retinal sensitivity is by regulating gap junctions throughout the neural retina. One key circuit regulated in this way is the "primary rod pathway," which is crucial for conveying the most sensitive rod signals to ganglion cells. The gap junction in question is known as connection no. 36, encoded by the *Gjd2* gene, which is significantly linked to myopia in GWAS studies (Chen et al. 2012; Solouki et al. 2010; van der Sande et al., 2022).

In mice, a subset of DACs receives a second source of glutamatergic excitatory ON input from intraretinal axons of ipRGCs, branching off their main axon *en route* to the optic nerve. This input can sustain light responses in these DACs even in the absence of functional rod and cone input, through melanopsin phototransduction by M1 ipRGCs and their glutamatergic synapses onto DACs (Munteanu et al., 2018). M1 cells themselves receive this unusual ON bipolar drive in the accessory ON sublayer. Thus, mouse DACs may receive the specialized ON drive not only directly from the bipolar cells themselves but also indirectly through their inputs from M1 cells. Mouse models indicate that ipRGCs play a role in emmetropization. Eliminating ipRGC photosensitivity (through melanopsin knockout) or killing ipRGCs (using diphtheria toxin) impacts myopigenesis in mice, at least partly through DACs (Chakraborty et al., 2022; Liu et al., 2022; Mazade et al., 2024). Surprisingly, dopamine release in the retina is apparently neither driven by nor dependent on melanopsin (Cameron et al., 2009). In fact, rods contribute much more than cones to the light-evoked release of dopamine (Pérez-Fernández et al., 2019).

The similarities in structure and function between M1 ipRGCs and DACs are remarkable. As already noted, both receive specialized ON channel input and are unusual among inner retinal neurons in encoding irradiance (luminance). They deploy their dendrites in the same narrow sublamina of the IPL—the accessory ON sublayer. Genetic manipulations that alter the stratification of DACs produce similar alterations in M1 ipRGCs (Matsuoka et al., 2011). Both are unusual among amacrine and ganglion cells in sometimes extending processes into the outer plexiform layer. Further, M1s and DACs reciprocally influence one another, through dopamine receptors on the M1 cells (Van Hook et al., 2012) and glutamatergic synapses from M1 axons onto the DACs (Zhang et al., 2008). Though some DACs exhibit transient light responses, sustained DACs encode light intensity just as ipRGCs do, through a mix of contributions from rods, cones, and melanopsin.

Diverse Roles of the ON Pathway in Luminance Coding and Myopia Development

Complete congenital stationary night blindness (cCSNB) is a genetic disorder that disrupts dim light vision, among other abnormalities. It is linked to mutations in genes required for signaling at the photoreceptor-to-ON-bipolar synapse. This specialized synapse inverts the sign of the voltage response to light, changing it from hyperpolarizing (OFF) in the rod and cone photoreceptors to depolarizing (ON) in the postsynaptic bipolar cells. The ON bipolar cell response (as reflected in the electroretinogram [ERG] b-wave) is perturbed in diverse mutations that disrupt this signaling process in ON bipolar cells, from photoreceptor synapse, with their metabotropic glutamate receptors through their depolarizing light response, reflecting an excitatory cation conductance through transient receptor potential M1 channels (Pardue & Peachey, 2014). All these mutations share a myopic phenotype and a severely disrupted b-wave (an ON-bipolar-cell-mediated ERG component). The consistent appearance of myopia in cCSNB across diverse genetic contexts provides strong evidence in favor of the ON pathway itself playing an integral role in the development of myopia (reviewed in Hendriks et al., 2017; Mazade et al., 2024; Zeitz et al., 2023).

A recent analysis suggests that the ON pathway is relatively understimulated in reading as compared to walking, perhaps a link to the protective effects of time spent outdoors on myopia prevalence (Poudel et al., 2023). Additionally, another study suggests ON pathways are less responsive in myopic eyes based on ERG recordings (Poudel et al., 2024), and this is supported by patch clamp recordings from myopic mouse eyes (Mazade & Pardue, 2023).

The ON pathway is of special relevance to both scotopic and short-wavelength sensitivity. In mammals, two distinct photoreceptor channels in the retina—for rods and for short-wavelength cones—share a unique dependence on the ON pathway. The most sensitive 'primary' rod pathway is entirely dependent on a dedicated bipolar type for scotopic vision—the rod bipolar cell (Demb & Singer, 2012). This is an ON type bipolar cell type, sharing the same 'sign-inverting' metabotropic glutamate receptors as cone bipolar cells of the ON type. Though rods have other ways of signaling, disruption of the rod bipolar signal will elevate the threshold for detecting light in dim conditions. cCSNB mutations that disrupt ON pathway signaling silence the rod bipolar cell's light response and have particularly severe impacts on dim-light vision. Likewise, there is a specific type of bipolar cell that appears to be the sole conduit of pure signals derived from the short-wavelength cones. This type appears conserved across mammalian retinas (Haverkamp et al., 2005). It too is an ON type bipolar cell. Thus, the "ON-channel defect" in congenital stationary night blindness should also be viewed as differentially impacting not only the sensitive rod vision but also the short-wavelength chromatic channel.

Several genes linked to high myopia are associated with the first synapse in the ON pathway linking rods and cones to ON bipolar cells. This involves a 'sign-inverting' metabotropic glutamate receptor (mGluR6), which regulates current flow through a transient receptor potential channel (Mazade et al., 2024; Zeitz et al., 2023). As mentioned above, another gene linked to myopigenesis is *Gjd2*, which codes for the gap junctional protein connexin 36. Connexin 36 gap junctions are required for signal transmission of the most sensitive ('primary') retinal rod pathways. They mediate the transmission of sensitive rod signals from AII amacrine cells to cone bipolar axon terminals in the IPL. Knockouts of connexin 36 are thus one mouse model of cCSNB (Demb & Singer, 2012; van der Sande et al., 2022). However, connexin 36 is expressed in diverse types of retinal neurons (Massey et al. 2003; van der Sande et al., 2022) and also in the RPE (Fadjukov et al., 2022), so the contribution of rod signaling defects to the myopigenic effects of *Gjd2* mutations remains to be determined.

Though the available data strongly implicate the ON channel, the OFF channel might also carry beneficial effects of time outdoors. There are diverse ways of selectively silencing the ON channel, but not so for the OFF. Is the present focus on the ON-channel contribution simply a reflection of this, or a real asymmetry? If the OFF channel were selectively silenced, would there be the same sort of effects as with ON defects because it would similarly disrupt ON/OFF balance? Mice whose OFF pathway was partially silenced through a *Vsx1* mutation had normal ocular development and blunted responses to form deprivation (Chakraborty et al., 2014). It would be very informative to know if the ON channel is necessary and sufficient for the effects of image properties on the sclera.

Evidence for Neural and Ocular Cell Populations in Eye-growth Regulation

The Brain

As noted above, numerous studies using optic-nerve crush to block retinal output indicate that higher-order visual processing in the brain is not required for the eye's response to myopigenic alterations in visual input (Choh et al. 2006; Gastinger et al., 2006; Troilo & Wallman, 1991; Troilo et al., 1987; Wildsoet & Wallman, 1995). Further, form-deprivation myopia can be induced in both chicks (McBrien et al., 1995) and tree shrews (Norton et al., 1994) after intravitreal injections of the sodium-channel blocker tetrodotoxin. Although subtle impacts of nerve crush on eye-growth regulation have been reported in mice, guinea pigs, and some species of non-human primates (Gong et al., 2020; McFadden & Wildsoet, 2020; Raviola & Wiesel, 1990), even these subtle impacts may ultimately be traceable to the retina. For example, severing the optic nerve triggers degeneration in most retinal ganglion cells, and likely compromises the central retinal artery, which supplies the inner retina (Flitcroft, 2012). In a more targeted manipulation, ganglion-cell spiking has been silenced with tetrodotoxin. This did not block the effects of form deprivation on refractive growth in chicks (McBrien et al., 1995; Wildsoet & Wallman, 1995) or tree shrews (Norton et al., 1994). Whether the link between eye and brain is disrupted by cutting optic axons or blocking their spiking, this will affect both eye movements and accommodation and thus the pattern of spatio-temporal contrast experienced by the retina.

In a related finding, Bitzer & Schaeffel (2006) found that visual stimulation that normally triggered myopia in chicks no longer did so if they were anesthetized by either of two methods. Glucagon-expressing amacrine cells that report the sign of defocus in their expression of an immediate-early-gene in intact alert animals failed to do so in anesthetized animals or in an *in vitro* preparation (Bitzer & Schaeffel, 2006). There are many possible explanations for these results, but they suggest that active, dynamic vision in a complex world is important for linking retinal images to eye growth, even if the key biological mechanisms lie within the eye. Together, the data strongly suggest that although some influence of central vision cannot be definitively ruled out, the main links between visual experience and eye growth lie within the eye itself and depend on retinal mechanisms.

There are a variety of possible mechanisms through which the brain may contribute to the regulation of ocular growth. First, the brain can modulate the retina by direct neural connectivity. Although the optic nerve carries signals almost exclusively from eye to brain in mammals, there are a few 'centrifugal' optic nerve fibers carrying signals from brain to retina. In primates, these comprise only a few hundred axons, arising mainly from small populations of hypothalamic neurons (Gastinger et al., 2006). This sparse, diffuse retinal innervation seems poorly suited to encoding spatial contrast or retinal location, but it could contribute to the representation of other stimulus features controlling eye growth such as luminance, for which detailed information about spatial structure is not essential.

A second opportunity for contributions from central visual mechanisms comes in the context of accommodation, through which the brain dynamically adjusts the optical power of the eye's crystalline lens under both reflexive and voluntary control, for example, by 'active vision' through gaze shifts to locations at different depths in extrapersonal space and by vergence-accommodation coupling in the 'near reflex.'

The brain's control over accommodation is exerted through the autonomic nervous system, which may contribute in other ways to the regulation of eye growth. For example, brainstem autonomic centers control choroidal blood flow through a nitric oxide signaling mechanism (Li et al., 2016; Reiner et al., 2018). Surgical interruption of the autonomic innervation of the chick eye alters normal circadian rhythms in eye growth and choroidal thickness, both of which have been linked to myopia mechanisms (Li et al., 2016; Nickla & Schroedl, 2019).

There are still more factors to consider. The brain's oculomotor system is responsible for making diverse patterns of voluntary and reflexive eye movements, both conjugate and vergence, and either fast or slow through the actions of the extraocular striated muscles. Accommodation and pupil diameter are dynamically regulated through intraocular smooth muscles. The patterns of these movements may differ between indoor and outdoor environments (see previous chapter).

Finally, whole-body movements through the world alter the structure and dynamics of the retinal image—for example the 'optic flow' that occurs during walking or driving. In this sense, the brain actively shapes the visual diet that the retina is exposed to. Beyond this, complex higher-level brain mechanisms govern decision-making, including whether to opt for an outdoor or indoor environment over the course of the day.

Still, the weight of evidence suggests that the effects of retinal images on eye growth are mostly an intrinsic regulatory function of the eye itself. If their outputs to the brain are not essential, are the RGCs themselves required for the process in some other way? ipRGCs make glutamatergic synapses onto DACs through intraretinal axons. Both ipRGCs and conventional RGCs are also linked to many diverse amacrine cell types through gap junctions. Blocking RGC spiking would presumably affect "centrifugal" (intraretinal) influences to some extent, but this had no effect on refractive development. Some role for ipRGCs in the effects of luminance on refractive development seems likely, as discussed above. On balance, though, there seems little compelling evidence that RGCs play a critical role in linking retinal images to scleral growth-control mechanisms. Certainly, RGCs are not required for other retinal cell types to encode luminance, spatial contrast, or wavelength.

Ganglion and Amacrine Cells

As discussed above, a luminance network involving both amacrine-cell (DACs) and ganglion-cell (ipRGC) components has been linked to the protective effects of daylight outdoors (Chakraborty et al., 2018, 2022; Feldkaemper & Schaeffel, 2013; Mutti et al. 2020; Zhou et al. 2017). New evidence implicating neuropsin (Opn5) in the protective effects of violet light appears to implicate RGCs as well, because within the retina this atypical opsin is apparently selectively expressed in ganglion cells (D'Souza et al., 2022). More generally, while the brain clearly relies on RGCs for information about the retinal image, it might not be the case that the brain's activity is involved in the mechanisms linking retinal images to eye growth.

For example, blocking nerve impulses in RGCs with the sodium-channel blocker tetrodotoxin stops communication between retina and brain but leaves the effects of image perturbation on eye growth intact (McBrien et al. 1995; Norton et al. 1994). In other words, while brain visual mechanisms are entirely dependent on RGCs for information about the retinal image, linkage with the brain is not necessary for the effects of visual experience on eye growth. Experimentally ablating various collections of chick retinal neurons by various means triggers changes in eye growth and alters the ocular response to defocus or blur (Bitzer & Schaeffel, 2004; Ehrlich et al., 1990; Fischer et al., 1997, 1998). Further, in chicks, specific retinal interneurons exhibit differential molecular responses to hyperopic and myopic defocus imposed *in vivo* (Fischer et al., 1999). These are a subtype of amacrine cell that expresses the insulin-related hormone glucagon.

Photoreceptors and Bipolar Cells

As mentioned earlier, mutations in genes disrupting retinal signaling in mice result have been found to result in myopia and/or effect dopamine levels (Nob [nyx]; Pardue et al., 2008; mGluR6 [Grm6]; Chakraborty et al., 2015); and Lrit3 and GPR179 (Mazade et al., 2024; Zeitz et al., 2023). Similarly, retinal degenerative diseases are frequently associated with high myopia in humans and mice (Hendriks et al., 2017; Park et al., 2013; see Chapter 5). Mutations disrupting signaling between photoreceptors and ON bipolar cells are also associated with myopia (Zeitz et al., 2023). The loss of rod function in transgenic mice prevents experimental myopia (Park et al., 2014), while the loss of cone function (Chakraborty et al., 2019) or melanopsin function (Chakraborty et al., 2022) caused increased myopic shifts.

Why In Vitro Models Are Poised to Advance This Field

Whatever the brain's role, if it were hypothesized that the eye can autonomously link retinal images to local changes in eye growth, the key biological processes would be narrowed to a small and accessible piece of tissue. The question from a neurobiological perspective is then, Which cells are critically involved in linking image data to scleral output? Current technology makes it relatively easy to monitor the excitability of many types of retinal neurons and how visual stimulus patterns alter retinal activity. In the context of myopigenesis, data from the chick model indicate that the scleral response to image manipulation can be remarkably fast—on the order of hours or less. Surprisingly, the one study that attempted to measure this found that lens defocus effects did not occur *in vitro*, nor in intact animals anesthetized by either of two different methods (Bitzer & Schaeffel, 2006). It seems important to try to develop a stronger empirical grounding for the idea that there is an autonomous ocular process of refractive growth. If myopigenesis could be captured in a dish, a wealth of imaging, electrophysiological, and pharmacological tricks could be used to corner the key biological processes.

Retinal Mechanisms for Encoding Defocus

Most retinal neurons are sensitive to spatial and temporal contrast. Tuning differs from one neuronal type to the next and is typically modulated by visual context. Blur reduces spatiotemporal contrast, which will reduce the responsiveness of most retinal cells. Thus, at least in this very general sense, the retina can encode blur. Hyperopic and myopic defocus of the retinal image similarly blur the image in the photoreceptor plane, but they exert opposite effects on eye growth. The eye detects and homeostatically minimizes defocus through differential eye growth (emmetropization). Thus, though defocus and blur share some features, they are not the same. Since the connection between eye and brain is not required for the differing effects of hyperopic and myopic defocus, the retina must encode the sign of defocus, but how?

There are cues in the visual image that might permit direct and real-time neural discrimination between myopic and hyperopic defocus, but such retinal neurons that can discriminate the sign of defocus have not yet been identified. The closest "defocus detector" neuron to be identified so far has been the finding that glucagonergic amacrine cells (GA cells) in chicks encode the sign of defocus in the levels of expression of ZENK (a.k.a. zif268 or Egr-1), an immediate early gene (ZENK [a.k.a. zif268; Egr-1]; Bitzer & Schaeffel, 2006; Brand et al., 2007). GA cells are killed by colchicine, which enhances axial eye growth, but not by other agents, such as quisqualate and ethylcholine mustard, that fail to have this effect despite killing many other amacrine cells (Fischer et al. 1999). This evidence implicates GA cells as key players in regulating chick eye growth.

However, these effects have not been reproduced in any *in vitro* experiments, nor when the chicks were anesthetized (Bitzer & Schaeffel, 2006). Thus, much remains uncertain about how these amacrine cells encode the sign of defocus and how these signals might engage scleral growth mechanisms. The relevance of this avian glucagon story for human emmetropization is therefore unclear. Mammals appear to lack a glucagon-expressing amacrine cell type, though a cell of similar function but lacking glucagon expression might exist (Mathis & Schaeffel, 2007).

The effects of defocus on eye growth may not require the presence of neurons carrying a real-time sign-of-defocus signal. Dynamics in accommodation and/or circadian rhythms in eye growth could also provide cues by modulating the responsiveness of contrast-sensitive retinal neurons on different time scales.

It seems important to know whether the key effects of defocus on eye growth can be recapitulated in an *in vitro* context where these other dynamic factors would play no role. In other words, a key unresolved question is whether the retina autonomously computes some internal representation of the sign of defocus from the retinal image (Schaeffel & Wildsoet, 2013).

In relation to evidence that nitric oxide (NO) may be a key retino-scleral signal (see below), it may also be relevant that the retina is one source of ocular nitric oxide synthase (NOS) (Lee et al., 2023). Very specific sets of amacrine cells express neuronal nitric oxide synthase (nNOS; Jacoby et al., 2018; Park et al., 2020).

Chromatic Mechanisms

As is mentioned above, LCA is a property of the retinal image that could be used to compute the sign of defocus (see Effects of Chromacity in Chapter 5). These experiments have shown that the spectral influence on myopia susceptibility is species-dependent. For instance, short-wavelength (blue) light slows eye growth and is protective for experimental myopia in chickens and guinea pigs (Foulds et al., 2013; Jiang et al., 2014; Liu et al., 2011; Long et al., 2009; Rohrer et al., 1992; Schaeffel et al., 1991; Seidemann & Schaeffel, 2002; Torii et al., 2017; Wang et al., 2011), but long wavelength (red) light has this effect in Rhesus monkeys and tree shrews (Gawne et al., 2017; Hung et al., 2018; Liu et al., 2014; She et al., 2023; Smith et al., 2015). Gawne & Norton (2020) have developed a model, based on opponent long-and short-wavelength-sensitive contrast channels, to explain how LCA could be read out by the nervous system to control eye growth. However, emmetropization is observed in chicks reared in quasi-monochromatic environments, so chromatic cues are apparently not necessary (Smith et al., 2015). In addition, the differences in chromatic sensitivity for eye growth between close mammalian species do not lend support for this to be an evolutionarily conserved pathway for refractive eye growth.

Short-wavelength light is abundant in daylight and is particularly effective in activating unconventional retinal opsins, namely melanopsin (Opn4) and neuropsin (Opn5), both of which have been linked to mechanisms of myopia (Chakraborty et al., 2022; D'Souza et al., 2021; Jiang et al., 2021; Linne et al., 2023). These experiments have implicated Opn5 in the protective effects of violet light (Jiang et al., 2021) and shown that violet light had a diurnal effect, with evening hours being the most protective in the mouse model. The protective effects of blue light in a mouse model were eliminated in a mouse with dysfunctional cones (Strickland et al., 2020).

Chromatic encoding in the retina is a cone-based process and operates best in daylight conditions. There are numerous types of wavelength-sensitive RGCs, with patterns that differ dramatically across myopia model organisms. All mammals share a blue-yellow opponent mechanism in the inner retina which seems well suited to some aspects of encoding LCA. Short-wavelength-cone-specific bipolar cells appear to be a conserved feature of mammalian retinal organization (Haverkamp et al., 2005), and they are a type of ON bipolar cell. Some of these contribute to conscious color vision (Dacey & Lee, 1994)

RETINA-TO-SCLERA SIGNALING CASCADE: THE ROLES OF THE RETINAL PIGMENT EPITHELIUM (RPE), CHOROID, AND SCLERA IN POSTNATAL OCULAR GROWTH AND MYOPIA DEVELOPMENT

Convincing evidence over the past 40 years indicates that postnatal eye growth is largely controlled by an intraocular retina-to-sclera chemical cascade (see Figure 6-10). This cascade is initiated by the quality of visual images on the retina, leading to molecular changes in the retina, the RPE and choroid, ultimately effecting changes in the sclera through scleral extracellular matrix synthesis and scleral biomechanics, resulting finally in eye shape. While many aspects of this cascade remain to be determined, discussed below are key findings that have elucidated some elements of this process.

RPE

The RPE has been implicated in refractive eye development, as it is located immediately adjacent to the retina, where it can relay any retina-derived growth regulatory signals to the choroid and sclera. The structure of the RPE consists of a single layer of pigmented cells that are interdigitated with the photoreceptor outer segments. The RPE has important functions for the regeneration of visual pigments and ionic transport (Strauss, 2005). Moreover, the RPE is known to be a major source of cytokines and growth factors (Strauss, 2005) and several studies have demonstrated differential expression of several genes in the RPE during changes in visually guided eye growth (Zhang et al., 2012, 2013, 2019).

Morphological changes have been reported in the RPE of experimental animals with induced myopia (Fleming et al., 1997; Harman et al., 1999; Lin et al., 1993). In chick and mammalian models of myopia, increases in the total area of the RPE layer were coupled with an increase in the surface area of individual RPE cells without increases in RPE cell number, as a mechanism of maintaining the coverage of the expanded globe (Fleming et al., 1997; Harman et al., 1999; Lin et al., 1993). Furthermore, in chick eyes allowed to recover from form-deprivation-induced myopia, significant edema and altered basal infoldings in the RPE along with thickening of Bruch's membrane were noted (Liang et al., 1996). Involvement of the RPE in refractive eye growth has also been implicated in co-culture experiments, in which the presence of the RPE stimulated a proliferation of scleral fibroblasts (Seko et al., 1994, 1997). Moreover, the presence of the RPE was required in eye cup preparations to mediate the effects of insulin on choroid thickening and scleral glycosaminoglycan (GAG) synthesis in eyes recovering from myopia (Sheng et al., 2013). Taken together, these animal studies indicate that the RPE may, at least in part, participate in the retina-to-sclera signaling cascade *in vivo* to regulate ocular growth postnatally.

Evidence for Choroidal Involvement

The choroid is a complex tissue, consisting of a rich blood supply, lymphatic vessels, stromal cells, intrinsic choroidal neurons, extravascular smooth muscle, and axons of sympathetic, parasympathetic, and sensory neurons (Nickla & Wallman, 2010). Of much interest are the choroidal changes associated with emmetropization and the control of postnatal ocular growth, as any retinal-derived scleral growth regulator must pass through the choroid, or act on the choroid to synthesize additional molecular signals that can subsequently act on the sclera to stimulate scleral extracellular matrix remodeling.

Several studies have characterized the choroidal changes associated with recovery and compensation for myopic defocus. In chickens, choroidal thickening (Wallman et al., 1995), increased choroidal permeability (Pendrak et al., 2000; Rada & Palmer, 2007), and increased choroidal blood flow (Fitzgerald et al., 2002; Jin & Stjernschantz, 2000) have been well documented during recovery from induced myopia. In guinea pigs, choroidal thinning is associated with lens-induced myopia (Yu et al. 2021) and form deprivation (FD; Chen et al. 2022, 2024). Choroidal thinning is accompanied by decreased blood vessel density and reduced choroidal blood flow (Che et al., 2024). Similar to chicks, recovery from form deprivation myopia is associated with choroidal thickening and increased choroidal vessel diameter (Chen et al., 2022). Additionally, during recovery or compensation to positive lenses, increases have been observed in the choroidal synthesis of interleukin 6 (IL-6) retinoic acid (Mertz & Wallman, 2000; Summers & Martinez, 2021; Troilo et al., 2006), the retinoic-acid synthesizing enzyme ALDH1a2 (Harper et al., 2016), ovotransferrin (Rada et al., 2001), and apolipoprotein A-I (Summers et al., 2016). Of these four, retinoic acid is the most promising candidate as a direct scleral growth regulator (discussed below).

In addition to the choroidal vascular and chemical changes associated with changes in ocular growth, the overall thickness of the choroid has been shown to be modulated in response to visual stimuli. Wallman et al. (1995) were the first to show that choroidal thickness is modulated in response to optical defocus in chickens, becoming thicker with myopic defocus (image in front of the retina), thereby pushing the retina forward toward the image plane, and thinner with hyperopic defocus (image behind the retina). Choroidal thickness changes have subsequently been demonstrated in mammalian models of myopia and in humans, although choroidal changes are small (< 50 micrometers) in primates, contributing to less than a 1 D change in refractive error (Troilo et al., 2000a). It has been suggested that the modulation of choroidal thickness is one mechanism to rapidly adjust the position of the retina closer to the focal plane, moving the retina proximally under conditions of myopic defocus, and distally with hyperopic defocus. It has also been suggested that choroidal thickness can mediate the scleral response. For example, if a thicker choroid provides a greater diffusional barrier to a stimulatory growth factor secreted by the retina or retinal pigment epithelium (Nickla & Wallman, 2010), or if it affords greater protection from stretching of the sclera by the intraocular pressure (van Alphen, 1961, 1986), then scleral growth might decrease after the choroid becomes thicker in myopic eyes. Choroidal thickening has been attributed to changes in the tonus of extravascular smooth muscle, possibly via inputs from both parasympathetic nitrergic and sympathetic adrenergic systems (Poukens et al., 1988), changes in choroidal vascular permeability (Pendrak et al., 2000; Rada & Palmer, 2007), altered transport of fluid from the retina across the RPE (Crewther et al., 2006), and increased synthesis and accumulation of Thyaluronic acid (Rada et al. 2010).

Changes in the Sclera

The elongation of the eye is closely related to the biomechanical properties of the sclera, which in turn are largely dependent on the composition of the scleral extracellular matrix. Therefore, an understanding of the cellular and extracellular events involved in the regulation of scleral growth and remodeling during childhood and young adulthood will provide future avenues for the treatment of myopia and its associated ocular complications.

The Highly Myopic Human Sclera

In highly myopic human eyes, the sclera undergoes significant thinning and gradually expands under the force of normal intraocular pressure. This thinner sclera and elongated globe put individuals at increased risk of serious disorders that can lead to blindness, such as retinal detachment, glaucoma, and macular degeneration (Pan et al., 2013; Qiu et al., 2013). Additionally, in myopia the tensile strength of the sclera is reduced, and the elasticity of the sclera is increased, especially at the posterior pole (Avetisov et al., 1983). The scleral stroma exhibits a more layered, lamellar structure, like that of the cornea (Curtin & Teng, 1958; Funata & Tokoro, 1990; McBrien et al., 1991). Scleral collagen fibril bundles are thinner as compared with those of emmetropic human eyes, and a preponderance of unusually small-diameter fibrils averaging below 60–70 nm can be found at the posterior pole of the sclera (Curtin & Teng, 1958; Curtin et al., 1979).

Researchers have also observed in the highly myopic eye abnormal collagen fibrils associated with an amorphous cementing substance and the presence of fissured or star-shaped fibrils (Curtin & Teng, 1958; Curtin et al., 1979, 1985). Together, these observations suggest a derangement of the growth and organization of the collagen fibrils in the highly myopic sclera, due to abnormal fibril formation, the accumulation of abnormal non-collagenous extracellular matrix material, and/or the presence of accentuated breakdown or catabolism of the sclera. As proof of concept, mice that lack the glycosylated proteins (proteoglycans) lumican and fibromodulin, or that have a mutation in the lumican gene (L199P) exhibit abnormal scleral collagen fibrils, overall scleral thinning, and increased axial length (Chakravarti et al., 2003; Song et al., 2016). It has been found that sulfated proteoglycans continue to be synthesized and accumulate in the human sclera throughout young adulthood (Rada et al., 2000a). This fact, together with the known functions of sulfated proteoglycans in collagen fibril assembly and organization, suggests that abnormal scleral proteoglycan biosynthesis in childhood and adolescent years may lead to disruption of the normal scleral extracellular matrix and abnormalities in ocular globe size and refraction, either as a result of an intrinsic defect or in response to the visual environment.

Given the important role of the sclera in controlling eye size and refraction, the association of genetic mutations in several scleral extracellular matrix components with the development of high myopia is not surprising. Genes that have been found to be responsible for myopia in association with other genetic syndromes include COL2A1 and COL11A1 for Stickler syndromes type 1 and 2 respectively (Annunen et al., 1999), lysyl-protocollagen hydroxylase for type VI Ehlers-Danlos syndrome (Heikkinen et al., 1997), COL18/A1 for Knobloch syndrome (Mahajan et al., 2010), and fibrillin for Marfan syndrome (Kainulainen et al., 1994; Paluru et al., 2003). Additionally, mutations in the gene, *LEPREL1*, encoding prolyl 3-hydroxylase 2, a gene responsible for collagen crosslinking, is associated with high myopia in Bedouin Israeli consanguineous kindred (Mordechai et al., 2011). Together, these conditions underscore the importance of extracellular matrix in maintaining scleral integrity, eye size, and refraction.

Scleral Changes in Experimental Myopia

Animal models of myopia have demonstrated an association between the development of induced myopia and recovery and significant changes in scleral collagen and proteoglycan synthesis, accumulation, and turnover (Norton & Rada, 1995; Rada et al., 1991, 2000b). In most vertebrates, an inner layer of cartilage and an outer fibrous layer comprise the sclera. However, in placental mammals (including humans and other primates such as the marmoset, macaque monkey, tree shrew, and mice), the entire sclera consists of the fibrous, type I collagen-dominated extracellular matrix, and the inner layer of cartilage that other vertebrates have is absent. Interestingly, the extracellular matrix molecules that were previously believed to be unique to cartilage, such as aggrecan, PRELP, and cartilage olimeric matrix protein (COMP), have been shown to be present in the mammalian sclera (Young et al., 2003), suggesting that cartilaginous components have been retained in the sclera through evolution and serve important biochemical and biomechanical functions (Coster et al., 1987; Johnson et al., 2006; Rada et al., 1997). In both mammals (Norton & Rada, 1995; Rada et al., 2000b) and birds (Gottlieb et al., 1990; Marzani & Wallman, 1997), the fibrous sclera thins and loses material as ocular elongation accelerates. In birds, increased growth of the cartilaginous layer of the sclera as the eye elongates is accompanied by an increase in dry weight and in the synthesis and accumulation of proteoglycans (Christensen & Wallman, 1991; Rada et al. 1991). At some level, all vertebrates probably use similar signaling mechanisms to control the sclera, but do so by controlling growth in the cartilage, where it is present, and by controlling remodeling in the fibrous sclera.

Similar to the scleral changes of the highly myopic human eye, described above, myopia development in nonhuman primates and tree shrews is associated with scleral thinning and changes in collagen fiber diameter and organization (Phillips et al., 2000; Rada et al., 2000b), and changes in biomechanical properties of the sclera associated with myopia development have been reported in tree shrews, guinea pigs, mice and chickens (Brown et al., 2022; Grytz & Siegwart, 2015; Hoerig et al., 2022; Lewis et al., 2014; McBrien et al., 2009). In tree shrews, the visco-elasticity in the sclera, as measured as the "creep rate" (continued elongation under a constant tension similar to that produced by intraocular pressure), was shown to increase significantly in form-deprived eyes relative to the contralateral control eye (Siegwart & Norton, 1999; Figure 6-11).

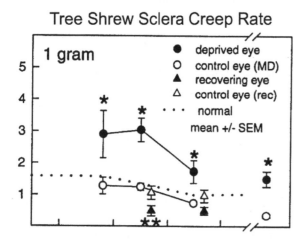

FIGURE 6-11 Creep rate of tree shrew scleral strips.
NOTES: Creep rate from deprived eyes (filled circles) and control eyes (open circles), and from eyes recovering from form deprivation myopia (filled triangles) and controls (open triangles) under 1 gram of tension. The data are plotted at the day of treatment when the creep rate was measured (visual experience). The dashed lines are the average creep rate of normal, untreated tree shrew sclera. Single asterisks indicate significant differences ($p < 0.05$) between the treated and control eye values. Double asterisks indicate significant differences between recovering and control eyes ($p < 0.05$).
SOURCE: Siegwart & Norton, 1999.

The increase in visco-elasticity would be expected to render the sclera more extensible, so that normal intraocular pressure may produce an enlargement of the vitreous chamber. Remarkably, when unrestricted vision in these animal subjects was restored (recovery), the scleral creep rate decreased rapidly and fell significantly below control levels within 2 days of removal of the diffuser, contributing to a recovery from myopia.

Nevertheless, the macromolecular changes in the sclera, directly responsible for mediating the increase in scleral creep rate during myopia development, have not been identified. Based on the minimal amount of time required to effect changes in scleral visco-elasticity in response to visual stimuli, it is reasonable to speculate that the synthesis and accumulation of smaller non-collagenous proteins may be altered in the sclera during visually guided ocular growth that may influence collagen fibril interactions and scleral biomechanics.

For example, changes in scleral cross-linking have been suggested to play a role controlling scleral visco-elasticity and ocular elongation. As mentioned above, mutations in prolyl-3-hydroxylase 2, an enzyme involved in collagen cross-linking, are associated with high-axial-grade myopia in an Israeli kindred (Mordechai et al., 2011). Using the tree shrew animal model of form deprivation myopia, McBrien and Norton (1994) demonstrated that prevention of collagen cross-linking, through the systemic administration of β-aminoproprionitrile (β-APN), resulted in markedly exaggerated elongation in myopic eyes as compared to myopic eyes treated with vehicle only. Interestingly, β-APN had no effect on contralateral control eyes, suggesting that additional scleral constituents are involved in restraining ocular elongation under normal visual conditions, even when scleral cross-linking is reduced. These results exemplify the dynamic nature of the sclera and compel investigation into the molecular basis of the visually driven changes in scleral biomechanics.

In the chick model, the outer fibrous layer of the sclera also undergoes remodeling during the development of myopia, as evidenced by an increased expression of matrix metalloproteinase-2 (MMP-2), decreased expression of tissue inhibitor of metalloproteinase (TIMP)-2, an endogenous inhibitor of MMP-2 (Rada & Brenza, 1995; Rada et al., 1999), decreased rate of proteoglycan synthesis (Marzani & Wallman, 1997; Rada et al., 1994), and overall thinning (Gottlieb et al., 1990). In contrast to the fibrous layer of chick sclera, the cartilaginous layer demonstrates increased synthesis and accumulation of DNA and of proteoglycans (Figure 6-12A; particularly of aggrecan) and overall thickening during the development of myopia (Christensen & Wallman, 1991; Rada et al., 1991, 1994).

In all species examined, the changes in scleral extracellular matrix synthesis and degradation are greatest at the posterior pole of the globe (Norton & Rada, 1995; Rada et al., 1994, 2000b), suggesting that these animal models of myopia accurately model the scleral changes associated with high myopia in humans. The localized response in the posterior sclera may be related to regional differences in the growth states of the scleral fibroblasts in this region or may be a reflection of a concentration of visually induced changes in the retina, choroid, and sclera along the visual axis. In chicks, tree shrews, and marmosets, scleral changes associated with myopia development are rapidly reversed when eyes are allowed to experience unrestricted vision from a prior period of form vision deprivation or when negative lens-induced defocus is discontinued (recovery). The slowed elongation of the vitreous chamber in the recovering eyes is associated with decreases in MMP-2 activity, increases in TIMP-2 activity, and increased proteoglycan synthesis in the fibrous sclera of marmosets and tree shrews (McBrien & Gentle, 2003; Rada et al., 2000b). In addition, GAG levels, which are reduced during myopia development by negative lenses, return to normal (Moring et al., 2007). In the posterior cartilaginous sclera of chicks, there is a rapid decrease in proteoglycan synthesis within hours following restoration of unrestricted vision (Figure 6-12 B; Summers Rada & Hollaway, 2011). In both chicks and tree shrews, changes in scleral GAG synthesis and levels during recovery occur prior to, or at least as early as, the most rapid deceleration in vitreous chamber elongation (Moring et al., 2007; Summers Rada & Hollaway, 2011), suggesting that changes in scleral extracellular matrix remodeling are responsible for changes in ocular elongation and refraction.

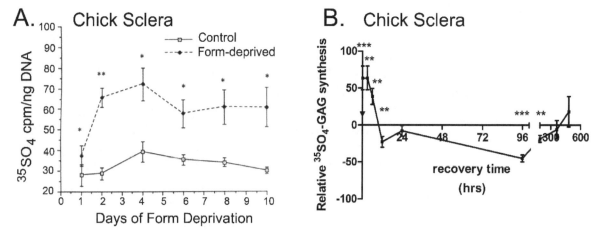

FIGURE 6-12 Changes in scleral proteoglycan synthesis during visually guided ocular growth.
NOTES: (A) Changes in 35S04-scleral proteoglycan synthesis during the development of form-deprivation myopia and (B) during recovery from induced myopia. Scleral proteoglycan synthesis rates are rapidly increased in response to form deprivation and rapidly decreased following removal of the occluder in response to the induced myopic defocus.
SOURCE: (A) Adapted from Rada et al., 1992; (B) Summers Rada & Hollaway, 2011.

Taken together, these animal studies demonstrate that scleral extracellular remodeling occurs rapidly in response to visual stimuli to adjust eye size and refraction. Identification of the visually driven signals within the eye responsible for the regulation of scleral remodeling would greatly aid in the understanding of the pathogenesis of myopia and likely lead to a viable anti-myopia therapy. While more work is needed to confirm these results in human sclera, a few studies indicate that alterations in scleral stiffness and extracellular matrix metabolism are present in the human sclera with increased axial length (reviewed in Boote et al., 2020; Harper & Summers, 2015; Katayama et al., 2021).

Chemical Mediators in the Retina-to-Sclera Signaling Cascade

As mentioned above, it is theorized that visually induced changes in ocular length are the result of a retina-to-choroid-to-scleral signaling cascade (or retino-scleral signaling pathways) that ultimately results in extracellular matrix remodeling of the scleral shell (Norton & Rada, 1995; Rada et al., 1991, 2000b). The exact members of this signaling cascade and how they interact have not yet been determined. Figure 6-12 summarizes the results of multiple investigations by many researchers that have identified key signaling molecules and pathways involved in the retina, RPE, choroid, and sclera.

Retinoic Acid

The vitamin A derivative, all-trans-retinoic acid (atRA) may be an important component for the control of postnatal ocular growth (McFadden et al., 2004; Mertz & Wallman, 2000; Seko et al., 1998; Troilo et al., 2006). Experimental treatment with atRA in guinea pigs, chickens, and mice resulted in larger eye size (Brown et al., 2023; Li et al., 2010; McFadden et al., 2004, 2006), but not always myopic refractive errors (McFadden et al., 2004). Molecular biological approaches have revealed that ocular atRA synthesis is regulated in response to visual stimuli exclusively though choroidal expression of the atRA synthesizing enzyme, retinaldehyde dehydrogenase 2 (RALDH2; Harper et al., 2016; Rada et al., 2012). While the source of atRA production was unknown, it was demonstrated in chicks and humans that RALDH2 is synthesized by a population of stromal cells, some of which are closely associated with blood vessels (Harper et al., 2015, 2016; Rada et al., 2012; Summers et al., 2020). In chicks, RALDH2 positive cells increased with recovery (Harper et al., 2016). Furthermore, RALDH2+ cells have been shown to co-localize with the intermediate filament vimentin (human) and collagen type I (chick). The presence of vimentin and collagen type I in RALDH2 positive cells suggests that RALDH2+ cells may resemble perivascular fibroblasts and suggests a potential role for retinoic acid in mediating some aspects of the choroidal response during recovery from induced myopia (Harper et al., 2016).

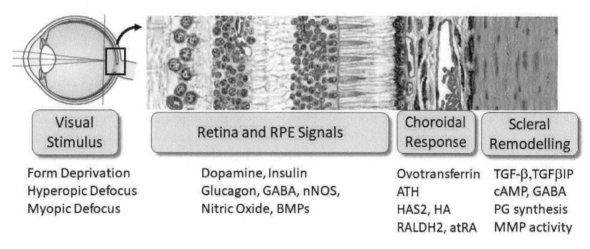

FIGURE 6-13 Schematic Diagram illustrating the retina-to-sclera signaling cascade regulating visually guided eye growth.
NOTES: The diagram summarizes the key tissue-specific signaling pathways found to be involved in visually guided eye development. Visual form deprivation and hyperopic optical defocus stimulate eye growth, whereas myopic defocus inhibits it. The retina processes information about optical defocus and converts this information into molecular signals, which are transmitted across the retina, RPE and choroid to the sclera via a multilayered signaling cascade. The signals generated by optical defocus cause remodeling of the sclera and adjust the growth rate of the posterior segment of the eye to match the optical power of the eye with its axial length.
SOURCE: Adapted from Summers et al., 2021.

Adenosine

Adenosine is one of the four nucleosides of DNA and RNA and is found abundantly in organic compounds. A role for adenosine in myopia was found with evidence that 7-methylxanthine (7-MX), a nonselective inhibitor of adenosine receptors and a metabolite of caffeine, influenced scleral collagen and proteoglycan content in rabbits (Trier et al., 1999). Many other studies have also shown that endogenous, exogenous, or genetic manipulation or adenosine can alter axial length (Beach et al., 2018; Liu et al., 2020; Smith et al., 2021; Srinivasalu et al., 2018). Treatment with 7-MX has been shown to reduce myopia progression in chicken, rabbits, guinea pigs, macaques, and children (Cui et al., 2011; Hung et al., 2018; Nie et al., 2012; Trier et al., 2008; Wang et al., 2014). However, oral 7-MX treatment in chickens and tree shrews showed minimal effects on lens defocus and no effect on form deprivation (Khanal et al. 2020; Liu et al., 2020; Wang et al., 2014).

Nitric Oxide

Evidence is now emerging that nitric oxide (NO) may play a significant role in the postnatal control of ocular growth and myopia development. *In vivo* administration of the nonspecific nitric oxide synthase inhibitor, L-NAME, inhibits the choroidal and scleral responses associated with recovery from induced myopia. Specifically, blockade of NO synthesis prevents choroidal thickening and choroidal IL6 synthesis in recovering chick eyes; it also disinhibits scleral proteoglycan synthesis, resulting in an increase in the rate of axial elongation in recovering eyes (Nickla & Wildsoet, 2004; Nickla et al., 2006; Summers & Martinez, 2021). Furthermore, administration of NO donors (PAPA-NONOate and sodium nitroprusside; SNP) as well as the NO precursor, l-arginine, slows the rate of ocular elongation and myopia in chicks and guinea pigs (Carr & Stell, 2016; McFadden, 2021). Additionally, NO has been shown to mediate the ocular growth-inhibiting properties of both the muscarinic receptor antagonist, atropine (Abdel-Messeih et al., 2017), and the dopamine agonist, quinpirole (Nickla et al., 2013).

Therefore, experts predict that NO is one of the earliest signaling events in the process of emmetropization, since administration of L-NAME immediately prior to recovery blocks the recovery-induced increase in IL6 observed following 6 hours of recovery (Summers & Martinez, 2021) as well as the change in choroidal thickening and axial elongation observed 7 hours after recovery (Nickla & Wildsoet, 2004). Taken together, these results suggest that NO acts to slow myopic eye growth, and inhibition of NO synthesis prevents recovery from induced myopia. While neither the cellular source of NO nor the target of NO mediating these effects on eye growth have been identified, it is possible that one or more cell populations in the choroid is a potential target of NO. This prediction is based on the observation that administration of L-NAME reduces choroidal concentrations of nitrate (Nickla et al., 2006) and that choroidal expression of interleukin 6 (IL6) is mediated by NO (Summers & Martinez, 2021).

CIRCADIAN RHYTHMS AND THE REGULATION OF POSTNATAL OCULAR GROWTH

Rhythms in Ocular Growth

Many studies over the past 50 years have suggested that circadian rhythms may play a role in the control of ocular growth (Jensen & Matson, 1957; Lauber & Kinnear, 1979; Lauber et al., 1961; Lauber & McGinnis, 1966; Lauber & Kivett, 1981). Initial work in chickens demonstrated that exposure to constant light or constant darkness resulted in excessive eye growth and corneal flattening, leading to the idea that emmetropization requires a normal light/dark cycle to synchronize ocular rhythms. Moreover, the growing eyes of chickens and monkeys demonstrated a diurnal rhythm in axial length: eyes grew faster during the day than during the night, while eyes that were deprived of form vision by translucent diffusers grew rapidly during both day and night (Nickla & Wildsoet, 1998a,b; Papastergiou et al., 1998; Weiss & Schaeffel, 1993) resulting in excessive overall elongation.

The rate of growth of the chicken eye is largely determined by the rate of synthesis of the extracellular matrix proteoglycan aggrecan by scleral chondrocytes (Rada et al., 1991, 1992, 1994). Because ocular growth shows diurnal fluctuations, it was predicted that scleral proteoglycan synthesis should also fluctuate in a diurnal pattern, and their phases should be correlated. To test this hypothesis, proteoglycan synthesis was measured in punches of sclera, dissected from normal or form-deprived chicken eyes in the morning, afternoon, or midnight, and cultured for 2 hours in radiolabeled sulfur. Results from these studies showed that proteoglycan synthesis was highest during the morning and lowest at midnight (Nickla et al., 1999). Moreover, the rhythm in scleral proteoglycan synthesis appears to be endogenous, as opposed to being light-driven, as it persists even when sclera are isolated and cultured over several days (Nickla et al., 1999, 2001). These results strongly support the observation that diurnal rhythms in scleral extracellular matrix synthesis underlie the diurnal rhythms in axial length in chicks. They demonstrate the existence of an endogenous clock in scleral chondrocytes, the first report of clocks in non-neuronal tissues in vertebrates.

There is also a rhythm in the thickness of the chicken choroid, with a peak at around midnight, coincident with the shortest axial length, and the relative phases of the rhythms in choroidal thickness and axial length change during experimentally induced changes in ocular growth rate, suggesting an influence of ocular rhythms on normal ocular growth and refraction (Nickla & Wildsoet, 1998a,b; Papastergiou et al., 1998). The human choroid exhibits a similar rhythm in thickness, with the choroid being significantly thicker at night and thinner in the daytime. These thickness changes, of about 20 μm, were significantly negatively correlated with systolic blood pressure (Usui et al., 2012).

Molecular Regulation of Ocular Circadian Rhythms

Genetic studies in humans and in animal models have implicated many genes and pathways involved in circadian rhythms (Hysi et al., 2020; Stone et al., 2024). Retinal levels of dopamine, a diurnally oscillating transmitter (discussed above), are decreased in form-deprived eyes, but only during the daytime when levels are normally highest. This suggests that form deprivation might constitute a type of "constant lighting condition" similar to constant light or darkness, leading to excessive axial elongation (Stone et al., 1989). Altered retinal expression of clock and circadian rhythm-related genes have been identified through experimental myopia in chickens and mice (Karouta et al., 2021; Riddel et al., 2016; Stone et al., 2011; Tkatchenko & Tkatchenko, 2021).

Specific visual alterations that experimentally induce refractive errors in chicks each alters the diurnal expression of clock and circadian rhythm genes (Stone et al., 2020). In mice, retinal-specific knockout of the clock gene *Bmal1* induces myopia (Stone et al., 2019); knockout of the melanopsin gene in the retina, a key modulator of circadian rhythms, alters normal eye development and augments experimental myopia (Chakroborty et al., 2022); and ablating intrinsically photosensitive retinal ganglion cells (ipRGCs), which contain melanopsin, suppresses myopia (Liu et al., 2022). In addition, findings from human genome-wide association studies have identified hundreds of specific genes and genetic loci associated with myopia and/or refractive error, including genes that point to genetic networks involving light sensitivity and circadian control (Fleming et al., 1997; Tedja et al., 2018).

Taken together, these experimental and clinical observations provide compelling evidence for the role of circadian rhythms in postnatal ocular growth regulation and myopia pathogenesis.

CONCLUSIONS

Conclusion 6-1: Retinal images regulate eye growth mainly through intrinsic regulatory functions of the eye itself. The entire retina—not only, or even primarily, the fovea—plays a critical role in this process.

Conclusion 6-2: The 'luminance network' of the retina provides a mechanistic link between the reduced time today's child spends outdoors and the increased incidence of myopia. This network, which encodes light intensity, includes dopaminergic amacrine cells and melanopsin-expressing intrinsically photosensitive retinal ganglion cells. It is uniquely dependent on some subset of channels within the retinal ON pathways, which have been implicated in myopia pathogenesis in diverse ways.

Conclusion 6-3: A closed feedback loop is essential for achieving precise homeostasis of eye growth. The specific contributions from candidate retinal image properties responsible for fine-tuning this process—such as defocus, blur, contrast (spatial, spectral, and temporal) and chromaticity—are currently unknown. The specific mechanisms through which these features are encoded by the retino-scleral signaling cascade are also unknown. More research is needed to determine how the retina encodes these image features and links them to refractive growth signals.

Conclusion 6-4: Animal models have provided important insights into potentially conserved processes controlling postnatal eye growth, such as visually driven signaling events in the retina, retinal pigment epithelium, and choroid that regulate the remodeling of the scleral extracellular matrix as well as eye size and refraction.

Conclusion 6-5: In infancy through adulthood, the sclera responds rapidly to visual stimuli by remodeling the extracellular matrix, altering biomechanical properties and changing eye shape and refraction.

Conclusion 6-6: Animal studies show that the quality of the peripheral retinal image— whether signed defocus, blur, contrast, or some other feature—is critical for emmetropization. For children, predicting the peripheral retinal image with optical interventions or environmental risk factors is more complicated than previously appreciated, due to individual and eccentricity-specific differences in optical aberrations and how they vary with eye shape. This problem arises from the lack of adequate eye models that link visual diet to image formation across the entire retina.

RECOMMENDATIONS

Recommendation 6-1: Funding agencies, including the National Institutes of Health, the National Science Foundation, the Department of Defense, and private

foundations, as well as industry, should seek to fund proposals across disciplines for both human and animal studies to investigate the mechanisms of emmetropization and myopia, including candidates for retino-scleral signaling, retinal neurons that detect the sign of defocus, the role of the choroid in regulating eye growth, the changes in the sclera that lead to axial elongation, gene–environment interactions, and the development of *in vitro* experimental models.

Recommendation 6-2: Funding agencies should target audacious proposals to foster the innovative, multidisciplinary research that is needed to fully harmonize our understanding of the visual information processing by the retina that leads to changes in scleral remodeling. Particular gaps in knowledge include the visual environment, ocular optics, retinal circuits, and signaling proteins involved in retino-scleral signaling.

Recommendation 6-3: The field of myopia research should adopt a retinocentric—in contrast to a foveocentric—approach.
- **For basic research, this means funding the development of eye models that can be readily tailored to individual variation ("personalized models") to link the visual diet to image formation across the entire retina.**
- **For industry, this means developing better technologies to measure 3D eye shape and assess the refractive state across the entire retina.**
- **For clinical researchers, this means guiding proposed optical treatments with a full understanding of the consequences for the peripheral retinal image.**

REFERENCES

Abbott, M. L., Schmid, K. L., & Strang, N. C. (1998). Differences in the accommodation stimulus response curves of adult myopes and emmetropes. *Ophthalmic Physiology Optics*, *18*(1), 13–20. https://doi.org/10.1046/j.1475-1313.1998.00294.x

Abdel-Messeih, P. L., Nosseir, N. M., & Bakhe, O. H. (2017). Evaluation of inflammatory cytokines and oxidative stress markers in prostate cancer patients undergoing curative radiotherapy. *Central European Journal of Immunology*, *42*, 68–72.

Aleman, A. C., Wang, M., & Schaeffel, F. (2018). Reading and Myopia: Contrast Polarity Matters. *Scientific Reports*, *8*(1), 10840. https://doi.org/10.1038/s41598-018-28904-x

Annunen, S., Korkko, J., Czarny, M., Warman, M. L., Brunner, H. G., Kaariainen, H., … Ala-Kokko, L. (1999). Splicing mutations of 54-bp exons in the COL11A1 gene cause Marshall syndrome, but other mutations cause overlapping Marshall/Stickler phenotypes. *American Journal of Human Genetics*, *65*, 974–983.

Aranda, M. L., & Schmidt, T. M. (2021). Diversity of intrinsically photosensitive retinal ganglion cells: circuits and functions. *Cellular and Molecular Life Sciences*, *78*(3), 889–907. https://doi.org/10.1007/s00018-020-03641-5

Ashby, R., McCarthy, C. S., Maleszka, R., Megaw, P., & Morgan, I. G. (2007). A muscarinic cholinergic antagonist and a dopamine agonist rapidly increase ZENK mRNA expression in the form-deprived chicken retina. *Experimental Eye Research*, *85*, 15–22.

Ashby, R. S., & Schaeffel, F. (2010). The effect of bright light on lens compensation in chicks. *Investigative Ophthalmology & Visual Science, 51*(10), 5247–5253. https://doi.org/10.1167/iovs.09-4689

Atchison, D. A., Li, S. M., Li, H., Li, S. Y., Liu, L. R., Kang, M. T., ... Wang, N. (2015). Relative peripheral hyperopia does not predict development and progression of myopia in children. *Investigative Ophthalmology & Visual Science, 56*(10), 6162–6170. https://doi.org/10.1167/iovs.15-17200

Atchison, D. A., Schmid, K. L., & Pritchard, N. (2006). Neural and optical limits to visual performance in myopia. *Vision Research, 46*(21), 3707–3722.

Avetisov, E. S., Savitskaya, N. F., Vinetskaya, M. I., & Iomdina, E. N. (1983). A study of biochemical and biomechanical qualities of normal and myopic eye sclera in humans of different age groups. *Metabolic Pediatric System Ophthalmology, 7*, 183–188.

Barlow, H. B., & Levick, W. R. (1969). Changes in the maintained discharge with adaptation level in the cat retina. *Journal of Physiology, 202*(3), 699–718. https://doi.org/10.1113/jphysiol.1969.sp008836

Bitzer, M., Kovacs, B., Feldkaemper, M., Schaeffel F. (2006). Effects of muscarinic antagonists on ZENK expression in the chicken retina. *Experimental Eye Research, 82*(3), 379–388. http://doi.org/10.1016/j.exer.2005.07.010

Bloomfield, S. A., & Völgyi, B. (2009). The diverse functional roles and regulation of neuronal gap junctions in the retina. *Nature Reviews. Neuroscience, 10*(7), 495–506. https://doi.org/10.1038/nrn2636

Bolz, M., Prinz, A., Drexler, W., & Findl, O. (2007). Linear relationship of refractive and biometric lenticular changes during accommodation in emmetropic and myopic eyes. *British Journal of Ophthalmology, 91*(3), 360–365. https://doi.org/10.1136/bjo.2006.099879

Boote, C., Sigal, I. A., Grytz, R., Hua, Y., Nguyen, T. D., & Girard, M. J. A. (2020). Scleral structure and biomechanics. *Progress in Retinal and Eye Research, 74*, 100773. https://doi.org/10.1016/j.preteyeres.2019.100773

Brand, C., Schaeffel, F., & Feldkaemper, M. P. (2007). A microarray analysis of retinal transcripts that are controlled by image contrast in mice. *Molecular Vision, 13*, 920–932.

Brown, D. M., Kowalski, M. A., Paulus, Q. M., Yu, J., Kumar, P., Kane, M. A., ... Pardue, M. T. (2022). Altered structure and function of murine sclera in form-deprivation myopia. *Investigative Ophthalmology & Visual Science, 63*(13), 13. https://doi.org/10.1167/iovs.63.13.13

Brown, D. M., Yu, J., Kumar, P., Paulus, Q. M., Kowalski, M. A., Patel, J. M., ... Pardue, M. T. (2023). Exogenous all-trans retinoic acid induces myopia and alters scleral biomechanics in mice. *Investigative Ophthalmology & Visual Science, 64*(5), 22. https://doi.org/10.1167/iovs.64.5.22

Bullimore, M. (2024). [Animal models of myopia: Lessons for the understanding of human myopia]. Commissioned Paper for the Committee on Focus on Myopia: Pathogenesis and Rising Incidence.

Cakmak, H. B., Cagil, N., Simavli, H., Duzen, B., & Simsek, S. (2010). Refractive error may influence mesopic pupil size. *Current Eye Research, 35*(2), 130–136.

Calver, R., Radhakrishnan, H., Osuobeni, E., & O'Leary, D. (2007). Peripheral refraction for distance and near vision in emmetropes and myopes. *Ophthalmic Physiology Optics, 27*, 584–593.

Campbell, M. C., Bunghardt, K., Kisilak, M. L., & Irving, E. L. (2012). Diurnal rhythms of spherical refractive error, optical axial length, and power in the chick. *Investigative Ophthalmology & Visual Science, 53*(10), 6245–6253. https://doi.org/10.1167/iovs.11-8844

Carkeet, A., Saw, S. M., Gazzard, G., Tang, W., & Tan, D. T. (2004). Repeatability of IOLMaster biometry in children. *Optometry and Vision Science, 81*(11), 829–834. https://doi.org/10.1097/00006324-200411000-00014

Carroll, J., Neitz, J., & Neitz, M. (2002). Estimates of L: M cone ratio from ERG flicker photometry and genetics. *Journal of Vision, 2*(8), 1–1. https://doi.org/10.1167/2.8.1

Chakraborty, R., Landis, E. G., Mazade, R., Yang, V., Strickland, R., Hattar, S., ... Pardue, M. T. (2022). Melanopsin modulates refractive development and myopia. *Experimental Eye Research, 214*, 108866. https://doi.org/10.1016/j.exer.2021.108866

Christensen, A. M., & Wallman, J. (1991). Evidence that increased scleral growth underlies visual deprivation myopia in chicks. *Investigative Ophthalmology & Visual Science, 32*, 2143–2150.

Cohen, Y., Peleg, E., Belkin, M., Polat, U., & Solomon, A. S. (2012). Ambient illuminance, retinal dopamine release and refractive development in chicks. *Experimental Eye Research, 103*, 33–40. https://doi.org/10.1016/j.exer.2012.08.005

Coletta, N. J., & Watson, T. (2006). Effect of myopia on visual acuity measured with laser interference fringes. *Vision Research, 46*(5), 636–651. https://doi.org/10.1016/j.visres.2005.05.025

Collins, M. J., Wildsoet, C. F., & Atchison, D. A. (1995). Monochromatic aberrations and myopia. *Vision Research, 35*(9), 1157–1163.

Cornell, B. (2016). Cladograms. https://old-ib.bioninja.com.au/standard-level/topic-5-evolution-and-biodi/54-cladistics/cladograms.html

Coster, L., Rosenberg, L. C., van der Rest, M., & Poole, A. R. (1987). The dermatan sulfate proteoglycans of bovine sclera and their relationship to those of articular cartilage. An immunological and biochemical study. *Journal of Biological Chemistry, 262*, 3809–3812.

Cottaris, N. P., Wandell, B. A., Rieke, F., & Brainard, D. H. (2020). A computational observer model of spatial contrast sensitivity: Effects of photocurrent encoding, fixational eye movements, and inference engine. *Journal of Vision, 20*(7), 17. https://doi.org/10.1167/jov.20.7.17

Curcio, C. A., Allen, K. A., Sloan, K. R., Lerea, C. L., Hurley, J. B., Klock, I. B., & Milam, A. H. (1991). Distribution and morphology of human cone photoreceptors stained with anti-blue opsin. *Journal of Comparative Neurology, 312*(4), 610–624. https://doi.org/10.1002/cne.903120411

Curcio, C. A., Sloan, K. R., Kalina, R. E., & Hendrickson, A. E. (1990). Human photoreceptor topography. *Journal of Comparative Neurology, 292*(4), 497–523.

Curtin, B. J. (1985). *The Myopias: Basic Science and Clinical Management*. Harper & Row.

Curtin, B. J., Iwamoto, T., & Renaldo, D. P. (1979). Normal and staphylomatous sclera of high myopia. An electron microscopic study. *Archives of Ophthalmology, 97*, 912–915.

Curtin, B. J., & Teng, C. C. (1958). Scleral changes in pathological myopia. *Transactions of the American Academy of Ophthalmology and Otolaryngology, 62*, 777–788.

Davies, L. N., & Mallen, E. A. H. (2009). Influence of accommodation and refractive status on the peripheral refractive profile. *British Journal of Ophthalmology, 93*, 1186–1190. https://doi.org/10.1136/bjo.2008.153130

Diether, S., & Schaeffel, F. (1997). Local changes in eye growth induced by imposed local refractive error despite active accommodation. *Vision Research, 37*(6), 659–668. https://doi.org/10.1016/s0042-6989(96)00224-6

Do, M. T. H. (2019). Melanopsin and the intrinsically photosensitive retinal ganglion cells: Biophysics to behavior. *Neuron, 104*(2), 205–226. https://doi.org/10.1016/j.neuron.2019.07.016

Dong, F., Zhi, Z., Pan, M., Xie, R., Qin, X., Lu, R., … Zhou, X. (2011). Inhibition of experimental myopia by a dopamine agonist: Different effectiveness between form deprivation and hyperopic defocus in guinea pigs. *Molecular Vision, 17*, 2824–2834.

Feldkaemper, M., & Schaeffel, F. (2013). An updated view on the role of dopamine in myopia. *Experimental Eye Research, 114*, 106–119. https://doi.org/10.1016/j.exer.2013.03.003

Fischer, A. J., Morgan, I. G., & Stell, W. K. (1999). Colchicine causes excessive ocular growth and myopia in chicks. *Vision Research, 39*(4), 685–697. https://doi.org/10.1016/s0042-6989(98)00178-3

Fledelius, H. C., Goldschmidt, E., Haargaard, B., & Jensen, H. (2014). Human parallels to experimental myopia? A literature review on visual deprivation. *Acta Ophthalmologica, 92*(8), 724–729. https://doi.org/10.1111/aos.12412

Fleming, P. A., Harman, A. M., & Beazley, L. D. (1997). Changing topography of the RPE resulting from experimentally induced rapid eye growth. *Visual Neuroscience, 14*, 449–461.

Flitcroft, D. I. (2012). The complex interactions of retinal, optical and environmental factors in myopia aetiology. *Progress in Retinal and Eye Research, 31*(6), 622–660. https://doi.org/10.1016/j.preteyeres.2012.06.004

Funata, M., & Tokoro, T. (1990). Scleral change in experimentally myopic monkeys. *Graefe's Archive for Clinical and Experimental Ophthalmology, 228*, 174–179.

Gan, J., Li, S.-M., Atchison, D. A., Kang, M.-T., Wei, S., He, X., … Wang, N. (2022). Association between color vision deficiency and myopia in Chinese children over a five-year period. *Investigative Ophthalmology & Visual Science, 63*(2), 2. https://doi.org/10.1167/iovs.63.2.2

Gastinger, M. J., Tian, N., Horvath, T., & Marshak, D. W. (2006). Retinopetal axons in mammals: Emphasis on histamine and serotonin. *Current Eye Research, 31*(7–8), 655–667. https://doi.org/10.1080/02713680600776119

Gawne, T. J., & Norton, T. T. (2020). An opponent dual-detector spectral drive model of emmetropization. *Vision Research, 173*, 7–20.

Gawne, T. J., Ward, A. H., & Norton, T. T. (2017). Long-wavelength (red) light produces hyperopia in juvenile and adolescent tree shrews. *Vision Research, 140*, 55–65.

Gottlieb, M. D., Joshi, H. B., & Nickla, D. L. (1990). Scleral changes in chicks with form-deprivation myopia. *Current Eye Research, 9*, 1157–1165. https://doi.org/10.3109/02713689009022297

Guillon, M., Dumbleton, K., Theodoratos, P., Gobbe, M., Wooley, C. B., & Moody, K. (2016). The effects of age, refractive status, and luminance on pupil size. *Optometry and Vision Science, 93*(9), 1093–1100.

Guo, S. S., Sivak, J. G., Callender, M. G., & Diehl-Jones, B. (1995). Retinal dopamine and lens-induced refractive errors in chicks. *Current Eye Research, 14*, 385–389. https://doi.org/10.3109/02713689508995475

Gwiazda, J., Grice, K., & Thorn, F. (1999). Response AC/A ratios are elevated in myopic children. *Ophthalmic & Physiological Optics: The Journal of the British College of Ophthalmic Opticians (Optometrists), 19*(2), 173–179. https://doi.org/10.1046/j.1475-1313.1999.00437.x

Hagen, L. A., Arnegard, S., Kuchenbecker, J. A., Gilson, S. J., Neitz, M., Neitz, J., & Baraas, R. C. (2019). The association between L:M cone ratio, cone opsin genes and myopia susceptibility. *Vision Research, 162*, 20–28. https://doi.org/10.1016/j.visres.2019.06.006

Harman, A. M., Hoskins, R., & Beazley, L. D. (1999). Experimental eye enlargement in mature animals changes the retinal pigment epithelium. *Visual Neuroscience, 16*(4), 619–628. https://doi.org/10.1017/s0952523899164022

Harper, A. R., Summers, J. A., Wang, X., Moiseyev, G., & Ma, J. X. (2016). Postnatal chick choroids exhibit increased retinaldehyde dehydrogenase activity during recovery from form deprivation induced myopia. *Investigative Ophthalmology & Visual Science, 57*, 4886–4897. https://doi.org/10.1167/iovs.15-18635

Harper, A. R., Wiechmann, A. F., Moiseyev, G., Ma, J. X., & Summers, J. A. (2015). Identification of active retinaldehyde dehydrogenase isoforms in the postnatal human eye. *PLoS One, 10*(4), e0122008. https://doi.org/10.1371/journal.pone.0122008

Hartline, H. K., & Ratliff, F. (1958). Spatial summation of inhibitory influences in the eye of Limulus, and the mutual interaction of receptor units. *Journal of General Physiology, 41*(5), 1049–1066. https://doi.org/10.1085/jgp.41.5.1049

Hartwig, A., Charman, W. N., & Radhakrishnan, H. (2011). Accommodative response to peripheral stimuli in myopes and emmetropes. *Ophthalmic & Physiological Optics, 31*(1), 91–99. https://doi.org/10.1111/j.1475-1313.2010.00783.x

Haverkamp, S., Wässle, H., Duebel, J., Kuner, T., Augustine, G. J., Feng, G., & Euler, T. (2005). The primordial, blue-cone color system of the mouse retina. *Journal of Neuroscience, 25*(22), 5438–5445. https://doi.org/10.1523/jneurosci.1117-05.2005

Heikkinen, J., Toppinen, T., Yeowell, H., Krieg, T., Steinmann, B., Kivirikko, K. I., & Myllyla, R. (1997). Duplication of seven exons in the lysyl hydroxylase gene is associated with longer forms of a repetitive sequence within the gene and is a common cause for the type VI variant of Ehlers-Danlos syndrome. *American Journal of Human Genetics, 60*, 48–56.

Hung, L.-F., Arumugam, B., She, Z., Ostrin, L., & Smith, E. L. III. (2018). Narrow-band, long-wavelength lighting promotes hyperopia and retards vision-induced myopia in infant rhesus monkeys. *Experimental Eye Research, 176*, 147–160.

Hysi, P. G., Choquet, H., Khawaja, A. P., Wojciechowski, R., Tedja, M. S., Yin, J., Simcoe, M. J., Patasova, K., Mahroo, O. A., Thai, K. K., Cumberland, P. M., Melles, R. B., Verhoeven, V. J. M., Vitart, V., Segre, A., Stone, R. A., Wareham, N., Hewitt, A. W., Mackey, D. A., Klaver, C. C. W., … Hammond, C. J. (2020). Meta-analysis of 542,934 subjects of European ancestry identifies new genes and mechanisms predisposing to refractive error and myopia. *Nature Genetics, 52*(4), 401–407. https://doi.org/10.1038/s41588-020-0599-0

Iuvone, P. M., Tigges, M., Fernandes, A., & Tigges, J. (1989). Dopamine synthesis and metabolism in rhesus monkey retina: Development, aging, and the effects of monocular visual deprivation. *Visual Neuroscience, 2*(6), 465–471. https://doi.org/10.1017/S0952523800006870

Iuvone, P. M., Tigges, M., Stone, R. A., Lambert, S., & Laties, A. M. (1991). Effects of apomorphine, a dopamine receptor agonist, on ocular refraction and axial elongation in a primate model of myopia. *Investigative Ophthalmology & Visual Science, 32*(6), 1674–1677. https://doi.org/10.1167/iovs.12-10126

Jackson, C. R., Ruan, G. X., Aseem, F., Abey, J., Gamble, K., Stanwood, G., Palmiter, R. D., Iuvone, P. M., & McMahon, D. G. (2012). Retinal dopamine mediates multiple dimensions of light-adapted vision. *Journal of Neuroscience, 32*(27), 9359–9368. https://doi.org/10.1523/JNEUROSCI.1770-12.2012

Jensen, L. S., & Matson, W. E. (1957). Enlargement of avian eye by subjecting chicks to continuous incandescent illumination. *Science, 125*(3248), 741. https://doi.org/10.1126/science.125.3248.741

Jiang, L., Zhang, S., Schaeffel, F., Xiong, S., Zheng, Y., Zhou, X., Lu, F., & Qu, J. (2014). Interactions of chromatic and lens-induced defocus during visual control of eye growth in guinea pigs (Cavia porcellus). *Vision Research, 94*, 24–32. https://doi.org/10.1016/j.visres.2013.10.020

Johnson, J. M., Young, T. L., & Rada, J. A. (2006). Small leucine rich repeat proteoglycans (SLRPs) in the human sclera: Identification of abundant levels of PRELP. *Molecular Vision, 12*, 1057–1066.

Kainulainen, K., Karttunen, L., Puhakka, L., Sakai, L., & Peltonen, L. (1994). Mutations in the fibrillin gene responsible for dominant ectopia lentis and neonatal Marfan syndrome. *Nature Genetics, 6*(1), 64–69. https://doi.org/10.1038/ng0194-64

Karouta, C., Kucharski, R., Hardy, K., Thomson, K., Maleszka, R., Morgan, I., & Ashby, R. (2021). Transcriptome-based insights into gene networks controlling myopia prevention. *The FASEB Journal, 35*(12), e21846. https://doi.org/10.1096/fj.202100376R

Katayama, H., Furuhashi, M., Umetsu, A., Hikage, F., Watanabe, M., Ohguro, H., & Ida, Y. (2021). Modulation of the physical properties of 3d spheroids derived from human scleral stroma fibroblasts (HSSFs) with different axial lengths obtained from surgical patients. *Current Issues in Molecular Biology, 43*(3), 1715–1725. https://doi.org/10.3390/cimb43030121

Kisilak, M. L., Bunghardt, K., Hunter, J. J., Irving, E. L., & Campbell, M. C. (2012). Longitudinal in vivo imaging of cones in the alert chicken. *Optometry and Vision Science: Official Publication of the American Academy of Optometry, 89*(5), 644–651. https://doi.org/10.1097/OPX.0b013e31825489df

Ko, G. Y. (2020). Circadian regulation in the retina: From molecules to network. *European Journal of Neuroscience/EJN. European Journal of Neuroscience, 51*(1), 194–216. https://doi.org/10.1111/ejn.14185

Kroger, R. H., Hirt, B., & Wagner, H. J. (1999). Effects of retinal dopamine depletion on the growth of the fish eye. *Journal of Comparative Physiology A, 184*(4), 403–412. https://doi.org/10.1007/s003590050334

Kuchenbecker, J. A., Neitz, J., & Neitz, M. (2014). Ethnic variation in the ratio of long- to middle-wavelength sensitive cones. *Investigative Ophthalmology & Visual Science, 55*(13), 4539. https://doi.org/10.1167/iovs.14-15726

Kuffler, S. W. (1953). Discharge patterns and functional organization of mammalian retina. *Journal of Neurophysiology, 16*(1), 37–68. https://doi.org/10.1152/jn.1953.16.1.37

Labhishetty, V., Cholewiak, S. A., & Banks, M. S. (2019). Contributions of foveal and non-foveal retina to the human eye's focusing response. *Journal of Vision, 19*(12), 18. https://doi.org/10.1167/19.12.18

Landis, E., Chrenek, M., Chakraborty, R., Strickland, R., Bergen, M., Yang, V., Iuvone, P., & Pardue, M. (2020). Increased endogenous dopamine prevents myopia in mice. *Experimental Eye Research, 193*, 107956. https://doi.org/10.1016/j.exer.2020.107956

Lauber, J. K., & Kinnear, A. (1979). Eye enlargement in birds induced by dim light. *Canadian Journal of Ophthalmology, 14*(3), 265–269.

Lauber, J. K., & Kivett, V. K. (1981). Environmental control of the rearing conditions and early preglaucomatous lesions in chicks. *Experimental Eye Research, 32*(5), 501–509. https://doi.org/10.1016/s0014-4835(81)80038-4

Lauber, J. K., & McGinnis, J. (1966). Eye lesions in domestic fowl reared under continuous light. *Vision Research, 6*(11-12), 619–626. https://doi.org/10.1016/0042-6989(66)90127-2

Lauber, J. K., Shutze, J. V., & McGinnis, J. (1961). Effects of exposure to continuous light on the eye of the growing chick. *Proceedings of the Society for Experimental Biology and Medicine, 106*(4), 871–872. https://doi.org/10.3181/00379727-106-26505

Leung, T.-W., Li, R. W., & Kee, C. S. (2021) Meridional anisotropy of foveal and peripheral resolution acuity in adults with emmetropia, myopia, and astigmatism. *Investigative Ophthalmology & Visual Science, 62*(10), 11. https://doi.org/10.1167/iovs.62.10.11

Li, C., Fitzgerald, M. E., Del Mar, N., & Reiner, A. (2016). Stimulation of Baroresponsive Parts of the Nucleus of the Solitary Tract Produces Nitric Oxide-mediated Choroidal Vasodilation in Rat Eye. *Frontiers in Neuroanatomy, 10*, 94. https://doi.org/10.3389/fnana.2016.00094

Li, C., McFadden, S. A., Morgan, I., Cui, D., Hu, J., Wan, W., & Zeng, J. (2010). All-trans retinoic acid regulates the expression of the extracellular matrix protein fibulin-1 in the guinea pig sclera and human scleral fibroblasts. *Molecular Vision, 16*, 689–697. https://www.ncbi.nlm.nih.gov/pmc/articles/PMC2855729/

Liang, H., Crewther, S. G., Crewther, D. P., & Pirie, B. (1996). Morphology of the recovery from form deprivation myopia in the chick. *Australian and New Zealand Journal of Ophthalmology, 24*(1), 41–44. https://doi.org/10.1111/j.1442-9071.1996.tb01486.x

Lin, T., Grimes, P. A., & Stone, R. A. (1993). Expansion of the retinal pigment epithelium in experimental myopia. *Vision Research, 33*(13), 1881–1885. https://doi.org/10.1016/0042-6989(93)90173-w

Liu, R., Hu, M., He, J. C., Zhou, X. T., Dai, J. H., Qu, X. M., Liu, H., & Chu, R. Y. (2014). The effects of monochromatic illumination on early eye development in rhesus monkeys. *Investigative Ophthalmology & Visual Science, 55*(3), 1901–1909. https://doi.org/10.1167/iovs.13-12276

Liu, A. L., Liu, Y. F., Wang, G., Shao, Y. Q., Yu, C. X., Yang, Z., Zhou, Z. R., Han, X., Gong, X., Qian, K. W., Wang, L. Q., Ma, Y. Y., Zhong, Y. M., Weng, S. J., & Yang, X. L. (2022). The role of ipRGCs in ocular growth and myopia development. *Science Advances, 8*(5), eabm9027. https://doi.org/10.1126/sciadv.abm9027

Liu, R., Qian, Y. F., He, J. C., Hu, M., Zhou, X. T., Dai, J. H., Qu, X. M., & Chu, R. Y. (2011). Effects of different monochromatic lights on refractive development and eye growth in guinea pigs. *Experimental Eye Research, 92*(6), 447–453. https://doi.org/10.1016/j.exer.2011.03.003

Llorente, L., Barbero, S., Cano, D., Dorronsoro, C., & Marcos, S. (2004). Myopic versus hyperopic eyes: axial length, corneal shape and optical aberrations. *Journal of Vision, 4*(4), 288–298. https://doi.org/10.1167/4.4.288

Long, Q., Chen, D. H., & Chu, R. Y. (2009). Illumination with monochromatic long-wavelength light promotes myopic shift and ocular elongation in newborn pigmented guinea pigs. *Cutaneous and Ocular Toxicology, 28*(4), 176–180. https://doi.org/10.1080/15569520902987094

Mahajan, V. B., Olney, A. H., Garrett, P., Chary, A., Dragan, E., Lerner, G., Murray, J., & Bassuk, A. G. (2010). Collagen XVIII mutation in Knobloch syndrome with acute lymphoblastic leukemia. *American Journal of Medical Genetics Part A, 152A*, 2875–2879. https://doi.org/10.1002/ajmg.a.33620

Mao, J. F., Liu, S. Z., Qin, W. J., & Xiang, Q. (2011). Modulation of TGFβ(2) and dopamine by PKC in retinal Müller cells of guinea pig myopic eye. *International Journal of Ophthalmology, 4*(4), 357–360. https://doi.org/10.3980/j.issn.2222-3959.2011.04.06

Marsack, J. D., Thibos, L. N., & Applegate, R. A. (2004). Metrics of optical quality derived from wave aberrations predict visual performance. *Journal of Vision, 4*(4), 322–328. https://doi.org/10.1167/4.4.8

Marzani, D., & Wallman, J. (1997). Growth of the two layers of the chick sclera is modulated reciprocally by visual conditions. *Investigative Ophthalmology & Visual Science, 38,* 1726–1739. https://doi.org/10.1007/s00417-022-05837-w

Mathis, U., Feldkaemper, M., Liu, H., & Schaeffel, F. (2023). Studies on the interactions of retinal dopamine with choroidal thickness in the chicken. *Graefe's Archive for Clinical and Experimental Ophthalmology, 261*(2), 409–425. https://doi.org/10.1007/s00417-022-05837-w

Mathis, U., & Schaeffel, F. (2007). Glucagon-related peptides in the mouse retina and the effects of deprivation of form vision. *Graefe's Archive for Clinical and Experimental Ophthalmology, 245*(2), 267-275. https://doi.org/10.1007/s00417-006-0282-x

Mazade, R., & Pardue, M. T. (2023). Rod pathway electrical activity is modulated in the myopic mouse. *Investigative Ophthalmology & Visual Science, 64*(8), 843.

McBrien, N. A., Cottriall, C. L., & Annies, R. (2001). Retinal acetylcholine content in normal and myopic eyes: a role in ocular growth control? *Visual Neuroscience, 18,* 571–580. https://doi.org/10.1017/S0952523801184035

McBrien, N. A., & Gentle, A. (2003). Role of the sclera in the development and pathological complications of myopia. *Progress in Retinal and Eye Research, 22,* 307–338. https://doi.org/10.1016/S1350-9462(02)00063-0

McBrien, N. A., & Millodot, M. (1986). The effect of refractive error on the accommodative response gradient. *Ophthalmic and Physiological Optics, 6*(2), 145–149. https://doi.org/10.1111/j.1475-1313.1986.tb01056.x

McBrien, N. A., Moghaddam, H. O., Reeder, A. P., & Moules, S. (1991). Structural and biochemical changes in the sclera of experimentally myopic eyes. *Biochemical Society Transactions, 19,* 861–865. https://doi.org/10.1042/bst0190861

McBrien, N. A., & Norton, T. T. (1994). Prevention of collagen crosslinking increases form-deprivation myopia in tree shrew. *Experimental Eye Research, 59,* 475–486. https://doi.org/10.1006/exer.1994.1134

McCarthy, C. S., Megaw, P., Devadas, M., & Morgan, I. G. (2007). Dopaminergic agents affect the ability of brief periods of normal vision to prevent form-deprivation myopia. *Experimental Eye Research, 84,* 100–107. https://doi.org/10.1016/j.exer.2006.09.008

McFadden, S. A., Howlett, M. H., & Mertz, J. R. (2004). Retinoic acid signals the direction of ocular elongation in the guinea pig eye. *Vision Research, 44,* 643–653. https://doi.org/10.1016/j.visres.2003.10.027

Mertz, J. R., & Wallman, J. (2000). Choroidal retinoic acid synthesis: a possible mediator between refractive error and compensatory eye growth. *Experimental Eye Research, 70,* 519–527. https://doi.org/10.1006/exer.1999.0807

Mirhajianmoghadam, H., Jnawali, A., Musial, G., Queener, H. M., Patel, N. B., Ostrin, L. A., & Porter, J. (2020). In vivo assessment of foveal geometry and cone photoreceptor density and spacing in children. *Scientific Reports, 10,* 8942. https://doi.org/10.1038/s41598-020-65645-2

Moring, A. G., Baker, J. R., & Norton, T. T. (2007). Modulation of glycosaminoglycan levels in tree shrew sclera during lens-induced myopia development and recovery. *Investigative Ophthalmology & Visual Science, 48,* 2947–2956. https://doi.org/10.1167/iovs.07-0083

Munteanu, T., Noronha, K. J., Leung, A. C., Pan, S., Lucas, J. A., & Schmidt, T. M. (2018). Light-dependent pathways for dopaminergic amacrine cell development and function. *eLife, 7,* e39866. https://doi.org/10.7554/eLife.39866

Muralidharan, G., Martínez-Enríquez, E., Birkenfeld, J., Velasco-Ocana, M., Pérez-Merino, P., & Marcos, S. (2019). Morphological changes of human crystalline lens in myopia. *Biomedical Optics Express, 10*(12), 6084–6095. https://doi.org/10.1364/BOE.10.006084

Mutti, D. O., Hayes, J. R., Mitchell, G. L., Jones, L. A., Moeschberger, M. L., Cotter, S. A., Kleinstein, R. N., Manny, R. E., Twelker, J. D., & Zadnik, K. (2007). Refractive error, axial length, and relative peripheral refractive error before and after the onset of myopia. *Investigative Ophthalmology & Visual Science, 48*, 2510–2519. https://doi.org/10.1167/iovs.06-0562

Mutti, D. O., Mitchell, G. L., Jones-Jordan, L. A., Cotter, S. A., Kleinstein, R. N., Manny, R. E., Twelker, J. D., Zadnik, K., & CLEERE Study Group. (2017). The response AC/A ratio before and after the onset of myopia. *Investigative Ophthalmology & Visual Science, 58*(3), 1594–1602. https://doi.org/10.1167/iovs.16-19093

Mutti, D. O., Mitchell, G. L., Sinnott, L. T., Jones-Jordan, L. A., Moeschberger, M. L., Cotter, S. A., Kleinstein, R. N., Manny, R. E., Twelker, J. D., Zadnik, K., & CLEERE Study Group. (2012). Corneal and crystalline lens dimensions before and after myopia onset. *Optometry and Vision Science: Official Publication of the American Academy of Optometry, 89*(3), 251–262. https://doi.org/10.1097/OPX.0b013e3182418213

Mutti, D. O., Sinnott, L. T., Mitchell, G. L., Jones-Jordan, L. A., Moeschberger, M. L., Cotter, S. A., Kleinstein, R. N., Manny, R. E., Twelker, J. D., & Zadnik, K. (2011). Relative peripheral refractive error and the risk of onset and progression of myopia in children. *Investigative Ophthalmology & Visual Science, 52*(1), 199-205. https://doi.org/10.1167/iovs.09-4826

Neitz, M., Balding, S. D., McMahon, C., Sjoberg, S. A., & Neitz, J. (2006). Topography of long- and middle-wavelength sensitive cone opsin gene expression in human and Old World monkey retina. *Visual Neuroscience, 23*(3-4), 379-385. https://doi.org/10.1017/S095252380623325X

Nickla, D. L., Jordan, K., Yang, J., & Totonelly, K. (2017). Brief hyperopic defocus or form deprivation have varying effects on eye growth and ocular rhythms depending on the time-of-day of exposure. *Experimental Eye Research, 161*, 132–142. https://doi.org/10.1016/j.exer.2017.06.003

Nickla, D. L., Lee, L., & Totonelly, K. (2013). Nitric oxide synthase inhibitors prevent the growth-inhibiting effects of quinpirole. *Optometry and Vision Science, 90*, 1167-1175. https://doi.org/10.1097/OPX.0000000000000046

Nickla, D. L., Rada, J. A., & Wallman, J. (1999). Isolated chick sclera shows a circadian rhythm in proteoglycan synthesis perhaps associated with the rhythm in ocular elongation. *Journal of Comparative Physiology A: Sensory, Neural, and Behavioral Physiology, 185*, 81-90. https://doi.org/10.1007/s003590050366

Nickla, D. L., & Schroedl, F. (2019). Effects of autonomic denervations on the rhythms in axial length and choroidal thickness in chicks. *Journal of Comparative Physiology A: Neuroethology, Sensory, Neural, and Behavioral Physiology, 205*(1), 139-149. https://doi.org/10.1007/s00359-018-01310-4

Nickla, D. L., & Wallman, J. (2010). The multifunctional choroid. *Progress in Retinal and Eye Research, 29*, 144-168. https://doi.org/10.1016/j.preteyeres.2009.12.002

Nickla, D. L., & Wildsoet, C. F. (2004). The effect of the nonspecific nitric oxide synthase inhibitor NG-nitro-L-arginine methyl ester on the choroidal compensatory response to myopic defocus in chickens. *Optometry and Vision Science, 81*, 111-118. https://doi.org/10.1097/00006324-200402000-00008

Nickla, D. L., Wildsoet, C., & Troilo, D. (2001). Endogenous rhythms in axial length and choroidal thickness in chicks: implications for ocular growth regulation. *Investigative Ophthalmology & Visual Science, 42*, 584-588. https://iovs.arvojournals.org/article.aspx?doi=10.1167/iovs.01-0185

Nickla, D. L., Wildsoet, C., & Wallman, J. (1998a). The circadian rhythm in intraocular pressure and its relation to diurnal ocular growth changes in chicks. *Experimental Eye Research, 66*, 183-193. https://doi.org/10.1006/exer.1997.0435

Nickla, D. L., Wildsoet, C., & Wallman, J. (1998b). Visual influences on diurnal rhythms in ocular length and choroidal thickness in chick eyes. *Experimental Eye Research, 66*, 163-181. https://doi.org/10.1006/exer.1997.0426

Nickla, D. L., Wilken, E., Lytle, G., Yom, S., & Mertz, J. (2006). Inhibiting the transient choroidal thickening response using the nitric oxide synthase inhibitor l-NAME prevents the ameliorative effects of visual experience on ocular growth in two different visual paradigms. *Experimental Eye Research*, 83, 456-464. https://doi.org/10.1016/j.exer.2006.01.017

Norton, T. T., & Rada, J. A. (1995). Reduced extracellular matrix in mammalian sclera with induced myopia. *Vision Research*, 35, 1271-1281. https://doi.org/10.1016/0042-6989(94)00220-E

Norton, T. T., & Siegwart, J. T. Jr. (2013). Light levels, refractive development, and myopia—speculative review. *Experimental Eye Research*, 114, 48-57. https://doi.org/10.1016/j.exer.2013.05.004

Ohngemach, S., Hagel, G., & Schaeffel, F. (1997). Concentrations of biogenic amines in fundal layers in chickens with normal visual experience, deprivation, and after reserpine application. *Visual Neuroscience*, 14, 493-505. https://doi.org/10.1017/S0952523800010909

Orr, J. B., Seidel, D., Day, M., & Gray, L. S. (2015). Is Pupil Diameter Influenced by Refractive Error? *Optometry and Vision Science*, 92(4), e106-e114. https://doi.org/10.1097/OPX.0000000000000481

Ostadimoghaddam, H., Yekta, A. A., Heravian, J., Azimi, A., Hosseini, S. M., Vatandoust, S., Sharifi, F., & Abolbashari, F. (2014). Prevalence of refractive errors in students with and without color vision deficiency. *Journal of Ophthalmic & Vision Research*, 9(4), 484–486. https://doi.org/10.4103/2008-322X.150828

Paluru, P., Ronan, S. M., Heon, E., Devoto, M., Wildenberg, S. C., Scavello, G., Holleschau, A., Mäkitie, O., Cole, W. G., King, R. A., & Young, T. L. (2003). New locus for autosomal dominant high myopia maps to the long arm of chromosome 17. *Investigative Ophthalmology & Visual Science*, 44(5), 1830–1836. https://doi.org/10.1167/iovs.02-0697

Pan, C. W., Cheung, C. Y., Aung, T., Cheung, C. M., Zheng, Y. F., Wu, R. Y., Mitchell, P., Lavanya, R., Baskaran, M., Wang, J. J., Wong, T. Y., & Saw, S. M. (2013). Differential associations of myopia with major age-related eye diseases: the Singapore Indian Eye Study. *Ophthalmology*, 120(2), 284–291. https://doi.org/10.1016/j.ophtha.2012.07.065

Papastergiou, G. I., Schmid, G. F., Laties, A. M., Pendrak, K., Lin, T., & Stone, R. A. (1998). Induction of axial eye elongation and myopic refractive shift in one-year-old chickens. *Vision Research*, 38, 1883-1888. https://doi.org/10.1016/S0042-6989(97)00326-5

Phillips, J. R., Khalaj, M., & McBrien, N. A. (2000). Induced myopia associated with increased scleral creep in chick and tree shrew eyes. *Investigative Ophthalmology & Visual Science*, 41, 2028-2034. https://iovs.arvojournals.org/article.aspx?doi=10.1016/S0042-6989(97)00326-5

Polans, J., Jaeken, B., McNabb, R. P., Artal, P., & Izatt, J. A. (2015). Wide-field optical model of the human eye with asymmetrically tilted and decentered lens that reproduces measured ocular aberrations. *Optica*, 2(2), 124–134. https://opg.optica.org/optica/fulltext.cfm?uri=optica-2-2-124&id=310933

Poudel, S., Jin, J., Rahimi-Nasrabadi, H., Dellostritto, S., Dul, M. W., Viswanathan, S., & Alonso, J. M. (2024). Contrast sensitivity of ON and OFF human retinal pathways in myopia. *Journal of Neuroscience*, 44(3). https://doi.org/10.1523/JNEUROSCI.0904-21.2021

Provis, J. M., Dubis, A. M., Maddess, T., & Carroll, J. (2013). Adaptation of the central retina for high acuity vision: cones, the fovea and the avascular zone. *Progress in Retinal and Eye Research*, 35, 63–81. https://doi.org/10.1016/j.preteyeres.2013.01.005

Qian, Y. S., Chu, R. Y., He, J. C., Sun, X. H., Zhou, X. T., Zhao, N. Q., Hu, D. N., Hoffman, M. R., Dai, J. H., Qu, X. M., & Pao, K. E. (2009). Incidence of myopia in high school students with and without red-green color vision deficiency. *Investigative Ophthalmology & Visual Science*, 50(4), 1598–1605. https://doi.org/10.1167/iovs.07-1362

Qiu, M., Wang, S. Y., Singh, K., & Lin, S. C. (2013). Association between myopia and glaucoma in the United States population. *Investigative Ophthalmology & Visual Science*, 54, 830-835. https://doi.org/10.1167/iovs.12-10251

Rada, J. A., Achen, V. R., Penugonda, S., Schmidt, R. W., & Mount, B. A. (2000). Proteoglycan composition in the human sclera during growth and aging. *Investigative Ophthalmology & Visual Science, 41*(7), 1639-1648. https://pubmed.ncbi.nlm.nih.gov/10845580/

Rada, J. A., Achen, V. R., Perry, C. A., & Fox, P. W. (1997). Proteoglycans in the human sclera: Evidence for the presence of aggrecan. *Investigative Ophthalmology & Visual Science, 38*(9), 1740-1751.

Rada, J. A., & Brenza, H. L. (1995). Increased latent gelatinase activity in the sclera of visually deprived chicks. *Investigative Ophthalmology & Visual Science, 36*(8), 1555-1565.

Rada, J. A., Hollaway, L. R., Lam, W., Li, N., & Napoli, J. L. (2012). Identification of RALDH2 as a visually regulated retinoic acid synthesizing enzyme in the chick choroid. *Investigative Ophthalmology & Visual Science, 53*(3), 1649-1662. https://doi.org/10.1167/iovs.08-2366

Rada, J. A., Matthews, A. L., & Brenza, H. (1994). Regional proteoglycan synthesis in the sclera of experimentally myopic chicks. *Experimental Eye Research, 59*(6), 747-760.

Rada, J. A., McFarland, A. L., Cornuet, P. K., & Hassell, J. R. (1992). Proteoglycan synthesis by scleral chondrocytes is modulated by a vision-dependent mechanism. *Current Eye Research, 11*(8), 767-782.

Rada, J. A., Nickla, D. L., & Troilo, D. (2000). Decreased proteoglycan synthesis associated with form deprivation myopia in mature primate eyes. *Investigative Ophthalmology & Visual Science, 41*(7), 2050-2058.

Rada, J. A., Perry, C. A., Slover, M. L., & Achen, V. R. (1999). Gelatinase A and TIMP-2 expression in the fibrous sclera of myopic and recovering chick eyes. *Investigative Ophthalmology & Visual Science, 40*(13), 3091-3099.

Rada, J. A., Thoft, R. A., & Hassell, J. R. (1991). Increased aggrecan (cartilage proteoglycan) production in the sclera of myopic chicks. *Developmental Biology, 147*(2), 303-312.

Rajavi, Z., Sabbaghi, H., Baghini, A., Yaseri, M., Sheibani, K., & Norouzi, G. (2015). Prevalence of color vision deficiency and its correlation with amblyopia and refractive errors among primary school children. *Journal of Ophthalmic & Vision Research, 10*(2), 130-138.

Reiner, A., Fitzgerald, M. E. C., Del Mar, N., & Li, C. (2018). Neural control of choroidal blood flow. *Progress in Retinal and Eye Research, 64*, 96-130. https://doi.org/10.1016/j.preteyeres.2017.12.001

Riddell, N., Giummarra, L., Hall, N. E., & Crewther, S. G. (2016). Bidirectional expression of metabolic, structural, and immune pathways in early myopia and hyperopia. *Frontiers in Neuroscience, 10*, 390.

Rohrer, B., Schaeffel, F., & Zrenner, E. (1992). Longitudinal chromatic aberration and emmetropization: Results from the chicken eye. *Journal of Physiology, 449*(1), 363-376.

Rohrer, B., Spira, A. W., & Stell, W. K. (1993). Apomorphine blocks form-deprivation myopia in chickens by a dopamine D2-receptor mechanism acting in retina or pigmented epithelium. *Visual Neuroscience, 10*(3), 447-453.

Romashchenko, D., Rosén, R., & Lundström, L. (2020). Peripheral refraction and higher order aberrations. *Clinical and Experimental Optometry, 103*(1), 86-94. https://doi.org/10.1111/cxo.12943

Roorda, A., & Williams, D. R. (1999). The arrangement of the three cone classes in the living human eye. *Nature, 397*(6719), 520-522. https://doi.org/10.1038/17383

Rossi, E. A., Roorda, A., & Do Cooper, R. (2007). Visual performance in emmetropia and low myopia after correction of high-order aberrations. *Journal of Vision, 7*(8), 14-14.

Rozema J. J. (2023). Refractive development I: Biometric changes during emmetropisation. *Ophthalmic & Physiological Optics: The Journal of the British College of Ophthalmic Opticians (Optometrists), 43*(3), 347–367. https://doi.org/10.1111/opo.13094

Rozema, J., Dankert, S., Iribarren, R., Lanca, C., & Saw, S. M. (2019). Axial growth and lens power loss at myopia onset in Singaporean children. *Investigative Ophthalmology & Visual Science, 60*(9), 3091-3099.

Saltarelli, D., Wildsoet, C., Nickla, D., & Troilo, D. (2004). Susceptibility to form-deprivation myopia in chicks is not altered by an early experience of axial myopia. *Optometry and Vision Science, 81*(2), 119-126. https://doi.org/10.1097/00006324-200402000-00010

Sampaio, L. de O., Bayliss, M. T., Hardingham, T. E., & Muir, H. (1988). Dermatan sulphate proteoglycan from human articular cartilage. Variation in its content with age and its structural comparison with a small chondroitin sulphate proteoglycan from pig laryngeal cartilage. *The Biochemical Journal, 254*(3), 757–764. https://doi.org/10.1042/bj2540757

Schaeffel, F., Bartmann, M., Hagel, G., & Zrenner, E. (1995). Studies on the role of the retinal dopamine/melatonin system in experimental refractive errors in chickens. *Vision Research, 35*(9), 1247-1264.

Schaeffel, F., Hagel, G., Bartmann, M., Kohler, K., & Zrenner, E. (1994). 6-Hydroxy dopamine does not affect lens-induced refractive errors but suppresses deprivation myopia. *Vision Research, 34*(2), 143-149.

Schaeffel, F., & Howland, H. C. (1991). Properties of the feedback loops controlling eye growth and refractive state in the chicken. *Vision Research, 31*(4), 717-734.

Schmid, K. L., & Wildsoet, C. F. (2004). Inhibitory effects of apomorphine and atropine and their combination on myopia in chicks. *Optometry and Vision Science, 81*(2), 137-147.

Seidemann, A., & Schaeffel, F. (2002). Effects of longitudinal chromatic aberration on accommodation and emmetropization. *Vision Research, 42*(20), 2409-2417.

Seko, Y., Shimizu, M., & Tokoro, T. (1998). Retinoic acid increases in the retina of the chick with form deprivation myopia. *Ophthalmic Research, 30*(6), 361-367.

Seko, Y., Tanaka, Y., & Tokoro, T. (1994). Scleral cell growth is influenced by retinal pigment epithelium in vitro. *Graefe's Archive for Clinical and Experimental Ophthalmology, 232*(9), 545-552.

___. (1997). Apomorphine inhibits the growth-stimulating effect of retinal pigment epithelium on scleral cells in vitro. *Cell Biochemistry and Function, 15*(3), 191-196.

She, Z., Ward, A. H., & Gawne, T. J. (2023). The effects of ambient narrowband long-wavelength light on lens-induced myopia and form-deprivation myopia in tree shrews. *Experimental Eye Research, 234*, 109593. https://doi.org/10.1016/j.exer.2023.109593

Sheng, C., Zhu, X., & Wallman, J. (2013). In vitro effects of insulin and RPE on choroidal and scleral components of eye growth in chicks. *Experimental Eye Research, 116*, 439-448.

Siegwart, J. T., Jr., & Norton, T. T. (1999). Regulation of the mechanical properties of tree shrew sclera by the visual environment. *Vision Research, 39*(3), 387-407.

Smith, E. L., III, Huang, J., Hung, L. F., Blasdel, T. L., Humbird, T. L., & Bockhorst, K. H. (2009). Hemiretinal form deprivation: evidence for local control of eye growth and refractive development in infant monkeys. *Investigative Ophthalmology & Visual Science, 50*(11), 5057–5069. https://doi.org/10.1167/iovs.08-3232

Smith, E. L., III, & Hung, L. F. (2000). Form-deprivation myopia in monkeys is a graded phenomenon. *Vision Research, 40*(4), 371–381. https://doi.org/10.1016/s0042-6989(99)00184-4

Smith, E. L., III, Hung, L. F., Arumugam, B., Holden, B. A., Neitz, M., & Neitz, J. (2015). Effects of long-wavelength lighting on refractive development in infant rhesus monkeys. *Investigative Ophthalmology & Visual Science, 56*(11), 6490-6500.

Smith, E. L., III, Hung, L. F., & Huang, J. (2009). Relative peripheral hyperopic defocus alters central refractive development in infant monkeys. *Vision Research, 49*(19), 2386-2392.

Smith, E. L., III, Hung, L. F., Huang, J., & Arumugam, B. (2013). Effects of local myopic defocus on refractive development in monkeys. *Optometry and Vision Science: Official Publication of the American Academy of Optometry, 90*(11), 1176–1186. https://doi.org/10.1097/OPX.0000000000000038

Smith, E. L., III, Hung, L. F., Huang, J., Blasdel, T. L., Humbird, T. L., & Bockhorst, K. H. (2010). Effects of optical defocus on refractive development in monkeys: evidence for local, regionally selective mechanisms. *Investigative Ophthalmology & Visual Science, 51*(8), 3864–3873. https://doi.org/10.1167/iovs.09-4969

Smith, E. L., III, Kee, C. S., Ramamirtham, R., Qiao-Grider, Y., & Hung, L. F. (2005). Peripheral vision can influence eye growth and refractive development in infant monkeys. *Investigative Ophthalmology & Visual Science, 46*(11), 3965-3972. https://doi.org/10.1167/iovs.05-0292

Sng, C. C., Lin, X. Y., Gazzard, G., Chang, B., Dirani, M., Lim, L., Selvaraj, P., Ian, K., Drobe, B., Wong, T. Y., & Saw, S. M. (2011). Change in peripheral refraction over time in Singapore Chinese children. *Investigative Ophthalmology & Visual Science, 52*(11), 7880-7887. https://doi.org/10.1167/iovs.11-7290

Stone, R. A., Lin, T., Laties, A. M., & Iuvone, P. M. (1989). Retinal dopamine and form-deprivation myopia. *Proceedings of the National Academy of Sciences, USA, 86*(2), 704-706.

Stone, R. A., McGlinn, A. M., Baldwin, D. A., Tobias, J. W., Iuvone, P. M., & Khurana, T. S. (2011). Image defocus and altered retinal gene expression in chick: Clues to the pathogenesis of ametropia. *Investigative Ophthalmology & Visual Science, 52*(8), 5765-5777. https://doi.org/10.1167/iovs.10-7131

Stone, R. A., McGlinn, A. M., Chakraborty, R., Lee, D. C., Yang, V., Elmasri, A., Landis, E., Shaffer, J., Iuvone, P. M., Zheng, X., Sehgal, A., & Pardue, M. T. (2019). Altered ocular parameters from circadian clock gene disruptions. *PLoS ONE, 14*(12), e0217111. https://doi.org/10.1371/journal.pone.0217111

Stone, R. A., Tobias, J. W., Wei, W., Schug, J., Wang, X., Zhang, L., Iuvone, P. M., & Nickla, D. L. (2024). Diurnal retinal and choroidal gene expression patterns support a role for circadian biology in myopia pathogenesis. *Scientific Reports, 14*, 533. https://doi.org/10.1038/s41598-023-07185-1

Strang, N. C., Winn, B., & Bradley, A. (1998). The role of neural and optical factors in limiting visual resolution in myopia. *Vision Research, 38*(12), 1713-1721. https://doi.org/10.1016/S0042-6989(97)00363-4

Summers, J. A., & Martinez, E. (2021). Visually induced changes in cytokine production in the chick choroid. *eLife, 10*, e59916. https://doi.org/10.7554/eLife.59916

Summers, J. A., Cano, E. M., Kaser-Eichberger, A., & Schroedl, F. (2020). Retinoic acid synthesis by a population of choroidal stromal cells. *Experimental Eye Research, 201*, 108252. https://doi.org/10.1016/j.exer.2020.108252

Summers, J. A., Schaeffel, F., Marcos, S., Wu, H., & Tkatchenko, A. V. (2021). Functional integration of eye tissues and refractive eye development: Mechanisms and pathways. *Experimental Eye Research, 209*, 108693. https://doi.org/10.1016/j.exer.2021.108693

Summers Rada, J. A., & Hollaway, L. R. (2011). Regulation of the biphasic decline in scleral proteoglycan synthesis during the recovery from induced myopia. *Experimental Eye Research, 92*(5), 394-400. https://doi.org/10.1016/j.exer.2011.03.004

Tedja, M. S., Wojciechowski, R., Hysi, P. G., Eriksson, N., Furlotte, N. A., Verhoeven, V. J. M., Iglesias, A. I., Meester-Smoor, M. A., Tompson, S. W., Fan, Q., Khawaja, A. P., Cheng, C. Y., Höhn, R., Yamashiro, K., Wenocur, A., Grazal, C., Haller, T., Metspalu, A., Wedenoja, J., Jonas, J. B., … Klaver, C. C. W. (2018). Genome-wide association meta-analysis highlights light-induced signaling as a driver for refractive error. *Nature Genetics*, *50*(6), 834–848. https://doi.org/10.1038/s41588-018-0127-7

Tideman, J. W. L., Polling, J. R., Vingerling, J. R., Jaddoe, V. W. V., Williams, C., Guggenheim, J. A., & Klaver, C. C. W. (2018). Axial length growth and the risk of developing myopia in European children. *Acta ophthalmologica*, *96*(3), 301–309. https://doi.org/10.1111/aos.13603

Tkatchenko, T. V., & Tkatchenko, A. V. (2021). Genome-wide analysis of retinal transcriptome reveals common genetic network underlying perception of contrast and optical defocus detection. *BMC Medical Genomics, 14*, 153. https://doi.org/10.1186/s12920-021-01022-w

Torii, H., Kurihara, T., Seko, Y., Negishi, K., Ohnuma, K., Inaba, T., Kawashima, M., Jiang, X., Kondo, S., Miyauchi, M., Miwa, Y., Katada, Y., Mori, K., Kato, K., Tsubota, K., Goto, H., Oda, M., Hatori, M., & Tsubota, K. (2017). Violet light exposure can be a preventive strategy against myopia progression. *EBioMedicine*, *15*, 210–219. https://doi.org/10.1016/j.ebiom.2016.12.007

Trier, K., Olsen, E. B., Kobayashi, T., & Ribel-Madsen, S. M. (1999). Biochemical and ultrastructural changes in rabbit sclera after treatment with. *British Journal of Ophthalmology, 83*, 1370–1375. https://doi.org/10.1136/bjo.83.12.1370

Troilo, D. (1998). Changes in Retinal Morphology following Experimentally Induced Myopia. In *Vision Science and Its Applications, Technical Digest Series* (pp. SuC.4). Optica Publishing Group.

Troilo, D., Nickla, D. L., Mertz, J. R., & Summers Rada, J. A. (2006). Change in the synthesis rates of ocular retinoic acid and scleral glycosaminoglycan during experimentally altered eye growth in marmosets. *Investigative Ophthalmology & Visual Science, 47*(4), 1768-1777. https://doi.org/10.1167/iovs.05-1229

Troilo, D., Nickla, D. L., & Wildsoet, C. F. (2000a). Choroidal thickness changes during altered eye growth and refractive state in a primate. *Investigative Ophthalmology & Visual Science, 41*(5), 1249-1258. https://doi.org/10.1016/j.ebiom.2016.11.021

Troilo, D., Nickla, D. L., & Wildsoet, C. F. (2000b). Form deprivation myopia in mature common marmosets (callithrix jacchus). *Investigative Ophthalmology & Visual Science, 41*(8), 2043–2049. https://pubmed.ncbi.nlm.nih.gov/10892841/

Usui et al., (2012) Circadian changes in subfoveal choroidal thickness and the relationship with circulatory factors in healthy subjects. *Investigative Ophthalmology & Visual Science*, Vol. *53,* 2300

van Alphen, G. W. (1961). On emmetropia and ametropia. *Optica Acta, 142*(Suppl), 1-92.

___. (1986). Choroidal stress and emmetropization. *Vision Research, 26*, 723-734. https://doi.org/10.1016/0042-6989(86)90068-3

Wagner, S., Zrenner, E., & Strasser, T. (2019). Emmetropes and myopes differ little in their accommodation dynamics but strongly in their ciliary muscle morphology. *Vision Research, 163*, 42-51. https://doi.org/10.1016/j.visres.2019.08.002

Walker, T. W., & Mutti, D. O. (2002). The effect of accommodation on ocular shape. *Optometry and Vision Science, 79*, 424–430.

Wallman, J., Gottlieb, M. D., Rajaram, V., & Fugate-Wentzek, L. A. (1987). Local retinal regions control local eye growth and myopia. *Science, 237*(4810), 73–77. https://doi.org/10.1126/science.3603011

Wallman, J., Wildsoet, C., Xu, A., Gottlieb, M. D., Nickla, D. L., Marran, L., Krebs, W., & Christensen, A. M. (1995). Moving the retina: choroidal modulation of refractive state. *Vision Research, 35*, 37-50. https://doi.org/10.1016/0042-6989(94)e0049-q

Wallman, J., & Winawer, J. (2004). Homeostasis of eye growth and the question of myopia. *Neuron, 43*(4), 447-468. https://doi.org/10.1016/j.neuron.2004.08.008

Walls, G. (1942). *The Vertebrate Eye and Its Adaptive Radiations*. The Cranbrook Press.

Wandell, B. A., Brainard, D. H., & Cottaris, N. P. (2022). Visual encoding: Principles and software. *Progress in Brain Research, 273*(1), 199–229. https://doi.org/10.1016/bs.pbr.2022.04.006

Wang, J., Candy, T. R., Teel, D. F., & Jacobs, R. J. (2008). Longitudinal chromatic aberration of the human infant eye. *Journal of the Optical Society of America A, 25*(9), 2263-2270. https://doi.org/10.1364/JOSAA.25.002263

Wang, F., Zhou, J., Lu, Y., & Chu, R. (2011). Effects of 530 nm green light on refractive status, melatonin, MT1 receptor, and melanopsin in the guinea pig. *Current Eye Research, 36*, 103–111.

Wang, X., Zhu, C., Hu, X., Liu, L., Liu, M., Yuan, Y., & Ke, B. (2022). Changes in Dimensions and Functions of Crystalline Lens in High Myopia Using CASIA2 Optical Coherence Tomography. *Ophthalmic Research, 65*(6), 712-721. https://doi.org/10.1159/000526246

Wang, Y., Bensaid, N., Tiruveedhula, P., Ma, J., Ravikumar, S., & Roorda, A. (2019). Human foveal cone photoreceptor topography and its dependence on eye length. *eLife, 8*, e47148. https://doi.org/10.7554/eLife.47148

Weiss, S., & Schaeffel, F. (1993). Diurnal growth rhythms in the chicken eye: Relation to myopia development and retinal dopamine levels. *Journal of Comparative Physiology A, 172*, 263-270. https://doi.org/10.1007/BF00216471

Wells-Gray, E., Choi, S., & Bries, A. (2016). Variation in rod and cone density from the fovea to the mid-periphery in healthy human retinas using adaptive optics scanning laser ophthalmoscopy. *Eye, 30*, 1135–1143. https://doi.org/10.1038/eye.2016.107

Whatham, A., Zimmermann, F., Martinez, A., Delgado, S., de la Jara, P. L., Sankaridurg, P., & Ho, A. (2009). Influence of accommodation on off-axis refractive errors in myopic eyes. *Journal of Vision, 9*(3), 1–13. https://doi.org/10.1167/9.3.14

White, J. M., & Wick, B. (1995). Accommodation in humans with juvenile macular degeneration. *Vision Research, 35*(6), 873–880.

Wildsoet, C. F., Atchison, D. A., & Collins, M. J. (1993). Longitudinal chromatic aberration as a function of refractive error. *Clinical and Experimental Optometry, 76*(4).

Witkovsky, P. (2004). Dopamine and retinal function. *Documenta Ophthalmologica: Advances in Ophthalmology, 108*(1), 17–40. https://doi.org/10.1023/b:doop.0000019487.88486.0a

Young, T. L., Guo, X. D., King, R. A., Johnson, J. M., & Rada, J. A. (2003). Identification of genes expressed in a human scleral cDNA library. *Molecular Vision, 9*, 508-514.

Zadnik, K., & Mutti, D. O. (1995). How applicable are animal myopia models to human juvenile onset myopia? *Vision Research, 35*, 1283-1288. https://doi.org/10.1016/0042-6989(94)00238-F

Zhang, L. Q., Cottaris, N. P., & Brainard, D. H. (2022). An image reconstruction framework for characterizing initial visual encoding. *eLife, 11*, e71132. https://doi.org/10.7554/eLife.71132

Zhang, Y., Liu, Y., Ho, C., & Wildsoet, C. F. (2013). Effects of imposed defocus of opposite sign on temporal gene expression patterns of BMP4 and BMP7 in chick RPE. *Experimental Eye Research, 109*, 98-106. https://doi.org/10.1016/j.exer.2013.01.004

Zhang, Y., Liu, Y., & Wildsoet, C. F. (2012). Bidirectional, optical sign-dependent regulation of BMP2 gene expression in chick retinal pigment epithelium. *Investigative Ophthalmology & Visual Science, 53*, 6072-6080. https://doi.org/10.1167/iovs.12-9864

Zhang, Z., Mu, J., Wei, J., Geng, H., Liu, C., Yi, W., Sun, Y., & Duan, J. (2023). Correlation between refractive errors and ocular biometric parameters in children and adolescents: A systematic review and meta-analysis. *BMC Ophthalmology, 23*(1), 472. https://doi.org/10.1186/s12886-023-03222-7

Zhang, Y., Phan, E., & Wildsoet, C. F. (2019). Retinal defocus and form-deprivation exposure duration affects RPE BMP gene expression. *Scientific Reports, 9*, 7332. https://doi.org/10.1038/s41598-019-43785-4

Zhao, X., Reifler, A. N., Schroeder, M. M., Jaeckel, E. R., Chervenak, A. P., & Wong, K. Y. (2017). Mechanisms creating transient and sustained photoresponses in mammalian retinal ganglion cells. *Journal of General Physiology, 149*(3), 335-353. https://doi.org/10.1085/jgp.201611720

Zheleznyak, L. (2023). Peripheral optical anisotropy in refractive error groups. *Ophthalmic and Physiological Optics, 43*(3), 435-444. https://doi.org/10.1111/opo.13104

Zheleznyak, L., Barbot, A., Ghosh, A., & Yoon, G. (2016). Optical and neural anisotropy in peripheral vision. *Journal of Vision, 16*(5), 1. https://doi.org/10.1167/16.5.1

Zheleznyak, L., Liu, C., & Winter, S. (2024). Differentiating positive from negative retinal defocus by peripheral chromatic optical cues. https://opg.optica.org/boe/fulltext.cfm?uri=boe-15-9-5098&id=554451

7
Current and Emerging Treatment Options for Myopia

This chapter focuses on clinical aspects of myopia: the treatments that are currently used and those that are being developed. The early parts of the chapter describe how the uncorrected blur associated with myopia can be treated. The chapter then transitions to the treatment of myopia progression. The foundations of the natural history of myopia are also described, so the reader may evaluate the efficacy of myopia progression treatments compared to myopic eye growth without intervention. Details from large-scale, randomized controlled clinical trials are included to provide examples of how myopia research is built, including cornerstone studies that laid the foundation for our current understandings in optical, pharmaceutical, and environmental interventions.

After touching on key perspectives of current treatment options from the International Myopia Institute[1] and the 2023 Cochrane review on myopia, the chapter transitions to emerging treatment options. The chapter does not attempt to be exhaustive, and instead aims to identify those treatments that hold the most promise (for more detail see Khanal et al., 2024). While treatment options are available for myopia onset and progression, the effect sizes remain small. This chapter includes theories on why current treatments are not more effective in order to stimulate new research areas. The goal of this chapter is to describe myopia and its progression in a manner that provides support for intervening, from considerations for funding and research directions to conversations about clinical care.

Over the last 100 years and especially in the last two decades, much work has been done to determine the natural growth of the eye, its excessive growth in nearsightedness (myopia), and subsequently how to slow down this natural myopia progression. Treatment of the myopic eye has historically centered on correcting the blurry distance vision associated with it. By the 1600s, it was discovered that concave lenses could help focus light onto the retina of a long (myopic) eye by diverting the light rays entering the eye (Frangenberg, 1991). Despite having clearer vision with glasses, however, the nearsighted eye continued to elongate, worsening the condition (Hou et al., 2018). Therefore, in the late 1900s researchers began to turn their focus toward slowing down this growth or myopia progression, at first in animals (Norton et al., 1977; Wallman et al., 1978; Wiesel & Raviola, 1977). In 2003, a multi-center clinical trial funded by the National Institutes of Health was the first to show that the myopic growth of the human eye could be slowed with an optical intervention in U.S. school-aged children (Gwiazda et al., 2003). Since then, in addition to correcting myopic blur, attempts at slowing the growth of the myopic eye have been explored using a variety of treatment options.

While being less myopic is beneficial, the preferred outcome would instead be the complete cessation of myopia progression (or better, the prevention of it altogether). If the length

---

[1]https://myopiainstitute.org

of the eye becomes excessive, the treatment may only partially reduce the risks of retinal detachment, myopic maculopathy, and glaucoma.

CURRENT TREATMENT OPTIONS FOR MYOPIA

Optical Treatments for Myopia

Glasses have been the mainstay for alleviating the side effect of blurry distance vision associated with myopia for hundreds of years and include a spectacle frame and lenses. The lens shape is concave, with the thinnest part of the lens in the middle, which helps the parallel rays of light entering the long eye diverge so they focus farther into the eye, preferably on the plane of the retina. The lens material was originally glass, which provides superior optics. Plastic lenses are used more often today due to their lighter weight. For children, plastic lenses are generally made of polycarbonate, a shatter-resistant material that protects the eyes of the child. Children may also have lenses made out of trivex, which makes lenses even thinner and lighter.

The most traditional lens design for treating the side effect of blur in myopia is single-vision, meaning there is one focusing power across the lens and not two, as in bifocals, and not a gradual increase in near power, as in progressive-addition lenses. Photochromic lenses, which change from light to dark and vice versa with changing ultraviolet (UV) light, do not significantly affect myopic blur in any way. Glasses can generally be worn by children of any age and require a proper fit so that the center and thinnest part of the lens sits directly in front of the eye's pupil.

Contact lenses began to be used in the United States in the 1930s. Today's contact lenses are plastic and offer more oxygen permeability than early glass versions (Moreddu, 2019). Contact lenses made of hard plastic are called rigid gas permeable (RGP) lenses. These lenses correct myopic blur in similar ways to glasses except that they are worn on the front surface of the eye, the cornea. RGP lenses also laid the foundation for orthokeratology, a system where RGP lenses are worn overnight and change the shape of the cornea enough to focus the light on the myopic retina so that vision is clear during the day without wearing the lenses. Soft contact lenses are made of a hydrogel material and were first FDA-approved in 1971. Unlike RGP contact lenses, which are custom fit to the shape of the cornea, soft contact lenses are generally 14 mm in diameter and drape over the approximately 12 mm diameter cornea. While contact lenses may be worn at any age, their use in myopic children generally starts at age 7 or 8 years, based on literature showing the safety of contact lenses in this age group (Chalmers et al., 2021; Sankaridurg et al., 2013; Walline et al., 2007, 2008, 2013).

Surgical Treatments for Myopia

Refractive Surgery

Refractive surgery is a term that describes any procedure that corrects the refractive error of the eye. The goal is to improve uncorrected visual acuity, thereby reducing dependency on glasses or contact lenses. One popular early refractive surgery was radial keratotomy. First introduced in the United States in 1978 (Bores, 1981), this procedure used deep radial incisions in the cornea to cause its flattening, thereby reducing its refractive power and moving the focus posteriorly to better match the longer myopic eye. In 1994, data were published showing the safety and efficacy of radial keratotomy, with 70% of participants reporting no need to wear vision correction 10 years after surgery (Waring et al., 1994). However, subsequent longer-term experience with radial keratotomy showed continued corneal flattening with progressive hyperopia and irregular astigmatisms, among other changes (Koosha et al., 2024). The procedure was gradually abandoned with the advent of more predictable excimer-based laser refractive surgery and the FDA approval of this laser refractive surgery in 1995.

Corneal surface ablations like photorefractive keratectomy were originally performed, followed by laser in situ keratomileusis (LASIK). For treatment of myopia, both procedures are used to flatten the cornea to reduce its refractive power. In 2002, the American Academy of Ophthalmology reported that LASIK was generally safe, effective, and predictable, especially in low to moderate myopia (Sugar et al., 2002). Since then, other refractive surgeries have been studied and developed, including variants of excimer surface ablation such as laser-assisted subepithelial keratectomy (LASEK) and femtosecond laser-based small-incision lenticule extraction (SMILE), which uses the femtosecond laser to precisely dissect a portion of the corneal stroma, which is then physically removed and causes a similar net flattening of the cornea. See Box 7-1 for more information about how optical corrections and refractive surgery do not alter risk for myopia complications.

BOX 7-1
Optical Corrections and Refractive Surgery Do Not Alter Risk for Myopia Complications

Despite refractive surgery's positive impact on minimizing dependency on glasses and contacts, it must be noted that refractive surgery corrects only the optical blur from the refractive error. Refractive surgery does not directly address presbyopia (loss of accommodation), and for those individuals who have lost accommodation due to age, reading glasses may still be needed after successful refractive surgery.

Perhaps most important to note is that the axially myopic eye remains physically long even after refractive surgery. So, while uncorrected vision is often much better following refractive surgery, the retina has still stretched from axial elongation of the eye and is still, as in any myopic eye, at increased risk for thinning, holes, and detachments (Haarman et al., 2020). This means that despite better uncorrected vision after refractive surgery, dilated eye exams are still important in addressing the potential ocular health risks associated with myopia.

Clear Lens Extraction

Clear lens extraction, also known as refractive lensectomy, is another surgical option to modify how light focuses on the retina. Clear lens extraction may be performed when corneal surgery is not possible. It is similar to cataract surgery whereby the human lens is removed; however, in clear lens extraction, the lens is removed in the general absence of cataract. Typically, a lens implant follows to correct distance vision. As with refractive surgery, the eye retains its original length. Reports in 1999 showed that individuals with high myopia who had clear lens extraction had nearly double the incidence of retinal detachments after seven years compared to those who did not have the surgery (Colin et al., 1999); however, later studies show better safety (Fernández-Vega et al., 2003; Srinivasan et al., 2016).

An important point is that clear lens extraction and corneal refractive surgery do not mitigate presbyopia. Because the crystalline lens is responsible for providing accommodation and the ability to see ranges from far to near, when the crystalline lens is removed in clear lens extraction and replaced with a distance-vision-correcting intraocular lens implant, reading glasses are required following the procedure to see near. Currently available intraocular lenses cannot accurately accommodate in response to demand like the natural human lens, though there are multi-focal, extended depth of focus, and intraocular lenses with hinged haptics to provide various degrees of vision (from distance to near).

Phakic Intraocular Lens Implantation

Phakic intraocular lens implantation may be a refractive surgery option in high myopia when the cornea is not well suited for a laser or surgical procedure. In this procedure, the human lens is left in the eye and an additional lens is placed inside the eye. The lens may be inserted into the front (anterior chamber) of the eye and supported by the iris or iris angle. It may also be placed in the space behind the iris and in front of the natural lens. There are risks associated with phakic intraocular lenses, primarily related to their proximity to structures in the eye, though in 2009 the American Academy of Ophthalmology reported that the short-term safety and efficacy are acceptable. Continued evaluation is required to determine long-term risk of complications and safety (Huang et al., 2009).

TREATMENT OPTIONS TO MITIGATE SIDE EFFECTS OF AN AXIALLY ELONGATED EYE

Because myopia is associated with increased risk of retinal pathology (Haarman et al., 2020), there may be occasions when it is important to consider preventive measures that maximize retinal health. In contrast to interventions that aim to slow down the growth of the eye, these approaches are designed to minimize risk to the eye once it has already become too long and myopic (see Table 7-1).

Surgical Treatments for Retinal Effects of Myopia

Prophylactic retinal procedures have been considered in patients with high myopia. However, there is no clear answer on the value of these preventative procedures. Pneumatic retinopexy involves a surgeon injecting an expanding gas bubble into the back of the eye in an effort to press the retina closer to the back of the eye. Laser retinopexy aims to avoid detached retina by more firmly attaching the retina using laser photocoagulation. Scleral buckle attempts to hold the retina in place, while a cryotherapy or laser is used to "tack" down the retina. The American Academy of Ophthalmology suggests that prophylactic retinal procedures be based on many factors including symptoms, extent of the condition including thinning, holes, or tears, and post-operative complication risk (Silva & Blumenkranz, 2013). It should also be noted that prophylactic retinal procedures do not alter the side effect of blur related to myopia. These procedures are intended to prevent retinal detachments, which can leave an individual blind if left untreated.

Pharmaceutical/Nutraceutical Treatments for Retinal Effects of Myopia

The macula is the area in the retina that is most involved in clear central vision. Lutein is a naturally occurring antioxidant found in the macular region that is thought to act as a filter of light, perhaps protecting the eye from sunlight damage. Lutein has been shown to provide benefit to the health of the macula since the Age-Related Eye-Disease Study 2 (AREDS2) was published in 2013 (Age-Related Eye Disease Study 2 Research Group, 2013). In age-related macular degeneration, the macula becomes fragile and functions more poorly as a result of aging-related pathological processes, such as chronic inflammation and lipid deposition, especially in those with a family history of this disease. In myopia, the macula can become fragile and function more poorly as a result of the retina stretching to accommodate the growth of the eye. In 2023, Yoshida et al. (2023) reported benefits of lutein supplements related to macular pigment optical density in highly myopic individuals in a randomized clinical trial. Because visual acuity, contrast sensitivity, and electroretinogram values were similar at 6 months between those who took lutein and those who took a placebo, further study in long-term and practical benefits is needed. However, lutein remains an emerging prophylactic management option for high myopia and its associated myopic maculopathy.

TABLE 7-1 Treatment Options for Myopia: Optical, Surgical, and Pharmaceutical/Nutraceutical

Treatment Options for *Myopia*	Optical	Surgical	Pharmaceutical/ Nutraceutical
For alleviating optical blur	Glasses Contact lenses Pinhole	Laser refractive surgery (e.g., photorefractive keratectomy/ LASIK/SMILE) Clear lens extraction Phakic intraocular lens implantation	None available
To mitigate the risks associated with an axially elongated eye		Prophylactic retinal procedures: - Retinopexy - Pneumatic - Laser - Retinal binding/scleral buckle	Lutein

SOURCE: Committee generated.

HISTORY OF MYOPIA PROGRESSION WITHOUT INTERVENTION

Longitudinal Studies on Growth of the Human Eye and Myopia Progression

While myopic eyes were being studied in animals in the mid to late 20th century, little information was available on the typical growth of myopia (without intervention) in U.S. children. However, two large-scale longitudinal observational studies in diverse groups of U.S. children have shaped what is known about the natural growth of the human eye and myopia progression. Longitudinal studies on myopia progression show that without intervention myopic eyes continue to elongate throughout childhood. These studies thus provide the rationale for other longitudinal studies that evaluate how significantly myopia progression can be slowed with intervention.

The CLEERE Study

In 1989, the Orinda Longitudinal Study of Myopia was launched, the first of its kind, aiming to investigate normal eye growth and the development of myopia. In 1997, the study added three clinical centers to assess the influence of ethnicity on normal ocular and refractive error development, and thenceforward became known as the Collaborative Longitudinal Evaluation of Ethnicity and Refractive Error (CLEERE; National Library of Medicine, 2005).

In 1997, the Correction of Myopia Evaluation Trial (COMET) was funded by the National Eye Institute as a large-scale, randomized controlled trial of myopic children. The 3-year randomized COMET study was extended to year five. After the fifth year, the COMET study participants were no longer asked to remain in their randomized lens assignment. The COMET study became a natural history study (typical growth of myopia without intervention) of myopia when it became known as COSMICC (Collaborative Observational Study of Myopia in COMET Children; National Library of Medicine, 2016).

CLEERE was a seminal myopia study conducted between 1989 and 2010 at five clinical sites in the United States. Designed as an observational cohort study of ocular development and myopia onset, it collected data on an ethnically diverse group of over 4,500 non-myopic children ages 6 through 11 years at baseline. The CLEERE study was funded by the National Eye Institute and provided a foundation for natural history elements of myopia incidence and predictive factors of myopia progression in U.S. children (Jones-Jordan et al., 2021; Kleinstein et al., 2012; Zadnik et al., 2015).

Key Findings from the CLEERE Study:

- The CLEERE study defined myopia as −0.75 D or more of myopia in each of the principal meridians.
- The age at which a child became myopic ranged from 7 to 16 years, with the largest number of children diagnosed at age 11.
- The incidence rate of new cases increased yearly until age 11, then decreased.
- Among all non-myopic children at baseline, 16.4% (749/4,556) became myopic during the school-aged years.
- The proportion of new cases of myopia differed by race in U.S. school-aged children:
  - 27.3% of Asian American children had new myopia during the time of the study, as did:
  - 21.4% of Hispanic children,
  - 14.5% of Native American children,
  - 13.9% of Black children, and
  - 11% of White children.

Predictors of myopia, when studied in 414 children with complete biometric and accommodative data who became myopic during the school-aged years, were elucidated. Factors associated with risk of myopia onset included having myopic parents, low amounts of time outdoors, high accommodative convergence-to-accommodation (AC/A) ratio (i.e., how much the eyes turn in when focusing power is changed), ocular components that resemble myopic eyes (long axial length, low lens power, relatively hyperopic retinal periphery), low amounts of hyperopia, and astigmatism. Despite these many risk factors, future myopia could be predicted best in non-myopic children by their current spherical equivalent refractive error alone. Optimal cut-points for predicting future myopia decreased in hyperopia with age. Six-year-old children who were at less than +0.75 D of hyperopia were at increased risk for developing myopia, followed by +0.50 D for children ages 7–8, +0.25 D for those ages 9–10, and plano at age 11. Children who remained farsighted by age 8 or 9 (and had no parents who were near-sighted) tended to avoid near-sightedness altogether.

The CLEERE study also found that myopia progression is a function of age as well as of race and ethnicity. Myopia progressed faster in younger children. Asian American children experienced statistically significantly faster myopia progression compared with Hispanic children (estimated 3-year difference of −0.46 D), Black children (−0.88 D), and Native American children (−0.48 D), but with a similar progression to that of White children (−0.19 D). Parental history of myopia, time spent reading, and time spent in outdoor/sports activities were not statistically significant factors in multivariate models.

The COSMICC Study

The Collaborative Observational Study of Myopia in COMET Children (COSMICC) was funded as a longitudinal, subsequent, observational cohort study by the National Eye Institute and provided a foundation for natural history elements of myopia progression in U.S. school-aged children. The COMET study had preceded the COSMICC study using the same participants. Nearly all COMET participants switched from either progressive-addition spectacle lenses or single-vision spectacle lenses to single-vision glasses or contact lenses. Of the original ethnically diverse group of 469 children, 362 (77%) were studied longitudinally to year 14, when the average age was 24.1 years (Scheiman et al., 2016).

Key Findings from the COMET/COSMICC Study:

- School-aged children living in the United States in the study progressed 0.50 D per year on average wearing single-vision glasses.
- Younger children progressed faster and developed a higher level of myopia despite myopia being similar to the older cohort at baseline.
- A higher level of education in the parent of a COMET child was associated with a higher level of myopia in the COMET child.
- The average age when myopia progression stopped was 15 years; 48% of children were stable at age 15 and 77% at age 18, but 4% were still experiencing myopia progression at age 24.
- The average amount of myopia at the end of myopia progression was −4.87 D.

CURRENT TREATMENT OPTIONS FOR SLOWING MYOPIA PROGRESSION

How Myopia Progression Occurs: A Recap

In U.S. population-based studies, most preschool children are farsighted (Borchert et al., 2011; Multi-Ethnic Pediatric Eye Disease Study Group, 2010; Wen et al., 2013). As discussed in Chapter 2, farsighted or hyperopic eyes have axial lengths that are too short for the optical power of the eye. As the child develops, the eye will become less hyperopic due primarily to growth in axial length that outpaces the decreases in optical power of the cornea and crystalline lens (Gordon & Donzis, 1985; Mutti et al., 2018). As the eye grows, the refractive error moves closer to zero diopters or "emmetropia," so this growth process is referred to as emmetropization. The eyes of most children never grow to reach a point of perfect emmetropia, leaving them slightly farsighted.

The mechanisms of emmetropization are not completely known, as discussed in Chapters 5 and 6. One theory is that retinal blur signals the eye to grow axially (front to back) and the system is fine-tuned by accommodation, the process by which the lens changes shape to focus near objects on the retina. However, if the eye of the preschool child fails to receive the internal signals to stop eye growth, it will continue to grow and axial length will become too long for the optics to compensate, creating blur on the retina and stimulating yet more axial growth. It is known that once a child's eye is nearsighted, the eye continues to grow, becoming more and more myopic throughout the school-age years, even when corrected (Gwiazda et al., 1993; Hou et al., 2018; Norton, 1999; Walline et al., 2020a; Wildsoet, 1997). This continuous process is called "myopia progression."

Early animal studies using chicks (Wallman et al., 1978), tree shrews, (Norton et al., 1977), and monkeys (Wiesel & Raviola, 1977) helped researchers discover that eye growth could be modulated. Eyelid closure or light scattering lenses applied to deprive the eye of form vision (a procedure known as form deprivation), were found to cause the eye to grow excessively and become highly myopic. Negative-powered lenses worn by an animal were shown to induce compensatory eye growth, leaving the animal myopic when the lenses were removed (Hung et al., 1995). Later research in monkeys showed that form-deprivation was also reversible (Qiao-Grider et al., 2004; Smith et al., 2002). If eye growth could be manipulated in animals, researchers wondered if eye growth could be slowed in humans. Thus, scientists began to investigate methods to slow myopic progression in children using a range of treatments, including optical methods (progressive-addition lenses, soft multifocal contact lenses, and orthokeratology rigid gas-permeable lenses) and pharmaceutical methods (atropine eye drops, pirenzepine eye drops).

OPTICAL TREATMENT TO SLOW HUMAN EYE GROWTH

Early Theories on Optical Mechanisms

Typically, children have very strong and accurate focusing systems for near work (Hofstetter, 1944). However, in the 1990s, Gwiazda et al. (1993) and Abbott et al. (1998) reported that some myopes were not very accurate at near visual. Animal research suggested that blurry vision may cause eye growth (Norton, 1999; Wildsoet, 1997). Researchers hypothesized that if vision could become clearer by using a lens that improves near visual focus, less blur may cause less eye growth. As mentioned earlier in this chapter, progressive-plus powered lenses used in a large-scale, national, multicenter, randomized clinical trial funded by the National Eye Institute did work to slow the growth of the eye (Gwiazda et al., 2003). Despite statistical significance, however, the effect was small and did not support widespread use of multifocal spectacle lenses. However, the study did show proof of concept that human eye growth could be slowed with optical interventions.

Clinical researchers went on to study other lens modalities based on experimental myopia studies in animals. Perhaps it wasn't near visual focus (accommodation), or lack thereof, driving eye growth. Two important concepts helped researchers refine this line of thinking. First, research suggested that blur on the retina could induce eye growth; however, it is now understood that the direction of the blur is important. When the direction of the blur is known (i.e., whether the focal point is in front of or behind the retina, myopic or hyperopic), this is known as defocus. Natural eye growth typically starts with an eye that is too short, where the optics land behind the back of the eye. The eye can alter its lens to focus the image on the retina, or it can grow. Based on animal experiments, it is theorized that blur caused by hyperopic defocus (image focused behind the retina) could be a driver of eye growth for emmetropization (Troilo et al., 2019). Second, Smith et al. (2017, 2009a) showed that the central retina may not be very important in eye growth. When the macula or central retina is compromised in animals, the remaining healthy peripheral retina can still slow and drive eye growth with various lens powers (Huang et al., 2011; Smith et al., 2007, 2009a).

Questions arose: How important is the peripheral retina to focus? And, if hyperopic defocus, in which the optics of the eye focus behind the retina, was a driver for eye growth, could myopic defocus, in which the optics of the eye focus in front of the retina, be a signal to slow down the growth of the eye? Further, if this relative myopic defocus occurred in the periphery, would the growing eye have a stronger stop signal? And how would fovea-driven accommodation change the peripheral refractive status? Glasses to treat myopia have historically ensured that light is focused on the back central part of the eye. This is accomplished with a single divergent lens power and allows the wearer to have clear central vision. However, because of the increasingly prolate (i.e., oval) shape of the growing myopic eye, the peripheral retina remains blurry. Progressive addition lenses that have increasingly strong near power may have worked in the COMET study by creating relative myopic defocus in the peripheral retina rather than the hypothesized impact on near focus. That said, the relative myopic defocus would have occurred only on the superior (top part of the) retina since progressive addition lenses are placed in the inferior (bottom part of the) view of the patient.

The Bifocal Lenses in Nearsighted Kids (BLINK) study attempted to answer the question: If putting the focal plane in front of the retina could be accomplished in all meridians of the peripheral retina, would eye growth slow down using multifocal soft contact lenses? These lenses were typically used for individuals over age 40 for near visual focus, making them readily commercially available. The optics of the soft contact lens include a center zone for clear central distance vision, while the periphery of the lens adds medium- and high-powered optics to help individuals see more clearly up close (Figure 7-1). However, in children who could see close-up just fine, it was reasoned that the lenses could create relative myopic defocus, thus creating a system where more of the retina is receiving a hypothetical stop signal. The results supported the theory underlying the study: there was a dose-response relationship between the level of peripheral myopic defocus and treatment efficacy (Walline et al., 2020b). Medium additional power slowed myopia progression relative to single-vision lenses, but not to a statistically significant degree. High additional power slowed down eye growth by 0.38 D over 3 years, which did differ statistically from the single vision lens option.

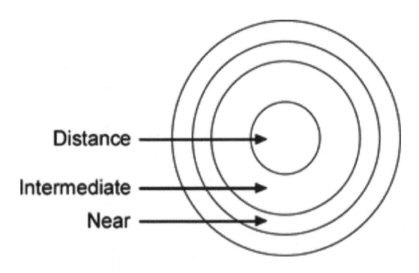

FIGURE 7-1 A schematic of the power distribution for a center-distance multifocal contact lens, such as used in the BLINK Study.
SOURCE: Adapted from Walline et al., 2017.

CORNERSTONE HUMAN STUDIES ON
SLOWING THE GROWTH OF THE HUMAN EYE

The Correction of Myopia Evaluation Trial (COMET)

COMET was the first large-scale, randomized clinical trial to show proof of concept that growth of the human eye could be slowed with an optical intervention (progressive-addition lenses in glasses). The researchers who created COMET, which was funded by the National Eye Institute and conducted in the United States, reasoned that blur on the retina causes growth of the eye (Norton, 1999; Wildsoet, 1997) and that some myopes had poor near-focusing skills (Abbott et al., 1998; Gwiazda et al., 1993). If near focus could be made more accurate, in this case by using a progressive-addition lens to provide gradually increasing reading power in the bottom of the child's spectacle lenses, it was hypothesized that near vision would become clearer, thus reducing retinal blur, and thus reducing human eye growth.

COMET investigators at four U.S. sites recruited a group of ethnically diverse children ages 6 to less than 12 years old who had low to moderate spherical-equivalent myopia, ranging from −1.25 D to −4.50 D by cycloplegic autorefraction. The average baseline age of the 469 children randomized was 9.3 years (+/− 1.3 years). Participants were randomized to either single-vision lenses or progressive-addition lenses at a 1:1 ratio. At year three, 462 of the 469 (98.5%) randomized participants were retained and evaluated. The COMET study group went on to publish 36 peer-reviewed journal articles between 2001 and 2018 (COMET Group, 2013; Gwiazda et al., 2002, 2011; Hou et al., 2018; Hyman et al., 2001).

The COMET study showed that the children who wore single-vision glasses had progressed in their myopia on average by −1.48 (±0.06) D (more nearsighted), while those wearing progressive-addition lenses had progressed by only -1.28 (±0.06) D. This difference of 0.20 (+0.08) D between the two groups was statistically significant (P = 0.004). Results were similar concerning change in axial length. Children wearing single-vision glasses had eye growth or axial elongation of 0.75 (+0.02) mm, and those wearing progressive-addition lenses had eye growth of 0.64 (+0.02) mm (See Figure 7-2.) This 0.11 (+0.03) mm difference between the two groups was also statistically significant (P = 0.0002). Importantly, this treatment effect was seen in the first year only; no additional treatment effect was seen in years two and three. COMET investigators deemed these treatment differences statistically different but not clinically meaningful. However, this was the first large-scale, prospective, multi-center, federally funded randomized clinical trial to show slowing of human eye growth by an optical intervention.

Key Findings from the COMET Study:

- Progressive-plus powered lenses slowed myopia progression, but only by 0.20 D over three years.
- Axial length growth was also slowed by 0.11 mm using the progressive-addition lens.
- These findings were deemed statistically significant but not enough to warrant a change in clinical practice.
- The treatment effect was seen only in the first year. No additional treatment effect was seen in years two and three.

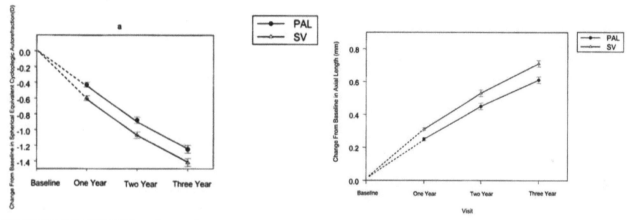

FIGURE 7-2 COMET study results.
NOTES: Progressive-Addition Lenses (PAL) had a treatment effect compared to single-vision lenses (SV). The treatment effect on both spherical equivalent refractive error and axial length was largely seen only in the first year of the study. Mean change in (A) spherical equivalent refractive error. (B) Mean increases in the axial length of eyes of children in the PAL and SVL groups at each annual visit. *Dashed lines* are included for illustrative purposes, to show the similarity of the two treatment groups at baseline. Error bars, SE.
SOURCE: Gwiazda et al., 2003.

The Bifocal Lenses in Nearsighted Kids (BLINK) Study

BLINK was a large-scale, multicenter, randomized control trial funded by the National Eye Institute to evaluate myopia progression in 294 children wearing single-vision, soft contact lenses vs. commercially available multifocal contact lenses. Children were ages 7 to 11 years at baseline with spherical equivalent myopia between −0.75 and −5.00 D and less than one diopter of astigmatism when recruited between 2014 and 2016 (Walline et al., 2017).

By 2010, peripheral positive lens defocus, when the focus of light is behind the peripheral retina, had been shown to induce central axial myopia in monkeys (Smith et al., 2009b, 2010).

Prior to this time, blur-inducing myopic growth was thought to be concentrated on the central retina. These studies were the first of their kind suggesting that the peripheral retina could mediate the axial length of the eye. If peripheral minus lens defocus could induce myopia, could peripheral myopic defocus (where the light is focused in front of the peripheral retina) minimize myopic progression? Animal studies suggested that this was true (Huang et al., 2012; Smith et al. 2013).

Human studies followed with a variety of optical interventions. Orthokeratology, a technique in which children wear rigid gas-permeable plastic (hard) contact lenses overnight to flatten the cornea, may work in this mechanism to minimize peripheral hyperopic defocus. MiSight contact lenses, the first soft contact lenses FDA-approved for treating myopia progression, were also suggested to put the focus of the light in front of the retina. These daily-disposable contact lenses use alternating concentric rings within the optics of the contact lens and may also work by taking advantage of relative myopic defocus.

BLINK investigators wondered if commercially available, standard, soft multifocal contact lenses could be used in U.S. children to create relative myopic defocus and reduce myopia progression over three years. Three groups were compared, each wearing a different type of contact lenses: single-vision, medium-add power, and high-add-power. As shown in Figure 7-3, the contact lenses choice altered the position of focused light on the peripheral retina. At year three, 292 of 294 (99%) randomized participants were retained and evaluated (Berntsen et al., 2023; Chandler et al., 2023; Gaume et al., 2022; Walline et al., 2013, 2020b).

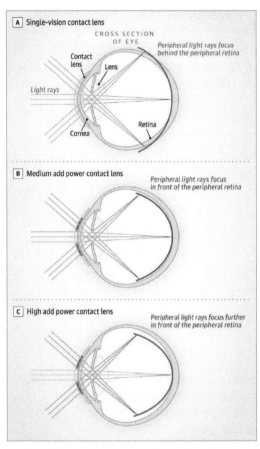

FIGURE 7-3 BLINK study rationale.
NOTE: In the BLINK study, three groups of children wore three different contact lenses that altered the peripheral focus to be either (A) behind the retina using single-vision lenses; (B) slightly in front of the peripheral retina using medium-add-power contact lenses; or (C) further in front of the peripheral retina using high-add-power contact lenses.
SOURCE: Walline et al., 2020b.

Key Findings from the BLINK Study:

- School-aged children living in the United States progressed −1.05 D over 3 years (average of −0.35 D per year) wearing single-vision contact lenses. Commercially available, soft multifocal contact lenses with a *high add* were able to slow myopia progression by 0.46 D over three years.
- There was no statistically significant difference between single-vision contact lenses and lenses with *medium add* powers.
- The number of adverse events were minimal, supporting the safety of soft contact lenses in children ages 7 to 11 years old.
- Nearly 5 years of multifocal contacts with an add power did not significantly affect the participants' ability to focus at near without the lens.

- Despite the theory of myopic peripheral defocus slowing myopia and the potential to induce peripheral defocus in a multifocal contact lens, most peripheral defocus metrics and defocus at most peripheral retinal loci accounted for little to no variance in the treatment effect of the +2.50 D addition lens. Thus, the mechanism of the treatment effect did not appear to be peripheral defocus or pupil size (Berntsen et al., 2023). (Also see Figure 7-4.)

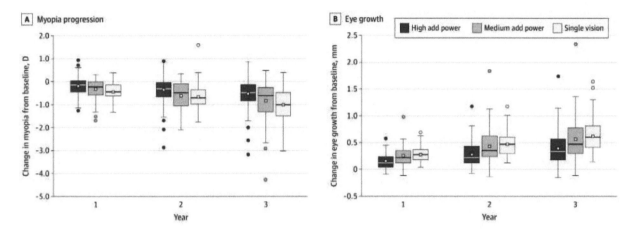

FIGURE 7-4 BLINK study results.
NOTE: Results of the BLINK study for refractive error change (A) and change in axial length; (B) High-add powers were able to slow myopia progression by 0.46 D and axial elongation by 0.23 mm over three years. There were no statistically significant differences between single-vision contact lenses and medium-add powers. See Figure 7-3 for description of the treatment groups.
SOURCE: Walline et al., 2020b.

CURRENT OPTICAL TREATMENTS FOR MYOPIA PROGRESSION AVAILABLE IN THE UNITED STATES

Currently, there are no spectacle options available in the United States for treatment of myopia progression (see treatment section below). However, in addition to the CooperVision Biofinity Multifocal, other contact lens options have been used to slow the growth of the eye (see Figure 7-5) and are based on the theory of providing relative peripheral myopic defocus.

The MiSight® contact lens by CooperVision, Inc., is the only soft contact lens option that is FDA-approved specifically for slowing the growth of the myopic eye. Long-term study results from large-scale, multicenter, national, longitudinal clinical research suggest that (a) myopia slows in children wearing these daily disposable contact lenses compared to children wearing single-vision contact lenses; (b) the benefit occurs even in later childhood; (c) the treatment effect continues to accrue beyond the initial year into subsequent years; and (d) although there is a rebound effect after use of the contact lenses is discontinued, it is not statistically significant (Chamberlain et al., 2022 Lumb et al., 2023).

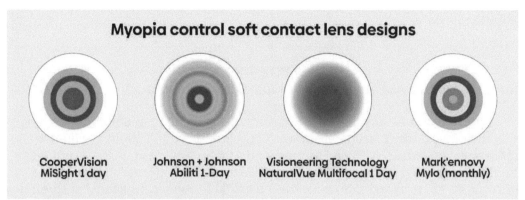

FIGURE 7-5 Myopia control soft contact lens designs.
NOTE: The MiSight 1 day contact lens by CooperVision is the only FDA-approved treatment option for myopia control currently available in the United States. Other contact lens companies are working toward such labeling. These soft contact lenses use concentric rings of variable optics to try and direct some of the light entering the eye to focus in front of the retina, rather than in focus with the retina, in hopes of serving as a partial stop signal for eye growth.
SOURCE: Figure reproduced from "How do myopia control soft contact lenses work?" Published on MyKidsVision.org with the permission of MyopiaProfile.com.

Additionally, orthokeratology rigid contact lenses also seem to take advantage of minimizing peripheral hyperopic defocus. As mentioned earlier, these lenses are worn at night to reshape the cornea by morning to minimize the need for glasses or contacts during the day. Because the cornea takes on the shape of the lens and is flattened, the optics of the eye are pulled in front of the retina. In a meta-analysis, orthokeratology was reported to slow down the axial-length growth of the eye on average by 0.25 mm over the course of 2 years (Wen et al., 2015). Ranking just below the use of high- and mid-concentration atropines, orthokeratology seems to provide the most effective treatment for slowing growth in axial length, according to the Cochrane Review from 2023 (Lawrenson et al., 2023).

BOX 7-2
What Is the Role of Astigmatism in Myopia Development and Treatment Options?

In a population-based study of U.S. preschoolers living in and around Los Angeles, California, the prevalence of astigmatism was 6% in non-Hispanic White children and 8% in Asian children (Wen et al., 2013); in Hispanic and African American children in the same area, the prevalence was higher at 17% and 13% respectively (Fozailoff et al., 2011). In a population-based study in and around Baltimore in 2013, myopic preschool children were 4.6 times more likely to have astigmatism than children without refractive error (McKean-Cowdin et al., 2011).

Astigmatism in children is often corneal or lenticular in origin. Infantile astigmatism is associated with myopia during the school-aged years (Gwiazda et al., 2000). From Gwiazda et al. (2000) through to CLEERE (Zadnik et al., 2015), against-the-rule astigmatism (astigmatism where the steepest curve lies near the 180-degree meridian) was associated with a higher risk of myopia onset. The mechanism for why against-the-rule astigmatism is more associated with myopia onset than with-the-rule astigmatism (a more common form of astigmatism, where the steepest curve lies near the 90-degree meridian) is unclear; however, neither is as predictive for myopia onset as spherical equivalent refractive error (Zadnik et al., 2015).

The role of astigmatism in myopia onset and progression is made more unclear as most randomized controlled treatment trials (the gold standard in research) often exclude participation by children with high astigmatism, in order to study a more homogenous eye type. Because this may limit well-studied treatment options and disproportionately affect racial and ethnic groups due to differences in astigmatism prevalence, further study of the role of astigmatism in myopia onset and progression treatments may be beneficial. That said, astigmatism is not emphasized in this report, since its influence on myopia development and progression appears to be limited.

PHARMACOLOGICAL TREATMENTS FOR MYOPIA PROGRESSION

Myopia has been associated with education, implicating a role for near work (see Chapter 5, Onset and Progression of Myopia). Thus, paralyzing the eye's focusing power even in one of the two eyes might reduce myopia progression (Luedde, 1932). In the mid-1960s and 1970s, atropine 1% was being studied, given its ability to paralyze the eye's focusing ability for near work. Atropine eye drops showed a treatment effect in the treated eye, but only while using the drop (Bedrossian, 1966, 1979; Brodstein et al., 1984). Later, studies using eye drop alternatives to atropine like cyclopentolate (Yen et al., 1989) and tropicamide (Shih et al., 1999) showed no treatment benefit, despite the ability of these alternatives to at least moderately paralyze the eye's ability to focus near objects (or increase pupil size). Taken together, these results suggested that atropine's beneficial effects on myopia were potentially due to another mechanism and not to the blocking of accommodation. Despite evidence that atropine eye drops could slow down the growth of the eye, side effects remained. Light sensitivity from the dilated pupil and near blur that accompanies the use of atropine makes daily use challenging and has the potential to increase the dropout rate in atropine studies. However, as the prevalence of myopia increased in the late 1900s, especially in Asia, the need for a treatment that effectively slowed myopia progression became urgent.

Early Theories on Pharmaceutical Mechanisms

Atropine Treatment

The mechanism to explain how atropine works on the eye remains unclear. Atropine is a nonselective muscarinic cholinergic antagonist. Thus, atropine's protective effects on myopia progression were expected to be due to inhibiting the effects of acetylcholine on muscarinic acethylcholine receptors, which are found on the smooth muscle fibers in the ciliary muscle that adjusts the lens shape during focusing. However, both historical and recent literature suggests that atropine's action on myopia is not related to action on muscarinic receptors, as atropine can also inhibit myopic eye growth in chicks, animals whose vision accommodation is mediated by nicotinic and not muscarinic receptors (McBrien et al., 2013; Stone et al., 1991). Also, ablating cholinergic retinal neurons did not alter the response to atropine (Fischer et al., 1998; Thomson et al., 2021; see review McBrien et al., 2013).

Atropine treatment has been associated with changes in choroidal thickness. However, evidence for a causal role is missing. Choroidal thickness has been shown to increase with atropine 1.0% in children (Jiang et al., 2021b; Zhang et al., 2016), with atropine 0.01% after 3 months (Wu et al., 2023), and in the LAMP study using various concentrations of low-dose atropine that were dose-dependent (Yam et al., 2022a). However, a recent meta-analysis found no significant effect with atropine 0.01% (Meng et al., 2023). Choroidal thickness has also been shown to be increased in myopic children treated with orthokeratology (Xiao et al., 2024), repeated low-level red therapy (Liu et al., 2024), multi-focal soft contact lenses (Peng & Jiang, 2023), and defocus-incorporated multiple-segment (DIMS) lenses (Chun, 2023). In addition, choroidal thickness changes have been observed in many animal studies in response to experimental myopia (Che, 2024; Chen et al., 2022; Jordan-Yu, 2021; Wallman, 1995) and when directly increasing choroidal thickness from intravitreal injections of atropine in chickens (Mathis et al., 2021). Collectively, this evidence does not support a causal relationship of atropine on choroidal thickness.

Another way atropine may have its anti-myopic effect is through dopamine, a neurotransmitter found in the retina and reported as a potential "stop" signal for myopic eye growth (Feldkaemper & Schaeffel, 2013; Stone et al., 1989; Zhou et al., 2017). Atropine has been shown to increase dopamine in the eye (Mathis et al., 2021; Schwahn et al., 2000; Zhu et al., 2022), particularly at high doses (Thomson et al., 2021). Studies investigating a potential causal role of atropine on dopamine release have been mixed, with dopamine receptor antagonists reducing atropine-induced choroidal thickening in response to flickering light in chickens (Mathis et al., 2023), while dopamine receptor antagonists did not block atropine's inhibition on myopia in chickens (Thomson et al., 2021). In addition, atropine reduced axial elongation in Lrp2-/- mice but did not alter dopamine or 3,4-dihydroxyphenylacetic acid (DOPAC) levels (van der Sande et al., 2023).

Other potential sites of action for atropine include vasoactive intestinal polypeptide (Wang et al., 2024), nitric oxide (Carr & Stell, 2016), and gamma-aminobutyric acid (GABA) (Barathi et al., 2014). More research is needed to evaluate the causal mechanisms of atropine, which may provide opportunities to optimize the treatment and reduce side effects.

Pirenzepine Ophthalmic Solution

The development of pirenzepine ophthalmic solution was an attempt to slow down the growth of the myopic eye using an alternative nightly eye drop. Atropine is a nonselective muscarinic antagonist that has affinity for all five acetylcholine receptor subtypes found in the retina. While this allowed the concentration of atropine to be effective in more diluted concentrations, side effects remain pervasive given its nonselective nature, affecting many parts of the eye. Pirenzepine is a more selective muscarinic receptor 1 (MR1) antagonist (Leech et al., 1995; Rickers & Schaeffel, 1995). In a 2003 study, pirenzepine was shown to be well tolerated in children (Bartlett et al., 2003). A 2008 report suggested that pirenzepine was effective for slowing refractive error progression but did not have a statistically significant effect on axial length (Siatkowski et al., 2008). Interestingly, animal experiments suggest a potential influence of pirenzepine on dopamine by increasing tyrosine hydroxylase expression in the retina (Qian et al., 2015).

An effective drug-based treatment for myopia would have the advantage of convenience, especially if the drug could be taken by mouth. Therefore, further research is needed to identify pharmacological agents that are more effective and have fewer adverse effects than current options.

CORNERSTONE ATROPINE STUDIES FOR MYOPIA PROGRESSION

Atropine Treatment of Myopia (ATOM) Study

ATOM was a cornerstone study that evaluated the effect of atropine 1% on myopia progression in a double-masked, randomized clinical trial. Children were from a single center in Singapore, ranging in age from 6 to 12 years old and with myopia ranging from -1.00 D to -6.00 D. Children were randomly assigned to two groups: the active treatment participants received atropine 1% eye drops in one eye and placebo drops in the fellow eye, while the control participants received placebo eye drops in each eye. At the end of the 2-year study, 346 of the 400 (86.5%) randomized participants were evaluated. The results of ATOM were published by Chua in 2006 and showed a very good treatment effect of 0.92 D in myopic refractive error at the end of year two ($-1.20 +0.69$ D in placebo-treated control eyes vs. -0.28 ± 0.92 D in atropine-treated eyes; P <0.001). Axial length was also nearly halted using atropine 1% with only 0.02 $+0.35$ mm growth in 2 years compared to 0.38 ±0.38 mm in the placebo-treated control eyes (Chua et al., 2006). Despite the treatment effect while using atropine, stopping the treatment caused a greater increase in myopia in atropine-treated eyes compared to placebo-treated eyes (-1.14 ± 0.80 D vs. -0.38 ± 0.39 D respectively, (P < 0.0001), with the atropine group almost catching up with the placebo group after stopping the atropine drops (Tong et al., 2009).

In children that were treated for two years and then untreated for one year, the treatment difference at year three between the atropine untreated group and the placebo untreated group diminished from 0.92 D to 0.28 D, almost negating the benefits of atropine's use. Additionally, although the overall treatment effect of atropine 1% remained better than placebo, the side effects of poor near visual acuity and light sensitivity remained. Further, it is unclear if accommodation skills and near visual acuity returned to normal after stopping atropine. As such, a need for an eye drop with fewer side effects was emerging.

Atropine Treatment of Myopia 2 (ATOM 2) Study

ATOM 2 was a second seminal study, evaluating the effect of atropine 0.5%, 0.1%, and 0.01% on myopia progression in a double-masked, randomized clinical trial. Investigators proposed that reducing the concentration of atropine 1% would result in less pupil dilation, better near vision, and less light sensitivity, while still slowing myopia progression. In 2012, ATOM 2 revealed the safety and efficacy of 0.5%, 0.1%, and 0.01% atropine applied over two years in 400 children from Singapore 6 to 12 years of age who had at least 2.00 D of myopia. The mean progression of myopia was not significantly different between the 0.5% and 0.1% groups (-0.30 ± 0.60D and -0.38 ± 0.60D). Both concentrations were more effective than the group treated with 0.01% (-0.49 ± 0.63D). However, the two stronger concentrations had statistically more side effects than the 0.01% atropine, which showed negligible changes in accommodative ability, near visual acuity, and pupillary size. Further, after stopping the treatment for one year, subjects on 0.5% atropine had significantly more rebound progression than those who had been on 0.1% and 0.01% atropine (Chia et al., 2014).

The ATOM 2 study was the first of its kind and limited by the lack of a control group, since 0.01% was initially chosen by investigators to serve as a possible placebo treatment. Regardless, given the lack of side effects and similar results, the atropine 0.01% became the new atropine of choice for the treatment of myopia progression for children living in East Asia (Chen & Yao, 2021; see Figure 7-6).

Key Clinical Findings from the ATOM and ATOM 2 studies:

- School-aged children living in Singapore experienced only 0.28 D of myopia progression in 2 years while treated with atropine 1% eye drops every evening, a treatment effect of 0.92 D. However, side effects of near blur, light sensitivity, and pupil dilation accompanied the atropine 1% use.
- After stopping the atropine 1% eye drop, myopia progressed more quickly than in children placed on placebo eye drops. This is called the rebound effect, and it reduced the treatment effect from 0.92 D on the eye drops at year two to 0.28 D off the eye drops at year 3.
- Lower concentrations of atropine have reasonably good treatment effects with less rebound. In 2016, atropine 0.01% showed a reasonably good treatment effect without the strong rebound effect.

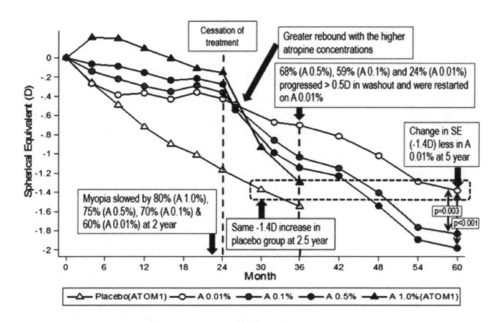

FIGURE 7-6 ATOM/ATOM 2 study results.
NOTE: The spherical equivalent refractive error plotted across time for the three atropine treatment groups (0.01%, 0.1%, and 0.5%) and placebo control.
SOURCE: Chia et al., 2016.

Low-Concentration Atropine for Myopia Progression (LAMP) Study

LAMP is a five-year, single-center, randomized clinical trial of atropine 0.05%, 0.025%, and 0.01% in children ages 4 to 12 years old living in Hong Kong. In year one, the authors found that the 0.05% atropine group had the largest reduction in myopic progression. While side effects were dose-dependent, they found that atropine was relatively well tolerated in all the groups. The Phase 2 report describes the second year of the study in which the atropine groups remained at the same concentrations, and the placebo group stopped using the placebo drop and started using 0.05% atropine. The authors suggested that 0.05% atropine is the most effective dose of atropine and side effects were well tolerated. Over three years, those in continued treatment continued to show dose-dependent effects (see Figure 7-7). Washout rebound was also concentration-dependent, but the differences in rebound myopia between 0.01%, 0.025%, and 0.05% were not significant (Yam et al., 2019, 2020, 2022b).

Key Findings from the LAMP Study:

- Children ages 4 to 12 years at baseline experienced the best treatment effect using 0.05% atropine compared to those using atropine 0.025% and 0.01%.
- Treatment benefit for myopic axial elongation was small at 0.05 mm at year one using atropine 0.01% in 2019.
- The success of low-dose atropine in children living in Asia prompted large-scale randomized clinical trials in non-Asian countries.

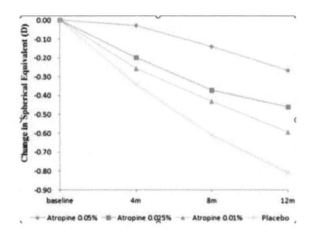

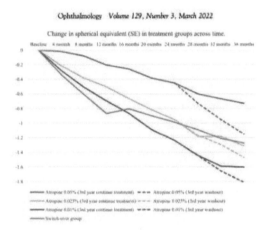

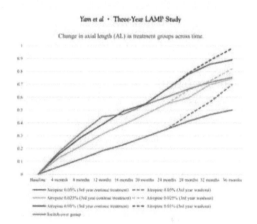

FIGURE 7-7 LAMP study results.
SOURCE: Yam et al., 2019.

CURRENT PHARMACEUTICAL TREATMENTS AVAILABLE IN THE UNITED STATES

The ATOM study results in 2006 (Chua et al., 2006) may be the impetus for atropine's widespread use for myopia control. A report of a recent survey completed by pediatric ophthalmologists worldwide suggests that over half the respondents treat myopia progression and that 70% prescribe atropine as their go-to treatment for myopia control (Zloto et al., 2018). While atropine 0.01% was the most popular concentration (Zloto et al., 2018), two large-scale, randomized clinical trials conducted in the United States reported marginal to no treatment effect using either atropine 0.01% or atropine 0.02% (Repka et al., 2023; Zadnik et al., 2023). The LAMP study of children with myopia in Hong Kong suggests that 0.05% may be the optimal concentration in Chinese children, balancing side effects and treatment effect (Yam et al., 2022b).

Studies suggest that the higher the concentration of atropine is, the better the treatment effect (Chia et al., 2012; Yam et al., 2022b)—often, but not always (Gong et al., 2017b; Zadnik et al., 2023). However, the side effects do seem to be consistently dose-dependent, with higher concentrations causing more light sensitivity, near blurred vision, and rebound growth after stopping use of the drops (Gong et al., 2017b; Yam et al. 2022b).

In summary, atropine is the only widely used pharmacological treatment for myopia progression. Yet, there remain many unanswered questions related to atropine. While long-term efficacy is not well studied, recently published data attempt to provide insight. Participants in the ATOM study were contacted 10 and 20 years after the conclusion of the original clinical trial. Despite atropine concentrations ranging from 0.01% to 1.0% demonstrating short-term efficacy during the clinical trial, these treatments did not have a long-term effect 10 and 20 years after treatment ended, at least in the sample of participants who could be re-contacted (Li et al., 2024). These results underscore a need for research that addresses how long atropine should be used, the ideal age for stopping treatment, and how to stop treatment. Research should also look at the long-term effect of prolonged accommodative paralysis on near visual acuity and accommodative amplitudes. Additionally, as atropine is studied, new delivery systems may be discovered along with ideal dosing cadences and/or day/night timing of the dose. Research in combination therapy, as described later in this chapter, such as atropine-plus orthokeratology or multifocal contact lenses, for example, would also be beneficial, especially in higher than 0.01% concentrations of atropine.

A better understanding of the causal mechanisms of atropine is needed. Using an intentionally integrated, multi-disciplinary approach could provide new therapeutic targets that increase efficacy while minimizing side effects for children. More studies are needed to identify the ideal dosing characteristics, including the concentration and cadence of more specific pharmaceuticals and potentially new delivery systems. In addition, longer studies are needed to determine how and when to end the intervention to provide the optimal effect with minimal rebound.

CONTEMPORARY SYSTEMATIC REVIEWS AND GLOBAL PERSPECTIVES

In the National Academies' (NRC, 1989) review on myopia, no treatment options were confirmed to slow down the naturally occurring growth of the human eye. Decades later, much evidence points to the value of attempting to control myopia progression. Two recent reports provide a rigorous summary of the current literature on myopia treatments and control, one authored by the Cochrane Living Systematic Review and Meta-Analysis author committee and the other by the International Myopia Institute. Both the International Myopia Institute and the Cochrane review and meta-analysis are internationally recognized, and together they provide a convergence of expertise on myopia that can provide a foundation for current and emerging treatment strategies. Figure 7-8 below highlights the results of a database search of the term "myopia" within research titles between 1842–2024.

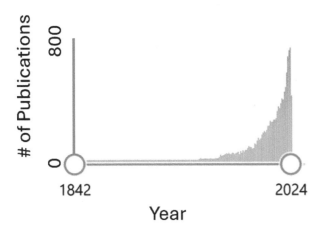

FIGURE 7-8 Frequency of the term "myopia" in research titles, by year, 1842–2024.
SOURCE: Committee generated based on PubMed database search performed July 2024.

Cochrane Living Systematic Review and Meta-Analysis

The *Cochrane Living Systematic Review and Meta-analysis* is the third Cochrane publication led by Jeff Walline since 2011 (Lawrenson et al., 2023; Walline et al., 2011, 2020a). The 2023 version was last updated in 2021. Stated objectives include the following:

- To assess the comparative efficacy of optical, pharmacological, and environmental interventions for slowing myopia progression in children using network meta-analysis;
- To generate a relative ranking of myopia control interventions according to their efficacy;
- To produce a brief economic commentary, summarizing the economic evaluations assessing myopia control interventions in children;
- To maintain the currency of the evidence using a living systematic review approach.

While the 2023 Cochrane review of myopia literature (Lawrenson et al., 2023) spans 265 pages, an important graphic from the review, representing a novel overview of myopia treatment options available today, is reproduced in Figure 7-9. The Cochrane review included 64 studies that randomized 11,617 children, aged 4 to 18 years. Studies were mostly conducted in China or other Asian countries (39 studies, 60.9%) and North America (13 studies, 20.3%). Searches included CENTRAL (which contains the Cochrane Eyes and Vision Trials Register); MEDLINE; Embase; and three trials registers. The search date was 26 February 2022. Randomized controlled trials (RCTs) of optical, pharmacological, and environmental interventions for slowing myopia progression in children aged 18 years or younger were included (Lawrenson et al., 2023).

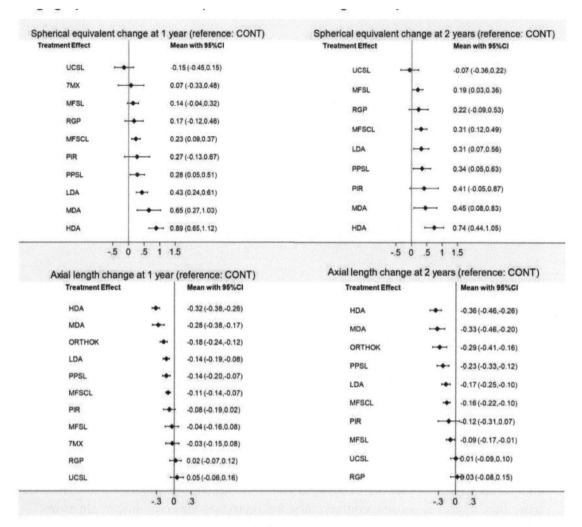

FIGURE 7-9 Cochrane Review of treatment effect of myopia.
NOTES: Estimates of effect from network meta-analyses for all treatments versus control for progression of myopia (based on spherical equivalent and axial length) at 1 and 2 years. Comparisons with control are less precise than direct meta-analyses due to the lack of directly comparative evidence. 7MX = 7-methylxanthing; HDA = high-dose atropine; LDA = low-dose atropine; MDA = moderate-dose atropine; MFSCL = multifocal soft contact lenses; MFSL = multifocal spectacle lenses; ORTHOK = orthokeratology; PIR = pirenzipine; PPSL = peripheral plus spectacle lenses; RGP = rigid gas-permeable contact lenses; UCSVL = undercorrected single vision spectacles.
SOURCE: Lawrenson et al., 2023.

Key Findings from the 2023 Cochrane Review of Myopia Treatment Effect on Myopia Progression:

- No treatment provides more than a 0.75 D treatment effect, on average, of less myopic progression of spherical equivalent refractive error over two years.
- No treatment on average provides more than a 0.37 mm treatment effect of reduced axial elongation over two years.

- After high- and mid-dose atropine pharmaceuticals, peripheral-plus spectacle lenses and orthokeratology contact lenses may be the most effective optical treatments.
- The treatment effect is not sustained in the second year for the pharmaceuticals even while on treatment, suggesting that the treatment effect is not as cumulative as would be ideal.
- Orthokeratology has the biggest treatment effect in the second year.
- Treatment effect for spherical equivalent refractive error and axial length are highly correlated.
- Under-correction or no correction may promote axial elongation and myopia progression.

The International Myopia Institute (IMI)

The IMI was created in 2015 when the World Health Organization and Brien Holden Vision Institute met to address increasing levels of myopia and the associated risk to sight. Experts from around the world have since provided a convergence of expertise in the formulation of evidence-based recommendations for "classification, patient management, and future research" (International Myopia Institute, 2024). IMI white papers and clinical summaries serve to broadly disseminate its perspectives to the general public as well as to "scientists, clinicians, policy makers, government and educators" in an effort to foster collaboration and shared knowledge.

The most recent citation of the IMI is the 2023 *IMI Digest* (Sankaridurg et al., 2023). Salient points from the 2023 abstract are quoted below. The committee believes this abstract provides a strong reflection of the state of myopia today and potential strategic future directions.

Key Findings from the 2023 IMI Digest:

Studies in animal models have continued to explore how wavelength and intensity of light influence eye growth and have examined new pharmacologic agents and scleral cross-linking as potential strategies for slowing myopia. In children, the term 'premyopia' is gaining interest with increased attention to early implementation of myopia control. Most studies use the IMI definitions of ≤ -0.5 diopters (D) for myopia and ≤ -6.0 D for high myopia, although categorization and definitions for structural consequences of high myopia remain an issue. Clinical trials have demonstrated that newer spectacle lens designs incorporating multiple segments, lenslets, or diffusion optics exhibit efficacy comparable to contact lens-based optical approaches. Clinical considerations and factors influencing efficacy for soft multifocal contact lenses and orthokeratology are discussed. Topical atropine remains the only widely accessible pharmacologic treatment. Rebound observed with higher concentration of atropine is less evident with lower concentrations or optical interventions. Overall, myopia control treatments show little adverse effect on visual function and appear generally safe, with longer wear times and combination therapies maximizing outcomes. An emerging category of light-based therapies for children requires comprehensive safety data to enable risk versus benefit analysis. Given the success of myopia control strategies, the ethics of including a control arm in clinical trials is heavily debated. (Sankaridurg et al., 2023, p. 1).

Global Trends in prescribing patterns: Despite the increasing levels of clinical activity in myopia control, single vision spectacles (32%) and contact lenses (7.5%) were still the most commonly prescribed methods of correction (although this is slowly decreasing), but myopic controlling spectacles are now being prescribed (15.2%) along with myopia controlling soft contact lenses (8.7%), orthokeratology (11.6%) and atropine therapy (7.2%; Wolffsohn, 2022).

EMERGING CLINICAL TREATMENT OPTIONS FOR MYOPIA PROGRESSION

There is still much to be learned about myopia and its progression. The COMET study, discussed earlier in the chapter, was the first large-scale, randomized clinical trial to show proof of concept that the growth of the human eye could be slowed by an optical intervention. Its results, published in 2003, showed a 0.20 D treatment benefit in spherical equivalent refractive error over 3 years, which was deemed statistically significant but not clinically meaningful. Since COMET results came out, over 20,000 new research articles have been published on myopia. Still, the treatment effects may be viewed as marginal at best despite two more decades of research.

Novel treatment options are required to advance the field of myopia control in more meaningful ways. Emerging treatment options, including new perspectives on time outdoors as well as optical, pharmaceutical, chromatic, and surgical strategies, are all reviewed in turn next.

Environmental Strategies

Time Outdoors Versus Near Work

Because the increasing prevalence of myopia is likely due, in large part, to the effects of environment, clinicians will be recommending modification of their pediatric patients' visual experience more and more as part of their care. Increased time outdoors will probably become a common recommendation. Restricting time spent engaged in near work seems more problematic and may have minimal benefit given the limited effect of near work on the rate of myopia progression (discussed in Chapter 5). The following reviews evidence on the effects of increased time outdoors on the risk of myopia onset and rate of progression.

In contrast to the controversy that surrounds the effects of near work on myopia, there is a broader consensus regarding the protective effects of more time outdoors (McBrien et al., 2009). Unlike studies of near work, both cross-sectional and longitudinal data show effects. In the cross-sectional perspective, children without myopia spend more time outdoors (Dirani et al., 2009; Jones-Jordan et al., 2011; Rose et al., 2008). More importantly, in the longitudinal perspective, emmetropic children who spend more time outdoors have a lower probability of becoming myopic (French et al., 2013b; Guggenheim et al., 2012; Jones et al., 2007; Zadnik et al., 2015).

The data on near work and time outdoors come from surveys of parents, so they are subject to criticism for recall bias and lack of detail. The failure to find effects for near work bring the utility of these surveys into question, yet these same parental surveys repeatedly detect the effects of time outdoors. Two important questions in this area of myopia research arise: (a) What is the mechanism by which time outdoors has this protective effect? and (b) Does this protective effect apply to the progressing myope in addition to the emmetropic child at risk for onset?

Effect of Time Outdoors on Onset Versus Progression

A meta-analysis conducted in 2017 concluded that the protective effects of time outdoors only apply to delaying or preventing myopia onset and not to slowing the rate of myopia progression (reviewed in Xiong et al., 2017). Xiong et al. (2017) analysis of six longitudinal studies showed a dose-response reduction in the probability of myopia onset with increased time outdoors. The asymptote of protection was reached at about 2 hours per day (Xiong et al., 2017). This amount of outdoor time parallels the recommendation from the International Myopia Institute (Jonas et al., 2021). The value of this meta-analysis is that it differentiated the incident myope from the prevalent myope and analyzed the effect of time outdoors in each group. It found no evidence for a dose-response relationship between time outdoors and myopia progression (Xiong et al., 2017).

Results from the Xiong et al. (2017) meta-analysis and the Orinda Longitudinal Study of Myopia suggest that 10 to 14 hours of outdoor time per week can substantially reduce the risk of myopia onset (Jones et al., 2007). In the analysis of CLEERE data, every additional hour of time outdoors reduced the odds of onset by 2–4% (Zadnik et al., 2015). CLEERE results also parallel the findings of Xiong's meta-analysis of progression. The rate of myopia progression showed no differences across quartiles of time outdoors (Jones-Jordan et al., 2012). There are exceptions, however. Wu et al. (2018b) found positive effects on both incidence and progression as the result of a program increasing time outdoors at school. Interestingly, the same investigators found effects only on incidence and no significant effects on progression in their earlier, 2013 report (Wu et al., 2013). Another exception is the findings from India in a study by Saxena et al. that spending more than 14 hours outdoors per week reduced the odds of showing some degree of myopic progression compared to having a stable myopic refractive error (Saxena et al., 2017).

At present, the evidence suggests that time outdoors is more effective in preventing or delaying myopia onset than in slowing its progression. Is the lack of effect on progression the result of myopic children spending less time outdoors? This behavior of spending lower amounts of time outdoors seems characteristic of myopic children but not to the extent that insufficient variation in behavior would invalidate the conclusion from this analysis. Jones-Jordan pointed out that even if time outdoors were restricted to the lower three of the four quartiles of time spent outdoors reported for emmetropic children, those representing the majority of the lowest amounts of outdoor time, there would still be detectable protective effects of more time outdoors against onset (Jones-Jordan et al., 2012). The lack of effect in slowing progression of myopia is therefore unlikely to be due to the tendency of myopic children to spend less time outdoors. That amount of time would still be sufficient to delay or prevent the onset of myopia in an emmetropic child.

Time Outdoors: What Is the Protective Mechanism?

Understanding the mechanism by which time outdoors exerts its protective effect would have tremendous benefit. Basic mechanisms underlying the physiology of eye growth would be revealed along with the possibility of controlling that growth (see Chapters 5 and 6 for discussion). Having children spend more time outdoors is an inexpensive intervention, and physical activity can have the collateral benefit of affecting rates of obesity, cardiovascular disease, and diabetes (Colberg et al., 2016). On the other hand, outdoor time can also have harmful effects on the health of the skin and eye with increased rates of cancer, cataract, and macular degeneration (Chawda & Shinde, 2022). Activation of the protective effects of time outdoors without exposure to higher energy short-wavelength light could preserve the benefits of time outdoors while avoiding harm. There are several candidate mechanisms for the protective effects of time outdoors (also see Chapter 5 on Onset and Progression). These are discussed next.

Ultraviolet Light

Time outdoors increases ultraviolet light exposure and cutaneous production of vitamin D (Barger-Lux & Heaney, 2002; Holick, 1995). Lower plasma levels of vitamin D show a linear relationship with more myopic refractive errors in European, East Asian, and American study samples (Choi et al., 2014; Guggenheim et al., 2014; Mutti & Marks, 2011; Tideman et al., 2016; Wolf et al., 2023; Yazar et al., 2014). The effect size is small, however, and the amount of variability is quite large by comparison. For example, the Western Australian Pregnancy Cohort (Raine) Study reported that a 100-nanomolar increase in circulating 25(OH)D3, an increase equal to nearly the entire range of serum values, would only be associated with a small difference in refractive error of 0.60 D (Yazar et al., 2014). Likewise, a Mendelian randomization analysis found that no significant effect on refractive error could be attributed to differences in circulating 25(OH)D (Cuellar-Pardita et al., 2017). An analysis of data from the Avon Longitudinal Study of Parents and Children (ALSPAC) performed by Guggenheim et al. (2014) concluded what most investigators in the field now see as the role of vitamin D in myopia: any associations between vitamin D and myopia are likely due to associations between time outdoors and myopia.

Flatter Dioptric Space

The outdoor environment presents the eye with a different set of viewing distances compared to indoors. Objects outdoors are more uniformly distant while objects indoors are at various and closer distances from the eye. Diopters of optical demand for clear vision are the inverse of the number of meters an object is from the eye. This optical environment may be thought of as the eye's dioptric space. Flitcroft presented one of the first analyses of indoor vs. outdoor dioptric space (Flitcroft, 2012). He characterized indoors as more varied in terms of dioptric stimuli in comparison to the relatively more flat, distant dioptric space outdoors. There are several challenges with attributing the protective effect of outdoors to its characteristically flat dioptric space. One is that peripheral myopia would seem to dominate the indoor scene during most near-work taking place indoors. A second is that the effects of defocus may be substantial in animal models, but these effects have not translated into substantial influences of refractive error development in either human infants or children.

Lastly, there is an implication of inferior-superior asymmetry along the vertical meridian in both defocus and therefore eye length in this analysis, one that is not found in human data. Nasal-temporal asymmetries are commonly found, but not meaningful inferior-superior asymmetry (Atchison et al., 2004, 2005, 2006; Mutti et al., 2019; Verkicharla et al., 2016). For example, vertical peripheral eye lengths at 30 degrees eccentricity in BLINK children only differed by 0.15 mm. Greater levels of myopia show the same differences in shape along the vertical meridian of the eye as well as along the horizontal meridian of the eye (i.e., lateral, or left to right); both become less oblate by the same amount as a function of increasing refractive error (Mutti et al., 2019; Verkicharla et al., 2016). Indoor and outdoor spaces may be different in many ways, dioptric space included, but any differences must also be relevant to the development of refractive error. The flatter dioptric space outdoors seems unlikely to be the source of protective effects. The accommodative system, however, needs to function differently in the flatter (outdoor) and steeper (indoor) dioptric spaces to optimize retinal image quality. For an account of the relative role of the periphery and fovea in accommodative effort, and its consequences for outdoor and indoor dioptric spaces, please see Chapter 6, Role of the Non-foveal Retina in Accommodation.

Absence of Near Work

Near work is seldom performed when outdoors, at least by children. The protective effects of time outdoors might be thought of as the protective effects of not engaging in near work. This view would depend on near work and time outdoors having a negative correlation, where more of one means less of the other. That assumption seems reasonable but, interestingly, most studies find that these are two independent factors with no negative correlation. For instance, Guggenheim et al. (2012) reported no significant correlation between these two variables in ALSPAC and they were also uncorrelated in the Orinda Longitudinal Study of Myopia (OLSM), CLEERE, and the Sydney Myopia Study (Jones et al., 2007; Rose et al., 2008; Zadnik et al., 2015).

Higher-Irradiance Sunlight

The more widely accepted hypothesis for the protective effects of time outdoors is that exposure to higher irradiance sunlight stimulates the release of dopamine from the retina, which, in turn, has an inhibitory effect on axial elongation (Norton et al., 2013; Rose et al., 2008; Stone et al., 1989). As discussed in detail in Chapter 6, retinal dopamine is secreted by amacrine cells stimulated through their connections with ON-bipolar cells. Intrinsically photosensitive retinal ganglion cells (ipRGCs) containing the photopigment melanopsin also provide excitatory input to sustained-firing dopaminergic amacrine cells through their own light-evoked responses (Zhang et al., 2008). Therefore, bright visible light increases retinal dopamine through stimulation of both traditional photoreceptors and nontraditional photosensitive ipRGCs. The release of dopamine may enhance and prolong the firing of melanopsin-driven responses in ipRGCs through the actions of cyclic adenosine monophosphate (cyclic AMP; Beaulieu et al., 2015; Sodhi & Hartwick, 2014).

Because ipRGCs project to the olivary pretectal nucleus, an area of the midbrain in the central nervous system that controls the reaction of the pupil of the eye to light, it has been hypothesized that evaluation of adaptive changes in pupillary responses to repeated light stimuli may represent an assay of this release of retinal dopamine. Results from this type of pupillometry support the hypothesis that non-myopic individuals produce more retinal dopamine in response to light stimulation. Less myopic refractive error in adults showed a linear correlation with greater pupillary constriction in response to repeated pulses of short-wavelength blue light and slower redilation following offset of the blue light stimuli (Mutti et al., 2020). Shorter axial lengths in children were correlated with slower redilation following offset of the blue light stimuli and faster pupillary escape in response to repeated pulses of long-wavelength red light. Interestingly, these responses related to axial length were only found in the summer months, a time when environmental light is more available, and not during winter months (Reidy et al., 2024). These findings suggest that more hyperopic/less myopic individuals may have a greater ability to take advantage of light exposure and its accompanying protective effect.

An important question for future research is whether any deficiencies in retinal responses to light exposure in children at risk for myopia onset are present early in life or develop along with the onset of myopia. A related question is this: If more and more children become myopic who could have avoided it by spending more time outdoors, does increasing their time outdoors now slow myopia *progression* in that subpopulation? Studies may begin to see effects of time outdoors on progression for this reason. Another issue is whether any deficiencies are intrinsic and unchanging or whether early behaviors may alter the ability of the retina to respond in a protective manner to environmental light. An analysis of ALSPAC data by Shah et al. showed positive effects in lowering the odds of future myopia onset between 10 and 15 years of age that were attributable to increased time outdoors as early as 3 years of age (Shah et al., 2017). Clearly, whatever the capabilities of the retina might be to respond in a beneficial manner to environmental light, that capability needs to be coupled with actual time outdoors in order produce protective effects.

International Examples of the Effects of Outdoor Time

Regardless of whether early exposure to more time outdoors changes retinal responses, early exposure may be a reasonable strategy simply on the basis of applying inhibitory influences on axial elongation over more years. Scandinavia and its uncharacteristic lower prevalence of myopia compared to other parts of Europe provides an interesting example (Hagen et al., 2018). Countries at northern latitudes may have a difference of as much as 13 hours in length of day between summer and winter. Extended darkness in winter does not sound consistent with obtaining protective effects from light exposure that would lower a national prevalence of myopia. Yet, Scandinavians seem to value whatever length of daylight is available. There is a cultural awareness of the need for light exposure in these countries, perhaps from the need to maintain adequate levels of vitamin D. This ethos is encapsulated in the word "friluftsliv" or "open-air living," a dedication to spending as much time outdoors as possible whatever the conditions. Babies are routinely left outdoors in strollers year-round as their parents shop or eat at cafes.

The Scandinavian example perhaps shows that even if sunlight is limited, following the recommendation of at least two hours per day, especially when experienced early in life, may be sufficient to have a positive effect on the prevalence of myopia. Taiwan also provides an encouraging example. Decades of increasing prevalence of myopia began to decline two years after schools in that country implemented a program encouraging 120 minutes per day of time outdoors (Wu et al., 2018a). Australia shares a similarly low prevalence of myopia, has an abundance of available sunlight, and a culture that values extended time spent in outdoor recreation. Australian children were reported to spend an average of 105 ± 42 min/day outdoors compared to 61 ± 40 min/day for children in Singapore (Read et al., 2018). These differences may in part account for the differences in myopia prevalence. The prevalence of myopia in teenagers in Singapore is on the order of 74% (Quek et al., 2004) while far fewer Australian teens are myopic (30%; French et al., 2013).

While studies support the hypothesis that myopia onset is prevented or delayed by spending time outdoors, many questions remain. For instance, determining the causal mechanisms for the protective effect of time outdoors could provide the opportunity to apply those key factors of the outdoor space while children are indoors. Numerous strategies are being considered: increased indoor illumination from larger windows, painting outdoor scenes on school walls, or having children look into devices delivering light to the eye with wavelengths anywhere from red to violet (Dolgin, 2024). If the protective mechanisms of time outdoors involve retinal dopamine release, investigations into other visual conditions that enhance retinal dopamine release, like retinal ON pathways, would be beneficial. Regardless of the mechanisms, encouraging children to spend more time outdoors, particularly early in life, could provide protective effects against myopia onset. However, due to the lack of evidence for time outdoors to slow myopia progression, it seems unlikely to serve as an effective adjunct to treatments aimed at slowing progression once children become myopic.

Optical Strategies for Mitigating Myopia Progression

Glasses for Slowing Myopia Progression

In addition to contact lenses for altering peripheral focus, emerging technology with "peripheral-plus spectacle lenses" shows promise in slowing axial growth of the eye. Unlike other treatment options that are used off-label in the United States (orthokeratology lenses, atropine, soft multi-focal lenses), these peripheral-plus spectacle lenses have been developed for the purpose of myopia control, although they are not yet FDA-approved and thus not commercially available in the country at this time. However, the lenses are available in Canada and in other parts of the world. While no studies have confirmed a treatment benefit in U.S. children, meta-analysis suggests that the treatment effect is fairly equal to if not more effective than that of contact lenses that attempt to control myopia (Lawrenson et al., 2023).

Three novel myopia-control spectacle options use peripheral myopic defocus as their mechanism. Each uses a lens as its base that provides a clear image centrally on the back of the eye. Additionally, surrounding a clear central zone of the lens, there is an overlay of "lenslets" that intend to create myopic defocus over much of the retina. The Hoya MiyoSmart® lens uses a zone of lenslets to provide myopic defocus over the mid-peripheral retina (Lam et al., 2020) (Figure 7-10). The Essilor Stellest® lens adopts a volume approach with a greater number of lenslets designed to create more dimensions of myopic defocus (Li et al., 2023a; Figure 7-11). Neither of these two lens designs seems to alter the focusing plane of the eye, likely because—unlike multifocal contact lenses—each convex lenslet forms a discrete image on the retina that cannot be fused to form a clear, continuous image.

For the ZEISS MyoCare® lens there is less longitudinal data, but the lens operates somewhat similarly in its attempt to create myopic defocus in the peripheral retina (Liu et al., 2023). Instead of using lenslets, this ZEISS lens is reported to create higher-order aberrations in the periphery as a signal to slow growth. SightGlass Vision DOT® is another spectacle lens design used to slow myopia; however, it uses reduced contrast, not myopic defocus, as its hypothesized mechanism is related to cone opsin photopigment defects (Rappon et al., 2022; see Chapter 5, Syndromic Myopia for more details). Similar to the dual focus spectacle lenses above, there is a clear zone in the spectacle lens at the center for maximum clarity in central vision. This requires careful measurement of the distance between the pupils and from the center of the pupil to the bottom of the frame.

There are several practical benefits to spectacles that may be able to slow the growth of the eye. First, glasses are the standard treatment option for children with myopia. Since the lenses seem to be well-tolerated (Gao et al., 2021; Lam et al., 2020; Rappon et al., 2022), the treatment is minimally different compared to wearing standard, vision-correcting spectacles. Additionally, these spectacles allow for greater powers of astigmatism to be corrected than some previous optical treatment options, which allows for more diversity in children who may benefit from wearing them. However, further study is required to determine the effect of peripheral refractive errors on road driving, as at least one early report suggests that the driving performance of young drivers may be impaired with the addition of myopia defocus (Ortiz-Peregrina et al., 2022).

In addition to the functional aspects of these lenses and their treatment effects, it may also be helpful to better understand how these lenses truly affect the peripheral retinal image. For example, it may be helpful to know if eccentricity from the macula toward the periphery of the retina is an important factor, in regard to the placement of the zone of defocus or reduced contrast. One study in rhesus monkeys suggests that myopia defocus in the near periphery can slow axial myopia, and that defocus beyond 20 degrees from the fovea does not (Smith et al., 2020). However, further studies are needed to confirm this result. Additionally, the effect of the corrective multifocal lens options on the amount of peripheral image quality—myopic defocus or contrast reduction—should be determined using a combination approaches: in situ optical bench measurements, on-eye evaluation with objective assays of optical quality (such as wavefront sensing and double-pass point spread function measurement), and wide-angle eye models. This may allow researchers to subsequently determine if these treatment options show an association that is consistent with their purported mechanism of action. At least one study showing treatment benefit using multifocal contact lenses with a high-add power suggested that peripheral defocus was not associated in a substantial manner with treatment benefit (Berntsen et al., 2023). (For more on evaluating the optical quality of these treatments and their mechanisms, also refer to the section below, "Mechanisms of Optical Treatments and their Limitations".)

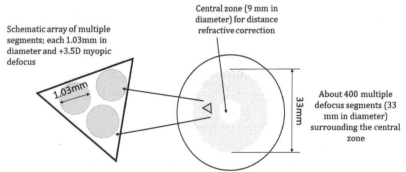

FIGURE 7-10 Schematic of the Defocus Incorporated Multiple Segments (DIMS) in the Hoya MiYOSMART lens.
SOURCE: Lam et al., 2020.

Visual stimuli are composed of luminance and chromatic information. The potential influence of luminance on myopia development was covered in the section on environment earlier in this chapter. Below, the committee considers the chromatic information in visual stimuli.

Longitudinal Chromatic Aberrations (LCA)

When light enters the eye, chromatic aberration causes the various wavelengths that make up the light to focus at different locations in the back of the eye. For light focused on the retina, long wavelengths (reds) are actually focused a little behind the retina, while short wavelengths (blues) are focused in front of the retina (Figure 7-11). There are several possible ways that such chromatic stimuli could be processed by the retina to provide signals about eye growth. While there are inter-species differences in the cone spectral types, the short-wavelength cones (S-cones) and their pathways are similar among mammals, implicating their role in the processing of LCA (Calkins, 2001). One hypothesis is that this LCA provides a cue for the eye to grow to emmetropia (Rucker & Wallman, 2009; see review in Troilo et al., 2019). If red light is in sharper focus than blue light, that could signal that the eye is too short and provide "grow" signals to elongate the eye. If blue light is focused more sharply than red, that could signal slowing of eye growth. A study with human participants reported that watching movies filtered to be in focus in the red plane for 45 minutes produced longer axial lengths in emmetropic participants, while young participants with myopia did not respond to the stimuli (Swiatczak & Schaeffel, 2022).

Many animal studies have investigated these effects by housing animals in monochromatic, narrowband lighting and have found significant effects on refractive development. Such experiments have been done using fish, chickens, guinea pigs, tree shrews, and rhesus monkeys. The studies conducted with fish (Kröger & Wagner, 1996), chickens (Foulds et al., 2013; Rohrer et al., 1992; Seidemann & Schaeffel, 2002; Shaeffel & Howland, 1991; Torii et al., 2017), and guinea pigs (Jiang et al., 2014; Liu et al., 2011; Long et al., 2009; Wang et al., 2011) have tended to support the LCA hypothesis, with short-wavelength light producing relative hyperopic refractive shifts and long-wavelength light producing relative myopia refractive shifts . Studies in other animals have shown the opposite effects, specifically in tree shrews (Gawne et al., 2017; She et al., 2023), and rhesus monkeys (Hung et al., 2018; Liu et al., 2014; Smith et al., 2015). Recently, a quantitative model has been developed to explain how LCA detection by the short- and long-wavelength sensitive cone photoreceptor types present in the tree shrew retina can decode the sign of defocus (Gawne et al., 2021). Notably, this LCA model of emmetropization provided predictions that were validated by experimental results (Khanal et al., 2023). Further study is necessary to clarify the role of LCA as a mechanism to drive refractive eye growth, especially due to the potentially conflicting differences in species, even among mammalian species.

Atypical Opsins: Opn3, Opn4, and Opn5

A second mechanistic hypothesis for short-wavelength light is detection through atypical opsins: Opn3, Opn4, and Opn5. These atypical opsins are all found in the retinal ganglion cells and have wavelength sensitivities ranging from 470–485, 480–485, and 350–450 nm, respectively (Guido et al., 2022; although see Emanuel & Do, 2023, for controversy about melanopsin wavelength sensitivity). Studies using mice with mutations in Opn3, Opn4, and Opn5 have demonstrated an influence on refractive development and/or myopia susceptibility (Chakraborty et al., 2022; Jiang et al., 2021a; Linne et al., 2023; Liu et al., 2022). Furthermore, the protective effect of violet light (360–400 nm) in wild-type mice was eliminated in a mouse without Opn5, and this effect was most prominent two hours prior to the end of the diurnal phase of the light cycle (Jiang et al., 2021a), demonstrating a causal effect of Opn5 and a diurnal effect of violet light exposure.

Emerging data in tree shrews also shows that short-wavelength light (420 nm) that activates OPN5 completely suppresses the expected myopia shift induced by experimental lens defocus (Grytz & Lang, 2023). Interestingly, the same wavelength that was found to be protective in mice (365 nm) was not protective in tree shrews, presumably due to lens absorbance. Modeling of lens transmittance indicated that wavelengths of 420 nm would be transmitted effectively through the tree shrew ocular lens and this wavelength inhibited myopia susceptibility.

Finally, violet light exposure in children using violet-light-emitting frames (360–400 nm at 310 μW/cm2) has also been shown to provide some benefit (change of 0.5 D in 24 weeks) (Torii et al., 2022).

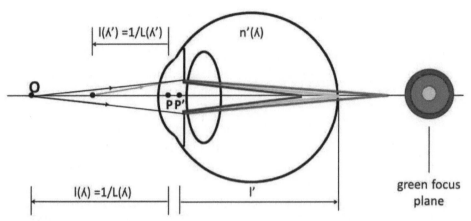

FIGURE 7-11 Illustration of longitudinal chromatic aberration in the eye.
NOTE: Rays of longer wavelength (red) are focused behind the retina and shorter wavelength rays (blue) are focused in front of the retina. As a consequence, the image of a point in the green focus plane is a focused on green, with halos in red and blue.
SOURCE: Vinas-Pena (2015). Reprinted with permission from the author.

Repeated Low-Level Red Light (RLRL) Therapy

RLRL was first reported as a treatment for slowing myopia progression in 2022 and has quickly become commercially available in several countries, but not the United States (Khanal et al., 2024). RLRL treatment generally consists of exposure to laser light (650 +/-10 nm; 1600 lux with a power of 0.29 mW for a 4-mm pupil) for 3 minutes, twice a day, 5 days per week (Jiang et al., 2022). Several randomized clinical trials have reported efficacy of RLRL in controlling myopia (Chen et al., 2022, 2023; Dong et al., 2023; Jiang et al., 2022; Lin et al., 2023; Tian et al., 2022; Xiong et al., 2021, 2022, 2023; Zhou et al., 2023). These studies have reported an impressive slowing of axial elongation and myopia refractive errors. For instance, one study found a 54% reduction in myopia over 12 months (He et al., 2023) and a decrease in myopia progression by –0.59 D in refractive error and 0.26 mm in axial elongation (Jiang et al., 2022). Some of the reported benefits of RLRL treatment include axial shrinkage of the globe in a minority of patients (Wang et al., 2023), which may involve effects of scleral myofibroblasts, as observed in an animal model (Phillips & McBrien, 2004).

While most reports of RLRL efficacy and safety have been positive, side effects include photosensitivity during treatment and temporary after-images with treatment (Deng et al., 2023; Tang et al., 2023; Wang et al., 2023). In addition, there appears to be a strong rebound effect when RLRL treatment is stopped (Chen et al., 2023; Xiong et al., 2022). A single case report of a 12-year-old with retinal damage after 5 months of RLRL therapy has raised concerns about the long-term safety of this treatment (Liu et al., 2024). Furthermore, bench testing of two RLRL therapy devices (Sky-n1201a and a Future Vision) found that the devices reached or exceeded the maximum permissible exposure after three minutes of continuous viewing (Ostrin & Schill, 2014). The mechanisms of RLRL treatment effects are not known and may include improved choroidal blood flow, nitric oxide signaling, mitochondrial effects via photobiomodulation, and/or reduction of scleral hypoxia (Zhou et al., 2023). Researchers agree that more research is needed to determine the mechanisms and evaluate the safety of RLRL for children (Salzano et al., 2023; Schaeffel & Wildsoet, 2024).

Structural and Surgical Strategies for Mitigating Myopia Progression

Scleral Cross Linking

The ultimate outcome of myopic eye growth is elongation of the ocular globe caused by remodeling of the sclera. This axial elongation involves changes in scleral biomechanics. Patients with high myopia can develop a posterior staphyloma in which the sclera thins and then develops an outpouching. Thus, one potential approach to treating progressive myopia has been to prevent the sclera from expanding using scleral cross-linking. Scleral cross-linking causes increased stiffness of the scleral tissue by forming new covalent bonds between collagen fibers and decreasing the space between fibers (Yasir et al., 2023).

There are multiple approaches to scleral cross-linking, and thus far the majority of studies on scleral cross-linking have been in animal models to demonstrate safety and feasibility. Studies in form-deprived rabbits and lens-defocus guinea pigs (Chen et al. 2023; Ding et al., 2021; Li et al., 2017; Liu et al., 2016) have shown that UV-A light and the photosensitizer riboflavin have the potential to increase the biomechanical strength of the sclera and slow the development of myopia. This approach requires the application of riboflavin to the targeted tissue and then exposure to UV-A light to create the chemical reaction. When feasibility studies were performed in human eyes with existing blindness (Li et al., 2023b), signs of inflammation or toxicity were observed, suggesting safety concerns. A limitation of this approach is reaching the most posterior globe, where changes in myopia are most prominent (Yasir et al., 2023).

Other cross-linking approaches have used Rose Bengal with green light, methylene blue with red light, and the non-photoactivated cross-linker genipin (Yasir et al., 2023). The approach with the least cytotoxicity appears to be low-level laser therapy using red or near-infrared light to penetrate deeper into the tissue (Yasir et al., 2023). Studies using RLRL therapy in myopic children found a benefit in controlling axial elongation (see section on RLRL above); however, it is not known currently whether the mechanism of action of RLRL is through scleral cross-linking. Importantly, some animal studies have reported potential risks associated with scleral cross-linking, such as increased intraocular pressure in genipin-treated guinea pigs (Guo et al., 2024). Repeated genipin injections in tree shrews caused degeneration of photoreceptors and retinal pigment epithelium (Hamdaoui et al., 2022). Therefore, additional studies are needed to develop scleral cross-linking methods that are both safe and effective.

Pharmacological and Combination Strategies

The only widely used pharmacological treatment for myopia progression is atropine, as described above. Its effectiveness in low doses in U.S. children necessitates further study. There are only a few emerging pharmacological strategies that have been tested in animal models and translated into the clinic. For instance, 7-MX, which blocks adenosine receptors and is a caffeine metabolite, has shown some benefit in rhesus monkeys with lens-induced myopia (Smith et al., 2021), but limited efficacy in clinical trials (Trier et al., 2023). (A full review of this treatment can be found in Khanal et al., 2024.)

When monotherapies provide incremental benefit to slow myopia progression, it makes sense to consider combination therapies. Any combination of optical (e.g., special contact lenses), pharmaceutical (typically low-dose atropine), environmental (more time outdoors), and structural (scleral cross-linking) could be considered, even up to a quadruple combination attempt. However, the typical combination studied thus far has been limited to dual therapies, including low-dose atropine with an optical intervention including soft contact lenses, orthokeratology, or special spectacle lenses. A review by Pucker (2023) and another by Cochrane (Lawrenson et al., 2023) suggest that some dual therapies may slow myopia progression more than monotherapies and that orthokeratology in combination with atropine 0.01% seems to have the largest treatment effect; however, the largest treatment benefit with dual therapy compared to monotherapy is 0.15 D per year. Some studies show a statistically significant difference between monotherapy and additive dual therapy; however, no combination shows a doubling effect between monotherapy and dual therapy (Pucker, 2023).

Research on combination therapies for myopia progression thus far has focused on using low-dose atropine (0.01%) with Asian children living in Asia. Concerning children in the United States, there is a study of atropine 0.01% in combination with multifocal contact lenses using a +2.50 add; however, that study showed no benefit in this combination (Jones et al., 2022). Future research is necessary to determine the effectiveness of combining treatments. It should be noted that if a monotherapy is not effective in treating myopia progression, a study of its combination with another effective (or ineffective) treatment is likely to suggest no benefit as well. As such, the effectiveness of the monotherapy must be proven first, especially in U.S. studies.

DECISIONS IN TREATMENT

For the optometrist and ophthalmologist considering the treatment of myopia progression, a thorough and ongoing review of myopia literature will be required. Despite modest advances in how much eye growth can be slowed, the preponderance of evidence suggests that treatment for myopia progression should at least be considered for all myopic children.

As the field of myopia progresses, it may be that treatment strategies will become specific to an individual patient. Myopia control methods do seem to slow the progression of myopia and its axial elongation. However, many questions remain. Is it standard of care? Are the treatment effects worth the cost of the treatment strategies? Do the treatment strategies require use throughout the school-aged years? Or beyond? And does the safety of the treatment outweigh the risk to the eye? It is questions like these that make treating for myopia progression sometimes difficult.

Care should be taken by the eye care professional to avoid suggesting to patients that a cure for myopia exists or that treatment effects will be more substantial than warranted by the evidence. The practitioner should offer an evidence-based approach to the treatment of myopia progression when discussing with patients and their families. Factors that identify who may benefit most from treatment or in whom myopia is more likely to progress are considered next.

Key Elements in the Decision to Pursue Myopia Control Treatment Options

- Once nearsighted, the eye tends to grow, especially between ages 7 and 16 years old. The average rate of progression in U.S. children is approximately 0.50 D per year; it may be faster in younger children.
- The average age of cessation in myopia progression is between 15 and 16 years. 75% of children with low to moderate myopia in the early school-aged years stop becoming more nearsighted at age 18; 4% are still growing more nearsighted at age 24.

- The preponderance of evidence suggests that myopia progression can be treated. While studies typically show 2- and 3-year results, clinical treatment is likely required to be much longer and may persist into early adulthood.
- Current treatment options have the following implications:
  - Atropine 0.01% may not be effective in U.S. children; higher doses may be required, but side effects and rebound effects should be considered.
  - Orthokeratology requires a larger pupil than the optical center for treatment to be effective.
  - Multifocal contact lenses for use in the treatment of myopia progression must have a center for distance and near power in the surround; the add power must be 2.50 D or higher.
- The only FDA-approved drug or device in the United States is the MiSight daily disposable contact lens.
- Special spectacles that use peripheral myopic defocus or contrast to attempt to slow down the progression of myopia are available in some parts of North America but are not FDA approved at this time and therefore not available in the United States.
- The largest treatment effect of any current treatment option is less than 0.75 D over two years. There is currently no cure for myopia progression.
- Past progression does not predict future progression. Delaying treatment until a criterion rate of progression is reached may not be ideal.
- Outdoor play seems to have a protective effect on myopia onset. Two hours per day or 14 hours per week may be enough to delay the onset of myopia.
- Under-correction is not ideal and may cause further progression, and overcorrection is likely to cause faster progression as well. The aim is to optimize acuity by providing an accurate refractive correction.
- Nearsighted eyes are at risk for retinal detachment, especially greater than - 6.00 D of myopia. Myopia greater than –5.00 D would benefit from annual dilated eye exams.
- Refractive error: +0.75 D or less hyperopia at age 6 is likely to progress. Consider low, non-myopic refractive error a risk factor in the younger ages.
- Age of patient at onset of myopia is important: The younger the child, the faster the nearsightedness seems to progress. Additionally, the more years a patient has myopia, the more myopia they are likely to have as an adult.

Ideal Characteristics of Treatments

As researchers continue to review evidence and attempt to push the field forward, the ideal characteristics of methods to slow the growth of the eye are starting to emerge. The following list of characteristics reflects the committee's view.

Accessibility and Inclusion

- Ideal solutions would show a meaningful effect on diverse groups of individuals on both spherical equivalent refractive error and axial length.
- Treatments should be done prior to onset to delay or prevent myopia.
- Their administration should be feasible for a child, working toward noninvasive and nonpainful delivery.

- The cadence of treatment should be timely and convenient for children and families.
- Cost-effectiveness must be prioritized to minimize health disparities.

Durability and Reliability of Effect

- New treatments should work toward having no rebound effect, prioritizing long-term data that show lasting effects into adulthood when myopic eyes may take on more cumulative risk.
- When monotherapies show effectiveness alone, it would be ideal if they showed added benefit when combined.
- Treatments with the most potential for success would likely affect multiple parts of the eye to increase the effect.
- They would also have been proven by robust bench or animal work with known and plausible mechanisms that support the translational research efficiently and frugally.
- Ideal treatments would also be FDA-approved to underscore the goal of systemic and ocular health and safety of the child.

WHY DON'T MYOPIA TREATMENTS WORK BETTER FOR CONTROLLING MYOPIA PROGRESSION?

Alternative Theories for Mechanisms

An unexpected feature of optical myopia control is that its effects seem limited in magnitude, limited in duration, and similar in magnitude across the underlying range of myopia progression and elongation. These issues were noted in an extensive recent review by Brennan et al. (2021). In clinical trials lasting at least 2–3 years, children in the intervention group typically experience only 0.50 D to 0.75 D less myopia progression, or 0.2 mm to 0.3 mm less axial elongation, than control subjects. A second characteristic is that treatment benefit is often greatest in the first year and may not continue to accrue past the second or third year of myopia control (Huang et al., 2016 Lawrenson et al., 2023).

The third characteristic is more than curious. It poses a potential challenge to the assumed underlying mechanism for optical myopia control: imposing a peripheral "STOP" signal of myopic defocus. An inhibitory signal, such as myopic defocus, might be expected to slow myopic changes in proportion to the underlying rate of change, the rate that would have occurred without treatment. A 50% treatment effect for a child with fast myopia progression should yield a greater treatment effect than a 50% treatment effect for a child changing more slowly. Proportional inhibition, one that is relative to the underlying untreated rate of change, should create skew in the distribution of refractive error and axial length for treated children. Notably, the distribution of refractive errors or axial lengths is strikingly similar between treated and control children (Charman & Radhakrishan, 2021). This overlap of treated and control distributions led Brennan et al. (2021) to conclude that this form of myopia control produces more of an offset between groups, an absolute treatment effect rather than a relative one.

Reconsidering the Role of Accommodation in Myopia Progression

The mechanism for optical myopia control should therefore be one that results in a discrete rather than a proportional treatment effect, that is randomly distributed, and that only accrues over a limited period of time. One such potential mechanism might be chronic relaxation of accommodation. The additional peripheral positive power in optical myopia control reduces the accommodative response of children (Cheng et al., 2019; Gong et al., 2017b). Chronic relaxation of the ciliary muscle may reduce the net force on the anterior segment of the eye, resulting in a less prolate/more oblate shape and a reduced axial length. The eye would essentially be redistributed into a relatively wider equatorial diameter with an accompanying shorter axial length. This is essentially the reverse of the proposed forces underlying the effect of accommodation on emmetropization (discussed in Chapter 5).

Chronically inhibiting accommodation might also be viewed as the reverse of the forces that created myopia in the first place, a reversal of the increase in tension in the anterior segment of the eye from a failure of crystalline lens stretch (discussed in Chapter 6). The near work habits of close working distance and uninterrupted periods of near work hypothesized to affect the rate of myopia progression represent prolonged accommodation. An increase in working distance and more frequent breaks from near work might be analogous to chronic reduction in accommodation. Future longitudinal studies investigating these factors should evaluate whether their effects are similar to or exceed those for myopia control. Modifying these behaviors may influence progression, but an interesting question is whether these strategies affect progression by a meaningful amount over a meaningful period of time or do they face the same limitations as current myopia control.

The pattern of peripheral eye growth during optical myopia control provides some support for this redistribution hypothesis. The pattern of eye expansion during myopic progression is characterized by axial elongation exceeding peripheral expansion. The eye becomes more prolate or less oblate. Optical myopia control results in more symmetric expansion between the central and peripheral retina. Peripheral eye length data from the BLINK study indicated that the treatment effect was greatest at the fovea and not in the periphery, as might be predicted with a center-distance contact lens. This pattern of inhibition of elongation meant multifocal contact lenses either neutralized or reversed the increase in retinal steepness seen with single-vision lenses.

Elongation during orthokeratology for myopia control also resulted in more symmetric expansion, expansion that was actually greater for the nasal retina than with single-vision spectacles by up to 0.21 mm (Huang et al., 2022). Peripheral refractive error, and indirect measure of eye shape, also showed more symmetric expansion during optical myopia control with DIMS specialty spectacles compared to single-vision correction (Zhang et al., 2020). Measurements of peripheral eye length beyond the $\pm 30°$ obtained from optical biometers would be useful for evaluating this hypothesis by determining how the shape of the eye is affected by accommodation during optical myopia control.

Furthermore, as reviewed in the section below on "Mechanisms of Optical Treatments and their Limitations," it remains unclear how existing and emerging treatments interact with each individual eye and modify the retinal image distribution as a function of eccentricity. Thus, this remains an important avenue for future research that will require not only individualized models of the eye's optics but also *in situ* characterization of the optical properties across a large field of view for the treatments.

Mechanisms of Optical Treatments and Their Limitations

To understand the purported mechanisms of treatment effects of optical corrections—spectacles or contact lenses—at least three parallel lines of inquiry are needed, along the lines of those conducted recently (Arias et al., 2023; Jaskulski et al., 2020; Papadogiannis et al., 2023; Sah et al., 2022). These are (a) *in situ* characterization of the optical performance of the corrective lens (Arias et al., 2023; Jaskulaki et al., 2020), (b) on-eye evaluation of visual performance with the corrective lenses (Papadogiannis et al., 2023), and (c) integration of the correction with eye models to evaluate retinal image quality (Sah et al., 2022). These need to be carried out with imposed variations in (at least) pupil size, retinal eccentricity, wavelength, and object distance (i.e., through focus characterization), since these variables capture the essential elements that vary in the visual diet through these corrective optics.

The optical characterization of the lenses *in situ* has been carried out using several techniques, including high-resolution aberrometry and high-dynamic range double-pass point-spread-function measurement. The utility of the point-spread-function measurement is to overcome the limitation imposed by the relatively sparse sampling imposed by the Shack Hartmann wavefront sensor with a finite number of lenslets. To effectively quantify optical quality at high spatial frequencies, as might be expected from multifocal optics such as the MiSight® and the spectacle lenses with repeating diffuse or defocus microstructures (DOT® and MiyoSmart® DIMS respectively), a point-spread-function, double-pass image *in vivo* and scatter quantification are required.

The differences in methods notwithstanding, the manipulation of optical contrast is uniformly evident in the periphery of a majority of these corrective lenses beyond the purported and intended change in the relative peripheral refraction. An open question that follows is the relative impact of optical defocus (magnitude, sign, dependence on eccentricity) vs. contrast as the driving mechanism in arresting eye growth with these treatments.

A few observations from prior studies are of note in this regard. When tested on an optical bench in situ, the DIMS lens exhibited increased sharpness and contrast in the periphery as compared to DOT and single-vision lenses (Arias et al., 2023). Under photopic conditions, the single-vision DIMS and DOT lenses all reduced contrast in the periphery, with the DOT lenses leading to the largest reduction. The DOT lens reduced contrast the most under mesopic lighting in the presence of glare sources in the Arias et al. (2023) study. The mechanism of contrast reduction is attributed to a pupil-size-dependent alteration in light scattering properties of the lenses, which have a clear zone in the center and periodic diffusing microstructures around the clear zone. The amount of scattered light at visual angles greater than 3 degrees was higher than that for standard elderly observers for these lenses.

Besides scattering, the DOT lenses were similar in their focusing properties to single-vision lenses, except for a diffraction pattern induced by the periodic microstructures. All lenses led to a hyperopic shift in the periphery when typical optical aberrations present in a myopic eye were incorporated into the measurement. This emphasizes the interaction inherent between these optical corrections and the native aberrations present in an eye, especially in the periphery. It also indicates the need for (c) above, i.e. integrating the corrections into realistic and individualized eye models to predict retinal image quality *in vivo* as a function of retinal eccentricity. In addition to the hyperopic shift, the DIMS lens led to a larger depth of focus compared to the other two, leading overall to sharper and higher contrast images through focus.

The lack of a defined peripheral myopic defocus was noted in the on-eye evaluation of other optical corrections: aspherical lenslets (Stellest®), defocusing lenslets (MiyoSmart®), and multifocal contact lenses (MiSight®; Papadogiannis et al., 2023). The fact that these devices have varying and insufficient efficacy indicates a mechanism besides peripheral myopic defocus mediating their treatment effects. Furthermore, relative peripheral refraction used to quantify optical quality is ill-defined because of the large depth of focus in the periphery attributed to the increased magnitude of higher-order aberrations and astigmatism. The horizontal progressive-addition (Perifocal®) was the only lens in this study noted to create a more myopic focus in the periphery (by ~1 D), but also to interact with the eye's aberrations, leading to an overall larger variability in its effect on peripheral image quality (Papadogiannis et al., 2023).

All four of these lenses were intended to create a myopic relative peripheral refraction with positive powered zones. However, the Stellest®, MiyoSmart®, and MiSight® treatments did not induce the intended myopic relative peripheral refraction. This seeming discrepancy can be attributed to the inability of classical paraxial eye models to capture the optical performance at greater retinal eccentricities that are important for myopic eye growth. For example, the effect of the large variation of optical power profiles across the pupil and at peripheral visual fields, as may be expected for the multifocal optical lens designs of these treatments, is not adequately captured by traditional foveocentric paradigms for measuring refraction (see Chapter 6 for an elaboration of foveocentric vs. retinocentric views of refractive error). Again, all lenses exhibited reductions in contrast in the peripheral retina, as evaluated from double-pass point-spread-function and peripheral acuity measurements. In the Papadogiannis et al. (2023) study, the MiSight contact lens led to the largest reduction in contrast. Reductions in contrast and shifts in image focus are two suggested mechanisms of action of these corrections, but it has been argued that changes in accommodative capacity altered by these corrections might be yet another plausible mechanism. Overall, the mechanisms by which optical corrections function in arresting abnormal eye growth remain incompletely understood.

The importance of native optical quality and its interaction with the corrective optics emerges as a unifying finding from the bench and on-eye evaluations. This suggests that treatments such as the Perifocal and MiSight lens, which are intended to function through changes in peripheral refraction, led to larger inter-subject variability and are in general more sensitive to the native optical quality. On the other hand, the repeating diffuse or defocusing lenslets seem to be more resilient to the native optical quality and tend to function through a general reduction in peripheral contrast. Overall, this further emphasizes the need for establishing eye models to fully evaluate the optical correction as a function of retinal eccentricity, pupil size, wavelength, and object distance.

Theories on Contributions of ON/OFF Pathway Dysfunction to Myopia Progression

Increasing evidence suggests that retinal ON and OFF pathways have different influences on refractive eye growth. Retinal ON and OFF pathways are parallel neural circuits in the retina that are activated when light stimulation increases or decreases, respectively. For instance, bright light stimulates the retinal ON pathway and stimulates retinal dopamine release, which is thought to be a "stop" signal for axial growth (see Chapter 6; reviewed in Hendriks et al., 2017; Mazade et al., 2024; Zeitz et al., 2023). Dopamine is a retinal neuromodulator that alters the neural connectivity of the retina under different lighting conditions by modulating the gap junction between retinal neurons. In addition, participants exposed to white text on a black background for 60 minutes, which disproportionally stimulates retinal ON pathways, exhibited increased choroidal thickness, while participants exposed to black text on a white background, stimulating retinal OFF pathways, had thinner choroids (Aleman et al., 2018). Finally, mutations in retinal ON pathways, such as in patients with congenital stationary blindness, result in myopia (reviewed in Hendriks et al., 2017; Mazade et al., 2024; Zeitz et al., 2023).

These results suggest that visual stimuli activating retinal ON pathways could provide a signaling cue that slows refractive eye growth and thus protects against myopia, while visual stimuli that activate retinal OFF pathways may be myopigenic. Furthermore, the myopic retina may develop an imbalance in the ON and OFF pathways. Functional measurements of the retina using the electroretinogram indicate a decreased b-wave amplitude in individuals with myopia, indicating some dysfunction at an early stage of the retinal ON pathways (Poudel et al., 2024). In addition, emerging data from mouse retinas exposed to lens-induced myopia have an imbalance of ON and OFF pathway activation in their inner retinal neurons, with ON pathway activation decreasing (Mazade & Pardue, 2023, 2024). These results suggest that imbalance of ON and OFF pathway stimulation in the visual diet could contribute to myopic eye growth and that these stimuli could alter the development of ON and OFF pathways in the myopic retina, which may further decrease the ability of the retina to process low contrast and regulate retinal illuminance in bright environments (Poudel et al., 2024).

As noted above, changes in contrast may be an integral component of defocus and optical corrections, as described in the section above, "Mechanisms of Optical Treatments and their Limitations." Contrast is detected jointly by the retinal ON and OFF pathways (see Chapter 6). Thus, if optical corrections for myopia control create a "rebalancing" of the ON and OFF retinal pathways, myopic growth signals in the eye may be diminished. However, if the eye is still experiencing myopigenic visual stimuli during treatment, then the drive for myopic eye growth may still be present and produce continued signaling for axial elongation and continued development of a retinal ON/OFF pathway imbalance in the retina, and thus a positive-feedback loop for continued myopia progression.

COST-EFFECTIVENESS OF TREATMENTS

Economic assessments of healthcare interventions aid evidence-based advocacy, policymaking, and patient care (Sorenson et al., 2008) by helping decision-makers to understand the quantity of resources required for treatment or prevention, to understand the value of treating or preventing the condition, and to weigh these considerations against other uses of the resources. The economic burden associated with myopia grows with its prevalence. In 2015, globally, uncorrected myopia cost \$244 billion, and myopic macular degeneration accounted for \$6 billion in potential productivity loss[2] (Khanal et al., 2024; Smith et al., 2009c). This may seem like a small amount given the size of the economy and the enormous impact of other conditions, but it becomes important to compare the burden with the cost of reducing it. Also, it is important to recognize that the data used in the estimate are from before 2015 and 2009, respectively. Since that time, the opportunities to be productive without vision correction have changed, the cost of vision correction has changed in ways other than just inflationary pressures, and the knowledge of long-term consequences and cost of treating them has also changed.

Direct Costs

Due to the increasing prevalence of myopia and the strain on healthcare resources, a reliable economic evaluation of myopia treatments is necessary to maximize benefits that can be obtained using the budget that is available. Data are sparse on the economic benefits of myopia

---

[2]All \$ figures are in USD, unless otherwise indicated.

treatments, such as the benefits of improved classroom behavior because of a child not losing attention, increased educational attainment or other skills that lead to higher incomes, and the monetary value of decreased incidence of later complications. In Singapore, the annual direct cost of treating myopia for teens before 2010 was $25 million (Lim et al., 2009) and $755 million for adults (Zheng et al., 2013); part of the reason for the disparate cost is that there are many more myopic adults than teens. The cost estimate for Singapore includes refractive surgery, glasses, contact lenses, solutions, and associated myopia visual impairment issues.

Lack of economic evaluation evidence may hamper decision-makers' abilities to make rapid decisions about allocating resources to myopia interventions (Fricke et al., 2023). The cost of myopia treatment varies significantly worldwide, but direct costs are the major contributor. A review of the literature review was published in 2021 with data from 2002 (Spain) to 2018 (Iran) and other studies in 2006, 2009, and 2013; the previously published cost figures do not appear to have been inflation-adjusted for the reviewer (Foo et al., 2021). In the United States, the annual direct costs range from $14 to $26 per capita over the entire population, with contact lenses being the most expensive item on a per-patient basis (Foo et al., 2021). In Singapore, the mean annual direct cost of myopia is approximately SGD$900 ($709) per patient. The major drivers of this cost are spectacles, contact lenses, and optometry services (Zheng et al., 2013). For Singaporean school children, the mean annual direct cost of myopia per student with myopia is SGD$221.68 ($148), with higher costs associated with higher family income and parental education levels (Lim et al., 2009).

Financial Burden and Cost-Effectiveness of Interventions

The cost of myopia treatment is a significant financial burden for patients and their families, and effective control methods are needed to alleviate these costs (Tang et al., 2021). There are now evidence-based standards of care for myopia globally (Gifford et al., 2019; Hendicott & Block, 2022; Németh et al., 2021; Saxena et al., 2023; Tapasztó et al., 2023). The 2023 Myopia Consensus Statement released by The World Society of Pediatric Ophthalmology and Strabismus states, "There is sufficient evidence to warrant the adoption of myopia prevention and control measures in clinical practice in children with progressive myopia of childhood" (World Society of Pediatric Ophthalmology & Strabismus, 2023). Despite the increasing recognition of myopia as a high-priority problem and the establishment of a task force by the American Academy of Ophthalmology (Modjtahedi et al., 2021), there are no formalized insurance or vision plan services that cover the costs of myopia treatments in the United States.

The cost-effectiveness of various myopia treatment options varies. In earlier years, Gwiazda (2009) and Chang & Joo (2012) pointed out limitations in available treatments and information on the treatments that were available; this included short-term benefits and side effects (Chang & Joo, 2012; Gwiazda, 2009). However, in 2021, Foo et al. suggested that myopia treatment and prevention costs are justified based on the opportunity to reduce the ongoing expenditures related to myopia. Discussions of the cost-effectiveness of myopia treatments are drawing more attention (Bullimore & Brennan, 2023; Vutipongsatorn et al., 2019). One systematic review noted that the annualized value of lifetime direct expenditures per patient for contact lenses in Iran ranged from $198.30 to $378.10 per patient, while the costs for spectacles and refractive procedures were $342.50 and $19.10, respectively (Foo et al., 2021). Lifetime direct costs for the three options are $9374, $5203, and $568. The authors of the original study from Iran (Mohammadi et al., 2018) note that a U.S. study (Javitt & Chiang, 1994) had reached similar conclusions about substantially lower lifetime costs for surgery in comparison with soft contact lenses.

As noted, the annual prevalence-based direct expenditures for myopia across the entire population were between $14 and $26 per capita in the United States, in comparison with $56 per capita in Iran and $199 per capita in Singapore. Hong et al. (2022) examined the cost-effectiveness of photorefractive myopia screening at age 11, administering atropine 0.01% eye drops for positive cases. They found that screening plus atropine eye drops saved seven lifelong blindness cases per 100,000 children and had an incremental cost-effectiveness ratio of NZ$1,590 (95% CI 1390, 1791) per quality-adjusted life-years gained, which is generally considered a good value.

In a recent systematic review, Agyekum et al. (2023a) evaluated the cost-effectiveness of interventions for myopia and its complications, including those for preventing myopia progression, correcting refractive error, and treating pathologic myopia using costs, quality-adjusted life-years, and incremental cost-effectiveness ratio as outcome measures. They found that low-concentration atropine (0.01%) and corneal refractive surgery were the most cost-effective treatments for myopia, and ranibizumab and conbercept were the most affordable treatments for pathological myopia, that is, for the more severe levels of myopia that have an adverse effect on the health of the eye.

Preventing myopia progression was reported to be more cost-effective than treating pathological myopia. For instance, the use of 0.01% atropine for myopia progression produced an incremental cost-effectiveness ratio of $1,001 per quality-adjusted life-year, as compared with $12,852 to $246,486 per quality-adjusted life-year for treating pathologic myopia. Although the cost-effectiveness of refractive surgery was low, 0.01% atropine was found to be more cost-effective due to lower treatment cost and the additional benefits of preventing myopia complications and related visual impairment.

More recently, a Markov model was used to perform an economic evaluation on the cost-effectiveness of 13 interventions for preventing myopia progression in children (Agyekum et al., 2023a). A comparison of the economic implications of 13 different treatments would have a great deal of value if it was understood how much society should be willing to spend to avoid a change in spherical equivalent or to shorten the axial length; unfortunately, that is not known. So, while the results are interesting, they are challenging to interpret and fail to rule out choices that are dominated (less effective and more expensive). In the future, this type of analysis should be replicated with a focus on a longer time period (over which the long-term complications for the myopic eye can be included) and the results should be converted to changes in quality-adjusted life years, as has been done in other studies. The cost of children spending time outdoors should include the opportunity cost of time, the potential risk to eye health, the risk of skin cancer, and risks to personal safety.

Apart from the evidence of effectiveness, evidence regarding the value proposition of interventions seems critical. To address this gap, Fricke et al. (2023) developed and modeled a system for assessing and comparing the lifetime financial expenses of active myopia management (i.e., use of treatments) against traditional myopia management (i.e. use of corrective lenses). In contrast to Agyekum et al. (2023b), who modeled cost-effectiveness options for a 10-year-old myope with varying levels of myopia, Fricke et al. (2023) presented data using an 8-year-old who presented with symptomatic –0.75D correction in both eyes in urban areas of Australia and China and was given the choice of active or traditional myopia management. Options for these managements were available in both nations, and the costs of all product kinds, essential appointment fees, and other relevant expenditures were calculated using data provided by important sources in both countries. The authors found that the lowest lifetime cost options were anti-myopia spectacles in Australia and low-dose atropine in China. The lifetime cost for traditional myopia management, with a 3% discount rate, was $7,437 (95% CI: $4,953 to $10,740) in Australia and $8,006 (95% confidence interval: $3,026 to $13,707) in China. The final level of myopia had the greatest impact on the lifetime costs of myopia in both countries. This type of work should be replicated for other countries with varying health care financing systems.

In summary, lifetime savings from reduced myopia often offset the upfront costs of myopia treatments in childhood. The use of low concentrations of atropine is cost-effective, but it requires the additional cost of correction with spectacles or contact lenses; 0.05% atropine can reduce myopia progression in children with acceptable side effects and can minimize adult myopia treatment costs (Agyekum et al., 2023b). Nevertheless, comprehensive economic reviews of myopia treatments and evidence of their cost-effectiveness are lacking. As childhood myopia is increasing in prevalence and severity worldwide, and multiple myopia treatments are now available, a robust and comprehensive analysis of the cost-effectiveness of myopia treatments will provide critical data for health policy decisions, thereby maximizing health outcomes with limited resources.

CONCLUSIONS

Conclusion 7-1: Treatment options for myopia progression have increased in the last 20 years, with clinical trials showing that axial growth of the human eye can be slowed down with optical and pharmaceutical intervention. Current treatments for myopia progression include multifocal optical corrections (orthokeratology, soft multi- and dual-focal contact lenses, peripheral refractive error spectacles) and atropine eye drops.

Conclusion 7-2: Atropine is the only pharmacological treatment for myopia progression widely available and used across the globe. Stronger concentrations of atropine produce better treatment effects but more side effects, including rebound effect. Atropine 0.01% is the mostly widely used; however, the treatment effects appear limited. The mechanism of action for atropine remains elusive, and long-term effects require more study.

Conclusion 7-3: While still an emerging treatment strategy, time outdoors is consistently reported to have a protective effect on myopia prevention, especially in the younger years. Studies indicate 2 hours per day may provide the needed amount of outdoor exposure, but exact recommendations for exposure time, time of day, luminance levels, and chromatic contributions have not been determined.

Conclusion 7-4: Current treatments for myopia progression have limited effects. The largest treatment effect of any published treatment option remains under 0.75 diopters over 2 years, based on recent systematic reviews. Some treatment options are effective in the first year and less effective in subsequent years. The reasons for this limited efficacy are unknown, but potential reasons include a role for accommodation, incomplete data on how optical corrections affect the retinal image, and factors that influence ON and OFF pathway balance. Further work is also needed to understand the mechanisms of action underlying the efficacy of optical treatments.

Conclusion 7-5: Current treatments stop working after cessation and can have a rebound effect with subsequent rapid eye growth. It is therefore unclear how and when treatment should be stopped, and if rapid eye growth during rebound is more detrimental to the eye than slow and steady growth without treatment. Ideal treatment options would show similar or accruing treatment effects with each year of use, without rebound effects.

Conclusion 7-6: Current literature suggests that combination therapy shows minimal to no additive effectiveness. However, studies have only used the minimally effective 0.01% concentration of atropine in combination with other treatments. Combination therapy should be studied using higher concentrations.

Conclusion 7-7: Clinical trials for myopia treatments have provided important insights into the progression of myopia. Predictors of myopia progression include a child's existing refractive error, age, sex, and ethnic identity. Past myopia progression does not predict future progression. Myopia tends to progress faster when onset is at younger ages, which may suggest early treatment of myopia in the preschool years. It is unclear whether treatments known to be effective for low to moderate myopia in school-aged children are effective in preschool-aged children, and also unclear whether treatments for low to moderate myopia in school-aged children are effective in high myopia or myopia associated with genetic and systemic disorders.

Conclusion 7-8: Treatment of myopia may be needed daily and to be undertaken for a decade or more. Therefore, safety of the treatment is paramount and new treatment options and interventions need to be carefully evaluated to determine any negative side effects.

Conclusion 7-9: The current state of knowledge of treatment options reflects our limited understanding of the fundamental mechanisms of eye length regulation and how treatments act to alter the progression—and perhaps even the onset—of the disease.

RECOMMENDATIONS

Recommendation 7-1: Funding agencies, foundations, and NGOs, including the National Institutes of Health, should support research to develop new treatment strategies for myopia (age at initiation and cessation, optimal treatment for a given population, efficacy of combination treatments, optimal timing for treatment combinations such as alternating vs. simultaneous, longer-term outcomes), as well as to determine the mechanisms that underlie current treatments. Progress in this area

needs intentionally integrated, multi-disciplinary research in basic and clinical vision science to understand the mechanisms by which therapies can control eye growth. Areas deserving urgent focus are listed here.

- Develop fundamental studies—potentially including animal models—of the mechanisms by which existing and new therapies affect eye growth.
- Perform research on the mechanisms of atropine action to determine the causes of treatment effects and side effects, thereby providing opportunities to optimize treatment efficacy in children and to develop novel pharmaceuticals with fewer side effects.
- Design studies to identify the ideal dosing characteristics of current and novel pharmaceuticals, including concentration and cadence, to slow eye growth.
- Develop new pharmaceutical options to provide structural scleral reinforcement, without creating dose-dependent side effects. Further research is needed to identify pharmacological agents that are more effective and have fewer adverse effects than current options.
- Determine optimal parameters for time outdoors, including duration per day, spectral distribution, time of day, and needed safety measures, to prevent or delay myopia onset. Such studies may create the opportunity to develop treatments for myopia that can be used indoors, independently of time outdoors.
- Combine bench and eye model studies of visual optics including the spectral composition of light, peripheral refractive characterization, and contrast to develop optical corrections for best visual performance and optical quality.
- Develop rigorous investigations of combination therapies.
- Conduct longer-term studies or assessments in adulthood to weigh the costs of myopia treatment against its benefits in terms of the ultimate amount of myopia and effects on ocular health.

Recommendation 7-2: Treatment safety is paramount, given that myopia control treatments are likely to be used throughout childhood and perhaps through young adulthood. Scientists should develop strategies to minimize short-term and long-term side effects.

Recommendation 7-3: Funding for multicenter randomized clinical trials should be directed toward longer-term human studies, starting at earlier ages on treatment and off treatment, to determine long-term benefit with respect to ultimate refractive error and ocular health.

REFERENCES

Abbott, M., Schmid, K. L., & Strang, N. C. (1998). Differences in the accommodation stimulus response curves of adult myopes and emmetropes. *Ophthalmic and Physiological Optics, 18*(1), 13–20. https://doi.org/10.1016/S0275-5408(97)00072-0

Age-Related Eye Disease Study 2 Research Group. (2013). Lutein + zeaxanthin and omega-3 fatty acids for age-related macular degeneration: The Age-Related Eye Disease Study 2 (AREDS2) randomized clinical trial. *JAMA, 309*(19), 2005–2015. https://doi.org/10.1001/jama.2013.4997

Agyekum, S., Chan, P. P., Adjei, P. E., Zhang, Y., Huo, Z., Yip, B. H. K., Ip, P., Wong, I. C. K., Zhang, W., Tham, C. C., Chen, L. J., Zhang, X. J., Pang, C. P., & Yam, J. C. (2023a). Cost-effectiveness analysis of myopia progression interventions in children. *JAMA Network Open, 6*(11), e2340986. https://doi.org/10.1001/jamanetworkopen.2023.40986

Agyekum, S., Chan, P. P., Zhang, Y., Huo, Z., Yip, B. H. K., Ip, P., Tham, C. C., Chen, L. J., Zhang, X. J., Pang, C. P., & Yam, J. (2023b). Cost-effectiveness analysis of myopia management: A systematic review. *Frontiers in Public Health, 11,* 1093836. https://doi.org/10.3389/fpubh.2023.1093836

Aleman, A. C., Wang, M., & Schaeffel, F. (2018). Reading and myopia: Contrast polarity matters. *Scientific Reports, 8*(1), 10840. https://doi.org/10.1038/s41598-018-28904-x

Arias, A., Ohlendorf, S., Artal, P., & Wahl, S. (2023). In-depth optical characterization of spectacle lenses for myopia progression management. *Optica, 10*, 594–603. https://doi.org/10.1364/OPTICA.486389

Ashby, R., Ohlendorf, A., & Schaeffel, F. (2009). The effect of ambient illuminance on the development of deprivation myopia in chicks. *Investigative Ophthalmology & Visual Science, 50*(11), 5348–5354. https://doi.org/10.1167/iovs.09-3419

Ashby, R. S., & Schaeffel, F. (2010). The effect of bright light on lens compensation in chicks. *Investigative Ophthalmology & Visual Science, 51*(10), 5247–5253. https://doi.org/10.1167/iovs.09-4689

Atchison, D. A., Jones, C. E., Schmid, K. L., Pritchard, N., Pope, J. M., Strugnell, W. E., & Riley, R. A. (2004). Eye shape in emmetropia and myopia. *Investigative Ophthalmology & Visual Science, 45*(10), 3380–3386. https://doi.org/10.1167/iovs.04-0292

Atchison, D. A., Pritchard, N., Schmid, K. L., Scott, D. H., Jones, C. E., & Pope, J. M. (2005). Shape of the retinal surface in emmetropia and myopia. *Investigative Ophthalmology & Visual Science, 46*(8), 2698–2707. https://doi.org/10.1167/iovs.04-1506

Atchison, D. A., Pritchard, N., & Schmid, K. L. (2006). Peripheral refraction along the horizontal and vertical visual fields in myopia. *Vision Research, 46*(9), 1450–1458. https://doi.org/10.1016/j.visres.2005.10.023

Atchison, D. A., & Smith, G. (2000). Chromatic aberrations. In *Elsevier eBooks* (pp. 180–193). https://doi.org/10.1016/b978-0-7506-3775-6.50021-3

Barathi, V. A., Chaurasia, S. S., Poidinger, M., Koh, S. K., Tian, D., Ho, C., Iuvone, P. M., Beuerman, R. W., & Zhou, L. (2014). Involvement of GABA transporters in atropine-treated myopic retina as revealed by iTRAQ quantitative proteomics. *Journal of Proteome Research, 13*(11), 4647–4658. https://doi.org/10.1021/pr500558y

Barger-Lux, M. J., & Heaney, R. P. (2002). Effects of above average summer sun exposure on serum 25-hydroxyvitamin D and calcium absorption. *The Journal of Clinical Endocrinology & Metabolism, 87*(11), 4952–4956. https://doi.org/10.1210/jc.2002-020636

Bartlett, J. D., Niemann, K., Houde, B., Allred, T., Edmondson, M. J., & Crockett, R. S. (2003). A tolerability study of pirenzepine ophthalmic gel in myopic children. *Journal of Ocular Pharmacology and Therapeutics, 19*(3), 271–279. https://doi.org/10.1089/108076803321908392

Beaulieu, J. M., Espinoza, S., & Gainetdinov, R. R. (2015). Dopamine receptors—IUPHAR review 13. *British Journal of Pharmacology, 172*(1), 1–23. https://doi.org/10.1111/bph.12906

Bedrossian, R. H. (1966). Treatment of progressive myopia with atropine. In Proceedings of the XX International Congress of Ophthalmology. Munich.

Bedrossian, R. H. (1979). The effect of atropine on myopia. *Ophthalmology, 86*(5), 713–719. https://doi.org/10.1016/s0161-6420(79)35455-0

Berntsen, D. A., Ticak, A., Sinnott, L. T., Chandler, M. A., Jones, J. H., Morrison, A., Jones-Jordan, L. A., Walline, J. J., Mutti, D. O., & BLINK Study Group. (2023). Peripheral defocus, pupil size, and axial eye growth in children wearing soft multifocal contact lenses in the BLINK Study. *Investigative Ophthalmology & Visual Science, 64*(14), 3. https://doi.org/10.1167/iovs.64.14.3

Borchert, M. S., Varma, R., Cotter, S. A., Tarczy-Hornoch, K., McKean-Cowdin, R., Lin, J. H., Wen, G., Azen, S. P., Torres, M., Tielsch, J. M., Friedman, D. S., Repka, M. X., Katz, J., Ibironke, J., Giordano, L., & Joint Writing Committee for the Multi-Ethnic Pediatric Eye Disease Study and the Balitmore Pediatric Eye Disease Study Groups. (2011). Risk factors for hyperopia and myopia in preschool children: The Multi-Ethnic Pediatric Eye Disease and Baltimore Pediatric Eye Disease studies. *Ophthalmology, 118*(10), 1966–1973. https://doi.org/10.1016/j.ophtha.2011.06.030

Bores, L. D., Myers, W., & Cowden, J. (1981). Radial keratotomy: An analysis of the American experience. *Annals of Ophthalmology, 13*(8), 941–948. https://pubmed.ncbi.nlm.nih.gov/7294635/

Brennan, N., Toubouti, Y., Cheng, X., & Bullimore, M. (2021). Efficacy in myopia control. *Progress in Retinal and Eye Research, 83*, 100923. https://doi.org/10.1016/j.preteyeres.2020.100923

Brodstein, R. S., Brodstein, D. E., Olson, R. J., Hunt, S. C., & Williams, R. R. (1984). The treatment of myopia with atropine and bifocals. A long-term prospective study. *Ophthalmology, 91*(11), 1373–1379. https://doi.org/10.1016/s0161-6420(84)34138-0

Bullimore, M. A., & Brennan, N. A. (2023). Juvenile-onset myopia-who to treat and how to evaluate success. *Eye, 38*(3), 450–454. https://doi.org/10.1038/s41433-023-02722-6

Calkins, D. J. (2001). Seeing with S cones. *Progress in Retinal Eye Research, 20*(3), 255–287. https://doi.org/10.1016/s1350-9462(00)00026-4

Carr, B. J., & Stell, W. K. (2016). Nitric oxide (NO) mediates the inhibition of form-deprivation myopia by atropine in chicks. *Scientific Reports, 6*(1), 9. https://doi.org/10.1038/s41598-016-0002-7

Chakraborty, R., Landis, E. G., Mazade, R., Yang, V., Strickland, R., Hattar, S., Stone, R. A., Iuvone, P. M., & Pardue, M. T. (2022). Melanopsin modulates refractive development and myopia. *Experimental Eye Research, 214*, 108866. https://doi.org/10.1016/j.exer.2021.108866

Chalmers, R. L., McNally, J. J., Chamberlain, P., & Keay, L. (2021). Adverse event rates in the retrospective cohort study of safety of pediatric soft contact lens wear: The ReCSS study. *Ophthalmic & Physiological Optics, 41*(1), 84–92. https://doi.org/10.1111/opo.12753

Chamberlain, P., Bradley, A., Arumugam, B., Hammond, D., McNally, J., Logan, N. S., Jones, D., Ngo, Cheryl, Peixoto-de-Matos, S., Hunt, C., & Young, G. (2022). Long-term effect of dual-focus contact lenses on myopia progression in children: A 6-year multicenter clinical trial. *Optometry and Vision Science, 99*(3), 204–212. https://doi.org/10.1097/OPX.0000000000001873

Chandler, M. A., Robich, M. L., Jordan, L. A., Mutti, D. O., Berntsen, D. A., Fenton, R., Day, E., & Walline, J. J. (2023). Accommodation in children after 4.7 years of multifocal contact lens wear in the BLINK study randomized clinical trial. *Optometry and Vision Science, 100*(7), 425–431. https://doi.org/10.1097/OPX.0000000000002040

Chang, D. J., & Joo, C. K. (2012). Current and future options for myopia treatment. *Journal of the Korean Medical Association, 55*(4). https://doi.org/10.5124/jkma.2012.55.4.362

Charman, W. N., & Radhakrishnan, H. (2021). Do optical treatments for the control of myopia progression produce proportional or absolute reductions in progression rates? *Ophthalmic & Physiological Optics, 41*, 192–197. https://doi.org/10.1111/opo.12750

Chawda, D., & Shinde, P. (2022). Effects of solar radiation on the eyes. *Cureus, 14*(1), e30857. https://doi.org/10.7759%2Fcureus.30857

Che, D., Qiao, D., Cao, Y., Zhang, Y., Zhou, Q., Tong, S., Miao, P., & Zhou, J. (2024). Changes in choroidal hemodynamics of form-deprivation myopia in Guinea pigs. *Biochemical and Biophysical Research Communications, 692*, 149348. https://doi.org/10.1016/j.bbrc.2023.149348

Chen, Z., Lv, X., Lai, L., Xu, Y., & Zhang, F. (2023). Effects of riboflavin/Ultraviolet-A(UVA) scleral crosslinking on the mechanical behavior of the scleral fibroblasts of lens-induced myopia guinea pigs. *Experimental Eye Research, 235*, 109618. https://doi.org/10.1016/j.exer.2023.109618.

Chen, C., & Yao, J. (2021). Efficacy and adverse effects of atropine for myopia control in children: A meta-analysis of randomized controlled trials. *Journal of Ophthalmology, 2021*. https://doi.org/10.1155/2021/4274572

Chen, Y., Xiong, R., Chen, X., Zhang, J., Bulloch, G., Lin, X., Wu, X., & Li, J. (2022). Efficacy comparison of repeated low-level red light and low-dose atropine for myopia control: A randomized controlled trial. *Translational Vision Science & Technology, 11*(10), 33. https://doi.org/10.1167/tvst.11.10.33

Cheng, X., Xu, J., & Brennan, N. A. (2019). Accommodation and its role in myopia progression and control with soft contact lenses. *Ophthalmic & Physiological Optics, 39,* 162–171. https://doi.org/10.1111/opo.12614

Chia, A., Chua, W. H., Cheung, Y. B., Wong, W. L., Lingham, A., Fong, A., & Tan, D. (2012). Atropine for the treatment of childhood myopia: Safety and efficacy of 0.5%, 0.1%, and 0.01% doses (atropine for the treatment of myopia 2). *Ophthalmology, 119*(2), 347–354. https://doi.org/10.1016/j.ophtha.2011.07.031

Chia, A., Chua, W. H., Wen, L., Fong, A., Goon, Y. Y., & Tan, D. (2014). Atropine for the treatment of childhood myopia: Changes after stopping atropine 0.01%, 0.1% and 0.5%. *American Journal of Ophthalmology, 157*(2), 451–457.e1. https://doi.org/10.1016/j.ajo.2013.09.020

Choi, J. A., Han, K., Park, Y. M., & La, T. Y. (2014). Low serum 25-hydroxyvitamin D is associated with myopia in Korean adolescents. *Investigative Ophthalmology & Visual Science, 55,* 2041–2047. https://doi.org/10.1167/iovs.13-12853

Chua, W. H., Balakrishnan, V., Chan, Y. H., Tong, L., Ling, Y., Quah, B. L., & Tan, D. (2006). Atropine for the treatment of childhood myopia. *Ophthalmology, 113*(12), 2285–2291. https://doi.org/10.1016/j.ophtha.2006.05.062

Chun, R. K. M., Zhang, H., Liu, Z., Tse, D. Y. Y., Zhou, Y., Lam, C. S. Y., & To, C. H. (2023). Defocus incorporated multiple segments (DIMS) spectacle lenses increase the choroidal thickness: a two-year randomized clinical trial. *Eye and Vision (London, England), 10*(1), 39. https://doi.org/10.1186/s40662-023-00356-z

Colberg, S. R., Sigal, R. J., Yardley, J. E., Riddell, M. C., Dunstan, D. W., Dempsey, P. C., Horton, E. S., Castorino, K., & Tate, D. F. (2016). Physical activity/exercise and diabetes: A position statement of the American Diabetes Association. *Diabetes Care, 39*(11), 2065–2079. https://doi.org/10.2337/dc16-1728

Colin, J., Robinet, A., & Cochener, B. (1999). Retinal detachment after clear lens extraction for high myopia: Seven-year follow-up. *Ophthalmology, 106*(12), 2281–2285. https://doi.org/10.1016/S0161-6420(99)90526-2

COMET Group. (2013). Myopia stabilization and associated factors among participants in the Correction of Myopia Evaluation Trial (COMET). *Investigative Ophthalmology & Visual Science, 54*(13), 7871–7884. https://doi.org/10.1167/iovs.13-12403

Cuellar-Partida, G., Williams, K. M., Yazar, S., Guggenheim, J. A., Hewitt, A. W., Williams, C., Wang, J. J., Kho, P. F., Saw, S. M., Cheng, C. Y., Wong, T. Y., Aung, T., Young, T. L., Tideman, J. W. L., Jonas, J. B., Consortium for Refractive Error and Myopia (CREAM), Mitchell, P., Wojciechowski, R., Stambolian, D., Hysi, P., … MacGregor, S. (2017). Genetically low vitamin D concentrations and myopic refractive error: A Mendelian randomization study. *International Journal of Epidemiology, 46*(6), 1882–1890. https://doi.org/10.1093/ije/dyx068

Deng, B., Li, W., Chen, Z., Zeng, J., & Zhao, F. (2023). Temporal bright light at low frequency retards lens-induced myopia in guinea pigs. *PeerJ, 11,* e16425. https://doi.org/10.7717/peerj.16425

Ding, H., He, M.-N., & Han, D. (2021). Protective effects of riboflavin-UVA-mediated posterior sclera collagen cross-linking in a guinea pig model of form-deprived myopia. *International Journal of Ophthalmology, 14*(3), 333–340. https://doi.org/10.18240/ijo.2021.03.01.

Dirani, M., Tong, L., Gazzard, G., Zhang, X., Chia, A., Young, T. L., Rose, K. A., Mitchell, P., & Saw, S. M. (2009). Outdoor activity and myopia in Singapore teenage children. *British Journal of Ophthalmology, 93*(8), 997–1000. https://doi.org/10.1136/bjo.2008.150979

Dolgin, E. (2024). A myopia epidemic is sweeping the globe. Here's how to stop it. *Nature, 629*(8014), 989–991. https://doi.org/10.1038/d41586-024-01518-2

Dong, J., Zhu, Z., Xu, H., & He, M. (2023). Myopia control effect of repeated low-level red-light therapy in Chinese children: A randomized, double-blind, controlled clinical trial. *Ophthalmology, 130(2),* 198–204. https://doi.org/10.1016/j.ophtha.2022.08.024

Emanuel, A. J., & Do, H. M. T. (2023). The multistable melanopsins of mammals. *Frontiers in Ophthalmology, 3.* https://doi.org/10.3389/fopht.2023.1174255

Feldkaemper, M., & Schaeffel, F. (2013). An updated view on the role of dopamine in myopia. *Experimental Eye Research, 114,* 106–119. https://doi.org/10.1016/j.exer.2013.02.007

Fernández-Vega, L., Alfonso, J. F., & Villacampa, T. (2003). Clear lens extraction for the correction of high myopia. *Ophthalmology, 110*(12), 2349–2354. https://doi.org/10.1016/S0161-6420(03)00794-2

Fischer, A. J., Miethke, P., Morgan, I. G., & Stell, W. K. (1998). Cholinergic amacrine cells are not required for the progression and atropine-mediated suppression of form-deprivation myopia. *Brain Research, 794*(1), 48–60. https://doi.org/10.1016/s0006-8993(98)00188-7

Flitcroft, D. I. (2012). The complex interactions of retinal, optical and environmental factors in myopia aetiology. *Progress in Retinal and Eye Research, 31*(6), 622–660. https://doi.org/10.1016/j.preteyeres.2012.06.004

Foo, L. L., Lanca, C., Wong, C. W., Ting, D., Lamoureux, E., Saw, S. M., & Ang, M. (2021). Cost of myopia correction: A systematic review. *Frontiers in Medicine, 8,* 718724. https://doi.org/10.3389/fmed.2021.718724

Foulds, W. S., Barathi, V. A., & Luu, C. D. (2013). Progressive myopia or hyperopia can be induced in chicks and reversed by manipulation of the chromaticity of ambient light. *Investigative Ophthalmology & Visual Science, 54*(12), 8004–8012. https://doi.org/10.1167/iovs.13-12476

Fozailoff, A., Tarczy-Hornoch, K., Cotter, S., Wen, G., Lin, J., Borchert, M., Azen, S., Varma, R., & Writing Committee for the MEPEDS Study Group. (2011). Prevalence of astigmatism in 6- to 72-month-old African American and Hispanic children: The Multi-ethnic Pediatric Eye Disease Study. *Ophthalmology, 118*(2), 284–293. https://doi.org/10.1016/j.ophtha.2010.06.038

Frangenberg, T. (1991). Perspectivist aristotelianism: Three case-studies of Cinquecento Visual Theory. *Journal of the Warburg and Courtauld Institutes, 54,* 137–158. https://doi.org/10.2307/751485

French, A. N., Morgan, I. G., Burlutsky, G., Mitchell, P., & Rose, K. A. (2013a). Prevalence and 5- to 6-Year Incidence and progression of Myopia and Hyperopia in Australian schoolchildren. *Ophthalmology, 120*(7), 1482–1491. https://doi.org/10.1016/j.ophtha.2012.12.018

French, A. N., Morgan, I. G., Mitchell, P., & Rose, K. A. (2013b). Risk factors for incident myopia in Australian schoolchildren: The Sydney adolescent vascular and eye study. *Ophthalmology,* 120(10), 2100–2108. https://doi.org/10.1016/j.ophtha.2013.02.035

Fricke, T. R., Sankaridurg, P., Naduvilath, T., Resnikoff, S., Tahhan, N., He, M., & Frick, K. D. (2023). Establishing a method to estimate the effect of antimyopia management options on lifetime cost of myopia. *The British Journal of Ophthalmology, 107*(8), 1043–1050. https://doi.org/10.1136/bjophthalmol-2021-320318

Gao, Y., Lim, E. W., Yang, A., Drobe, B., & Bullimore, M. A. (2021). The impact of spectacle lenses for myopia control on visual functions. *Ophthalmic & Physiological Optics, 41*(6), 1320–1331. https://doi.org/10.1111/opo.12878

Gaume Giannoni, A., Robich, M., Berntsen, D. A., Jones-Jordan, L. A., Mutti, D. O., Myers, J., Shaw, K., Walker, M. K., Walline, J. J., & BLINK Study Group. (2022). Ocular and nonocular adverse events during 3 years of soft contact lens wear in children. *Optometry and Vision Science, 99*(6), 505–512. https://doi.org/10.1097/OPX.0000000000001902

Gawne, T. J., Grytz, R., & Norton, T. T. (2021). How chromatic cues can guide human eye growth to achieve good focus. *Journal of Vision, 21*(5), 11. https://doi.org/10.1167/jov.21.5.11

Gawne, T. J., Ward, A. H., & Norton, T. T. (2017). Long-wavelength (red) light produces hyperopia in juvenile and adolescent tree shrews. *Vision Research, 140,* 55–65.

Gifford, K. L., Richdale, K., Kang, P., Aller, T. A., Lam, C. S., Liu, Y. M., Michaud, L., Orr, J. B., Rose, K. A., Saunders, K. A., Saunders, K. J., Seidel, D., Tideman, J. W. L., & Sankaridurg, P. (2019). IMI—Clinical management guidelines report. *Investigative Ophthalmology & Visual Science, 60*(3), M184–M203. https://doi.org/10.1167/iovs.18-25977

Gong, Q., Janowski, M., Luo, M., Wei, H., Chen, B., Yang, G., & Liu, L. (2017a). Efficacy and adverse effects of atropine in childhood myopia: A meta-analysis. *JAMA Ophthalmology, 135*(6), 624–630. https://doi.org/10.1001/jamaophthalmol.2017.1091

Gong, C. R., Troilo, D., & Richdale, K. (2017b). Accommodation and phoria in children wearing multifocal contact lenses. *Optometry and Vision Science, 94*, 353–360. https://doi.org/10.1097/OPX.0000000000001044

Gordon, R. A., & Donzis, P. B. (1985). Refractive development of the human eye. *Archives of Ophthalmology, 103*, 785–789. https://doi.org/10.1001/archopht.1985.01050060045020

Grytz, R. & Lang, R. (2023, December 5). Workshop on the Rise in Myopia: Exploring Possible Contributors and Investigating Screening Practices, Policies, and Programs. National Academies of Sciences, Engineering, and Medicine. Washington, DC, USA. https://www.nationalacademies.org/event/41360_12-2023_workshop-on-the-rise-in-myopia-exploring-possible-contributors-and-investigating-screening-practices-policies-and-programs

Guggenheim, J. A., Northstone, K., McMahon, G., Ness, A. R., Deere, K., Mattocks, C., Pourcain, B. S., & Williams, C. (2012). Time outdoors and physical activity as predictors of incident myopia in childhood: A prospective cohort study. *Investigative Ophthalmology & Visual Science, 53*(6), 2856–2865. https://doi.org/10.1167/iovs.11-9091

Guggenheim, J. A., Williams, C., Northstone, K., Howe, L. D., Tilling, K., St Pourcain, B., McMahon, G., & Lawlor, D. A. (2014). Does vitamin D mediate the protective effects of time outdoors on myopia? Findings from a prospective birth cohort. Investigative *Ophthalmology & Visual Science, 55*(12), 8550–8558. https://doi.org/10.1167/iovs.14-15839

Guido, M. E., Marchese, N. A., Rios, M. N., Morera, L. P., Diaz, N. M., Garbarino-Pico, E., & Contin, M. A. (2022). Non-visual opsins and novel photo-detectors in the vertebrate inner retina mediate light responses within the blue spectrum region. *Cellular and Molecular Neurobiology, 42*(1), 59–83. https://doi.org/10.1007/s10571-020-00997-x

Guo, L., Tao, J., Guo, Z., Tong, Y., Chen, S., Zhao, X., & Hua, R. (2024). Morphological and vascular evidence of glaucomatous damage in myopic guinea pigs with scleral crosslinking. *Scientific Reports, 14*(1), 298. https://doi.org/10.1038/s41598-023-48461-2

Gwiazda, J. (2009). Treatment options for myopia. *Optometry and Vision Science, 86*(6), 624–628. https://doi.org/10.1097/OPX.0b013e3181a6a225

Gwiazda, J., Deng, L., Dias, L., Marsh-Tootle, W., & COMET Study Group. (2011). Association of education and occupation with myopia in COMET parents. *Optometry and Vision Science, 88*(9), 1045–1053. https://doi.org/10.1097/OPX.0b013e31822171ad

Gwiazda, J., Hyman, L., Hussein, M., Everett, D., Norton, T. T., Kurtz, D., Leske, M. C., Manny, R., Marsh-Tootle, W., & Scheiman, M. (2003). A randomized clinical trial of progressive addition lenses versus single vision lenses on the progression of myopia in children. *Investigative Ophthalmology & Visual Science, 44*(4), 1492–1500. https://doi.org/10.1167/iovs.02-0816

Gwiazda, J., Grice, K., Held, R., McLellan, J., & Thorn, F. (2000). Astigmatism and the development of myopia in children. *Vision Research, 40*(8), 1019–1026. https://doi.org/10.1016/s0042-6989(99)00237-0

Gwiazda, J., Marsh-Tootle, W. L., Hyman, L., Hussein, M., Norton, T. T., & COMET Study Group. (2002). Baseline refractive and ocular component measures of children enrolled in the correction of myopia evaluation trial (COMET). *Investigative Ophthalmology & Visual Science, 43*(2), 314–321. https://pubmed.ncbi.nlm.nih.gov/11818372/

Gwiazda, J., Thorn, F., Bauer, J., & Held, R. (1993). Myopic children show insufficient accommodative response to blur. *Investigative Ophthalmology & Visual Science, 34*, 690–694. https://pubmed.ncbi.nlm.nih.gov/8449687/

Haarman, A. E. G., Enthoven, C. A., Tideman, J. W. L., Tedja, M. S., Verhoeven, V. J. M., & Klaver, C. C. W. (2020). The complications of myopia: A review and meta-analysis. *Investigative Ophthalmology & Visual Science, 61*(4), 49. https://doi.org/10.1167/iovs.61.4.49

Hagen, L. A., Gjelle, J. V. B., Arnegard, S., Pedersen, H. R., Gilson, S. J., & Baraas, R. C. (2018). Prevalence and possible factors of myopia in Norwegian adolescents. *Scientific Reports, 8*(1), 13479. https://doi.org/10.1038/s41598-018-31790-y

Hamdaoui, M. E., Levy, A. M., Stuber, A. B., Girkin, C. A., Kraft, T. W., Samuels, B. C., & Grytz, R. (2022). Scleral crosslinking using genipin can compromise retinal structure and function in tree shrews. *Experimental Eye Research, 219,* 109039. https://doi.org/10.1016/j.exer.2022.109039

He, X., Wang, J., Zhu, Z., Xiang, K., Zhang, X., Zhang, B., Chen, J., Yang, J., Du, J., Niu, C., Leng, M., Huang, J., Liu, K., Zou, H., He, M., & Xu, X. (2023). Effect of repeated low-level red light on myopia prevention among children in China with premyopia: A randomized clinical trial. *JAMA Network Open, 6*(4), e239612. https://doi.org/10.1001/jamanetworkopen.2023.9612

Hendicott, P., & Block, S. S. (2022). How the World Council of Optometry produced new guidelines for myopia management. *Community Eye Health, 35*(117), 21–22. https://www.ncbi.nlm.nih.gov/pmc/articles/PMC10061246/

Hendriks, M., Verhoeven, V. J. M., Buitendijk, G. H. S., Polling, J. R., Meester-Smoor, M. A., Hofman, A., RD5000 Consortium, Kamermans, M., Ingeborgh van den Born, L., & Klaver, C. C. W. (2017). Development of refractive errors—What can we learn from inherited retinal dystrophies? *American Journal of Ophthalmology, 182,* 81–89. https://pubmed.ncbi.nlm.nih.gov/28751151/

Hofstetter, H. W. (1944). A comparison of Duane's and Donders tables of the amplitude of accommodation. *American Journal of Optometry and Archives of American Academy of Optometry, 21*(7), 345–363. https://journals.lww.com/optvissci/citation/1944/09000/a_comparison_of_duane_s_and_donders__ta bles_of_the.1.aspx

Holick, M. F. (1995). Environmental factors that influence the cutaneous production of vitamin D. *The American Journal of Clinical Nutrition, 61*(3), 638S–645S. https://doi.org/10.1093/ajcn/61.3.638s

Hong, C. Y., Boyd, M., Wilson, G., & Hong, S. C. (2022). Photorefraction screening plus atropine treatment for myopia is cost-effective: A proof-of-concept Markov analysis. *Clinical Ophthalmology, 16,* 1941–1952. https://doi.org/10.2147/OPTH.S362342

Hou, W., Norton, T. T., Hyman, L., Gwiazda, J., & COMET Group (2018). Axial elongation in myopic children and its association with myopia progression in the Correction of Myopia Evaluation Trial. *Eye & Contact Lens, 44*(4), 248–259. https://doi.org/10.1097/ICL.0000000000000505

Huang, D., Schallhorn, S. C., Sugar, A., Farjo, A. A., Majmudar, P. A., Trattler, W. B., & Tanzer, D. J. (2009). Phakic intraocular lens implantation for the correction of myopia: A report by the American Academy of Ophthalmology. *Ophthalmology, 116*(11), 2244–2258. https://doi.org/10.1016/j.ophtha.2009.08.018

Huang, J., Hung, L. F., & Smith, E. L., 3rd (2011). Effects of foveal ablation on the pattern of peripheral refractive errors in normal and form-deprived infant rhesus monkeys (Macaca mulatta). *Investigative Ophthalmology & Visual Science, 52*(9), 6428–6434. https://doi.org/10.1167/iovs.10-6757

Huang, J., Hung, L. F., & Smith, E. L., 3rd (2012). Recovery of peripheral refractive errors and ocular shape in rhesus monkeys (Macaca mulatta) with experimentally induced myopia. *Vision Research, 73,* 30–39. https://doi.org/10.1016/j.visres.2012.09.002

Huang, J., Wen, D., Wang, Q., McAlinden, C., Flitcroft, I., Chen, H., Saw, S. M., Chen, H., Bao, F., Zhao, Y., Hu, L., Li, X., Gao, R., Lu, W., Du, Y., Jinag, Z., Yu, A., Lian, H., Jiang, Q., Yu, Y., … Qu, J. (2016). Efficacy Comparison of 16 Interventions for Myopia Control in Children: A Network Meta-analysis. *Ophthalmology, 123*(4), 697–708. https://doi.org/10.1016/j.ophtha.2015.11.010

Huang, X. L., Ding, C., Chen, Y., Chen, H., & Bao, J. (2022). Orthokeratology reshapes eyes to be less prolate and more symmetric. *Contact Lens & Anterior Eye, 45*(4), 101532. https://doi.org/10.1016/j.clae.2021.101532

Hung, L. F., Arumugam, B., She, Z., Ostrin, L., & Smith, E. L., 3rd. (2018). Narrow-band, long-wavelength lighting promotes hyperopia and retards vision-induced myopia in infant rhesus monkeys. *Experimental Eye Research, 176,* 147–160. https://doi.org/10.1016/j.exer.2018.07.004

Hung, L. F., Crawford, M. L., & Smith, E. L. (1995). Spectacle lenses alter eye growth and the refractive status of young monkeys. *Nature Medicine, 1*(8), 761–765. https://doi.org/10.1038/nm0895-761

Hyman, L., Gwiazda, J., Marsh-Tootle, W. L., Norton, T. T., Hussein, M., & COMET Group (2001). The Correction of Myopia Evaluation Trial (COMET): Design and general baseline characteristics.

Jaskulski, M., Singh, N. K., Bradley, A., & Kollbaum, P. S. (2020). Optical and imaging properties of a novel multi-segment spectacle lens designed to slow myopia progression. *Ophthalmic & Physiological Optics, 40*(5), 549–556. https://doi.org/10.1111/opo.12725

Javitt, J. C., & Chiang, Y. P. (1994). The socioeconomic aspects of laser refractive surgery. *Archives of Ophthalmology, 112*(12), 1526–1530. https://doi.org/10.1001/archopht.1994.01090240032022

Jiang, X., Pardue, M. T., Mori, K., Ikeda, S. I., Torii, H., D'Souza, S., Lang, R. A., Kurihara, T., & Tsubota, K. (2021a). Violet light suppresses lens-induced myopia via neuropsin (OPN5) in mice. *Proceedings of the National Academy of Sciences of the United States of America, 118*(1). https://doi.org/10.1073/pnas.2018840118

Jiang, L., Zhang, S., Schaeffel, F., Xiong, S., Zheng, Y., Zhou, X., Lu, F., & Qu, J. (2014). Interactions of chromatic and lens-induced defocus during visual control of eye growth in guinea pigs (*Cavia porcellus*). *Vision Research, 94,* 24–32. https://doi.org/10.1016/j.visres.2013.10.020

Jiang, Y., Zhang, Z., Wu, Z., Sun, S., Fu, Y., & Ke, B. (2021b). Change and recovery of choroid thickness after short-term application of 1% atropine gel and its influencing factors in 6-7-year-old children. *Current Eye Research, 46*(8), 1171–1177. https://doi.org/10.1080/02713683.2020.1863431

Jiang, Y., Zhu, Z., Tan, X., Kong, X., Zhong, H., Zhang, J., Xiong, R., Yuan, Y., Zeng, J., Morgan, I. G., & He, M. (2022). Effect of repeated low-level red-light therapy for myopia control in children: A multicenter randomized controlled trial. *Ophthalmology, 129*(5), 509–519. https://doi.org/10.1016/j.ophtha.2021.11.023

Jonas, J. B., Ang, M., Cho, P., Guggenheim, J. A., He, M. G., Jong, M., Logan, N. S., Liu, M., Morgan, I., Ohno-Matsui, K., Pärssinen, O., Resnikoff, S., Sankaridurg, P., Saw, S. M., Smith, E. L., 3rd, Tan, D. T. H., Walline, J. J., Wildsoet, C. F., Wu, P. C., Zhu, X., … Wolffsohn, J. S. (2021). IMI prevention of myopia and its progression. *Investigative ophthalmology & visual science, 62*(5), 6. https://doi.org/10.1167/iovs.62.5.6

Jones, J. H., Mutti, D. O., Jones-Jordan, L. A., & Walline, J. J. (2022). Effect of combining 0.01% atropine with soft multifocal contact lenses on myopia progression in children. *Optometry and Vision Science, 99*(5), 434–442. https://doi.org/10.1097/OPX.0000000000001884

Jones, L. A., Sinnott, L. T., Mutti, D. O., Mitchell, G. L., Moeschberger, M. L., & Zadnik, K. (2007). Parental history of myopia, sports and outdoor activities, and future myopia. *Investigative Ophthalmology & Visual Science, 48*(8), 3524–3532. https://doi.org/10.1167/iovs.06-1118

Jones-Jordan, L. A., Mitchell, G. L., Cotter, S. A., Kleinstein, R. N., Manny, R. E., Mutti, D. O., Twelker, J. D., Sims, J. R., Zadnik, K., & CLEERE Study Group. (2011). Visual activity before and after the onset of juvenile myopia. *Investigative Ophthalmology & Visual Science, 52*(3), 1841–1850. https://doi.org/10.1167/iovs.09-4997

Jones-Jordan, L. A., Sinnott, L. T., Chu, R. H., Cotter, S. A., Kleinstein, R. N., Manny, R. E., Mutti, D. O., Twelker, D. J., & Zadnik, K. (2021). Myopia progression as a function of sex, age, and ethnicity. *Investigative Ophthalmology & Visual Science, 62*(10), 36. https://doi.org/10.1167/iovs.62.10.36

Jones-Jordan, L. A., Sinnott, L. T., Cotter, S. A., Kleinstein, R. N., Manny, R. E., Mutti, D. O., Twelker, J. D., Zadnik, K., & CLEERE Study Group (2012). Time outdoors, visual activity, and myopia progression in juvenile-onset myopes. *Investigative Ophthalmology & Visual Science, 53*(11), 7169–7175. https://doi.org/10.1167%2Fiovs.11-8336

Jordan-Yu, J. M., Teo, K. Y. C., Chakravarthy, U., Gan, A., Tan, A. C. S., Cheong, K. X., Wong, T. Y., & Cheung, C. M. G. (2021). Polypoidal choroidal vasculopathy features vary according to subfoveal choroidal thickness. *Retina, 41*(5), 1084–1093. https://doi.org/10.1097/iae.0000000000002966

Khanal, S., Harrington, S., & Tomiyama, E. (2024). [Treatment of childhood myopia]. Commissioned Paper for the Committee on Focus on Myopia: Pathogenesis and Rising Incidence.

Khanal, S., Norton, T. T., & Gawne, T. J. (2023). Limited bandwidth short-wavelength light produces slowly-developing myopia in tree shrews similar to human juvenile-onset myopia. *Vision Research, 204,* 108161. https://doi.org/10.1016/j.visres.2022.108161

Kinoshita, N., Konno, Y., Hamada, N., Kanda, Y., Shimmura-Tomita, M., Kaburaki, T., & Kakehashi, A. (2020). Efficacy of combined orthokeratology and 0.01% atropine solution for slowing axial elongation in children with myopia: A 2-year randomised trial. *Scientific Reports, 10*(1), 12750. https://doi.org/10.1038/s41598-020-69710-8

Kleinstein, R. N., Sinnott, L. T., Jones-Jordan, L. A., Sims, J., & Zadnik, K. (2012). New cases of myopia in children. *Archives of Ophthalmology, 130*(10), 1274–1279. https://doi.org/10.1001/archophthalmol.2012.1449

Koosha, N., Riazi, M. S., Janfaza, P., Mohammadbeigy, I., Rahimi, A., Mehri, K., Mohsen, P., & Peyman, A. (2024). Laser vision correction after radial keratotomy: A systematic review and meta-analysis. *Journal of Cataract & Refractive Surgery, 50*(7), 767–776.https://doi.org/10.1097/j.jcrs.0000000000001426

Kröger, R. H. H., & Wagner, H. J. (1996). The eye of the blue acara (*Aequidens pulcher*, Cichlidae) grows to compensate for defocus due to chromatic aberration. *Journal of Comparative Physiology A, 179*(6), 837–842. https://doi.org/10.1007/bf00207362

Lam, C. S. Y., Tang, W. C., Tse, D. Y., Lee, R. P. K., Chun, R. K. M., Hasegawa, K., Qi, H., Hatanaka, T., & To, C. H. (2020). Defocus incorporated multiple segments (DIMS) spectacle lenses slow myopia progression: A 2-year randomized clinical trial. *British Journal of Ophthalmology, 104*(3), 363–368. https://doi.org/10.1136/bjophthalmol-2018-313739

Lawrenson, J. G., Shah, R., Huntjens, B., Downie, L. E., Virgili, G., Dhakal, R., Verkicharla, P. K., Li, D., Mavi, S., Kernohan, A., Li, T., Walline, J. J. (2023). Interventions for myopia control in children: A living systematic review and network meta-analysis. *The Cochrane Database of Systematic Reviews, 2*(2), CD014758. https://doi.org/10.1002/14651858.CD014758.pub2

Leech, E. M., Cottriall, C. L., & McBrien, N. A. (1995). Pirenzepine prevents form deprivation myopia in a dose-dependent manner. *Ophthalmic & Physiological Optics, 15*(5), 351–356. https://pubmed.ncbi.nlm.nih.gov/8524553/

Li, X., Huang, Y., Yin, Z., Liu, C., Zhang, S., Yang, A., Drobe, B., Chen, H., & Bao, J. (2023a). Myopia control efficacy of spectacle lenses with aspherical lenslets: Results of a 3-year follow-up study. *American Journal of Ophthalmology, 253,* 160–168. https://doi.org/10.1016/j.ajo.2023.03.030

Li, Yu, Qi, Y., Sun, M., Zhai, C., Wei, W., & Zhang, F. (2023b). Clinical feasibility and safety of scleral collagen cross-linking by riboflavin and ultraviolet A in pathological myopia blindness: A pilot study. *Ophthalmology and Therapy, 12*(2), 853–866. https://doi.org/10.1007/s40123-022-00633-5

Li, Y., Yip, M., Ning, Y., Chung, J., Toh, A., Leow, C., Liu, N., Ting, D., Schmetterer, L., Saw, S. M., Jonas, J. B., Chia, A., & Ang, M. (2024). Topical atropine for childhood myopia control: The atropine treatment long-term assessment study. *JAMA Ophthalmology, 142*(1), 15–23. https://doi.org/10.1001/jamaophthalmol.2023.5467

Li, T., Zhou, X., Li, B., & Jiang, B. (2017). Effect of MT3 on retinal and choroidal TGF-β2 and HAS2 expressions in form deprivation myopia of guinea pig. *Journal of Ophthalmology.* https://doi.org/10.1155/2017/5028019

Lim, M. C., Gazzard, G., Sim, E. L., Tong, L., & Saw, S. M. (2009). Direct costs of myopia in Singapore. *Eye, 23*(5), 1086–1089. https://doi.org/10.1038/eye.2008.225

Linne, C., Mon, K. Y., D'Souza, S., Jeong, H., Jiang, X., Brown, D. M., Zhang, K., Vemaraju, S., Tsubota, K., Kurihara, T., Pardue, M. T., & Lang, R. A. (2023). Encephalopsin (OPN3) is required for normal refractive development and the GO/GROW response to induced myopia. *Molecular Vision, 29,* 39–57. https://www.ncbi.nlm.nih.gov/pmc/articles/PMC10243678/

Liu, R., Hu, M., He, J. C., Zhou, X. T., Dai, J. H., Qu, X. M., Liu, H., & Chu, R. Y. (2014). The effects of monochromatic illumination on early eye development in rhesus monkeys. *Investigative Ophthalmology & Visual Science, 55*(3), 1901–1909. https://doi.org/10.1167/iovs.13-12276Liu, S., Li, S., Wang, B., Lin, X., Wu, Y., Liu, H., Qu, X., Dai, J., Zhou, X., & Zhou, H. (2016). Scleral cross-linking using riboflavin UVA irradiation for the prevention of myopia progression in a guinea pig model: Blocked axial extension and altered scleral microstructure. *PloS One, 11*(11), e0165792. https://doi.org/10.1371/journal.pone.0165792

Liu, A. L., Liu, Y. F., Wang, G., Shao, Y. Q., Yu, C. X., Yang, Z., Zhou, Z. R., Han, X., Gong, X., Qian, K. W., Wang, L. Q., Ma, Y. Y., Zhong, Y. M., Weng, S. J., & Yang, X. L. (2022). The role of ipRGCs in ocular growth and myopia development. *Science Advances, 8*(19), eabm9027. https://doi.org/10.1126/sciadv.abm9027

Liu, R., Qian, Y. F., He, J. C., Hu, M., Zhou, X. T., Dai, J. H., Qu, X. M., & Chu, R. Y. (2011). Effects of different monochromatic lights on refractive development and eye growth in guinea pigs. *Experimental Eye Research, 92*(6), 447–453. https://doi.org/10.1016/j.exer.2011.03.003

Liu, Z., Sun, Z., Du, B., Gou, H., Wang, B., Lin, Z., Ren, N., Pazo, E. E., Liu, L., & Wei, R. (2024). The effects of repeated low-level red-light therapy on the structure and vasculature of the choroid and retina in children with premeyopia. *Ophthalmology and Therapy, 13*, 729–759. https://doi.org/10.1007/s40123-023-00875-x

Liu, X., Wang, P., Xie, Z., Sun, M., Chen, M., Wang, J., Huang, J., Chen, S., Chen, Z., Wang, Y., Li, Y., Qu, J., & Mao, X. (2023). One-year myopia control efficacy of cylindrical annular refractive element spectacle lenses. *Acta Ophthalmologica, 101*(6), 651–657. https://doi.org/10.1111/aos.15649

Long, Q., Chen, D. H., & Chu, R. Y. (2009). Illumination with monochromatic long-wavelength light promotes myopic shift and ocular elongation in newborn pigmented guinea pigs. *Cutaneous and Ocular Toxicology, 28*(4), 176–180. https://doi.org/10.3109/15569520903178364

Luedde, W. H. (1932). Monocular cycloplegia for the control of myopia. *American Journal of Ophthalmology, 15*, 603–610. https://doi.org/10.1016/S0002-9394(32)90282-7

Lumb, E., Sulley, A., Logan, N. S., Jones, D., & Chamberlain, P. (2023). Six years of wearer experience in children participating in a myopia control study of MiSight® 1 day. *Contact lens & anterior eye, 46*(4), 101849. https://doi.org/10.1016/j.clae.2023.101849

Mathis, U., Feldkaemper, M., Liu, H., & Schaeffel, F. (2023). Studies on the interactions of retinal dopamine with choroidal thickness in the chicken. *Graefes Archive for Clinical and Experimental Ophthalmology, 261*(2), 409–425. https://doi.org/10.1007/s00417-022-05837-w

Mathis, U., Feldkaemper, M. P., & Schaeffel, F. (2021). Effects of single and repeated intravitreal applications of atropine on choroidal thickness in alert chickens. *Ophthalmic Research, 64*(4), 664–674. https://doi.org/10.1159/000515755

Mazade, R., & Pardue, M. T. (2023). Rod pathway electrical activity is modulated in the myopic mouse. *Investigative Ophthalmology & Visual Science, 65*(8). https://iovs.arvojournals.org/article.aspx?articleid=2786113

Mazade, R., & Pardue, M. T. (2024). Inhibition to the rod pathway is modulated in lens-induced myopic mice. *Investigative Ophthalmology & Visual Science, 65*(7), https://iovs.arvojournals.org/article.aspx?articleid=2796960&resultClick=1

Mazade, R., Palumaa, T., & Pardue, M. T. (2024). Insights Into Myopia from Mouse Models. *Annual review of vision science*, 10.1146/annurev-vision-102122-102059. Advance online publication. https://doi.org/10.1146/annurev-vision-102122-102059

McBrien, N. A., Morgan, I. G., & Mutti, D. O. (2009). What's hot in myopia research-the 12th international myopia conference, Australia, 2008. *Optometry and Vision Science, 86*(1), 2–3. https://doi.org/10.1097/opx.0b013e3181940364

McBrien, N. A., Stell, W. K., & Carr, B. (2013). How does atropine exert its anti-myopia effects? *Ophthalmic & Physiological Optics, 33*(3), 373–378. https://doi.org/10.1111/opo.12052

McKean-Cowdin, R., Varma, R., Cotter, S. A., Tarczy-Hornoch, K., Borchert, M. S., Lin, J. H., Wen, G., Azen, S. P., Torres, M., Tielsch, J. M., Friedman, D. S., Repka, M. X., Katz, J., Ibironke, J., Giordano, L., & Multi-Ethnic Pediatric Eye Disease Study and the Baltimore Pediatric Eye Disease Study Groups. (2011). Risk factors for astigmatism in preschool children: The multi-ethnic pediatric eye disease and Baltimore pediatric eye disease studies. Ophthalmology, 118(10), 1974–1981. https://doi.org/10.1016/j.ophtha.2011.06.031

Meng, Q. Y., Miao, Z. Q., Liang, S. T., Wu, X., Wang, L. J., Zhao, M. W., & Guo, L. L. (2023). Choroidal thickness, myopia, and myopia control interventions in children: a Meta-analysis and systematic review. International Journal of Ophthalmology, 16(3), 453–464. https://doi.org/10.18240/ijo.2023.03.17

Modjtahedi, B. S., Abbott, R. L., Fong, D. S., Lum, F., Tan, D., & Task Force on Myopia. (2021). Reducing the global burden of myopia by delaying the onset of myopia and reducing myopic progression in children: The Academy's Task Force on Myopia. Ophthalmology, 128(6), 816–826. https://doi.org/10.1016/j.ophtha.2020.10.040

Mohammadi, S. F., Alinia, C., Tavakkoli, M., Lashay, A., & Chams, H. (2018). Refractive surgery: The most cost-saving technique in refractive errors correction. International Journal of Ophthalmology, 11(6), 1013–1019. https://doi.org/10.18240/ijo.2018.06.20

Moreddu, R., Vigolo, D., & Yetisen, A. K. (2019). Contact Lens Technology: From fundamentals to applications. Advanced Healthcare Materials, 8(15). https://doi.org/10.1002/adhm.201900368

Multi-Ethnic Pediatric Eye Disease Study Group. (2010). Prevalence of myopia and hyperopia in 6- to 72-month-old African American and Hispanic children: the multi-ethnic pediatric eye disease study. Ophthalmology, 117(1), 140–147. https://doi.org/10.1016/j.ophtha.2009.06.009

Mutti, D. O., & Marks, A. R. (2011). Blood levels of vitamin D in teens and young adults with myopia. Optometry and Vision Science, 88(3), 377–382. https://doi.org/10.1097%2FOPX.0b013e31820b0385

Mutti, D. O., Mulvihill, S. P., Orr, D. J., Shorter, P. D., & Hartwick, A. T. E. (2020). The effect of refractive error on melanopsin-driven pupillary responses. Investigative Ophthalmology & Visual Science, 61(8), 22. https://doi.org/10.1167%2Fiovs.61.12.22

Mutti, D. O., Sinnott, L. T., Lynn Mitchell, G., Jordan, L. A., Friedman, N. E., Frane, S. L., & Lin, W. K. (2018). Ocular component development during infancy and early childhood. Optometry and Vision Science, 95(10), 976–985. https://doi.org/10.1097%2FOPX.0000000000001296

Mutti, D. O., Sinnott, L. T., Reuter, K. S., Walker, M. K., Berntsen, D. A., Jones-Jordan, L. A., Walline, J. J., & Bifocal Lenses In Nearsighted Kids (BLINK) Study Group. (2019). Peripheral refraction and eye lengths in myopic children in the Bifocal Lenses in Nearsighted Kids (BLINK) study. Translational Vision Science & Technology, 8(5), 17. https://doi.org/10.1167%2Ftvst.8.2.17

MyKidsVision. (n.d.). How do myopia control soft contact lenses work? https://www.mykidsvision.org/knowledge-centre/how-do-myopia-control-soft-contact-lenses-work

Myopia Profile. (n.d.). Biofinity® multifocal. https://www.myopiaprofile.com/product/biofinity

National Library of Medicine. (2005). The Collaborative Longitudinal Evaluation of Ethnicity and Refractive Error (CLEERE) Study. https://clinicaltrials.gov/study/NCT00000169#study-overview

National Library of Medicine. (2016). Correction of Myopia Evaluation Trial (COMET). https://clinicaltrials.gov/study/NCT00000113?term=COMET%20myopia&rank=1

National Research Council (1989). Myopia: Prevalence and Progression. Washington, DC: The National Academies Press. https://doi.org/10.17226/1420.

Németh, J., Tapasztó, B., Aclimandos, W. A., Kestelyn, P., Jonas, J. B., De Faber, J. H. N., Januleviciene, I., Grzybowski, A., Nagy, Z. Z., Pärssinen, O., Guggenheim, J. A., Allen, P. M., Baraas, R. C., Saunders, K. J., Flitcroft, D. I., Gray, L. S., Polling, J. R., Haarman, A. E., Tideman, J. W. L., Wolffsohn, J. S., … Resnikoff, S. (2021). Update and guidance on management of myopia. European Society of Ophthalmology in cooperation with International Myopia Institute. European Journal of Ophthalmology, 31(3), 853–883. https://doi.org/10.1177/1120672121998960

Nickla, D. L., & Totonelly, K. (2011). Dopamine antagonists and brief vision distinguish lens-induced- and form-deprivation-induced myopia. *Experimental Eye Research, 93*(6), 782–785. https://doi.org/10.1016/j.exer.2011.08.001

Norton, T. (1999) Animal models of myopia: learning how vision controls the size of the eye. *ILAR Journal, 40*(2), 59–77. https://doi.org/10.1093/ilar.40.2.59

Norton, T. T., Casagrande, V. A., & Sherman, S. M. (1977). Loss of Y-cells in the lateral geniculate nucleus of monocularly deprived tree shrews. *Science, 197*(4305), 784–786. https://doi.org/10.1126/science.887922

Norton, T. T., & Siegwart, J. T., Jr. (2013). Light levels, refractive development, and myopia–A speculative review. *Experimental Eye Research, 114*, 48–57. https://doi.org/10.1016/j.exer.2013.05.004

Ortiz-Peregrina, S., Casares-López, M., Castro-Torres, J. J., Anera, R. G., & Artal, P. (2022). Effect of peripheral refractive errors on driving performance. *Biomedical Optics Express, 13*(10), 5533–5550. https://doi.org/10.1364/BOE.468032

Ostrin, L., & Schill, A. (2014) Red light instruments for myopia exceed safety limits. *Ophthalmic and Physiological Optics, 44*(2), 241–248. https://doi.org/10.1111/opo.13272

Papadogiannis, P., Börjeson, C., & Lundström, L. (2023). Comparison of optical myopia control interventions: effect on peripheral image quality and vision. *Biomedical Optics Express, 14*(7), 3125–3137. https://doi.org/10.1364/BOE.486555

Peng, T., & Jiang, J. (2023). Efficiency and related factors of multifocal soft contact lenses in controlling myopia. *Eye & Contact Lens, 49*(12), 535–541. https://doi.org/10.1097/ICL.0000000000001043

Phillips, J. R., & McBrien, N. A. (2004). Pressure-induced changes in axial eye length of chick and tree shrew: significance of myofibroblasts in the sclera. *Investigative Ophthalmology & Visual Science, 45*(3), 758–763. https://doi.org/10.1167/iovs.03-0732

Poudel, S., Jin, J., Rahimi-Nasrabadi, H., Dellostritto, S., Dul, M. W., Viswanathan, S., & Alonso, J. M. (2024). Contrast sensitivity of ON and OFF human retinal pathways in myopia. *The Journal of Neuroscience: The Official Journal of the Society for Neuroscience, 44*(3), e1487232023. https://doi.org/10.1523/JNEUROSCI.1487-23.2023

Pucker, A. D. (2023) Understanding options for combination myopia management. *Ophthalmology Times, 48*(5). https://www.ophthalmologytimes.com/view/understanding-options-for-combination-myopia-management

Qian, L., Zhao, H., Li, X., Yin, J., Tang, W., Chen, P., Wang, Q., & Zhang, J. (2015). Pirenzepine inhibits myopia in guinea pig model by regulating the balance of MMP-2 and TIMP-2 expression and increased tyrosine hydroxylase levels. *Cell Biochemistry and Biophysics, 71*(3), 1373–1378. https://doi.org/10.1007/s12013-014-0359-9

Qiao-Grider, Y., Hung, L. F., Kee, C.-s., Ramamirtham, R., & Smith, E. L., 3rd. (2004). Recovery from form-deprivation myopia in rhesus monkeys. *Investigative Ophthalmology & Visual Science, 45*(10), 3361–3372. https://doi.org/10.1167/iovs.04-0080

Quek, T. P. L., Chua, C. G., Chong, C. S., Chong, J. H., Hey, H. W., Lee, J., Lim, Y. F., & Saw, S. (2003). Prevalence of refractive errors in teenage high school students in Singapore. *Ophthalmic and Physiological Optics/Ophthalmic & Physiological Optics, 24*(1), 47–55. https://doi.org/10.1046/j.1475-1313.2003.00166.

Rappon, J., Neitz, J., Neitz, M., Chung, C., & Chalberg, T. W. (2022). Two-year effectiveness of a novel myopia management spectacle lens with full-time wearers. *Investigative Ophthalmology & Visual Science, 63*(7), 408. https://iovs.arvojournals.org/article.aspx?articleid=2779016

Read, S. A., Vincent, S. J., Tan, C., Ngo, C., Collins, M. J., & Saw, S. (2018). Patterns of daily outdoor light exposure in Australian and Singaporean children. *Translational Vision Science & Technology, 7*(3), 8. https://doi.org/10.1167/tvst.7.3.8

Reidy, M. G., Hartwick, A. T. E., & Mutti, D. O. (2024). The association between pupillary responses and axial length in children differs as a function of season. *Scientific Reports, 14*(1), 598. https://doi.org/10.1038/s41598-024-51199-0

Repka, M. X., Weise, K. K., Chandler, D. L., Wu, R., Melia, B. M., Manny, R. E., Kehler, L. A. F., Jordan, C. O., Raghuram, A., Summers, A. I., Lee, K. A., Petersen, D. B., Erzurum, S. A., Pang, Y., Lenhart, P. D., Ticho, B. H., Beck, R. W., Kraker, R. T., Holmes, J. M., Cotter, S. A., ... Pediatric Eye Disease Investigator Group. (2023). Low-dose 0.01% atropine eye drops vs placebo for myopia control: A randomized clinical Trial. *JAMA Ophthalmology, 141*(8), 756–765. https://doi.org/10.1001/jamaophthalmol.2023.2855

Rickers, M., & Schaeffel, F. (1995). Dose-dependent effects of intravitreal pirenzepine on deprivation myopia and lens-induced refractive errors in chickens. *Experimental Eye Research, 61*(4), 509–516. https://doi.org/10.1016/s0014-4835(05)80147-2

Rohrer, B., Schaeffel, F., & Zrenner, E. (1992). Longitudinal chromatic aberration and emmetropization: Results from the chicken eye. *Journal of Physiology, 449*(1), 363–376. https://doi.org/10.1113/jphysiol.1992.sp019090

Rose, K. A., Morgan, I. G., Ip, J., Kifley, A., Huynh, S., Smith, W., & Mitchell, P. (2008). Outdoor activity reduces the prevalence of myopia in children. *Ophthalmology, 115*(8), 1279–1285. https://doi.org/10.1016/j.ophtha.2007.12.019

Rucker, F. J., & Wallman, J. (2009). Chick eyes compensate for chromatic simulations of hyperopic and myopic defocus: Evidence that the eye uses longitudinal chromatic aberration to guide eye-growth. *Vision Research, 49*, 1775–1783. https://doi.org/10.1016/j.visres.2009.04.014

Sah, R. P., Jaskulski, M., & Kollbaum, P. S. (2022). Modelling the refractive and imaging impact of multi-zone lenses utilised for myopia control in children's eyes. *Ophthalmic & Physiological Optics, 42*(3), 571–585. https://doi.org/10.1111/opo.12959

Salzano, A. D., Khanal, S., Cheung, N. L., Weise, K. K., Jenewein, E. C., Horn, D. M., Mutti, D. O., & Gawne, T. J. (2023). Repeated low-level red-light therapy: The next wave in myopia management? *Optometry and Vision Science, 100*(12), 812–822. https://doi.org/10.1097/OPX.0000000000002083

Sankaridurg, P., Chen, X., Naduvilath, T., Lazon de la Jara, P., Lin, Z., Li, L., Smith, E. L., 3rd, Ge, J., & Holden, B. A. (2013). Adverse events during 2 years of daily wear of silicone hydrogels in children. *Optometry and Vision Science, 90*(9), 961–969. https://doi.org/10.1097/OPX.0000000000000017

Sankaridurg, P., Berntsen, D., Bullimore, M., Cho, P., Flitcroft I., Gawne, T.J., Gifford, K. L., Jong, M., Kang, P., Ostrin, L.A., Santodomingo-Rubido, J., Wildsoet, J., Wolffsohn, J.S. (2023) IMI 2023 Digest. *Investigative Ophthalmology & Visual Science, 64*(6), 7. https://doi.org/10.1167/iovs.64.6.7

Saxena, R., Vashist, P., Tandon, R., Pandey, R. M., Bhardawaj, A., Gupta, V., & Menon, V. (2017). Incidence and progression of myopia and associated factors in urban school children in Delhi: The North India Myopia Study (NIM Study). *PloS One, 12*(12), e0189774. https://doi.org/10.1371/journal.pone.0189774

Saxena, R., Sharma, P., & Pediatric Ophthalmology Expert Group. (2020). National consensus statement regarding pediatric eye examination, refraction, and amblyopia management. *Indian journal of ophthalmology, 68*(2), 325–332. https://doi.org/10.4103/ijo.IJO_471_19

Schaeffel, F., & Howland, H. C. (1991). Properties of the feedback loops controlling eye growth and refractive state in the chicken. *Vision Research, 31*(4), 717–734. https://doi.org/10.1016/0042-6989(91)90011-s

Schaeffel, F., & Wildsoet, C. F. (2024). Red light therapy for myopia: Merits, risks and questions. *Ophthalmic & Physiological Optics*, 10.1111/opo.13306. Advance online publication.

Scheiman, M., Gwiazda, J., Zhang, Q., Deng, L., Fern, K., Manny, R. E., Weissberg, E., & Hyman, L. (2016) Longitudinal changes in corneal curvature and its relationship to axial length in the Correction of Myopia Evaluation Trial (COMET) cohort, *Journal of Optometry, 9*(1), 13–21., https://doi.org/10.1016/j.optom.2015.10.003

Schwahn, H. N., Kaymak, H., & Schaeffel, F. (2000). Effects of atropine on refractive development, dopamine release, and slow retinal potentials in the chick. *Visual Neuroscience, 17*(2), 165–176. https://doi.org/10.1017/s0952523800171184

Seidemann, A., & Schaeffel, F. (2002). Effects of longitudinal chromatic aberration on accommodation and emmetropization. *Vision Research, 42*(20), 2409–2417. https://doi.org/10.1016/s0042-6989(02)00262-6

Shah, R. L., Huang, Y., Guggenheim, J. A., & Williams, C. (2017). Time outdoors at specific ages during early childhood and the risk of incident myopia. *Investigative Ophthalmology & Visual Science, 58*(3), 1158–1166. https://doi.org/10.1167%2Fiovs.16-20894

She, Z., Ward, A. H., & Gawne, T. J. (2023). The effects of ambient narrowband long-wavelength light on lens-induced myopia and form-deprivation myopia in tree shrews. *Experimental eye research, 234*, 109593. https://doi.org/10.1016/j.exer.2023.109593.

Shih, Y. F., Chen, C. H., Chou, A. C., Ho, T. C., Lin, L. L., & Hung, P. T. (1999). Effects of different concentrations of atropine on controlling myopia in myopic children. *Journal of Ocular Pharmacology and Therapeutics, 15*(1), 85–90. https://doi.org/10.1089/jop.1999.15.85

Siatkowski, R. M., Cotter, S. A., Crockett, R. S., Miller, J. M., Novack, G. D., Zadnik, K., & U.S. Pirenzepine Study Group. (2008). Two-year multicenter, randomized, double-masked, placebo-controlled, parallel safety and efficacy study of 2% pirenzepine ophthalmic gel in children with myopia. *Journal of AAPOS, 12*(4), 332–339. https://doi.org/10.1016/j.jaapos.2007.10.014

Silva, R. A., & Blumenkranz, M. S. (2013). Prophylaxis for retinal detachment. *American Academy of Ophthalmology, The Ophthalmic News and Education Network.* https://www.aao.org/education/current-insight/prophylaxis-retinal-detachments

Smith, E. L., 3rd, Arumugam, B., Hung, L. F., She, Z., Beach, K., & Sankaridurg, P. (2020). Eccentricity-dependent effects of simultaneous competing defocus on emmetropization in infant rhesus monkeys. *Vision Research, 177*, 32–40. https://doi.org/10.1016/j.visres.2020.08.003

Smith, E. L., 3rd, Huang, J., Hung, L. F., Blasdel, T. L., Humbird, T. L., & Bockhorst, K. H. (2009a). Hemiretinal form deprivation: Evidence for local control of eye growth and refractive development in infant monkeys. *Investigative Ophthalmology & Visual Science, 50*(11), 5057–5069. https://doi.org/10.1167/iovs.08-3232

Smith, E. L., 3rd, Hung, L. F., & Huang, J. (2009b). Relative peripheral hyperopic defocus alters central refractive development in infant monkeys. *Vision Research, 49*(19), 2386–2392. https://doi.org/10.1016/j.visres.2009.07.011

Smith, E. L., 3rd, Hung, L. F., Arumugam, B., Holden, B. A., Neitz, M., & Neitz, J. (2015). Effects of long-wavelength lighting on refractive development in infant rhesus monkeys. *Investigative Ophthalmology & Visual Science, 56*(11), 6490–6500. https://doi.org/10.1167%2Fiovs.15-17025

Smith, E. L., 3rd, Hung, L. F., Huang, J., & Arumugam, B. (2013). Effects of local myopic defocus on refractive development in monkeys. *Optometry and Vision Science, 90*(11), 1176–1186. https://doi.org/10.1097/OPX.0000000000000038

Smith, E. L., 3rd, Hung, L. F., Huang, J., Blasdel, T. L., Humbird, T. L., & Bockhorst, K. H. (2010). Effects of optical defocus on refractive development in monkeys: Evidence for local, regionally selective mechanisms. *Investigative Ophthalmology & Visual Science, 51*(8), 3864–3873. https://doi.org/10.1167/iovs.09-4969

Smith, E. L., 3rd, Hung, L. F., Kee, C. S., & Qiao, Y. (2002). Effects of brief periods of unrestricted vision on the development of form-deprivation myopia in monkeys. *Investigative Ophthalmology & Visual Science, 43*(2), 291–299. https://pubmed.ncbi.nlm.nih.gov/11818369/

Smith, E. L., 3rd, Hung, L. F., She, Z., Beach, K., Ostrin, L. A., & Jong, M. (2021). Topically instilled caffeine selectively alters emmetropizing responses in infant rhesus monkeys. *Experimental Eye Research, 203*, 108438. https://doi.org/10.1016/j.exer.2021.108438

Smith, E. L., 3rd, Ramamirtham, R., Qiao-Grider, Y., Hung, L. F., Huang, J., Kee, C. S., Coats, D., & Paysse, E. (2007). Effects of foveal ablation on emmetropization and form-deprivation myopia. *Investigative Ophthalmology & Visual Science, 48*(9), 3914–3922. https://doi.org/10.1167/iovs.06-1264

Smith, T. S., Frick, K. D., Holden, B. A., Fricke, T. R., & Naidoo, K. S. (2009c). Potential lost productivity resulting from the global burden of uncorrected refractive error. *Bulletin of the World Health Organization, 87*(6), 431–437. https://doi.org/10.2471/blt.08.055673

Sodhi, P., & Hartwick, A. T. (2014). Adenosine modulates light responses of rat retinal ganglion cell photoreceptors through a cAMP-mediated pathway. *Journal of Physiology, 592*(18), 4201–4220. https://doi.org/10.1113%2Fjphysiol.2014.276220

Sorensen, L., Gyrd-Hansen, D., Kristiansen, I. S., Nexøe, J., & Nielsen, J. B. (2008). Laypersons' understanding of relative risk reductions: Randomised cross-sectional study. *BMC Medical Informatics and Decision Making, 8*(1). https://doi.org/10.1186/1472-6947-8-31

Srinivasan, B., Leung, H.Y., Cao, H., Liu, S., Chen, L., & Fan, A.H. (2016). Modern phacoemulsification and intraocular lens implantation (refractive lens exchange) is safe and effective in treating high myopia. *Asia-Pacific Journal of Ophthalmology, 5*(6), 438–444. https://doi.org/10.1097/APO.0000000000000241

Stone, R. A., Lin, T., & Laties, A. M. (1991). Muscarinic antagonist effects on experimental chick myopia. *Experimental Eye Research, 52*(6), 755–758. https://doi.org/10.1016/0014-4835(91)90027-c.

Stone, R. A., Lin, T., Laties, A. M., & Iuvone, P. M. (1989). Retinal dopamine and form-deprivation myopia. *Proceedings of the National Academy of Sciences, 86*(18), 704–706. https://doi.org/10.1073/pnas.86.2.704

Sugar, A., Rapuano, C. J., Culbertson, W. W., Huang, D., Varley, G. A., Agapitos, P. J., de Luise, V. P., & Koch, D. D. (2002). Laser in situ keratomileusis for myopia and astigmatism: safety and efficacy: A report by the American Academy of Ophthalmology. *Ophthalmology, 109*(1), 175–187. https://doi.org/10.1016/s0161-6420(01)00966-6

Swiatczak, B., & Schaeffel, F. (2022). Myopia: why the retina stops inhibiting eye growth. *Scientific Reports, 12*(1), 21704. https://doi.org/10.1038/s41598-022-26323-7

Tang, J., Liao, Y., Yan, N., Dereje, S., Wang, J., Luo, Y., Wang, Y., Zhou, W., Wang, X., & Wang, W. (2023). Efficacy of repeated low-level red-light therapy for slowing the progression of childhood myopia: A systematic review and meta-analysis. *American Journal of Ophthalmology, 252*. https://doi.org/10.1016/j.ajo.2023.03.036

Tang, N., Zhao, X., Chen, J., Liu, B., & Lu, L. (2021). Changes in the choroidal thickness after macular buckling in highly myopic eyes. *Retina, 41*(9), 1858. https://doi.org/10.1097/IAE.0000000000003125

Tapasztó, B., Flitcroft, D. I., Aclimandos, W. A., Jonas, J. B., De Faber, J. H. N., Nagy, Z. Z., Kestelyn, P. G., Januleviciene, I., Grzybowski, A., Vidinova, C. N., Guggenheim, J. A., Polling, J. R., Wolffsohn, J. S., Tideman, J. W. L., Allen, P. M., Baraas, R. C., Saunders, K. J., McCullough, S. J., Gray, L. S., Wahl, S., … SOE Myopia Consensus Group. (2023). Myopia management algorithm. Annexe to the article titled Update and guidance on management of myopia. European Society of Ophthalmology in cooperation with International Myopia Institute. *European Journal of Ophthalmology*. https://doi.org/10.1177/11206721231219532

Thomson, K., Kelly, T., Karouta, C., Morgan, I., & Ashby, R. (2021). Insights into the mechanism by which atropine inhibits myopia: Evidence against cholinergic hyperactivity and modulation of dopamine release. *British Journal of Pharmacology, 178*(22), 4501–4517. https://doi.org/10.1111/bph.15629

Tian, L., Cao, K., Ma, D. L., Zhao, S. Q., Lu, L. X., Li, A., Chen, C. X., Ma, C. R., Ma, Z. F., & Jie, Y. (2022). Investigation of the efficacy and safety of 650 nm low-level red light for myopia control in children: A randomized controlled trial. *Ophthalmology and Therapy, 11*(6), 2259–2270. https://doi.org/10.1007/s40123-022-00585-w

Tideman, J. W., Polling, J. R., Voortman, T., Jaddoe, V. W., Uitterlinden, A. G., Hofman, A., Vingerling, J. R., Franco, O. H., & Klaver, C. C. (2016). Low serum vitamin D is associated with axial length and risk of myopia in young children. *European Journal of Epidemiology, 31*(5), 491–499. https://doi.org/10.1007/s10654-016-0128-8

Tong, L., Huang, X. L., Koh, A. L., Zhang, X., Tan, D. T., & Chua, W. H. (2009). Atropine for the treatment of childhood myopia: Effect on myopia progression after cessation of atropine. *Ophthalmology, 116*(3), 572–579. https://doi.org/10.1016/j.ophtha.2008.10.020

Torii, H., Kurihara, T., Seko, Y., Negishi, K., Ohnuma, K., Inaba, T., Kawashima, M., Jiang, X., Kondo, S., Miyauchi, M., Miwa, Y., Katada, Y., Mori, K., Kato, K., Tsubota, K., Goto, H., Oda, M., Hatori, M., & Tsubota, K. (2017). Violet Light Exposure Can Be a Preventive Strategy Against Myopia Progression. *EBioMedicine, 15*, 210–219. https://doi.org/10.1016/j.ebiom.2016.12.007

Torii, H., Mori, K., Okano, T., Kondo, S., Yang, H. Y., Yotsukura, E., Hanyuda, A., Ogawa, M., Negishi, K., Kurihara, T., & Tsubota, K. (2022). Short-term exposure to violet light emitted from eyeglass frames in myopic children: A randomized pilot clinical trial. *Journal of Clinical Medicine, 11*(20), 6000. https://doi.org/10.3390/jcm11206000

Trier, K., Cui, D., Ribel-Madsen, S., & Guggenheim, J. (2023). Oral administration of caffeine metabolite 7-methylxanthine is associated with slowed myopia progression in Danish children. *British Journal of Ophthalmology, 107*(10), 1538–1544. https://doi.org/10.1136/bjo-2021-320920

Troilo, D., Smith, E. L., 3rd, Nickla, D. L., Ashby, R., Tkatchenko, A. V., Ostrin, L. A., Gawne, T. J., Pardue, M. T., Summers, J. A., Kee, C. S., Schroedl, F., Wahl, S., & Jones, L. (2019). IMI - Report on experimental models of emmetropization and myopia. *Investigative Ophthalmology & Visual Science, 60*(3), M31–M88. https://doi.org/10.1167/iovs.18-25967

van der Sande, E., Polling, J. R., Tideman, J. W. L., Meester-Smoor, M. A., Thiadens, A. A. H. J., Tan, E., De Zeeuw, C. I., Hamelink, R., Willuhn, I., Verhoeven, V. J. M., Winkelman, B. H. J., & Klaver, C. C. W. (2023). Myopia control in Mendelian forms of myopia. *Ophthalmic & Physiological Optics: The Journal of the British College of Ophthalmic Opticians (Optometrists), 43*(3), 494–504. https://doi.org/10.1111/opo.13115

Verkicharla, P. K., Suheimat, M., Schmid, K. L., & Atchison, D. A. (2016). Peripheral refraction, peripheral eye length, and retinal shape in myopia. *Optometry and Vision Science, 93*(9), 1072–1078. https://doi.org/10.1097/opx.0000000000000905

Vutipongsatorn, K., Yokoi, T., & Ohno-Matsui, K. (2019). Current and emerging pharmaceutical interventions for myopia. *British Journal of Ophthalmology, 103,* 1539–1548. https://doi.org/10.1136/bjophthalmol-2018-313798

Walline, J. J., Gaume Giannoni, A., Sinnott, L. T., Chandler, M. A., Huang, J., Mutti, D. O., Jones-Jordan, L. A., Berntsen, D. A., & BLINK Study Group. (2017). A randomized trial of soft multifocal contact lenses for myopia control: Baseline data and methods. *Optometry and Vision Science, 94*(9), 856–866. https://doi.org/10.1097%2FOPX.0000000000001106

Walline, J. J., Greiner, K. L., McVey, M. E., & Jones-Jordan, L. A. (2013). Multifocal contact lens myopia control. *Optometry and Vision Science, 90*(11), 1207–1214. https://doi.org/10.1097/opx.0000000000000036

Walline, J. J., Jones, L. A., Rah, M. J., Manny, R. E., Berntsen, D. A., Chitkara, M., Gaume, A., Kim, A., & Quinn, N. (2007). Contact Lenses in Pediatrics (CLIP) study: Chair time and ocular health. *Optometry and Vision Science, 84*(9), 896–902. https://doi.org/10.1097/opx.0b013e3181559c3c

Walline, J. J., Jones, L. A., Sinnott, L., Manny, R. E., Gaume, A., Rah, M. J., Chitkara, M., & Lyons, S. (2008). A randomized trial of the effect of soft contact lenses on myopia progression in children. *Investigative Ophthalmology & Visual Science, 49*(11), 4702. https://doi.org/10.1167/iovs.08-2067

Walline, J. J., Lindsley, K., Vedula, S. S., Cotter, S. A., Mutti, D. O., & Twelker, J. D. (2011). Interventions to slow progression of myopia in children. *The Cochrane Database of Systematic Reviews*, (12), CD004916. https://doi.org/10.1002/14651858.cd004916.pub3

Walline, J. J., Lindsley, K. B., Vedula, S. S., Cotter, S. A., Mutti, D. O., Ng, S. M., & Twelker, J. D. (2020a). Interventions to slow progression of myopia in children. *The Cochrane Database of Systematic Reviews, 1*(1), CD004916. https://doi.org/10.1002/14651858.cd004916.pub4

Walline, J. J., Walker, M. K., Mutti, D. O., Jones-Jordan, L. A., Sinnott, L. T., Giannoni, A. G., Bickle, K. M., Schulle, K. L., Nixon, A., Pierce, G. E., Berntsen, D. A., & BLINK Study Group (2020b). Effect of high add power, medium add power, or single-vision contact lenses on myopia progression in children: The BLINK randomized clinical trial. *JAMA, 324*(6), 571–580. https://doi.org/10.1001/jama.2020.10834

Wallman, J., Turkel, J., & Trachtman, J. (1978). Extreme myopia produced by modest change in early visual experience. *Science, 201*(4362), 1249–1251. https://doi.org/10.1126/science.694514

Wallman, J., Wildsoet, C., Xu, A., Gottlieb, M. D., Nickla, D. L., Marran, L., Krebs, W., & Christensen, A. M. (1995). Moving the retina: choroidal modulation of refractive state. *Vision Research, 35*(1), 37–50. https://doi.org/10.1016/0042-6989(94)e0049-q

Wang, W., Jiang, Y., Zhu, Z., Zhang, S., Xuan, M., Chen, Y., Xiong, R., Bulloch, G., Zeng, J., Morgan, I. G., & He, M. (2023). Clinically significant axial shortening in myopic children after repeated low-level red light therapy: A retrospective multicenter analysis. *Ophthalmology and Therapy, 12*(2), 999–1011. https://doi.org/10.1007/s40123-022-00644-2

Wang, Y., Li, L., Tang, X., Fan, H., Song, W., Xie, J., Tang, Y., Jiang, Y., & Zou, Y. (2024). The role of vasoactive intestinal peptide (VIP) in atropine-related inhibition of the progression of myopia. *BMC Ophthalmology, 24*(1), 41. https://doi.org/10.1186/s12886-024-03309-9

Wang, F., Zhou, J., Lu, Y., & Chu, R. (2011). Effects of 530 nm green light on refractive status, melatonin, MT1 receptor, and melanopsin in the guinea pig. *Current Eye Research, 36*(2), 103–111. https://doi.org/10.3109/02713683.2010.526750

Waring, G. O., 3rd, Lynn, M. J., & McDonnell, P. J. (1994). Results of the prospective evaluation of radial keratotomy (PERK) study 10 years after surgery. *Archives of Ophthalmology, 112*(10), 1298–1308. https://doi.org/10.1001/archopht.1994.01090220048022

Wen, D., Huang, J., Chen, H., Bao, F., Savini, G., Calossi, A., Chen, H., Li, X., & Wang, Q. (2015). Efficacy and acceptability of orthokeratology for slowing myopic progression in children: A systematic review and meta-analysis. *Journal of Ophthalmology, 2015*, 360806. https://doi.org/10.1155/2015/360806

Wen, G., Tarczy-Hornoch, K., McKean-Cowdin, R., Cotter, S. A., Borchert, M., Lin, J., Kim, J., Varma, R., & Multi-Ethnic Pediatric Eye Disease Study Group. (2013). Prevalence of myopia, hyperopia, and astigmatism in non-Hispanic white and Asian children: Multi-ethnic pediatric eye disease study. *Ophthalmology, 120*(10), 2109–2116. https://doi.org/10.1016/j.ophtha.2013.06.039

Wiesel, T. N., & Raviola, E. (1977). Myopia and eye enlargement after neonatal lid fusion in monkeys. *Nature, 266*(5597), 66–68. https://doi.org/10.1038/266066a0

Wildsoet, C. F. (1997). Active emmetropization: Evidence for its existence and ramifications for clinical practice. *Ophthalmic & Physiological Optics, 17*, 279–290. https://pubmed.ncbi.nlm.nih.gov/9390372/

Wolf, A. T., Klawe, J., Liu, B., & Ahmad, S. (2023). Association between serum vitamin D levels and myopia in the National Health and Nutrition Examination Survey (2001-2006). *Ophthalmic Epidemiology, 31*(3), 229–239. https://doi.org/10.1080/09286586.2023.2232460World Society of Pediatric Ophthalmology & Strabismus. (2023). *Myopia consensus statement 2023.* https://www.wspos.org/swdcore/uploads/WSPOS-Myopia-Consensus-Statement-2023-1.pdf

Wolffsohn, J. S., Whayeb, Y., Logan, N. S., & Weng, R. (2023). IMI—Global Trends in Myopia Management Attitudes and Strategies in Clinical Practice—2022 Update. *Investigative Ophthalmology & Visual Science, 64*(6), 6. https://doi.org/10.1167/iovs.64.6.6

Wu, J., Gong, H., Li, H., Liang, J., Zhang, X., Yang, H., Liu, X., Zhang, G., Cheng, G., Bai, G., & Zhang, H. (2023). Changes in choroidal thickness in myopic children with 0.01% atropine: Evidence from a 12-month follow-up. *Photodiagnosis and Photodynamic Therapy, 42*, 103528. https://doi.org/10.1016/j.pdpdt.2023.103528

Wu, P. C., Chang, L. C., Niu, Y. Z., Chen, M. L., Liao, L. L., & Chen, C. T. (2018a). Myopia prevention in Taiwan. *Annals of Eye Science, 3*, 12. https://aes.amegroups.org/article/view/4010/4715

Wu, P. C., Chen, C. T., Lin, K. K., Sun, C. C., Kuo, C. N., Huang, H. M., Poon, Y. C., Yang, M. L., Chen, C. Y., Huang, J. C., Wu, P. C., Yang, I. H., Yu, H. J., Fang, P. C., Tsai, C. L., Chiou, S. T., & Yang, Y. H. (2018b). Myopia Prevention and Outdoor Light Intensity in a School-Based Cluster Randomized Trial. *Ophthalmology, 125*(8), 1239–1250. https://doi.org/10.1016/j.ophtha.2017.12.011

Wu, P. C., Tsai, C. L., Wu, H. L., Yang, Y. H., & Kuo, H. K. (2013). Outdoor activity during class recess reduces myopia onset and progression in school children. *Ophthalmology, 120*(5), 1080–1085. https://doi.org/10.1016/j.ophtha.2012.11.009

Xiang, F., He, M., & Morgan, I. G. (2012). Annual changes in refractive errors and ocular components before and after the onset of myopia in Chinese children. *Ophthalmology, 119*(7), 1478–1484. https://doi.org/10.1016/j.ophtha.2012.01.017

Xiao, J., Pan, X., Hou, C., & Wang, Q. (2024). Changes in subfoveal choroidal thickness after orthokeratology in myopic children: A systematic review and meta-analysis. *Current Eye Research.* https://doi.org/10.1080/02713683.2024.2310618

Xiong, F., Mao, T., Liao, H., Hu, X., Shang, L., Yu, L., Lin, N., Huang, L., Yi, Y., Zhou, R., Zhou, X., & Yi, J. (2021). Orthokeratology and low-intensity laser therapy for slowing the progression of myopia in children. *BioMed Research International.* https://doi.org/10.1155/2021/8915867 .

Xiong, S., Sankaridurg, P., Naduvilath, T., Zang, J., Zou, H., Zhu, J., Lv, M., He, X., & Xu, X. (2017). Time spent in outdoor activities in relation to myopia prevention and control: A meta-analysis and systematic review. *Acta Ophthalmologica, 95*(6), 551–566. https://doi.org/10.1111/aos.13403

Xiong, R., Zhu, Z., Jiang, Y., Wang, W., Zhang, J., Chen, Y., Bulloch, G., Yuan, Y., Zhang, S., Xuan, M., Zeng, J., Morgan, I. G., & He, M. (2022). Sustained and rebound effect of repeated low-level red-light therapy on myopia control: A 2-year post-trial follow-up study. *Clinical & Experimental Ophthalmology, 50*(9), 1013–1024. https://doi.org/10.1111/ceo.14149

Xiong, R., Zhuoting, Z., Jiang, Y., Wang, W., Zhang, J., Chen, Y., Bulloch, G., Yuan, Y., Zhang, S., Xuan, M., Zeng, J., & Morgan, I. G. (2023). Longitudinal changes and predictive value of choroidal thickness for myopia control after repeated low-level red-light therapy. *Ophthalmology, 130*(3), 286–296. https://doi.org/10.1016/j.ophtha.2022.10.002.

Yam, J. C., Jiang, Y., Lee, J., Li, S., Zhang, Y., Sun, W., Yuan, N., Wang, Y. M., Yip, B. H. K., Kam, K. W., Chan, H. N., Zhang, X. J., Young, A. L., Tham, C. C., Cheung, C. Y., Chu, W. K., Pang, C. P., & Chen, L. J. (2022a). The association of choroidal thickening by atropine with treatment effects for myopia: Two-year clinical trial of the Low-Concentration Atropine For Myopia Progression (LAMP) Study. *American Journal of Ophthalmology,* 237, 130–138. https://doi.org/10.1016/j.ajo.2021.12.014

Yam, J. C., Jiang, Y., Tang, S. M., Law, A. K. P., Chan, J. J., Wong, E., Ko, S. T., Young, A. L., Tham, C. C., Chen, L. J., & Pang, C. P. (2019). Low-Concentration Atropine for Myopia Progression (LAMP) study: A randomized, double-blinded, placebo-controlled trial of 0.05%, 0.025%, and 0.01% atropine eye drops in myopia control. *Ophthalmology, 126*(1), 113–124. https://doi.org/10.1016/j.ophtha.2018.05.029

Yam, J. C., Li, F. F., Zhang, X., Tang, S. M., Yip, B. H. K., Kam, K. W., Ko, S. T., Young, A. L., Tham, C. C., Chen, L. J., & Pang, C. P. (2020). Two-year clinical trial of the Low-Concentration Atropine for Myopia Progression (LAMP) study: Phase 2 report. *Ophthalmology, 127*(7), 910–919. https://doi.org/10.1016/j.ophtha.2019.12.011

Yam, J. C., Zhang, X. J., Zhang, Y., Wang, Y. M., Tang, S. M., Li, F. F., Kam, K. W., Ko, S. T., Yip, B. H. K., Young, A. L., Tham, C. C., Chen, L. J., & Pang, C. P. (2022b). Three-year clinical trial of Low-Concentration Atropine for Myopia Progression (LAMP) study: Continued versus washout: Phase 3 report. *Ophthalmology, 129*(3), 308–321. https://doi.org/10.1016/j.ophtha.2021.10.002

Yasir, Z. H., Sharma, R., & Zakir, S. M. (2023). Scleral collagen cross linkage in progressive myopia. *Indian Journal of Ophthalmology.* https://doi.org/10.4103/IJO.IJO_1392_23.

Yazar, S., Hewitt, A. W., Black, L. J., McKnight, C. M., Mountain, J. A., Sherwin, J. C., Oddy, W. H., Coroneo, M. T., Lucas, R. M., & Mackey, D. A. (2014). Myopia is associated with lower vitamin D status in young adults. *Investigative Ophthalmology & Visual Science, 55*(7), 4552–4559. https://doi.org/10.1167/iovs.14-14589

Yen, M. Y., Liu, J. H., Kao, S. C., & Shiao, C. H. (1989). Comparison of the effect of atropine and cyclopentolate on myopia. *Annals of Ophthalmology, 21*(5), 180–187. https://pubmed.ncbi.nlm.nih.gov/2742290/

Yoshida, T., Takagi, Y., Igarashi-Yokoi, T., & Ohno-Matsui, K. (2023). Efficacy of lutein supplements on macular pigment optical density in highly myopic individuals: A randomized controlled trial. *Medicine, 102*(12), e33280. https://doi.org/10.1097/MD.0000000000033280

Zadnik, K., Schulman, E., Flitcroft, I., Fogt, J. S., Blumenfeld, L. C., Fong, T. M., Lang, E., Hemmati, H. D., Chandler, S. P., & CHAMP Trial Group Investigators. (2023). Efficacy and safety of 0.01% and 0.02% atropine for the treatment of pediatric myopia progression over 3 years: A randomized clinical trial. *JAMA Ophthalmology, 141*(10), 990–999. https://doi.org/10.1001/jamaophthalmol.2023.2097

Zadnik, K., Sinnott, L. T., Cotter, S. A., Jones-Jordan, L. A., Kleinstein, R. N., Manny, R. E., Twelker, J. D., Mutti, D. O., & Collaborative Longitudinal Evaluation of Ethnicity and Refractive Error (CLEERE) Study Group. (2015). Prediction of juvenile-onset myopia. *JAMA Ophthalmology, 133*(6), 683–689. https://doi.org/10.1001/jamaophthalmol.2015.0471

Zeitz, C., Roger, J. E., Audo, I., Michiels, C., Sánchez-Farías, N., Varin, J., Frederiksen, H., Wilmet, B., Callebert, J., Gimenez, M., Bouzidi, N., Blond, F., Guilllonneau, X., Fouquet, S., Léveillard, T., Smirnov, V. M., Vincent, A., Héon, E., Sahel, J., . . . Picaud, S. (2023). Shedding light on myopia by studying complete congenital stationary night blindness. *Progress in Retinal and Eye Research, 93,* 101155. https://doi.org/10.1016/j.preteyeres.2022.101155

Zhang, H. Y., Lam, C. S. Y., Tang, W. C., Leung, M., & To, C. H. (2020). Defocus incorporated multiple segments spectacle lenses changed the relative peripheral refraction: A 2-Year randomized clinical trial. *Investigative Ophthalmology & Visual Science, 61*(5), 53. https://doi.org/10.1167/iovs.61.5.53

Zhang, D. Q., Wong, K. Y., Sollars, P. J., Berson, D. M., Pickard, G. E., & McMahon, D. G. (2008). Intraretinal signaling by ganglion cell photoreceptors to dopaminergic amacrine neurons. *Proceedings of the National Academy of Sciences, 105*(37), 14181–14186. https://doi.org/10.1073/pnas.0803893105

Zhang, X. J., Zhang, Y., Kam, K. W., Tang, F., Li, Y., Ng, M. P. H., Young, A. L., Ip, P., Tham, C. C., Chen, L. J., Pang, C. P., & Yam, J. C. (2023). Prevalence of Myopia in Children Before, During, and After COVID-19 Restrictions in Hong Kong. *JAMA network open, 6*(3), e234080. https://doi.org/10.1001/jamanetworkopen.2023.4080

Zhang, Z., Zhou, Y., Xie, Z., Chen, T., Gu, Y., Lu, S., & Wu, Z. (2016). The effect of topical atropine on the choroidal thickness of healthy children. *Scientific Reports, 6,* 34936. https://doi.org/10.1038/srep34936

Zheng, Y. F., Pan, C. W., Chay, J., Wong, T. Y., Finkelstein, E., & Saw, S. M. (2013). The economic cost of myopia in adults aged over 40 years in Singapore. *Investigative Ophthalmology & Visual Science, 54*(12), 7532–7537. https://doi.org/10.1167/iovs.13-12795

Zhou, L., Tong, L., Li, Y., Williams, B. T., & Qiu, K. (2023). Photobiomodulation therapy retarded axial length growth in children with myopia: Evidence from a 12-month randomized controlled trial evidence. *Scientific Reports, 13*(1), 3321. https://doi.org/10.1038/s41598-023-30500-7

Zhou, X., Pardue, M. T., Iuvone, P. M., & Qu, J. (2017). Dopamine signaling and myopia development: What are the key challenges. *Progress in Retinal and Eye Research, 61,* 60–71. https://doi.org/10.1016/j.preteyeres.2017.06.003Zloto, O., Wyganaski-Jaffe, T., Farzavandi, S., Gomez-de-Liaño, Sprunger, D., Mezer, E. (2018). Current trends among pediatric ophthalmologists to decrease myopia progression—An international perspective. *Graefe's Archive for Clinical and Experimental Ophthalmology, 256*(12), 2457–2466. https://doi.org/10.1007/s00417-018-4078-6

Zhu, Q., Goto, S., Singh, S., Torres, J. A., & Wildsoet, C. F. (2022). Daily or Less Frequent Topical 1% Atropine Slows Defocus-Induced Myopia Progression in Contact Lens-Wearing Guinea Pigs. *Translational Vision Science & Technology, 11*(3), 26. https://doi.org/10.1167/tvst.11.3.26

8

Identifying Children with Myopia and the Links to Treatment: Methods and Barriers

This chapter focuses on medically underserved populations of children and their families that face health disparities, specifically racial and ethnic minority groups, people with lower socioeconomic status, rural communities, and children with disabilities. Sexual and gender minority groups were not included because a quick search yielded no studies on the topic. The chapter, like the rest of this report, focuses on myopia, though it should be noted that childhood visual problems in need of detection extend beyond myopia to other refractive errors, amblyopia, and amblyogenic risk factors (see Box 8-1).

Myopia can be identified through vision screening and comprehensive eye exams. Vision screenings for children may occur in pediatric primary care practices, schools, and community-based settings and are either targeted to medically underserved populations or provided universally to all children. Vision screenings offer a cost-effective way to evaluate key elements of vision in many children. Comprehensive eye exams, by contrast, evaluate the full picture of eye health for each child, are provided by doctors of optometry and ophthalmology where available in local communities, and generally incur higher costs.

The barriers to identifying and treating myopia are vast. To start with, myopia is a condition that most often begins early in life (Kleinstein et al., 2012) when children are unable to articulate that their distance vision is blurry or even realize that blurry vision is not normal. Community- or school-based vision screenings may help identify children with myopia who need a full comprehensive eye exam and a prescription for glasses from an eye care professional. However, if identified myopia is left untreated the vision screening will have had no impact for those children. Furthermore, vision screening by itself fails to establish an "eye care home" for the child with myopia, a lifelong condition that worsens throughout childhood (Houet al., 2018). Comprehensive eye exams for all children may increase the likelihood that a child with myopia will be detected, provided with glasses, and monitored by an eye doctor. However, comprehensive eye exams for all children may not be feasible for reasons including shortages in the supply of eye care professionals, especially pediatric eye care professionals in the United States where 90% of counties do not have a pediatric ophthalmologist (Walsh et al., 2023) and nearly 25% of counties do not have an optometrist (Feng et al., 2020). The provision of a prescription for glasses after a comprehensive eye exam either triggered by vision screening or booked independently may be helpful. However, research suggests that glasses are often unavailable and even when dispensed may not be worn or replaced if broken or lost (Ethan et al., 2010; Nishimura et al.,2024).

Even in ideal models with long-term case-management and cohesive multidisciplinary collaboration, several barriers exist to identifying and treating myopia and its progression: finances, lack of awareness, and logistics such as transportation. Vision screening and comprehensive eye exams are informed by a range of policies and recommendations across states and professional associations. This range of policies and recommendations, compounded by poor strategies to ensure follow-up, make surveillance challenging. The outcome of this is often inadequate vision care and follow-up with eye care professionals. In short, there is a critical need for novel, effective strategies to ensure adequate detection and management of childhood myopia.

BOX 8-1
Other Childhood Visual Problems Besides Myopia That Deserve Attention

Although the focus of this National Academies report is myopia, childhood visual problems in need of detection extend beyond myopia to other refractive errors, amblyopia, and amblyogenic risk factors. Other refractive errors include hyperopia (far-sightedness), astigmatism (cornea and/or lens non-spherical irregularity), and anisometropia (unequal refractive error between the paired two eyes). In early childhood, hyperopia and astigmatism are more common than myopia, but by middle childhood myopia is the most common refractive error.

Amblyopia is reduced visual acuity, typically in a structurally normal eye, that results from perturbation in visual experience in one eye relative to the other, providing poor binocular input to the visual cortex early in life. Factors that may lead to the development of amblyopia include unequal focus between the eyes (anisometropia), non-straight paired eye alignment (strabismus), and inability to form a clear image because of a high refractive error, as examples. Although less common than refractive error, amblyopia occurs in 3–5% of the population in the United States. It can be effectively treated or prevented before about age 8 years (Holmes & Levi, 2018). After this early neurodevelopmentally sensitive period, it is still possible to improve visual impairment due to amblyopia, but not to the same degree as would be the case in early childhood, and amblyopia remains as a lifelong impairment (Scheiman, 2005).

Amblyogenic conditions other than refractive error that can be due to structural ocular changes include childhood cataracts or glaucoma, corneal cloudiness, vitreous hemorrhage, optic nerve maldevelopment, and significant eyelid droop (ptosis) that covers the pupil, among others.

MODELS FOR IDENTIFYING AND TREATING MYOPIA

Comprehensive Eye Exams

A comprehensive eye exam generally refers to a detailed eye exam that is provided by an eye care professional (optometrist or ophthalmologist) and is the highest standard of care for children's vision (American Optometric Association & Carey, 2018). Comprehensive eye exams often occur in a doctor's office, involve multiple assessments and, usually, the use of dilating eye drops. Assessments in a comprehensive eye exam include ocular history, external inspection of the eye structures, distance visual acuity, ocular motility assessment (ability to move the eyes in specified directions), cross cover test (to check for eye misalignment), corneal light reflex, red reflex, pupil examination, ophthalmoscopy (examination of the back of the eye with a special instrument), instrument-based screening (if needed), and color vision (American Optometric Association, 2017). The multiple tests included in a comprehensive eye exam are described in the chapter on diagnosis (see Chapter 4). Comprehensive eye exams can detect not only myopia but also other refractive errors, amblyopia, and risk factors for amblyopia.

While dilating eye drops are not required in a comprehensive eye exam, they are almost universally recommended in national practice policies for children, because they are likely to enhance the ability to evaluate and diagnose eye and vision problems in children (American Optometric Association, 2017; Flitcroft, 2019; Hutchinson et al., 2023; Saxena et al., 2020). The use of dilating eye drops helps knock out the child's dynamic focusing system and provides a more stable and precise measure of refractive error and glasses prescription for any discovered myopia. It is also essential for detecting hyperopia in children, because hyperopia can be masked easily by the child's focusing ability. Dilation also helps doctors evaluate the health of the eye by increasing and stabilizing the size of the pupil so that the retina can be visualized.

Even for children who are asymptomatic or at low risk, the American Optometric Association recommends comprehensive eye exams, the first between 6 and 12 months of age, then at least once between ages 3 and 5 years, then before first grade, and then every one to two years thereafter (Table 8-1; see Table 8-5 for recommendations from other professional associations). Comprehensive eye exams can be more expensive than vision screening; however, they involve a broader evaluation of a child's vision, eye health, and refractive error; follow-up eye care may also be better (Ekdawi et al., 2021).

TABLE 8-1 Recommended Eye Examination Frequency for the Pediatric Patient per the American Optometric Association

Examination Interval		
Patient Age	**Asymptomatic/ Low Risk**	**At-risk**
Birth through 2 years	At 6 to12 months of age	At 6 to 12 months of age or as recommended
3 through 5 years	At least once between 3 and 5 years of age	At least once between 3 and 5 years of age or as recommended
6 through 18 years	Before first grade and annually thereafter	Before first grade and annually, or as recommended, thereafter

NOTES: The American Optometric Association Clinical Practice Guidelines provide more information on other eye and vision disorders and their risk factors. (For more information about the practical guidelines, see https://www.aoa.org/practice/clinical-guidelines/clinical-practice-guidelines?sso=y.) SOURCE: American Optometric Association, 2017.

Vision Screening

Vision screening generally refers to an abbreviated evaluation of vision and is important for the early detection of vision loss in children who may not have had a comprehensive eye exam. Vision screening aims to identify common vision disorders and facilitate diagnosis and treatment through referrals to eye care providers (optometrists and ophthalmologists). It can be conducted by persons other than eye doctors (e.g., school nurses, trained volunteers) in primary care practices, as a school-based universal screening program, as a community-based program (e.g., at a shopping mall, summer camp, or mobile eye unit), or as a targeted program at sites selected to address a high level of need. Vision screenings may be instrument-based, such that an automated device measures refractive error. Instrument-based screenings may also pick up eye turns and structural issues, including droopy lids and cataracts, and instrument-based screening can be used as early as infancy. For older children, vision screening usually includes a measure of distance visual acuity by having the child view letters or pictures of decreasing size one eye at a time. Some vision screenings also include assessments of eye alignment, stereoscopic 3D depth perception, color vision, and/or near acuity. Vision screening, as an abbreviated evaluation, will not obtain identical results to a comprehensive eye exam. The rate of false positive and false negative screening results varies as a function of the type of vision screening tool used, the age of the child, the referral cut-offs, and the visual impairment. The amount of time needed for each type of vision screening test varies significantly based on the type of tool used. Compared to acuity tests, vision screening with instrument-based tools (e.g., autorefractors or photoscreeners) is quick (less than a minute for newer models) and requires minimal cooperation from the child (Donahue & Nixon, 2016; Donahue et al., 2016a; Loh & Chaing, 2018). Nevertheless, because of their cost and clinical practice recommendations, instrument-based devices are used less often compared to visual acuity tests and physical examination of the eye (Hoover et al., 2023; Oke et al., 2023).

Data on the prevalence of vision screening are often based on small samples of the population that are not representative of the general population, that lack standardized definitions, or that depend on parental[1] reports. An example of data based on parental reporting comes from a large nationwide survey of parents in 2018 and 2019, in which 14% of all U.S. children were reported by their caregivers to have received a vision test in the prior year in school, 28% in pediatric primary care clinics, and 34% in eye clinics (Child and Adolescent Health Measurement Initiative). Figures based on this national survey reflect parental *awareness* that the child had been screened and may, therefore, underestimate the actual amount of screening. Also, prior to 2021, no national survey has measured whether parents followed up when screening results indicated a referral to an eye doctor was warranted.

Measured Benefits of Vision Screening

Vision screening with follow-up eye care with an eye care professional (optometrist or ophthalmologist) to diagnose and treat vision impairment has been shown to have positive impacts on many aspects of a child's development. In the Baltimore City public schools, a randomized controlled trial of 2,304 students in grades 3 to 7 found that universal vision screening with the provision of needed prescription glasses for uncorrected refractive errors improved academic achievement in reading over the next year (Harewood et al., 2024; Killeen et al., 2023). A review of nine studies, six of them randomized controlled trials (RCTs) and all of them of satisfactory or good quality (Pirindhavellie et al., 2023) revealed that getting glasses improved children's math and literacy scores, school behaviors (focusing, practice), and mental health and quality-of-life scores, and it also decreased anxiety, with small effects in each case

---

[1]Throughout this report, the term "parent" is used to denote any adult in the position of primary caregiver to a child and not restricted to biological parent.

(see also Lee et al, 2023; Muhammad & Tumin, 2022; Shin & Finnegan, 2009; Simon et al., 2007). Three of the studies were conducted in the United States.

Vision Screening in Primary Care Practice

In primary care practice, vision screening (including ocular risk assessments and visual acuity measurements) is provided as part of routine preventive screenings and assessments at well-child visits, starting from infancy and continuing through adolescence (Bright Futures & American Academy of Pediatrics, 2022; Donahue et al., 2016a). Well-child visits are preventive healthcare assessments recommended throughout childhood in pediatric primary care. These well-child visits are scheduled to require about 15–20 minutes on average and include a vision screening and assessments of a child's medical history.

Vision screenings as part of well-child visits are usually conducted by support staff, such as medical assistants, but the onus is on the primary care clinicians to refer the child to an eye care provider when needed, and to explain to the parent(s) the importance of taking the child for a comprehensive eye exam. If the primary practice provider has an autorefractor, the vision screening for myopia and other refractive errors can take less than a minute. If it involves acuity charts, it will take 5–15 minutes, depending on the age and cooperation of the child.

The Centers for Medicaid & Medicare Services (CMS) provides three different Current Procedural Terminology (CPT) codes for billing insurance for vision screening, specifically CPT 99173 (visual acuity test using optotypes or charts), 99174 (instrument-based screening with off-site analysis) and 99177 (instrument-based screening with on-site analysis).

Vision Screening as a Universal Program at School

One strategy for detecting all children with myopia (and other visual problems) is universal vision screening at school. Elementary schoolchildren are a "captive" population, which makes it possible to provide them with universal access to this first step in eye care. School-based programs at the very minimum usually include a visual acuity measurement and referral to a community eye care provider. Other models have included the use of on-site comprehensive eye exams by eye care professionals (optometrist or ophthalmologist).

Vision Screening Methodologies and Their Applicability

To detect myopia, vision screening programs can use distance visual acuity or photoscreeners (a type of instrument-based tool). The same tools can be used in primary care practices, community-based screening, and targeted screening programs. In the following sections, the methodology behind the successful use of each tool as part of vision screening is described along with its general applicability.

Using Distance Visual Acuity

A survey of screening in school-aged children in 18 countries on five continents found that all programs used some form of distance visual acuity test, and for 44% of countries this was the only test (Chen et al., 2019), perhaps because it is the cheapest. Similarly, distance visual acuity is the most common test in mandated vision screening in the United States (Wahl et al., 2021). There are variations in which symbols are used on the acuity chart, both across countries and across states. Consensus guidelines from the U.S. Committee on Vision and the International Council of Ophthalmology specify that the letters, numbers, or pictures must be of more-or-less equal legibility, with the same number of items on each line and the items spaced horizontally by the width of each symbol and vertically by the width of the symbols in the next line. The sizes should decrease by approximately 0.1 log units across lines and the symbols should be black on a white background (reviewed in Chaplin & Bradford, 2011). These requirements are fulfilled by Sloan letters, LEA numbers, Tumbling Es with crowding bars, HOTV with proportional spacing or crowding bars, Cambridge crowded acuity, and LEA symbols with proportional spacing.

Acuity must be tested monocularly (one eye at a time) with the child situated at a specified distance away from the symbols (typically 10 or 20 feet). This is because the myopic child might have different refractive errors in the two eyes and because the child may well be able to read the test items at a close distance but fail as they become fuzzy at further distances. There is a marked drop-off in distance acuity with increasing myopia, at least up to −2.0 D (Kleinstein et al., 2021). For younger children, the test is more effective at a closer distance, such as 5 feet, and can be turned into a matching game such that the child points to the letter/symbol on a chart they are holding that matches the one the experimenter is pointing to on the distant test chart (Kulp et al., 2022). For children ages 4–6 years, this can usually be done successfully with letter charts; for younger children, charts with icons for common objects can work better. The Tumbling E chart and Allen picture cards are other options, but they can lead to errors because young children confuse left and right (Tumbling E) or the test can overestimate acuity (Tumbling E and Allen picture cards; reviewed in Chaplin & Bradford, 2011). Children's distance visual acuity can be tested as young as 3 years of age if they are given a matching card instead of being asked to name the letters and if the testing distance is reduced to 5 feet (Kulp et al., 2022). However, many will be untestable (27% at age 3 vs. 8% at age 4 according to Hered & Wood, 2013) and 4- and 5-year-olds are easier to test. Moreover, overall sensitivity and specificity are higher at age 5 than at age 4 (Nishimura et al., 2020).

The test chart must be illuminated by good lighting, and distractions such as another child being tested nearby need to be avoided. Finishing monocular tests of both eyes typically takes less than 10 minutes for a 4- to 6-year-old child and less time for older children. The advantage of distance acuity testing is that the charts are inexpensive; the disadvantages are the need for a well-lighted space in the school, which can be scarce, and the duration of the test. To detect amblyopia, as opposed to myopia, the symbols/letters need to be "crowded," meaning surrounded by other symbols/letters or bars (Lalor et al., 2016). This is because many amblyopes can read single letters and have difficulty only when the letters are embedded in print among other letters.

In a sample of 6,017 Chinese children ages 4 to 15 years who were screened at school, a well-designed chart (Early Treatment Diabetic Retinopathy Study or ETDRS) and a cut-off of 6/7.5 for children ages 7 and older was accurate in detecting children with −0.5D of myopia or worse by cycloplegic retinoscopy (sensitivity 91.7% and 95.6% for children ages 7–12 years and 13–15 years, respectively; specificity, 80.3% and 85.4%, respectively). For younger children, that cutoff yielded a sensitivity of 86.5% and a specificity of 51.2%. Specificity improved with a cutoff of 6/9.5 to 84.7%, but then sensitivity dropped to 67.3%; 31.8% of the sample proved to be myopic (Wang et al., 2022).

Using Photoscreeners

Photoscreeners such as the Spot (Welch Allyn) and the Plusoptix devices are faster but more expensive than visual acuity charts. In September 2020, 17 U.S. states permitted the optional use of some type of instrument-based device for screening, especially if the child is young or unable to complete acuity screening (Wahl et al., 2021). Photoscreeners work by shining a point of infrared light into both eyes off the fixating axis and estimating the refractive error by how well focused is the red reflex that returns from the retina. For school screening, the devices are used without cycloplegia, leading to a possible underestimation of hyperopia (which a child can partially overcome by accommodation) or a slight overestimation of myopia (because the child is focusing hard on the fixation point). Nevertheless, the devices are quite accurate in detecting higher levels of myopia and measuring astigmatism.

Values obtained from the Spot and Plusoptix photoscreeners are highly correlated (Peterseim et al., 2014). Screening typically takes less than a minute and requires only that the child view a fixation attractor in the center of the device (Modest, 2017). The Spot will generally work in any lighting, and it was successful in screening 99.10% of 4,811 children ages 4–5 years in one study, while the PlusoptiX, which requires a darkened space in order to detect the pupil accurately, was successful with only 95.8% of the same children (Nishimura et al., 2019, 2020). In primary care settings, more children were screened successfully with a photoscreener (the Spot; 90%) than with the combination of distance visual acuity and a preschool test of 3D stereoscopic vision (54%), with the largest difference found among 3-year-olds (Modest, 2017). Similarly, the Spot (89.9% successful) and PlusoptiX (73.8% successful) were able to screen most of the 84 children who could not be assessed with the Lea symbols acuity test or the Stereo butterfly test in a preschool screening program for Michigan 3-to-5-year-olds (Musch et al., 2022). Children who are untestable should be referred, because they are more likely to have a vision problem than those who pass screening (Maguire & Vision in Preschool Study Group., 2007).

These screening tools have been used successfully with lay personnel given minimal training (Kulp et al., 2022). Besides screeners, help is needed to fetch and return children to the classroom and to manage the flow between screening stations. Referral values differ with the age of the child because the average eye changes with development from being hyperopic in early childhood to being emmetropic during primary school. The referral cutoff for myopia usually begins around −1.5 D to −3.0 D during the early period when most children are hyperopic and decreases to −0.5 D to −1.0 D when the child is older than 7 years (see, for example, Arnold et al, 2022; Donahue et al., 2016a; Grossman et al., 2017). An unanswered question is whether a child who is already emmetropizing before primary school should be referred for longitudinal screening or regular visits to an eye care professional because this may be a sign of emerging myopia (see Chapter 5). Enough is now known to be concerned about the child showing *any* myopia before age 7 and to recommend that they have regular follow-up with a comprehensive eye exam (see Box 5-2 in Chapter 5 on Onset and Progression).

Sensitivity and Specificity

The literature gives values for the sensitivity, specificity, and positive predictive value for screening for amblyopia and refractive errors using distance visual acuity, photoscreeners, or both, for children of different ages. The outcome depends on the referral cutoff: a strict cutoff increases sensitivity, resulting in fewer missed eye problems, but it also decreases specificity, allowing more false positives. Constant software updates make it difficult to compare studies precisely. A meta-analysis of 21 studies involving 5,022 children found no significant difference in sensitivity or specificity in detecting all types of refractive error between the Spot and Plusoptix, either in the entire population or in the 10 studies involving 3,221 children under age 7

(Zhang et al., 2019). The results were similar for studies conducted in the United States and in Asia.

Table 8-2 gives the sensitivity and specificity of the Spot and Plusoptix photoscreeners for detecting myopia with different cutoffs. Although there are several studies giving these values for hyperopia and astigmatism, or any type of refractive error, there are fewer for myopia, and those are mainly from China, perhaps because of higher prevalence or concern. A study of French children seen for follow-up in an eye clinic found a correlation of 0.91 between the refractive error value obtained by the Plusoptix and the value obtained by cycloplegic retinoscopy for the 14 myopic children, who were between 18 and 86 months old, with 90% of values within 1.0 D of each other (Payerols et al., 2016).

TABLE 8-2 Sensitivity and Specificity of Photoscreeners Against Cyclopleged Retinoscopy for the Detection of Myopia

Study; Photoscreener	Type of Sample	Age Range (mean years)	Country	Number of Children	Cut-off for Myopia (diopters) (worse than)	Sensitivity	Specificity
Qian et al., 2019; Spot	Eye hospital screening or check-up	4–6 (5.2)	China	113	−1.5 in any meridian	93.5%	90.3%
Mu et al., 2016; Spot	Eye hospital screening or check-up	4–7 (5.7)	China	168	−1.5 in any meridian	85.6%	79.65%
Yan et al. 2015: Plusoptix	Patients at eye hospital	2–14 (6.2)	China	178	−3.0 in any meridian	85.7%	94.7%

SOURCE: Committee generated.

Community-Based Screening

Another model is to offer vision screening in places where parents often take their children, like shopping malls, summer camps, or community events, where one captures great numbers of children at one time. The screening can be conducted in an empty store space, in an office, in a portable van, or at an after-school program. While the tools used are the same as in screening in schools, the coverage will not be universal. However, the presence of parent(s) means that the results and their importance can be conveyed immediately, and any questions answered. Community-based screening is often conducted by volunteer groups such as the Lions Club. Follow-up rates with eye care providers for individuals screened in these programs is often low unless effective follow-up strategies are used, such as the use of portable equipment to conduct on-the-spot follow-up comprehensive eye exams for those who fail screening (Asare et al., 2017; Donahue et al., 2006).

Targeted Screening

A general finding from universal school screening is that children from medically underserved neighborhoods are more likely to "fail" screening and be referred for a comprehensive eye exam. Children from medically underserved populations are often less likely to have a family doctor or attend well-child visits. The advantage of targeted screening is that resources are allocated where there is the greatest need and the total cost is less than offering screening in every school (Abdus & Selden, 2022; Asare al., 2022). The tools used are the same as for universal screening in schools.

For example, after photoscreening of 14,000 children in all grades (elementary through high school) in 58 schools in three Virginia school districts, the referral rate correlated with the percentage of economically disadvantaged students in each school (Kruszewski et al., 2023). Similarly, in vision screening of 71,000 4- to 5-year-old children in Queensland, Australia, using distance acuity and a photoscreener, more children from more disadvantaged areas were referred and more of them were also untestable (Harris et al., 2023). Likewise, a study of 4,365 children screened at ages 4–5 in Tayside, Scotland, with distance acuity and an orthoptist's assessment of binocularity, found that children living in the most disadvantaged area (worst 20%) were 1.4 times as likely to be referred for failed screening as those in the other areas combined; those who had been rated as at-risk near birth because of family instability were 3 times as likely to be referred as children from families labelled stable (O'Colmain et al, 2016).

Targeted screening can also be implemented as part of a community-based program run as an after-school program, like those offered by the Boys and Girls Clubs in the United States, as a student-run clinic, or at community health centers including federally qualified health centers (Register, 2010). An example of a vision screening community event is Philadelphia's one-day Give Kids Sight Day, held each year on a college campus. Approximately 1,200 children ages 19 and under receive free eye care (Dotan et al., 2015). The program targets uninsured or underinsured children. Free student-run clinics overseen by faculty eye care professionals include one in Indianapolis, which partners with Indiana University's School of Optometry to provide vision screening services and referrals to the local county hospital for care (Scheive et al., 2022). Another student-run clinic in Philadelphia provides comprehensive eye exams monthly within a long-term homeless shelter (Henstenburg et al., 2019).

Community health centers in the United States are federally funded facilities that serve the healthcare needs of medically underserved communities through an integrated care model in a team-based practice setting (Lam et al., 2019; McNamara & Polse, 2019). U.S. community health centers also enhance patient acceptance of care and the coordination of care for overall health. The cost of care in U.S. community health centers is based on a sliding fee scale or free, thus overcoming financial barriers faced by most families in medically underserved communities. Even though community health centers are an ideal place for providing vision care service to high-risk populations, only 32% of such centers in the United States provide vision care services (Woodward et al., 2024).

VISION CARE POLICIES IN THE UNITED STATES

The detection of myopia in children is heavily influenced by the U.S. insurance structure and state mandates for comprehensive eye exams or vision screenings. When insurance covers the assessment and/or treatment, some barriers are removed. When some form of vision assessment is mandated, even medically underserved children are likely to get some type of service.

The Affordable Care Act of 2010 requires that all individual, small group, or state-based health insurance plans cover well-child visits and vision care services for children which is one of 10 Essential Health Benefits (Centers for Medicare & Medicaid Services, n.d.b; National Academies of Sciences, Engineering, and Medicine, 2012; Prevent Blindness, 2020). However, the *type* of coverage mandated for pediatric vision care is decided by each state. Forty-two states cover annual comprehensive eye exams and one pair of prescription glasses per year (Centers for Medicare & Medicaid Services, n.d.b; Prevent Blindness, 2020). Children with Medicaid are entitled to coverage for comprehensive health screenings, including well-child checkups, as part of the federally required Early and Periodic Screening, Diagnostic and Treatment (EPSDT) benefit (Centers for Medicare & Medicaid Services). In some states, Medicaid also covers comprehensive eye exams and a pair of prescription glasses per year (National Academies, 2016).

Guidelines and Mandates

A few states in the United States require that children have a comprehensive eye exam before entering school, but adherence with this mandate is not universal. For example, Illinois, Kentucky, and Nebraska require that proof of an eye exam be submitted in the first year in which the child is enrolled, although the details of the requirement differ as to how quickly that proof is due and whether it must be conducted by an optometrist or ophthalmologist (Kentucky), other types of physicians (Illinois and Nebraska), or clinic staff (physician's assistants or advanced practice nurses in Nebraska; Kentucky Department of Education, 2024; State of Illinois, 2024; U.S. Preventative Services Task Force et al., 2022). A 2022-2023 report published by the State of Illinois showed that only 62% (68,349/110,054) of children were reported by schools to have adhered to the mandate (Illinois State Board of Education, 2024). Most states require vision screening instead of a comprehensive eye exam.

A survey of data from September to October 2020 found that 24 states mandated vision screening at school, 9 states mandated that the child must undergo vision screening in the community and produce proof of screening for the school system or other authorities, and 8 states required both, with the details depending on the grade level. Four states (Missouri, Montana, New Hampshire, and South Carolina) only recommended vision screening but did not mandate it. Six states (Alabama, Idaho, North Dakota, South Dakota, Wisconsin, and Wyoming) had no vision screening requirements or recommendations (Wahl et al., 2021). However, at least one state (Alabama) has line-item state funding without a state mandate (State of Alabama, 2024). All states with a vision screening mandate required that the screening be done before or during kindergarten. Some required additional screening in middle school (59%) and/or high school (37%). (See Figure 8-1; Prevent Blindness, 2023.)

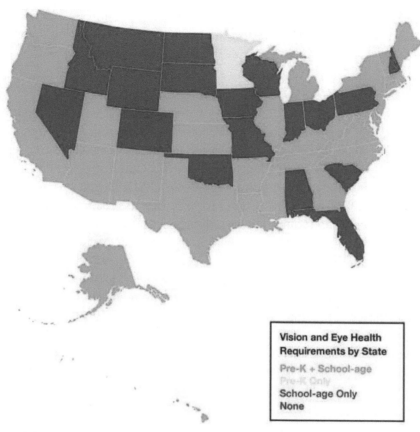

FIGURE 8-1 Vision assessment requirements by state for children.
NOTE: The figure shows whether any kind of assessment is mandated by each state (e.g., screening and referral when indicated or comprehensive eye exam). The colors indicate the school ages at which the screening is required.
SOURCE: Prevent Blindness, 2022.

However, funding to conduct screenings is just as important as legislated requirements. A mandate without funding may not be effective, whereas state funding can be effective even without a mandate. For example, Sight Savers America offers screening in 15 states, including Alabama (which has no legislated requirements) and South Carolina (where vision screening is only recommended). In some states, like Alabama, the program includes not only vision screening with the Plusoptix photoscreener but also follow-up care involving a case manager for every child referred for a comprehensive eye exam (Sight Savers America, 2020); over 75% of children who are referred see an eye care professional and receive any prescribed treatment (Sight Savers America, 2020). Of public-school children in Alabama, 60.2% are eligible for free and reduced lunch, which is higher than the national average of 53.3% in 2022–2023 (National Center for Education Statistics, n.d.).

Some consensus exists among vision screening guidelines on the importance of screening and criteria for the identification of vision disorders. Vision screening for children as a preventive strategy for detecting refractive errors, amblyopia, and risk factors for amblyopia is recommended by the World Health Organization (2007); the American Academy of Ophthalmology (American Academy of Ophthalmology Pediatric Ophthalmology/Strabismus Panel, 2018); the American Academy of Pediatrics (AAP), the American Association for

Pediatric Ophthalmology and Strabismus, and the U.S. Preventive Services Task Force (2017). Recommended assessments include a red reflex test, external inspection of the ocular structures, pupil examination, corneal light reflex, cover test, instrument-based screening to detect refractive errors and, where possible, visual acuity (Table 8-3; Donahue & Nixon, 2016).

Age and Recommended Tools

The American Academy of Pediatrics provides the *Bright Futures Recommendations for Preventive Pediatric Health Care,* which includes recommendations for the assessments that should be done at different ages. They include recommendations for visual acuity screening at various ages (see Table 8-3; American Academy of Pediatrics Committee on Practice and Ambulatory Medicine and Section on Ophthalmology et al., 2003; Bright Futures & American Academy of Pediatrics, 2022). Visual acuity charts for children are recommended as soon as children are capable of cooperating (which is typically age 3 to 4 years). Instrument-based screening is recommended for children 12 months to 3 years to detect risk factors that may lead to vision impairment from amblyopia (amblyopia risk factors; Donahue et al., 2016a). This starting age for visual acuity screening results from the combined facts that younger children cannot be tested reliably with acuity charts and that amblyopia treatment is more effective before about age 8. Instrument-based screening is recommended as an alternative to visual acuity assessments for children ages 3 to 5 years who are unable or unwilling to complete visual acuity screening or who have developmental delays or neurodevelopmental disorders, such as attention deficit hyperactivity disorder (ADHD) or autism spectrum disorder (ASD; Donahue et al., 2016a). Referrals to eye care providers for comprehensive eye examination are recommended if any component of the vision screening is abnormal (Donahue et al., 2016a; Donahue & Nixon, 2016). The American Academy of Pediatric Ophthalmology and Strabismus provides referral criteria for instrument-based screening to detect amblyopia risk factors including myopia (Table 8-4; Donahue & Nixon, 2016). Other organizations such as the American Academy of Pediatrics provide referral cutoffs for visual acuity screening with letter or symbol charts (Donahue et al., 2016a).

TABLE 8-3 Periodicity Schedule for Vision Assessment in Infants, Children, and Young Adults

Assessment	Newborn–6 mo	6–12 mo	1–3 y	4–5 y	6 y and older
Ocular history	x	x	x	x	x
External inspection of lids and eyes	x	x	x	x	x
Red reflex testing	x	x	x	x	x
Pupil examination	x	x	x	x	x
Ocular motility assessment	—	x	x	x	x
Instrument-based screening[a] when available	—	[b]	x	x	[c]
Visual acuity fixate and follow response	x[f]	x	x	—	—
Visual acuity age-appropriate optotype[d] assessment	—	—	x[e]	x	x

[a]Current Procedural Terminology code 99174.

[b]The American Academy of Ophthalmology (AAO) has recommended instrument-based screening at age 6 mo. However, the rate of false-positive results is high for this age group, and the likelihood of ophthalmic intervention is low. A future AAO policy statement will likely reconcile what appears to be a discrepancy.

[c]Instrument-based screening at any age is suggested if unable to test visual acuity monocularly with age-appropriate optotypes.

[d]Current Procedural Terminology code 99173.

[e]Visual acuity screening may be attempted in cooperative 3-y-old children.

[f]Development of fixating on and following a target should occur by 6 months of age; children who do not meet this milestone should be referred.

SOURCE: Committee on Practice and Ambulatory Medicine et al., 2016. Reproduced with permission from *Pediatrics, 137*, 28–30, © 2016 by the American Academy of Pediatrics.

TABLE 8-4 Refractive Error Cutoffs for Amblyopia Risk Factor Targets Recommended by the American Association for Pediatric Ophthalmology and Strabismus

Refractive Risk Factor Targets[a]				
Age, months	**Astigmatism**	**Hyperopia**	**Anisometropia**	**Myopia**
12–30	>2.0 D	>4.5 D	>2.5 D	>−3.5 D
31–48	>2.0 D	>4.5 D	>2.0 D	>−3.0 D
>48	>1.5 D	>3.0 D	>1.5 D	>−1.5 D

Nonrefractive Amblyopia Risk Factor Targets[b]	
All ages	Manifest strabismus >8 prism D in primary position
	Media opacity >1 mm

NOTE: D = diopters, PD = prism diopters.

[a]Additional reporting of sensitivity to detect greater-magnitude refractive errors is encouraged.

[b]For all ages.

SOURCE: Donahue et al., 2013.

BARRIERS TO ACCESSING VISION HEALTH SERVICES IN CHILDREN

In summarizing barriers to vision care, a modified version of Andersen's Behavioural Model of Health Services Use was utilized to conceptualize the factors that influence access to vision health services for children (Aday & Andersen, 1974, 1981; Andersen, 1968, 1995; Andersen & Davidson, 2007). The model emphasizes the importance of both contextual and individual factors that influence access (see Box 8-2). Andersen's Behavioural Model of Health Services Use was chosen because it is one of the most widely accepted frameworks for understanding the factors informing access to health care (Aday & Andersen, 1974, 1981; Andersen, 1968, 1995; Andersen & Davidson, 2007). Applying the framework to vision care, an example would be a child with myopia who is screened in school but whose myopia is not detected because of a screening tool with low sensitivity (contextual characteristic). Treatment for their myopia will be delayed (health behavior) which could in turn lead to a mistrust of (predisposing characteristics) and lack of patient/family satisfaction (outcomes) with vision screening programs. Another example is a child with low socioeconomic status (predisposing characteristics) whose family is unable to afford health insurance (enabling resources) and therefore the parents will be less likely to afford or to believe that a comprehensive eye exam (health behavior) is a good value for the money they have to spend; as a result, that child may go without a comprehensive eye exam (health behavior).

BOX 8-2
A Conceptual Framework for Understanding the Barriers to Accessing Vision Care Services for Children

A modified version of the Behavioral Model of Health Services Use was used to conceptualize the factors that influence access to vision health services (vision screening, or comprehensive eye exams) for children (Aday & Andersen, 1968, 1974, 1981; Andersen, 1995; Andersen & Davidson, 2007). The model emphasizes the importance of both contextual and individual factors that influence access (Figure 8-2).

Contextual characteristics are macro- and meso-level factors beyond the child (micro-level) that influence the child's ability to access vision health services. That is, contextual characteristics are factors in the health system and external environment. Examples include health plans, family units, national healthcare systems, and provider-related and neighborhood factors (Andersen & Davidson, 2007). Children impacted by these factors are either members or residents of these units.

Individual-level characteristics influencing access to vision health services may be predisposing characteristics, enabling resources, and need.

- *Predisposing characteristics* are pre-existing conditions that indirectly influence a child's ability to access vision health services. These include a child's family social structure, health beliefs, and demographic factors.
- *Enabling resources* support or hinder a child's access to vision health services. The social determinants of health consist of both predisposing and enabling factors.
- *Need* represents the conditions that a child, caregiver (perceived need), or a child's health provider (based on professional judgement and objective measurements, 'evaluated need') has identified as needing medical attention and thus resulting in accessing vision health services. Perceived need is determined largely by a child's (or their caregiver's) own perceptions of the importance and magnitude of their vision and eye health. Evaluated need on the other hand, informs the type and amount of treatment given to a child after they consult with a vision care provider (Andersen, 1995; Andersen & Davidson, 2007).

Health behavior includes the actual process of accessing or utilizing vision health services that may influence a child's vision health outcomes. These vision health outcomes are a function of a child's *perceived* and *evaluated health status* and how they feel (satisfaction) about vision health services received. These outcomes influence whether they access vision health services in the future. For example, a caregiver who believes their child has poor vision based on the result of an eye examination by an eye care provider or a vision screening test will feel the need for and likely take action on follow-up appointments for treatment.

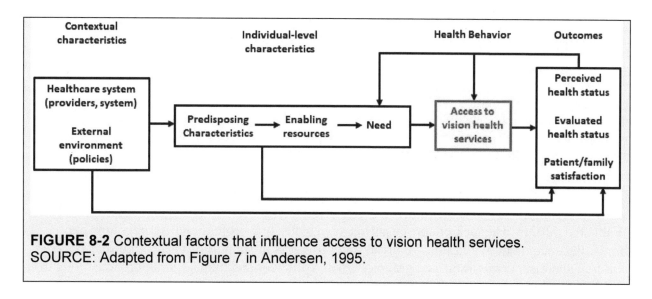

FIGURE 8-2 Contextual factors that influence access to vision health services.
SOURCE: Adapted from Figure 7 in Andersen, 1995.

CONTEXTUAL BARRIERS TO ACCESSING VISION HEALTH SERVICES IN CHILDREN

Contextual Barriers to Vision Screening

Contextual barriers to receiving vision screening include a lack of consensus on the importance and process of vision screening, lack of funding to conduct vision screening, concerns about the accuracy of vision screening tests, instrument malfunction, and limited statewide surveillance of preventive services under the Early and Periodic Screening, Diagnostic and Treatment (EPSDT) Medicaid benefit (Ambrosino et al., 2023; American Optometric Association, 2017; Brener et al., 2007; Donahue & Baker, 2015; Donahue & Nixon, 2016; Donahue et al., 2011, 2016a; Grossman et al., 2017; Levinson, 2010; Lillvis et al., 2020; U.S. Preventative Services Task Force et al., 2017; Wahl et al., 2021).

Lack of Consensus on Importance and Process of Vision Screening

Lack of consensus on the importance and process of vision screening (i.e., types of assessments performed, target age groups, and referral criteria) between states and professional organizations may hinder access to vision screening for children.

Some consensus among professional associations and expert groups has been reached on the importance of routine vision screening of children at risk of myopia progression and other vision disorders (American Academy of Pediatrics, 2003; U.S. Preventative Services Task Force, 2017). This is evidenced by a joint policy statement (published in 2003 and renewed in 2016) supporting early vision screening for children 3 to 5 years and endorsed by the American Academy of Pediatrics (AAP), The American Association for Pediatric Ophthalmology and Strabismus (AAPOS), the American Academy of Ophthalmology (AAOphth), and the American Association of Certified Orthoptists (AACO; Donahue, 2016; Donahue et al., 2016a). The United States Preventive Services Taskforce (USPSTF) also supports the need for vision screening for children aged 3 to 5 years (Donahue et al., 2011; Grossman et al., 2017; Jonas et al., 2017; see Table 8-5). The American Academy of Optometry (AAOpt) endorses the need for both vision screenings and comprehensive eye exams to ensure the early detection and treatment of vision disorders in childhood (Ciner et al., 2016; Kulp et al., 2016).

There is a lack of consensus among professional groups on the criteria used for referral to eye care professionals, as well as the extent to which such referral is facilitated. AAPOS provides referral thresholds designed for identifying amblyopia risk factors, not myopia. Using the AAPOS thresholds for referral may miss myopia because a child with *any* myopic refraction before age 6–7 years needs regular follow-up for myopia that is likely increasing with age (Donahue & Nixon, 2016; Grossman et al., 2017).

Vision screening requirements also vary by state (see Figure 8-1) and do not align with professional guidelines (Ambrosino et al., 2023; Wahl et al., 2021). Children might not receive vision screening if they live in a state without vision screening requirements (Lillvis et al., 2020; Wahl et al., 2021). The lack of consensus between states and professional associations may hinder the enactment of additional policies and programs in support of vision care services for children and discourage interested groups such as volunteer and humanitarian organizations from providing vision screening services.

Photoscreening, as described earlier, has been validated as a tool that provides high sensitivity to detect vision disorders in children with ASD (McCurry et al., 2013; Miller et al., 2012; Singman et al., 2013). It is an ideal tool to screen children with ASD and other special healthcare needs because of its unintimidating, largely automated technique, which requires minimal cooperation of the child. Despite this evidence, current vision screening guidelines from the AAP and other professional pediatric and eye care associations do not provide guidance on vision screening for children with ASD (Donahue & Nixon, 2016). Policies to encourage the routine use of photoscreening tools for children at high risk of developing vision disorders are critical to reduce disparities in the provision of vision screening for children. These policies should also address the meager reimbursements by insurance payers in primary care practice for instrument-based vision screening.

TABLE 8-5 A Comparison of Vision Screening Recommendations by Professional Societies in the United States

Professional Organization	Vision Disorder	Target Age	Screening Interval	Setting / Personnel
American Academy of Family Physicians (AAFP) Note: AAFP endorses the screening recommendations of the U.S. Preventive Services Task Force; see American Academy of Family Physicians (n.d.)	Amblyopia, strabismus, anisometropia, astigmatism, hyperopia, myopia	6 mo–5 y	Not specified	Primary care clinic/ family physician, medical assistants or other technicians
Joint policy statement by American Academy of Pediatrics, American Academy of Ophthalmology, American Association for Pediatric Ophthalmology and Strabismus, & American Association of Certified Orthoptists (Donahue et al., 2016)	Eye tracking disorders, ocular media opacities, strabismus, pupils, refractive error	Newborn–6 y	Newborn–6 mo, 6–12 mo, 1–3 y, 4–5 y, 6 y and older	Primary care clinic/ pediatrician, medical assistant or other technicians
American Association for Pediatric Ophthalmology and Strabismus (American Association for Pediatric Ophthalmology and Strabismus, n.d.; Arnold et al., 2022)	Eye tracking disorders, retinoblastoma, strabismus, chronic tearing, refractive error	Newborn–5 y	Newborn–12 mo, 12–36 mo, 36 mo–5 y, and repeat screening every 1–2 y after age 5	During eye exam
American Academy of Ophthalmology (Hutchison et al., 2023)	Refractive error (myopia, hyperopia, astigmatism), amblyopia, strabismus, cerebral visual impairment including traumatic brain injury, cataract, retinitis of prematurity, congenital glaucoma, retinoblastoma, pediatric	Newborn–18 y	Newborn–6 mo; 6–12 mo; 1–3 y; 3–4 y; 4–5 y; every 1–2 y after age 5	Primary care clinic or community setting/ physicians, nurses, other health care providers, and lay individuals specifically trained to perform vision screening

uveitis, vision, ocular alignment, and the presence of ocular structural abnormalities

Organization	Conditions Screened	Ages	Frequency	Setting
Joint Policy Statement by the American Academy of Ophthalmology & American Association for Pediatric Ophthalmology and Strabismus (Simon et al., 2016)	amblyopia, strabismus, refractive errors, high-priority on myopia	3–5 y	Not Specified	Community and school screening programs; primary care clinic
American Academy of Optometry (American Academy of Optometry, 2016)	Significant refractive error, amblyopia, strabismus, and observable external ocular disease, color vision deficits	Newborn to < 3 y; preschool; school age	Not Specified	Not specified
National Center for Children's Vision and Eye Health & National Association of School Nurses (Cotter et al., 2015; National Center for Children's Vision and Eye Health, 2016)	visual impairment—acuity, alignment	Newborn; preschool and up	Neonatal; every month before 6 mo, every 3 mo before 3 y, and every year thereafter	Primary care clinic (well-child visits)
United States Preventive Services Task Force (Donahue et al., 2011; Jonas et al., 2017; United States Preventive Services Task Force et al., 2017)	Strabismus, refractive errors, and ocular media opacity; risk factors for vision disorders such as family history in a first-degree relative, prematurity, low birth weight, maternal substance abuse, maternal smoking during pregnancy, and low	3–5 y	At least once between ages 3–5 y	Primary care setting/pediatrician, family physician, medical assistants and other technicians

	levels of parental education		
World Health Organization (World Health Organization, 2024)	**Newborn:** infections, congenital and/or acquired conditions; **Preschool age:** reduced visual acuity, amblyopia, strabismus; infection/inflammation; **School-age:** same as preschool except comprehensive eye exam included	All ages	Newborn once; early childhood (3–5 y old) once, later childhood (5–18 y old) every 1–2 y, middle to late adulthood (> 60 y old)	Primary care clinic or school program

SOURCE: Adapted from Harewood et al., 2024.

Lack of Funding to Conduct Vision Screenings

Most states mandate some kind of vision screening, but that mandate is ineffective if funds are not allocated to conduct the screening or to allow effective follow-up with a comprehensive eye exam when warranted. Community-based vision care programs require significant resources, which often negatively impacts their sustainability. Also, instrument-based tools may cost a couple thousand dollars up-front to purchase and bring ongoing maintenance costs, which may make them cost-prohibitive to some programs. In addition, resources need to be sufficient so each child can receive vision screening on a regular basis (Harewood et al., 2024).

Concerns About Accuracy of Screening Methods and Equipment Malfunction

Newer instrument-based vision screening tools developed over the past decade have higher sensitivity and thus lower rates of false negative screening tests. Because of concern about false positive and false negative results, vision screening providers might not refer a child who has vision impairment ('under referral') or might refer children that do not have vision impairment ('over-referral').

Another concern is that vision screening programs that rely on instrument-based tools may experience interruptions if the tool malfunctions, which can often occur with instrument-based tools. When this happens, not all the children scheduled to be screened that day or in the near future may receive the service. This problem can be overcome by having back-up instruments, although their cost may prohibit the extra purchase.

Limited Statewide Surveillance of Preventive Healthcare Services

Statewide surveillance of preventive healthcare services, especially under Medicaid's EPSDT program, is important to ensure that low-income children get evidence-based services such as vision screening (Centers for Medicare & Medicaid Services, n.d.a). The EPSDT program requires that vision screening be provided at "reasonable" intervals decided by the States. However, a 2010 examination of nine states (Arkansas, Florida, Idaho, Illinois, Missouri, North Carolina, Texas, Vermont, and West Virginia) by the Office of Inspector General, Department of Health and Human Services, revealed that 60% of children had not received any vision screening (Levinson, 2010; Prevent Blindness, 2020). The nine states indicated they did not monitor the utilization of specific preventive care services (Levinson, 2010). Beginning in 2024, The Center for Medicaid Services will require all states to report annually on the Core Set of Children's Health Care Quality Measures (Department of Health and Human Services, 2023). However, vision screening and well-child visits in the third, fourth, fifth, and sixth year of life are not included in the core set, even though well-child visits in the first 30 months of life and oral evaluation (dental services) are included (Centers for Medicare & Medicaid Services, 2024; Department of Health and Human Services, 2023).

Contextual Barriers to Vision Screening in Pediatric Primary Care

Contextual barriers to accessing vision screening for children in well-child visits in pediatric primary care include limited physician knowledge of and attitudes about vision screening, perceptions of insufficient time in the clinic workflow, inadequate reimbursement for vision screening, limited number of appointments for well-child visits, and long travel distance to nearest primary care provider (Guagliardo, 2004; Hered & Wood, 2013; Kemper & Clark, 2006; Marsh-Tootle et al., 2012). Each barrier is discussed in turn, next.

Limited Physician Knowledge

Pediatrician survey responses across three states (Alabama, South Carolina, and Illinois) showed that poorer knowledge and attitudes about preschool vision screening among pediatricians was associated with less likelihood of conducting good pediatric vision screening (Marsh-Tootle et al., 2010). The screener or provider's lack of self-efficacy with and confidence in vision screening may result in non-referral to an eye care specialist for treatment after an abnormal vision screening test (Anzeljc et al., 2019; Kimel, 2006; Wall et al., 2002). Primary care physicians receive minimal training in the identification and management of myopia and other vision impairment (Hartmann et al., 2006). Limited knowledge in ophthalmology topics may result in over-referral or under-referral of children after vision screening tests.

Perception of Insufficient Visit Time

A potential factor that impedes access to vision screening in pediatric primary care includes provider perceptions of insufficient time to complete recommended assessments in a well-child visit (Hered & Wood, 2013; Kemper & Clark, 2006; Marsh-Tootle et al., 2012). In a single well-child visit, all recommended assessments (per Bright Futures Schedule) are expected to be completed (Bright Futures & American Academy of Pediatrics, 2022; Donahue & Nixon, 2016; Donahue et al., 2016a). When pressed for time, providers may decide to exclude tests (such as vision screening) with meager reimbursement that they perceive to be less of a priority based on a child's medical history or their initial assessments of the child. This is most likely to occur in community or private clinics that run on a fee-for-service model in which the practitioner's reimbursement for the screening service is tied to how many children they see (Fairbrother et al., 2001).

Inadequate Reimbursement

Related to a perceived lack of time for vision screening in well-child visits, inadequate practitioner reimbursement of services rendered is a significant deterrent for pediatric primary care providers to conduct vision screening (Hered & Wood, 2013; Kemper & Clark, 2006). This is especially problematic considering the high up-front and maintenance costs of instrument-based screening tools, which may be in themselves prohibitive especially for small pediatric primary care practices (Miller et al., 2012). Reimbursement amounts range between an average of $4 for acuity (chart-based) screening and a median of $24 for instrument-based screening depending on insurance type (Oke et al., 2023). The amount reimbursed varies by state. For comparison, reimbursement for applying fluoride varnish in well-child visits (CPT 99188, which is also a comparatively quick process but with no high-cost equipment) is reimbursed at $14 for Medicaid and up to as much as $35 in commercial plans as of 2019 (Kim et al., 2020). Commercial plans have higher rates of reimbursement for vision screening (CPT code 99177) in the Northeast, West, and parts of the South than the Midwest (Hillrom, 2020). With the increased use of instrument-based screening for young children, the rate of reimbursement for this form of screening has steadily declined since 2013 (Oke et al., 2023). The decision to reimburse may depend on the child's age and whether or not reimbursement is bundled in the global code for well-child visits. Preventive care services such as vision screening provided under Medicaid's

EPSDT program are reimbursed at a global rate, and no additional reimbursement is allowed when vision screening is included.

Longer Distance to Providers

Longer distances to health care providers are a recognized barrier to healthcare access in the United States (Guagliardo, 2004). An estimated 1 million children live in areas without access to primary care physicians (Shipman et al., 2011). The number of primary care physicians per 10,000 residents varies across U.S. regions (Guagliardo, 2004). The Northeast, West Coast, Hawaii, Mountain West, and Upper Midwest report higher numbers of primary care physicians per 10,000 residents, as compared with the Great Plains, Lower Mississippi Delta, and Southeast (Guagliardo, 2004). Further variation in the availability of primary care physicians exists between rural and urban regions, with a lower prevalence of primary care physicians in rural areas (Guagliardo, 2004). There is also an uneven distribution of pediatric primary care professionals across the United States, especially as it relates to urban vs rural communities, which leads to significant disparities in access to primary care for children (Drescher & Domingue, 2023; Shipman et al., 2011). Children living in areas with fewer pediatric primary care physicians are six times less likely to have access to primary care than children living in areas with higher numbers of pediatric primary care physicians (Shipman et al., 2011).

Contextual Barriers to Vision Screening in Schools and Communities

Contextual barriers to accessing vision screening in schools or other community settings include variability in state requirements for vision screening in school; limitations due to space, school schedules and calendars; problematic consent processes for children to participate in vision screening; poor communication about the program; and parent socioeconomic barriers (Kimel, 2006; Vongsachang et al., 2020; Wahl et al., 2021). Each of these barriers is discussed in turn in this section.

Variability in State Requirements

There is variability among state requirements with regard to school vision screening. Some children may not get vision screening because they live in states where it is not a requirement or a funding priority (Kindle & Spencer, 2019; State of Alabama, 2024). Even among states that have mandates for vision screening in schools, access is not uniform because private schools are not obligated to adhere to state-mandated vision screening policies (Berntsen & Walline, 2023; Davidson et al., 2016; Nowroozzadeh, 2016; Wolffsohn et al., 2019; Zadnik et al., 2015).

Limited Space or Scheduling Time

Vision screening sessions organized in schools or other community settings are often limited by the availability of space for screening, school schedules, and calendars (Vongsachang et al., 2020). Vision screenings can only be performed when school is in session, on specific days, and during specific hours dictated by school administration. Also, vision screening may require rooms that are large enough to measure distance visual acuity, and in the case of instrument-based tests sufficiently dark rooms with no distractions. There may not be a space available that meets these requirements. Children may also miss out on screening if they are absent from school on a scheduled day and the screeners do not return to pick up previously absent children. In one Canadian program conducted in a variety of communities (rural and urban; high-needs and non-high needs), on average 6.9% of eligible children missed screening because they were absent from school (range across 43 schools, 1.5–14.3%; Nishimura et al., 2020).

Complex Parent/Guardian Consent Process

The consent process in school-based screening programs may hinder access to vision screening for school children (Vongsachang et al., 2020). Consent forms are usually sent home with children for parents to grant permission for their child to participate in vision screening and other preventive care activities. Children may forget to pass on consent forms or lose them before they get home. Parents are often required to read, sort and complete several consent and information slips at a time. Therefore, they may lose or forget to complete consent forms. School-based screening programs are typically free with no out-of-pocket or insurance requirements (Vongsachang et al., 2020). Parents may not be aware of this and therefore not provide consent if they believe their children are not eligible for free service (Vongsachang et al., 2020). Parents with socioeconomic barriers may particularly struggle to keep up with consent forms and other permission slips for school-based screening.

Contextual Barriers to Comprehensive Eye Exams and Treatment

Barriers to comprehensive eye exams and treatment include poor provider-patient communication of results of a vision test, low reimbursement rates for rendering eye care, low supply of eye care specialists willing to see children, lack of affordable prescription glasses and poor compliance with wear (Anzeljc et al., 2019; Feng et al., 2020; Hartmann et al., 2006; Kemper et al., 2003; Kimel, 2006; Killeen et al., 2021; Kodjebacheva et al., 2015; Lee et al., 2012, 2023; Saydah et al., 2020; Varadaraj et al., 2019; Vongsachang et al., 2020; Wall et al., 2002; Williams et al., 2013).

Poor Communication with Parents

Poorly communicating the results of a vision screening test or comprehensive eye exam may prevent access to treatment (Kimel, 2006; Williams et al., 2013). Children may not get follow-up comprehensive eye exams because their parents did not understand or know their children had an abnormal vision screening test requiring a comprehensive eye exam (Kimel, 2006; Williams et al., 2013), which in turn may be the result of a lost 'pink slip' (referral slip) in a school screening (Vongsachang et al., 2020). In well-child visits, where pediatric primary care providers have direct access to parents or caregivers, providers may not have clearly communicated the importance of follow-up care to parents, or parents may not have understood the importance due to language barriers or lack of language concordance with providers (Williams et al., 2013).

For instance, in a study by Frazier et al. (2009), Hispanic immigrant parents reported that they had not sought eye care for their children because of a lack of information about the importance of eye care for children along with language barriers. Interviews in the Midwest with parents whose children attended high-needs schools in kindergarten through Grade 5 revealed financial concerns (31%), including an apparent concern that Medicaid exams and glasses were substandard, and logistical barriers (difficulty scheduling, 22%) as reasons for not receiving an eye exam after failing vision screening; other reasons included appointments being too far in the future [16%]; Kimel, 2006; see Wang et al., 2023 for similar Canadian data). After initial diagnosis and starting treatment, breakdown in communication may also occur between eye care providers and parents whose children need regular follow-ups with eye care professionals.

Low Reimbursement Rates

Reimbursement rates for vision care services are a barrier to accessing treatment from eye care professionals, who are less likely to see patients with Medicaid insurance than those with private insurance (Biviji et al., 2024; Lee et al., 2018). This may be because of the lower reimbursement associated with Medicaid insurance compared to private insurance (Blanchard et al., 2008). Households with lower incomes may be unable to afford higher-premium commercial health insurance plans, such as preferred provider organization (PPO) plans which give more flexibility to see eye care specialists even outside of their network.

Low Access to Eye Care Professionals

Access to eye care professionals is also limited by low availability, especially in rural and low-income communities, despite an increasing demand for eye care providers (optometrists and ophthalmologists) in the United States (Berkowitz et al., 2024; Feng et al., 2020; Kodjebacheva et al., 2015; Lee et al., 2007, 2023; Siegler et al., 2024). Data from the National Center for Health Workforce Analysis (NCHWA) indicates that across 38 medical and surgical specialties, ophthalmology is projected to have the second worst rate of workforce adequacy (projected supply over projected demand), a rate of 70%, by the year 2035 (Berkowitz et al. 2024). From 2020 to 2035, a 12% decline in supply of ophthalmologists and a 24% increase in demand are expected, indicating a workforce adequacy of just 30% overall, including a 77% vs. 29% workforce adequacy in metro versus nonmetro geographies, respectively (Berkowitz et al. 2024). Importantly, despite identifying nearly 600 pediatric optometrists and just over 1,000 pediatric ophthalmologists in the United States, 96.4% of U.S. counties had neither a pediatric optometrist nor a pediatric ophthalmologist (Siegler et al., 2024). Additionally, counties with neither type of pediatric eye care specialist had the lowest mean household incomes (Siegler et al., 2024).

The density of pediatric ophthalmologists in the United States has decreased significantly since the early to mid-2000s, with little possibility of improvement given the fact that fewer residents are pursuing pediatric ophthalmology fellowships (Lee et al., 2023; Simon et al., 2007). The lower number of pediatric ophthalmologists results in less access to specialist eye care, longer wait times, and longer travel times, especially for children living in rural parts of the United States (Kodjebacheva et al., 2015; Simon et al., 2007). States with the lowest number of pediatric ophthalmologists include North and South Dakota, Delaware, Idaho, and Wyoming (Lee et al., 2023). Increases in the density of optometrists from 1990 to 2017 have resulted in adequacy (100%) of optometrists, but an 89% workforce inadequacy is expected by 2035 under the reduced barriers demand scenario (Berkowitz et al., 2024; Feng et al., 2020).

Similar inadequacies of 60% are expected in the optician workforce by 2035 (Berkowitz et al., 2024). The Health Workforce Simulation Model from the National Center for Health Workforce Analysis describes the demand for physicians under 2 scenarios which include the reduced barriers scenario. The reduced barriers scenario estimates the number of physician full-time equivalents (FTEs) required if populations who historically faced barriers to accessing health care services demonstrated care use patterns comparable to populations perceived to have fewer barriers to accessing care. Therefore, this scenario describes the implications for physician demand if policies and programs are implemented to reduce access-based disparities to healthcare services (Berkowitz et al., 2024).

This maldistribution of eye care professionals in the United States, especially for rural communities, leads to significant disparities in access to primary and specialist eye care for children (Drescher & Domingue, 2023; Shipman et al., 2011). Less access to specialist care leads to poor vision health outcomes, especially for children with asymptomatic conditions such as myopia and amblyopia, which require early identification and treatment to slow myopia progression and prevent irreversible vision loss, respectively (Lee et al., 2023). An area where the supply of eye care providers is particularly low is in community health centers (Shin & Finnegan, 2009). In a policy brief by Shin and Finnegan published in 2009, seven out of 10 community health centers were reported to not have on-site eye care professionals to provide comprehensive eye exams because of an inability to afford the required space and equipment and/or difficulties creating business plans, designing an appropriate space for eye examinations, and creating an inventory of necessary equipment for eye examinations (Shin & Finnegan, 2009).

High Cost of Prescription Glasses and Compliance with Wear

The cost of prescription glasses is a barrier to treatment for myopia, especially for children with low socioeconomic status (Kemper et al., 2003; Killen et al., 2021; Kodjebacheva et al., 2015; Saydah et al., 2020; Varadaraj et al., 2019). When that barrier is eliminated and its removal is communicated clearly to parents, more children receive treatment. For example, a summer program for children in inner-city Philadelphia that comprised vision screening, immediate follow-up, and two pairs of free glasses if needed found that most parents (64%) came because the program included free glasses (Dotan et al., 2015). (Most [77%] of the children receiving the glasses were myopic.) Concern about the affordability of glasses can also lead parents to not book the referral appointment.

Children who are provided free glasses to correct their myopia, when compared to children for whom the glasses must be purchased by the parents, are more likely to be found wearing glasses and have increased academic performance even with imperfect compliance with glasses wear (Ethan et al., 2010; Ma et al., 2014). A systematic review of randomized controlled trials, mostly conducted in China, provides evidence from 11 studies that children are 2.45 times more likely (odds ratio of 2.45) to be wearing prescribed glasses at an unexpected follow-up visit if they are provided at no charge than if the parents only received a letter with the prescription (Wu et al., 2023). The effect was smaller with longer follow-up time (odds ratio of 2.30 after 6–12 months vs. 3.18 with earlier follow-up). Compliance was higher when the refractive error was higher or visual acuity was poorer. Nevertheless, in some of the RCTs, less than half the children who received free glasses were wearing them at follow-up.

INDIVIDUAL-LEVEL BARRIERS

Predisposing Characteristics Hindering Access to Vision Screening, Comprehensive Eye Exams, and Treatment for Children

Predisposing characteristics that may hinder access to vision screening and treatment include a child's age, race, ethnicity, mental and physical disabilities, sex, and social determinants of health. Parental factors include parental health beliefs, mistrust and misconceptions, and mental and physical disabilities (Antonio-Aguirre et al., 2024; Asare et al., 2022; Child and Adolescent Health Measurement Initiative, 2024; Elam et al., 2022; Frazier et al., 2009; Hoover et al., 2023; Killeen et al., 2023; Kimel, 2006; Kodjebacheva et al., 2011, 2015; Muhammad & Tumin, 2022; Qui et al., 2014; Rajesh et al., 2023; Repka et al., 2023; Sharma et al., 2016; Swanson et al., 2020; Varadaraj et al., 2019; Vongsachang et al., 2020; Williams et al., 2013). In this section we report race and ethnicity categories as used in the original articles.

Child's Age

Younger children are less likely than older children to get vision screening, comprehensive eye exams, or treatment, regardless of socioeconomic status (Antonio-Aguirre et al., 2024; Hoover et al., 2023; Killeen et al., 2023; Muhammad & Tumin, 2022; Repka et al., 2023) Based on nationally representative data from the 2018 and 2019 National Survey of Children's Health, parents reported that only 7% of children under age 6 received a vision test in school, 28% in primary care, and 10.2% in eye clinics (Table 8-6; Child and Adolescent Health Measurement Initiative, 2024). From the age of 5 years, when children are usually enrolled in school, they have more structured visual tasks (reading, writing, drawing, etc.) and therefore are more likely to recognize and seek help for any impaired vision. Vision screening is also more likely to be offered in the child's school or checked as part of a well-child visit for school-aged children. Many eye care providers do not offer appointments for young children. For example, a study of every eye care practice (ophthalmologists and optometrists) that could be identified in Arizona (over 1,000 eye care practices) found that only 41% would accept children under the age of 6 years (Biviji et al., 2024).

TABLE 8-6 Proportion of Children Receiving Vision Tests (by Setting) and No Vision Testing Based on Parental Report, From the National Survey of Children's Health 2018–2019

Age (years)		Setting for Vision test (%)			No Vision Testing
		School	Primary Care	Eye Clinic	
0–5	Row %	6.7	27.8	10.2	58.7
	CI	5.9–7.5	26.5–29.2	9.4–11.0	57.2–60.2
	Sample count	1,250	4,867	1,978	9,299
	Population estimate	1,564,386	6,503,574	2,383,714	13,726,380
6–11	Row %	22.7	33.9	38.7	23.5
	Confidence interval	21.5–24.0	32.5–35.3	37.3–40.2	22.1–24.9
	Sample count	4,583	5,953	7,466	3,889
	Population Estimate	5,572,228	8,299,418	9,479,673	5,752,331
12–17	Row %	11.0	22.4	51.6	25.8
	Confidence interval	10.1–11.9	21.2–23.6	50.1–53.0	24.5–27.1
	Sample count	2,594	5,230	13,323	6,131
	Population estimate	2,731,975	5,580,245	12,846,902	6,425,703

NOTES: Rows do not add up to 100% because vision testing could be reported in more than one location and this is not an exhaustive list of settings for vision testing. CI = confidence interval.
SOURCE: Data obtained from interactive data query of the National Survey of Children's Health (https://www.childhealthdata.org).

Racial and Ethnic Disparities

There are racial and ethnic disparities in accessing vision screening, comprehensive eye exams, and treatment (Antonio-Aguirre et al., 2024; Kodjebacheva et al., 2011; Stults et al., 2024; Varadaraj et al., 2019). A retrospective study, undertaken with data from electronic health records linked to census data for over 20,000 children aged 3 years with a well-child visit to the Palo Alto Medical Foundation in Northern California, reported lower rates of vision screening for Black and Hispanic children compared with Asian and White children (Asian, 73.1%; Black, 58.5%; Hispanic, 63.5%; White,74.3%; $p < 0.001$; Stults et al., 2024). The only options for race and ethnicity in the electronic health record used were Asian, Black, Hispanic, White, other (American Indian, Multiracial, Native Hawaiian, and Other Race not further specified), and unknown. Another study using nationally representative and population-based survey data of randomly sampled households (U.S. Census Bureau, 2023) reported that compared to non-Hispanic White children, Hispanic children and those from other non-Hispanic groups (Asian, American Indian or Alaska Native, Native Hawaiian, other Pacific Islanders, and those with two or more races) in the United States are less likely to get vision screening (Antonio-Aguirre et al., 2024). However, after adjusting for key sociodemographic characteristics (specifically, age, children with disabilities, healthcare visits in the past 12 months, insurance type, primary household language, parents' education, and household income) there is no difference in the likelihood of vision screening or comprehensive eye exams among these groups (Antonio-Aguirre et al., 2024).

Race is a social construct without genetic or biological association (Williams & Eberhardt, 2008). Therefore, this discrepancy in the association between race, ethnicity, and the likelihood of vision screening before adjusting for sociodemographic characteristics suggests that socioeconomic disadvantage related to the history of colonization, racial and ethnic discrimination, and the existence of a social gradient of power and privilege explain most of the disparities in access to vision screening experienced by members of minority racial or ethnic groups (Antonio-Aguirre et al., 2024; Elam et al., 2022; Furtado et al,, 2023; Hamm et al., 2021). This has been demonstrated for many other health outcomes and highlights the importance of considering both race, ethnicity and socioeconomic factors to understand health disparities (Robert Wood Johnson Foundation Commission to Build a Healthier America, 2009).

There are also disparities in the receipt of treatment for vision impairment. Children 12 years and older who are Mexican American or non-Hispanic Black have considerably higher odds of having inadequate refractive correction when they have poor vision compared to non-Hispanic White children, with the biggest disparity observed in children 12 to 19 years of age, according to data from NHANES 2005 to 2008 (Qiu et al., 2014). This was determined by measuring the proportion of children with poor visual acuity (worse than 20/40 with any refractive correction the child already had) that could be improved (to 20/40 or better with a first or better pair of glasses), that is, the proportion of children with uncorrected and under-corrected refractive error (Qui et al., 2014). Also, among first-grade children, Non-Hispanic Black/African American and Latino children are more likely than Non-Hispanic White children to not have prescription glasses despite having poor vision, as determined in a comprehensive eye exam by an ophthalmologist (adjusted odds ratios of 1.75 and 1.50 respectively adjusting for school, age, sex, and year; Kodjebacheva et al., 2011). (Options for race and ethnicity were non-Hispanic White, Latino, Non-Hispanic Black/African American, Asian/Pacific Islander, and other or mixed races/ethnicities.)

Furthermore, some instrument-based tools have problems screening children with dark irises, which may contribute to Black and Asian children having a lower likelihood of successful vision screening (Vaughan et al., 2010). The challenge with colored irises is especially problematic, because it perpetuates inequities in access for non-White populations, which have and are projected to continue to have the highest number of vision impairment cases through 2060 (Varma et al., 2017). The inequity will continue whenever vision screening is based solely on instrument screening. It also provides an additional justification for facilitating follow-up with a full comprehensive eye exam for children who cannot be screened.

Similar disparities are evident in treatment for strabismus. Using the American Academy of Ophthalmology's database known as the Intelligent Research In Sight (IRIS) Registry, which includes data on patient visits from electronic health records, Black, Hispanic, and Asian children with strabismus are found to be less likely to receive strabismus surgery, with a longer delay between diagnosis and surgery compared with White children after adjusting for insurance status (Rajesh et al., 2023; Repka et al., 2023). The IRIS Registry version used for the analysis provided a single variable for race and only had patient race categories of White, Black or African American, Asian, and other. While these findings regarding delays in receiving strabismus surgery may be partially explained by the variability by race and ethnicity in the incidence of refractive amblyopia risk factors, this may also reflect the under-diagnosis of amblyopia in non-White groups relative to the actual prevalence of strabismus (exotropia). Also, regardless of insurance status, Black children had a higher probability of experiencing residual amblyopia with strabismus (exotropia), compared to White children (Rajesh et al., 2023).

Children with Disabilities

Despite an increased risk for eye disease, children with disabilities such as those with autism spectrum disorder (ASD), Down Syndrome, or behavioral problems are less likely to get vision screening or comprehensive eye exams and are more likely to have unmet vision needs (Guo et al., 2022; Haller et al., 2022; Heslin et al., 2006; Hoover et al., 2023; Kimel, 2006; Silverstein et al., 2021; Swanson et al., 2020). Children with ASD have lower rates of vision screening at well-child visits than children who have not been diagnosed with ASD (Swanson et al., 2020). This is especially evident among young and Black children with ASD (Swanson et al., 2020). Non-Hispanic Black children with ASD also have lower rates of vision screening compared to non-Hispanic White children with ASD after adjusting for insurance, sex, developmental delays, and geographic region (Hoover et al., 2023).

Sex

Sex is associated with access to vision care (Antonio-Aguirre et al., 2024; Asare et al., 2022; Hoover et al., 2023). Male children are significantly less likely to get vision screening in well-child visits than females after adjusting for insurance type, race, ethnicity, ASD, developmental delays, sex, and geographic region (Hoover et al., 2023). Both referrals to eye care providers after an abnormal vision screening test and visits to an eye doctor are more likely in female than in male children (Antonio-Aguirre et al., 2024). However, this observation may be due to the higher prevalence of vision disorders in females compared to males (Vitale et al., 2008; Xiao et al, 2015).

Social Determinants of Health and Interrelated Factors

Social determinants of health are "the conditions in the environments where people are born, live, learn, work, play, worship, and age that affect a wide range of health, functioning, and quality-of-life outcomes and risks" (Healthy People 2030, n.d.; WHO, 2024a). Socioeconomic status, a social determinant of health, is a measure of an individual or family's economic and social position in relation to others in society measured by income, education and occupation. Socioeconomic status of children is informed by their parents' highest level of education, income, and employment (Dutton & Levine, 1989). Socioeconomic status and other social determinants of health such as household language may hinder access to vision screening, care, and treatment, including the use of prescription glasses in children (Adler et al., 1994, 2019; Antonio-Aguirre et al., 2024; Asare et al., 2022; Elam et al., 2022; Kimel, 2006; Sharma et al., 2016; Vongsachang et al., 2020; Williams et al., 2013).

Data from the 2021 National Survey of Children's Health indicate that social determinants of health continue to affect access to vision care in the United States (Antonio-Aguirre et al., 2024). Based on parental report, only 53% of children had a vision screening in the past 2 years. Children were less likely to have had vision screening—with odds adjusted for age, race, ethnicity, sex, special needs, health care visit in the last 12 month, insurance type, primary household language, parents' education, and household income—if they were younger than 3 years, had no insurance, did not have special health needs, had no health visits in the last year, had parents without more than high school education, or lived in a household with lower income (< 200% of the federal poverty level).

Referrals to eye care providers after an abnormal vision screening test were *more* likely for older children (aged 6 to 17 years vs 5 and under), female children, any ethnicity other than non-Hispanic White, and children with special needs, lower income (< 200% of the federal poverty level), or a primary language other than English. These factors were confounded by the odds of having had a visit to the eye doctor: that occurred for only 38.6% of the children and was more likely for older children (aged 3 to 17 vs. under 3), female children, special-needs children, children with a health visit in the last year, when there was some form of health insurance, and when English was the primary language. At every point, children with no health insurance were less likely to get vision screening or a visit to an eye doctor.

Parents with low health literacy, less education, or language barriers are less likely to understand the process of consenting to their children getting vision screening (Vongsachang et al., 2020). In focus groups on eye care undertaken with Hispanic immigrant parents, the parents reported a lack of knowledge about health care coverage for eye exams (Frazier et al., 2009). Low health literacy hinders access to vision health services for children. Parents with higher levels of education may have higher health literacy and may be more likely to be employed and have higher income. Parents with low socioeconomic status may find it particularly difficult to get permission to be absent from work to attend clinic appointments during the day (Kimel, 2006; Williams et al., 2013; Wolf et al., 2021).

Related to difficulties with permissions to be absent from work, parents may have competing priorities preventing them from attending appointments for well-child visits and comprehensive eye exams (Kimel, 2006). These competing priorities may be related to concerns about basic needs such as food and housing, household structure (single-family homes, multiple child households, foster care), multiple jobs, and precarious work (Kimel, 2006). Parents may have precarious jobs or other unpredictability in their schedules and therefore be unable to schedule appointments further than 1–2 weeks in advance or may have difficulties getting appointments within the preferred time frame (Kimel, 2006; Kodjebacheva et al., 2011). They also may not have flexibility in their work schedules to attend clinics for health care visits during work hours.

Related to unpredictable schedules and competing priorities, parents report difficulties with remembering scheduled appointments (Kimel, 2006). Also, parents with low health literacy may face increased challenges with scheduling appointments with eye care professionals (Collins et al., 2022b; Dudovitz et al., 2015; Kemper et al., 2006; Kimel, 2006). These challenges may lead to missed preventive care visits for children. Structural racism may indirectly contribute to such social disadvantages in racial and ethnic minoritized populations (Elam et al., 2022).

Parental Health Beliefs and Mistrust of Health Care Systems

Parents may develop a mistrust in vision screening because of high false-positive rates (Couser & Smith-Marshall, 2011; Frazier et al., 2009; Zhou et al., 2023). They may doubt the accuracy of vision screening results, question the safety of the vision screening process, or entertain fears about their children's inclusion in research studies without their permission (Kimel et al., 2006; Vongsachang et al., 2020). Some parents question whether the screening personnel are licensed or qualified (especially in school screening programs) or may be uncomfortable sharing personal information on consent forms (Vongsachang et al., 2020). Other parents may have mistrust in a school vision screening program if vision impairment they are already aware of is not detected in a vision screening test (Kimel, 2006). A survey of patients in a free clinic in Michigan showed that prior negative experiences with the health care system and subsequent lack of trust in the health care system were reasons for not acquiring glasses (Killeen et al., 2023). More than one-third of parents in the Midwest who have children in kindergarten through Grade 5 in a high-needs school did not follow up by booking an eye exam because they did not believe the results of the vision screening (38%) or did not believe the child needed a follow-up exam (29%; Kimel, 2006).

Parents with Mental and/or Physical Disabilities

Parents with physical or mental disabilities may be unable to offer consent for their children to attend vision screenings or may have trouble scheduling referrals (or follow-through with follow-up eye exams) because of their disability (Kimel, 2006).

Enabling Factors Hindering Access to Vision Screening, Comprehensive Eye Exams, and Treatment for Children

Enabling factors that present barriers to accessing vision care in U.S. children include type and lack of health insurance, household income, transportation, and household structure (Antonio-Aguirre et al., 2024; Centers for Medicare & Medicaid Services, n.d.; Killeen et al., 2023; Kimel, 2006; Kodiebacheva et al., 2015; Muhammad & Tumin, 2022; Newacheck, Hughes, & Stoddard, 1996; Prevent Blindness, 2020; Rajesh et al., 2023; Repka et al., 2023; Swanson et al., 2020; Syed et al., 2013; Williams et al., 2013; Zhang et al., 2012).

Type and Lack of Health Insurance and Household Income

In the 2018 to 2020 National Survey of Children's Health, parents reported that uninsured children were 41% less likely to get a vision test in pediatric primary care compared to children with private insurance, after adjusting for sex, race and ethnicity, household language, preventive health visit in the past year, and having special health care needs (Killeen et al., 2023). Similarly, children with public insurance were 24% less likely to get vision screening in pediatric primary care compared to children with private insurance, after adjusting for race, ethnicity, ASD diagnosis, developmental delays, sex, and geographic region (Killeen et al., 2023; Swanson et al., 2016). Data from the IRIS Registry demonstrate that Medicaid recipients have much lower chances than other patients of being successfully treated for amblyopia and are more likely to have residual amblyopia, after adjusting for key variables such as age, sex, race and ethnicity (Rajesh et al., 2023; Repka et al., 2023). A "secret shopper" survey conducted on over 1,000 ophthalmologist and optometrist practices in Arizona found that up to 74% of practices did not accept children covered by Arizona's Medicaid program, the Arizona Health Care Cost Containment System (Biviji et al., 2024).

Even when a child has insurance, co-pays for well-child visits and comprehensive eye exams, disparities in accessing vision care for children remain (Zhang et al., 2012). This is evident in studies conducted in Canada, where disparities in access to comprehensive eye exams remain for children with low socioeconomic status despite universal health coverage (Asare et al., 2022; Jin & Trope, 2011). One such study, conducted in Ontario, Canada, with linked health administrative and demographic data for children under the age of 8 years, found that children with high socioeconomic status were 43% more likely to have had a comprehensive eye examination than children with low socioeconomic status despite universal health insurance covering the cost (Asare et al., 2022). Similarly, in the United States, even among those with health insurance, children from low-income households are less likely to access eye care services by an eye care professional compared to children from high-income households (Asare et al., 2022; Kimel, 2006; Stein et al., 2016).

Despite requirements by the Affordable Care Act for health plans to cover pediatric vision care services, co-pays may be required in older, "grandfathered" health plans that existed prior to the enactment of the Affordable Care Act. Co-pays may also be required in short-term plans (less than 12 months), federal employee plans, some government plans, and membership plans like faith-based cost-sharing services (Center for Consumer Information Insurance Oversight, 2022; Prevent Blindness, 2020). People who work for larger companies (more than 100 employees) or who are self-insured are not covered by Essential Health Benefits of the Affordable Care Act (Center for Consumer Information Insurance Oversight, 2022). In addition, there is variation among states in the benefit for the provision of eye glasses (Center for Consumer Information Insurance Oversight, 2022; Prevent Blindness, 2020).

Transportation

Longer travel distances to healthcare providers, especially for children living in rural (as compared with urban) communities, are exacerbated for children who do not have a reliable form of transportation (Kimel, 2006; Kodjebachva et al., 2015; Newacheck et al., 1996; Syed et al, 2013). This is typically experienced by children experiencing poor social determinants of health (Syed et al., 2013).

Household Structure

Households with multiple children, single parents, or foster-care situations present unique circumstances which may prevent access to comprehensive eye exams and compliance with treatment for children. Coordinating schedules for large families can be difficult or even impossible in such households. Also, single parents may lack a shared caregiver and be overwhelmed with work and family responsibilities. The lack of a consistent home can also lead to difficulties scheduling appointments because caregivers may not know where a child will be on any given day (Kimel, 2006).

Factors Related to Need that Hinder Access to Vision Screening, School Screening, Comprehensive Eye Exams, and Treatment for Children

Factors related to perceived and evaluated need include false positive and negative tests, low health literacy, cultural beliefs, and mistrust of vision screening results (Kimel, 2006; Vongsachang et al., 2020).

False Positive and Negative Screening Tests

False positive and negative vision screening tests impact a patient's decision to seek eye care. They cause a false sense of security or psychological stress and result in unnecessary use of resources.

Low Health Literacy, Cultural Beliefs and Mistrust of Vision Screening Results

Parents with low health literacy may not understand pediatric vision disorders such as myopia and the impact of delayed vision care and poor vision on learning, and therefore fail to understand the urgency of vision care for their children (Kimel, 2006; Vongsachang et al., 2020). In focus groups with Hispanic immigrant parents to discuss eye care, parents noted that the higher frequency with which children wore glasses in the United States compared to their home countries was worrisome and likely due to something potentially harmful in the environment (Frazier et al., 2009). Alternatively, or in addition, parents may lack a cultural acceptance of prescription glasses and therefore not believe that their children need them (Frazier et al., 2009).

Many Native populations mistrust healthcare services, which together with a lack of cultural safety (which is an inability to safely practice cultural traditions within Western medical settings) contribute to vision disparities (Burn et al., 2021). Barriers based on personal and cultural beliefs, together with poor health literacy, have been shown to disproportionally impact racial and ethnic minority populations (Burn et al., 2021; Yashadhana et al., 2020).

Physicians can help improve access to vision care by following recommendations like those in Box 8-3, which increase the efficiency of screening and leave time for explaining the results and encouraging the follow-up and continuing care that are needed once an eye problem is identified.

BOX 8-3
10 Clinical Practices to Improve Vision Care Access, Adherence, and Continuity

1. Successful screening tools can be inexpensive and low-tech (visual acuity testing using optotypes) or more expensive and higher tech (instrument-based). Increasing access to care should be based on local resources available.
2. If a child fails an in-office screening, refer and follow up.
3. Both referral and follow up care should be case managed and confirmed.
4. If a child has had a previous vision screening and passed, repeat screening in office. If failed, refer and follow up. If a child has had a previous vision screening and failed, do not rescreen. If a child fails, believe it. Utilize time to encourage follow up care.
5. Avoid passing a previously failed screening. False negatives are the worst outcome.
6. If a child has an eye doctor or wears glasses or has a history of wearing glasses, do not rescreen. Utilize time to encourage follow up care with the same eye doctor. Underscore that the eye doctor should take care of the eyes and vision.
7. A physical exam of the eyes is likely not enough. Children who are myopic can often function quite well and may have no clinically observable signs of myopia.
8. Developmental delay constitutes a failed vision screening. Children with special needs fail by history alone. Conversely, high myopia discovered in a comprehensive eye exam may be a dysmorphic feature that contributes to conditions of broader developmental delay.
9. If glasses do not appear to help the child, encourage glasses wear and regular follow up with the eye doctor. Blur despite glasses indicates amblyopia. Children who not wear glasses at a young age and who have amblyogenic factors may never have clear vision.
10. If a child is seen by an eye doctor who doesn't dilate the child's eyes, choose another eye doctor.

Consequences of Poor Communication of Test Results and False Results

Families' experiences with vision health services, whether vision screening or a comprehensive eye exam, impact their future use of vision health services. Therefore, barriers to future use of vision health services include poor communication of results of a vision test, false positive and negative vision screening results, and patient and family dissatisfaction with services received.

Poor communication of results of a vision screening or comprehensive eye exam by the service provider to the child or family may give parents the false perception that their child has good vision (perceived health status) and therefore hinder follow-up care for treatment of vision impairment. On other occasions, the parents may perceive that any prescribed treatment is all that is needed with no call for follow-up.

A false positive or negative vision screening result may lead to under-referral or over-referral. As a result of false positive and negative tests, parents may lack confidence in or not be satisfied with vision screening tests. Children or families that are not confident in or satisfied with the care received might not consent to future vision screenings or may not attend follow-up appointments with an eye care provider.

BARRIERS TO RESEARCH TO ACCESS TO PEDIATRIC VISION SCREENING, COMPREHENSIVE EYE EXAMS, AND TREATMENT

Despite recent calls to action by the World Health Organization and the Lancet Commission on Global Eye Health (Burton et al., 2021) for increased research on improved access to vision care for children, there are significant barriers to conducting research on access to vision screening, comprehensive eye exams, and treatment (Burton et al., 2021; WHO, 2019). These barriers include poor data collection for surveillance, limited funding to conduct research, ethical concerns about randomized trials, and poor representation of minoritized populations in research.

Lack of Data Collection for Surveillance

Variability in vision screening policy mandates across U.S. states hinders the collection of standardized surveillance data for research that could inform the development of programs and policies. Similarly, the collection of standardized data is hindered by the poor collection of data on sociodemographic factors such as race vs ethnicity and sex vs. gender.

Limited Funding

There is limited funding to conduct research on the topic of access to care and pediatric populations (Arnold et al., 2018a; Pober et al., 2001; Sung et al., 2003). Few foundations have shown interest in funding population-based research, and when they are interested, the funding is often relatively minimal. For this reason, researchers compete for mainstream funding from federal institutions that have historically favored basic science and adult research (Arnold et al., 2018a; Hunter, 2013; Marzolf et al., 2017; O'Hara, 2016). One of the implications of limited funding for population-based research in the vision-care space is the plethora of cross-sectional, observational studies and secondary data studies that, while important, are limited in the conclusions and impact they can make. Longitudinal and randomized studies are needed to determine the long-term impacts of interventions in populations. However, research funding to conduct such important studies is limited.

Ethical Concerns Regarding the Conduct of Randomized Trials in Children

Randomized trials are essential for determining the efficacy of interventions to improve access to care for children and ultimately to improve health outcomes. However, these studies are rare because of limited funding and, when they do occur, are not adequately powered (Donahue et al., 2013; Jonas et al., 2017). Historically, there has been significant reluctance by caregivers, health care providers, educators, and institutional review boards to include children in clinical trials because of concerns about harming them by withholding treatment from control groups (Arnold et al., 2022; Rajalakshmi & Rajeshwari, 2019; Wahl et al., 2021). The International Myopia Institute (IMI) suggested that it remained ethical to randomize to control in its 2021 statement (Jong et al., 2021). In its 2023 digest, the IMI suggests (Sankaridurg et al., 2023):

> Ultimately, ethical questions are best answered region by region, with the availability of on-label myopia control modalities and the prevailing standard of

care being key considerations. Alternative clinical trial designs have been summarized in the "Study Design" section (Bullimore et al., 2023), including using a virtual control group based on previous studies (Chamberlain et al., 2021 2023), comparison with established treatments, or a time-to-treatment-failure (survival analysis) approach (Sankaridurg et al., 2019). (p. 17)

The National Eye Institute supports randomized clinical trials as a gold standard, suggesting that randomization reduces bias and provides a rigorous tool to examine cause-effect relationships between an intervention and outcome. This is because the act of randomization balances participant characteristics (both observed and unobserved) between the groups allowing attribution of any differences in outcome to the study intervention. This is not possible with any other study design. (Hariton & Locascio, 2018). Ultimately, the decision to randomize lies within the potential participant following a judicious informed consent process (Sankaridurg et al., 2023).

Poor Representation of Ethnic and Minority Populations

Marginalized population groups such as ethnic and minority populations and those with lower socioeconomic status are underrepresented in research, and the consequent lack of data can result in compounding health inequities (Bodack et al., 2010; Jones-Jordan et al., 2010; Morrison, 1998). Without representative data including all population groups, especially the most vulnerable and marginalized, interventions designed to address barriers to care will not be as effective as they could otherwise be. Numerous reasons are given for the lack of adequate representation of these key populations, including difficulties accessing specific population groups based on their geographic location, e.g., Native American children living on reserves; limited availability of researchers; significant resources required to translate research documents; and mistrust in research because of negative studies focused on racial and ethnic minorities in history (Wallace et al., 2018). These reasons for nonparticipation of marginalized populations are likely to be continuing problems limiting the inclusion of ethnic and minority groups in population-based research unless specific efforts are made to overcome these barriers.

STRATEGIES RECOMMENDED TO OVERCOME BARRIERS

Offering Parental Opt-outs Rather than Consent

One strategy for handling low rates of parental consent for vision screening is to send parents a letter describing what will happen at school during a vision screening and telling them how to opt their child *out* of the screening (Foe & Larson, 2016; Tigges, 2003). A Canadian vision screening project for children ages 4–6 in a variety of geographic locations had an average opt-out rate of 4% when an opt-out model was used and of 8% when active consent was required, but 22% of parents in the latter case failed to return the consent form and hence prevented the screening of their child (Nishimura et al., 2020).

School Visits to Promote Parental Consent

Another strategy that has been recommended to overcome barriers associated with low rates of parental consent is for a member of the vision screening team to make visits to the class and school to promote the project to principals, teachers, and students (O'Donnell et al., 1997; Secor-Turner et al., 2010; Wolfenden et al., 2009). Other strategies include providing incentives to teachers and students (Ji et al., 2006; O'Donnell et al., 1997; Secor-Turner et al., 2010; Wolfenden et al., 2009), choosing a time of school year with high attendance and few distractions (Detty, 2012), and providing translation services to address literacy and language barriers (Vongsachang et al., 2020).

In-School Follow-Up

Critical to the success of universal vision screening (or any other form of screening) is that referred children go to an eye care professional for follow-up treatment of any eye problem discovered and for continuing care. To promote follow-up, some universal screening programs have brought an eye care professional into the school with portable optometry equipment (Chu et al., 2015; Hark et al., 2018; Hendler et al., 2016; Silverstein et al., 2021; Williams et al., 2013). Any glasses that are ordered are usually also dispensed at the school. The reasoning is that the school is a familiar and trusted space, the program can do the scheduling and check on compliance, and that the wearing of dispensed glasses can be encouraged by the child's teacher. Such hybrid school-based programs are highly successful, because they eliminate financial, geographic, and transportation barriers to care and because they reduce mistrust (Collins et al., 2022b; Diao et al., 2016; Peterseim et al., 2015 Simon et al., 2007).

The Wills on Wheels Mobile Eye Unit provided in-school follow-up comprehensive eye exams for children enrolled in low-income schools (where more than 80% of students had a household income below $19,090 for a family of three or $23,050 for a family of four) that were referred from the National Football League Philadelphia Eagles Eye Mobile vision screening program. Through this initiative, completed follow-up eye exams increased from 53% prior to its implementation to 62%.

The See Well to Learn Program in San Francisco, CA, provides autorefractor screening in local Head Start preschool programs, comprehensive exams in a mobile van, and two pairs of glasses for children that need them (Sabharwal et al., 2021). Similarly, Vision for Baltimore uses a mobile van to provide vision screenings, comprehensive eye exams, and prescription glasses for elementary and middle school children in Baltimore public schools who require them. On-site school-based vision centers make vision care and eye care professionals part of the child's wellness team by bringing care closer to students attending local schools at minimal to no cost to families. These centers, which are more permanent than mobile vans, are established within the school or where the school district provides a trusted and safe space. Another advantage of these onsite vision centers is the ability for them to coordinate resources and expertise to support students (Collins et al., 2022b Lyons et al., 2011). They also make it more likely that the child's teacher will become aware of the child's need to wear glasses, so that the teacher can encourage compliance. When the teacher is asked to monitor compliance daily, as in the See Well to Learn Program, 64%–77% of children wore their glasses at least half the day during the 28 weeks after they received the glasses (Sabharwal et al., 2021).

Social workers and facilitators have been used by some vision screening programs to assist children who fail a vision screening test to receive follow-up care with an eye care professional (Hamm et al., 2021; Hark et al., 2018; Silverstein et al., 2021). In one study, a social worker assisted parents in scheduling appointments, in obtaining necessary referrals, and in reviewing insurance coverage with the family, which resulted in a 72% adherence rate for completing the eye exam (Silverstein et al., 2021).

Additional strategies recommended to improve adherence with follow-up care include providing no-cost care, offering transportation assistance, implementing email/text reminders, and collecting multiple forms of contact information to ensure effective patient outreach (Hark et al., 2018; Kimel, 2006). For the Philadelphia-based Give Kids Sight Day, a social worker helped ensure accurate contact information was collected, arranged follow-up appointments with eye care professionals, assisted with insurance enrollment, and provided transportation vouchers, reducing many of the commonly cited barriers to completing follow-up care (Dotan et al., 2015). Even after a comprehensive eye exam and prescription of glasses for myopia, the system may break down if the glasses are not worn. See Box 8-4 for the most common reasons such glasses may not be worn.

BOX 8-4
Adherence with Wearing Prescribed Glasses Is Low

Reasons for not wearing the glasses that were dispensed, as reported in both the United States (Dhirar et al., 2020) and China (Congdon et al., 2008), where the incidence of myopia is higher are:

- broken or lost glasses
- wearing the glasses only on special occasions.
- Misunderstanding about the importance of adherence with wearing prescribed glasses perpetuate thoughts that glasses:
    - are not needed
    - could make vision worse, and/or
    - could cause teasing.

These results indicate that any successful treatment for myopia will have to also involve a change in societal attitudes about the importance of diagnosis and treatment.

No-Cost Eye Glasses

Providing glasses at no cost—and ensuring that parents know that will happen in advance—is another effective strategy for reducing barriers. A systematic review of randomized controlled trials, mostly conducted in China, provides evidence from 11 studies that children are 2.45 times more likely to be wearing prescribed glasses at an unexpected follow-up visit if they were provided at no charge than if the parents only received a letter with the prescription (Wu et al., 2023). The effect is smaller with longer follow-up time (odds ratio 2.30 after 6–12 months versus 3.18 with earlier follow-up). Compliance was higher when the refractive error was higher or visual acuity was poorer. Nevertheless, in some of the RCTs, less than half the children who received free glasses were wearing them at follow-up.

One of the studies from China used an interesting comparison relevant to the sustainability of programs offering free glasses: parents in three intervention groups were offered free glasses, but those in two of them were allowed to purchase upgraded glasses (scratch-proof lenses and popular frames) for either $15 or $30, the 25th and 75th percentile of the average cost of purchased glasses at the time (Wang et al., 2017). More revenue was generated when the glasses were not free (control group) or upgrades could be purchased. However, an unannounced visit to the classrooms revealed that only 18%–32% of children were wearing the prescribed glasses, with no difference between children from groups given the upgrade voucher and the control group. However, the results are likely not generalizable to the United States because at least 97% of parents in each group went to the county hospital to obtain the prescribed glasses even though the county hospital was at a median distance of 27 km from the township of residence. No program in the United States reaches that level of compliance.

A study included in the systematic review (Wu et al., 2023) included children in grades 1 and 2 in New York City public schools serving low-income neighborhoods (Ethan et al., 2010). All schools received the state-mandated vision screening. Children were included if they had failed vision screening the year before and if the parents did not opt out after receiving a letter about the program (less than 1% of parents opted out). Parents of children who failed screening in the four control schools received a letter indicating that they should take the child for an eye exam. Children in the four intervention schools who failed the state screening received a non-cyclopleged optometric examination (comprehensive eye exam) and, if needed, two pairs of glasses, one for the teacher to keep and one to wear. In addition, teachers received instruction on children's visual problems and were asked to "lend" the second pair of glasses when needed. Observations during an unexpected visit to the classroom revealed that 47% of the children prescribed glasses were wearing them in the intervention group compared to 19% in the control group. Some students relied on the loaner glasses all the time at school because the "home" glasses had been lost or broken and not replaced.

An ideal design for vision screening and facilitated follow-up, therefore, should include easy and inexpensive access to comprehensive eye exams for those who fail screening—either by bringing an optometrist into the school or helping with booking at a community provider. It should also include provision of two pairs of subsidized glasses, one of which is kept with the teacher at school, who is made aware of the child's need to wear glasses for near and/or far work. Broken and lost glasses should be replaced promptly.

However, even with two pairs of free glasses, a program for mostly Native American 8- to 14-year-olds found that 67% were not wearing their glasses a year later, mostly because the glasses were lost (45%) or broken (35%; Messer et al., 2012). Other reasons given were not liking the glasses (15%), thinking they were not needed (2%), and having left them at home (2%). Nevertheless, over 90% of the students reported that the glasses helped them to see more clearly, whether or not they were wearing them (98% vs. 94%). Those with worse acuity were more likely to be wearing their glasses: children were 60% more likely to be wearing their glasses with each line of decreased acuity. Similarly, a comparison of glasses wearing after 1 year in states with programs involving just a referral letter and programs adding free comprehensive eye exams and glasses revealed low compliance overall (27% of children needing glasses were wearing them) with no difference between programs but better compliance when visual acuity was poorer (Manny et al., 2012). In another study, 66% of children in second or third grade who had been given two pairs of glasses after a comprehensive eye exam at school needed replacement glasses before the 1-year follow-up, with nearly half of these students needing replacements two or three times (Huang et al., 2019). Vision Screening programs that go a step further to collaborate with parents to address children's concerns about discomfort or adaptation have demonstrated improvement in compliance rates and in encouraging children from low-income families to wear glasses (Perez et al., 2022).

Economic Evaluations

To overcome the barriers related to funding for universal vision screening programs, economic evaluations are needed to inform resource allocation and policy decisions. These economic evaluations should include a determination of the cost-effectiveness of various vision care models to detect myopia compared to standard of care. In a study examining the cost-effectiveness of providing on-site exams in detecting amblyopia, relatively similar follow-up rates were observed when students who failed a screening were referred to a community provider (59% following up) compared to those who underwent a comprehensive eye exam through an onsite mobile clinic (55%; Lowry & de Alba, 2016; Ross & Stein, 2016). Given that the mobile clinic had a higher cost per case of amblyopia, community-based eye care was deemed more cost-effective. However, the follow-up rate for the mobile clinic was low due to challenges with parental consent. Implementing modifications to improve consent rates could increase the cost-effectiveness of a mobile clinic in detecting amblyopia.

To inform the conduct of economic evaluation of vision care models for myopia, studies on the impact of myopia on quality of life are needed. There is evidence that myopia can negatively impact the quality of life of both children with myopia and their parents for reasons that depend on the type of optical correction (e.g., glasses, contact lenses, refractive surgery). The impact of myopia control treatments on quality of life warrants further study, using instruments specifically developed for this population and condition (Lipson et al., 2022). Studies are also needed on the impact of untreated myopia on quality of life.

Improved Vision Screening Criteria for Myopia

The natural history of myopia development necessitates consistent vision screening throughout the school-age years to identify early onset and progression of myopia. During this period, 23.4% of children in the CLEERE study developed myopia (–0.50D or worse) (Kleinstein et al., 2012). The highest percentage of new cases occurred at age 11, with the onset spanning ages 7 to 16 years. Given the progressive nature of childhood and adolescent myopia, screening examinations encompassing visual acuity are recommended every 1 to 2 years (Hutchinson et al., 2023). Though the average prevalence of myopia is low among children younger than 5 years, it is critical that individuals with risk factors for myopia be identified early to encourage better vision health outcomes. Treatment interventions for delaying the onset of myopia and reducing myopia progression in childhood are available (see chapter 7 on Treatment). Therefore, a targeted strategy of periodic screening and evaluation of children at risk for myopia progression would address the problem of myopia as well as other ocular conditions. This could result in fewer visual disabilities and reduced risk of visual impairment (Bullimore & Brennan, 2019), ultimately alleviating the burden on the entire health care system.

Integrated Data Systems to Improve Surveillance of Children with Myopia

The success of a vision screening program is determined by ensuring that children are screened for vision impairment and that those identified receive follow-up comprehensive eye exams and treatment. Policies directed at addressing this issue can increase the effectiveness of screening programs. One recommended approach has been the implementation of an integrated data system for reporting screening and exam results (Brody et al., 2007; Collins et al., 2022a; Hartmann et al., 2015; Shakarchi & Collins, 2019). The Centers for Disease Control and Prevention's Vision Health Initiative (VHI) in collaboration with NORC at the University of Chicago developed The Vision and Eye Health Surveillance System (VEHSS) in 2015 to leverage data sources on vision and eye health to better understand the scope of vision loss, eye disorders, and eye care services in the United States (Rein et al., 2018). The current data on childhood myopia in VEHSS is from claims (Medicare, Medicaid, Managed Vision Care, and commercial medical insurance) and the IRIS Registry, which includes data from electronic health records of ophthalmology practices in the United States. Available vision services data such as vision screening is from national survey data.

Expanding VEHSS to include standardized statewide surveillance data on patient demographics, vision care services (i.e., vision screening, comprehensive eye exams), referrals to eye care providers, and diagnoses of vision disorders for children would not only enhance care integration and communication but also enable monitoring and development of strategic interventions to ensure that follow-up care is received. Such an expanded, national vision surveillance system would support public health efforts to understand if efforts are meeting set targets (Lee et al., 2012).

INNOVATIVE APPROACHES TO ADDRESS BARRIERS TO VISION CARE SERVICES

Innovative approaches for vision screening using smartphones have been introduced over the last decade. These innovations include Peek Vision (Rono et al., 2018), which measures acuity, and GoCheckKids (Arnold et al., 2018b), which measures not only visual acuity but also acts as a photoscreener to detect abnormal refractive errors and other vision problems. These applications are used around the world in remote locations and, in some cases, by parents instructed on their use at home, an innovation that proved useful during COVID-19 (e.g., Davara et al., 2022; reviewed in Thirunavukarasu et al., 2023; Painter et al., 2021). Some of these innovative smartphone applications are integrated with software aimed at encouraging follow-up with an eye care professional. Voluntary organizations such as Sight Savers America are also promoting integrated care (screening using conventional tools and facilitated follow-up) in some U.S. locales.

Peek Vision Foundation

In 2018, Peek Vision Foundation launched what they called a "dynamic social enterprise" with the goal of "vision and eye health for all" (Rono et al., 2018). As part of his PhD project, ophthalmologist Dr. Andrew Bastawrous saw the challenges facing Kenya, where the number of vision problems was high, and the number of resources was low. He set out to create the "eye-phone" to identify individuals with poor vision, using smart phones to allow increased access to screening, even in the most remote places. (See Figure 8-3.)

Software		
⊡	Eye health screening	Our smartphone app, Peek Capture, with its clinically-validated vision test, allows task shifting of screening to health workers closer to the communities they serve, increasing screening coverage, improving service efficiency and facilitating programme equity.
	User management	With our Peek Admin web-based administration platform, programme managers control who accesses what data.
	Notifications	Programme managers and IT leads are provided with tailored alerts, directing them to where their attention is needed.
	SMS referral reminders	Our referral reminders tool allows Peek-powered programmes to drive greater adherence to referral by automatically contacting patients or their contacts via SMS, in their preferred language, as their appointment date approaches.
	Messaging optimisation	Our messaging platform introduces democratised optimisation tools, standard in the web-industry, to the eye care sector. These tools allow programmes to tailor their messaging to their specific audience and achieve better referral adherence in their setting.
	Up-to-date monitoring	Programme managers can view data in near real-time, allowing them to act quickly to resolve issues and lower barriers.
	Reports	Our software produces regular, in-depth reporting, configured to meet the needs of the individual Peek-powered programme.
	Workflow configuration	Our software is highly configurable, capable of matching the unique practitioner workflows and patient pathways of every Peek-powered programme.
	Data Security	We are industry leaders in applying data security and privacy to digital health in The Global South. We employ leading industry standards in our approach, keeping your data safe and secure.
Support Services		
	Programme Design Service	We offer a proven solution built on rigorous scientific evidence and a comprehensive approach that supports programmes from planning through evaluation.
	Software user training	Our training and support team utilise a blend of self-directed and instructor-led training to achieve rapid software user proficiency.
	Data Insights Service	We provide unparalleled visibility of programme operation, highlighting opportunities to improve efficiency and equity.

FIGURE 8-3 Peek-Powered Program features.
SOURCE: Bastawrous & Peek Vision, n.d.

The first step in Peek's smartphone-based system is acuity testing, which can be conducted by a health worker or teacher. The screen displays tumbling Es and the child is asked to point in the direction in which the E is pointing. A built-in algorithm quickly determines the sizes that are needed to obtain a threshold. It requires minimal training to use it. The Es are surrounded by a box to create crowding, which improves accuracy of the visual acuity measurement. Comparisons of Peek results to conventional acuity testing have demonstrated good comparability in adults and children (e.g., Bastawrous et al., 2015; Bhaskaran et al., 2022), with better comparability than that found for many of the other smartphone acuity testing apps available (reviewed in De Samanta et al., 2023). However, in a study with children in Paraguay, Peek tended to overestimate acuity compared to a pediatric ophthalmologist's measurement with a Snellen chart (de Venecia et al., 2018). Only 31% of assessed acuity values agreed exactly, but 59% were within one step and 71% within two steps. One reason may be the higher probability of guessing 1 of 4 directions correctly by chance with Tumbling Es, vs. 1 of 26 letters with standard letter charts.

Importantly, results of Peek acuity applications are integrated with a system for scheduling and encouraging follow-up for children referred for a full comprehensive eye exam. In a recent clustered randomized controlled trial, this integrated system was used in 25 schools in Kenya (Rono et al., 2018). Parents of children who could not see the 20/40 letters after the teacher tested acuity with the Peek system received a picture of how blurry the child's vision is and repeated SMS messages about how to take the child for follow-up. Similar messages went to the child's teacher and the hospital to which the child was referred. The comparison was 25 schools in which the teacher tested with a conventional Tumbling E chart and, if the child could not see the 20/40 letters, sent a standard referral letter home. Within the next 8 weeks, only 22% of parents in the standard group brought their children to the hospital for follow-up, compared to 54% of parents in the integrated Peek system group.

The Peek Vision program reports that about five million individuals had been screened with their system in community, school, and workplace settings between 2018 to 2022. More than 20% of them were identified as needing eye care, and more than half of those identified were seen by an eye care specialist.[2] The number of people screened each year is now increasing rapidly around the world.[3]

GoCheckKids

GoCheckKids is a vision screening system that works only via iPhone both to test visual acuity with Sloan letters with crowding bars and to do photoscreening to detect children in need of a referral to an eye doctor. It is being used in schools, Head Start programs, and physicians' offices in the United States and Europe. The photoscreening capabilities of GoCheckKids have been tested extensively with children (as well as adults) and involve taking a flash picture of the eye in a darkened room while the iPhone is surrounded by a black flash-concentrating case and the child is fixating the screen 6 meters away. The appearance of the reflected red reflex (Bruckner's reflex) is used to judge whether the child has a referrable refractive error or other visual problem. Judgments can be made remotely by an expert or immediately through AI-powered algorithms. GoCheckKids measurements are eligible for reimbursement under photoscreening billing codes provided by the Centers for Medicare and Medicaid Services, (CPT 99174, CPT 99177) and the system works with a subscription model rather than as a capital purchase.

Studies of the photoscreening app with young children indicate good sensitivity and specificity for amblyopia risk factors compared to findings of a gold-standard cyclopleged eye exam (76% and 85%, respectively, with expert grading, 65% and 83%, with automatic grading; Arnold et al., 2018b), although comparisons are less favorable for children under 1 year of age (positive predictive value of only 26%; Law et al., 2020). Overall, values for sensitivity and specificity of the photoscreening app for detecting amblyopia risk factors compare favorably to those reported for the conventional Spot and Plusoptix photoscreeners (Sopeyin et al., 2021). One limitation is that, at least with young children, slightly more than 10% of images from the GoCheckKids device cannot be scored, mostly because of lack of fixation (Arnold et al., 2018b). A limitation of the GoCheckKids system is its lack of compatibility with other smartphone systems besides the iPhone. However, this is limitation is mitigated by its use of a subscription service which includes an iPhone device with the necessary software.

---

[2]For more information, see https://peekvision.org/our-impact

[3]See https://peekvision.org/wp-content/uploads/2023/11/Peek-Vision-Brochure.pdf

Sight Savers America—Alabama

Although the State of Alabama does not have a mandate to provide vision care to children, it has had an annual line item in the budget for statewide vision screening and comprehensive follow-up eye care for public school kindergarten, second, and fourth grades since 2004 (Prevent Blindness, 2022). After competitive re-evaluation in 2021 and 2022, Sight Savers America remained the sole recipient of allocated state funding for Alabama's comprehensive follow-up eye care program. A 501(c)(3) nonprofit program since 1997, Sight Savers America has reached over 750,000 children with case management support for comprehensive dilated eye exams, eyeglasses, medications, surgeries, and other eye care treatments[4] (Sight Savers America, 2024). Sight Savers America helps coordinate care and establish an eye care home for on-going vision needs for over 50,000 children each year from Alabama, Texas, Louisiana, Mississippi, Georgia, and South Carolina.

Children who fail the vision screening step are assigned a case specialist, who helps manage care throughout the multistep process from consent and vision screening to the establishment of an eye care home and long-term treatment. Case specialists use motivational health coaching techniques to educate parents about vision screening and the importance of obtaining a comprehensive dilated eye examination for children who fail screenings to facilitate compliance. Personnel from Sight Savers America help those who qualify obtain Medicaid insurance, which will provide an annual comprehensive eye exam to the child. For medically underserved families, transportation and prescribed treatments are provided at no cost to the families. Data on the success of this integrated approach is provided annually on the program's website and to state personnel. State-allocated funds are leveraged with private financial gifts and gifts in-kind.

The capture rate for comprehensive eye examination following vision screening has been reported in the United States to be roughly 39% in primary care pediatric practices (Hered & Wood, 2013; Sight Savers America, 2024). Sight Savers America reports that through their integrated, case-managed eye care program, 71% of children who were reached following failed vision screening received a comprehensive eye exam (Sight Savers America, 2024). Sight Savers attributes their cost-effectiveness and success to using a quick vision screening tool, individual case managers, and a network of eye care providers who increase their patient base and help with costs by donating prescription glasses and discounting comprehensive eye exams when necessary.

The following three tables summarize contextual (Table 8-7), individual-level (Table 8-8), and research (Table 8-9) barriers, potential actors and strategies to overcome barriers to vision screening, comprehensive eye exams and treatment for myopia and other refractive errors in children.

---

[4]For more information, see https://sightsaversamerica.org/eye-care

TABLE 8-7 Summary of Contextual Barriers, Potential Actors and Strategies to Overcome Barriers to Vision Screening, Comprehensive Eye Exams and Treatment for Myopia and Other Refractive Errors in Children

Barrier	What Can Be Done?	Who Can Help?
A lack of consensus on the importance and conduct of vision screening	Engage in consensus building to develop standardized vision screening guidelines for myopia	• National professional associations (AAP, AAFP, AAOpt, AOA AAOphth, AAOMD, AAPOS, NMA, AMA) • USPSTF • DHHS
A lack of funding for vision screening programs	1. Prioritize and fund universal vision screening and continuing eye care 2. Where resources are limited, target screening to medically underserved populations 3. Conduct economic evaluations to determine cost-effective vision care models to inform policy decisions and resource allocation 4. Conduct studies on the impact of myopia and vision impairment on quality of life to support fund raising efforts, program planning and policy efforts 5. Provide guidance for state health systems and schools on how to secure Medicaid dollars through Healthy Schools Campaign	• Local, state, and national funding agencies (NIH, AHRQ, PCORI, CDC, RPB, etc.) • DHHS • Researchers (health economists, health services, and others)
Concerns about the accuracy of vision screening tests	Increase education on conducting effective and frequent vision screenings and the variability in accuracy of instrument-based screening devices and gain consensus on referral criteria	• Eye care providers, public health officials • National professional associations (AAP, AAFP, AAOpt, AOA AAOphth, AAPOS, NMA, AMA)
Instrument malfunction, availability	1. Utilize resources maximally using visual acuity testing if limited and instrument-based if more readily available 2. Consider philanthropic gifts-in-kind to targeted areas in the community that would increase availability 3. Research and promote innovations to reduce cost, increase availability including with smartphones	• Industry and device manufacturers • Local, state, and national funding agencies (NIH, AHRQ, CDC, Research to Prevent Blindness [RPB], etc.)

Barrier	Recommendation	Responsible Parties
Limited statewide surveillance of preventive services under the Early and Periodic Screening, Diagnostic and Treatment (EPSDT) Medicaid benefit	• Create formal surveillance policy and procedures at the state level, including prospective artificial intelligence tactics and electronic data entry. • Vision screening and well-child visits at ages 3, 4, and 6 years should be included in the Core Set of Children's Health Care Quality Measures	• Device manufacturers • National Institutes of Health • DHHS (The Centers for Medicare & Medicaid Services (CMS)) • CDC (Vision Health Initiative)

Pediatric Primary Care

Barrier	Recommendation	Responsible Parties
Perceptions of insufficient time in the clinic workflow	Research to understand clinic workflow, develop and implement strategies to overcome barriers	• Industry and device manufacturers • Researchers (implementation science, health services, qualitative and others)
Inadequate reimbursement for vision screening	Reimbursement for vision screening is low and should not be bundled into the global code of well-child visits	• The Centers for Medicare & Medicaid Services • Health insurance companies • Local, state, and national funding agencies (NIH, AHRQ, CDC, RPB, etc.)
Limited number of appointments for well-child visits, especially in resource-deprived communities	1. Develop pipeline programs to improve primary care workforce 2. Create incentives to attract foreign medical graduates to improve primary care workforce	National professional associations (AAP, AAFP, AAOpt, AAOphth, AAPOS, NMA)
Long travel distance to nearest primary care provider	1. Develop pipeline programs to improve primary care workforce 2. Create incentives to attract foreign medical graduates to improve primary care workforce	National professional associations (AAP, AAFP, AAOpt, AAOphth, AAPOS, NMA)

School and Community Vision Screening

Barrier	Recommendation	Responsible Parties
Variability in state requirements for vision screening in schools	Develop national standardized guidelines for vision screening	• DHHS • State departments of education • School boards
Limitations due to space, school schedules, and calendars	• Consider time of school year for screening • Developing effective screening protocols in small spaces	• DHHS • National and state departments of education • Organizers of screening programs including public health units, schools and volunteer groups

Barrier	Recommended actions	Potential responsible parties
		- NASN - Industry and device manufacturers - Local, state, and national funding agencies (NIH, AHRQ, CDC, RPB, etc.) - Researchers (implementation science, health services, public health, and others)
Problematic consent processes for children to participate in vision screening	1. Send parents a letter describing what will happen at school during a vision screening, including how to opt their child out of the screening 2. Make visits to the class and school to promote programs to principals, teachers, and students 3. Provide incentives to teachers and students to increase return of consent forms 4. Use translation services to address literacy and language barriers	- State departments of education - Organizers of screening programs including public health units, schools, and volunteer groups - NASN
Poor communication about the program	- Use multiple forms of contact information to ensure effective patient outreach - Development of effective communication strategies about the importance of vision screening and comprehensive eye exams	- State departments of education - National professional associations (AAP, AAFP, AAOpt, AOA, AAOphth, AAPOS, NMA, AMA) - Organizers of screening programs including public health units, schools and volunteer groups - NASN - NACHW - Local, state, and national funding agencies (NIH, AHRQ, CDC, RPB, etc.) - Researchers (public health, implementation science, qualitative researchers, and others)
Parent socioeconomic barriers	- Fund local programs to address barriers to access for vision care in medically underserved and health-disparity populations - Use social workers, community health workers, or patient navigators in underserved communities to support parents with consent processes for participation in school-based programs	- Local, state, and national funding agencies (NIH, AHRQ, PCORI, CDC, RPB, etc.) - DHHS

Comprehensive Eye Exams and Treatment

303

Barrier	Strategies	Stakeholders
Lack of follow-up with eye care professional	1. Deploy integrated or hybrid models that bring eye care professional into the school with portable optometry equipment 2. Use social workers, community health workers, or patient navigators to help schedule appointments and provide reminders 3. Offer no-cost comprehensive eye exams and glasses 4. Provide transportation assistance 5. Send email or text reminders about appointments 6. Develop collaborative efforts amongst stakeholders 7. Develop effective, innovative programs to ensure follow-up care with eye care professionals 8. Engage in public education to improve awareness and vision health literacy	• DHHS • Industry and device manufacturers • State departments of education • National professional associations (AAP, AAFP, AAOpt, AOA, AAOphth, AAPOS, NMA, AMA) • NACHW • Local, state, and national funding agencies (NIH, AHRQ, CDC, RPB, etc.) • Researchers (implementation scientists, health services, public health and others)
Poor provider–patient communication of results of a vision test	Offer physician continuing culturally sensitive training, refresher training/courses, and changes to medical curricula	National professional associations (AAP, AAFP, AAOpt, AOA, AAOphth, AAPOS, NMA, AMA)
Low reimbursement rates for rendering eye care	Increase rates of reimbursement for rendering eye care	• Centers for Medicare & Medicaid Services • Health insurance companies
Low supply of eye care specialists willing to see children	1. Support pipeline programs to improve pediatric eye care workforce 2. Create incentives to attract foreign medical graduates 3. Conduct continuing education for optometrists and ophthalmologists not specializing in pediatrics	National professional associations (AAP, AAFP, AAOpt, AOA AAOphth, AAPOS, NMA, AMA, ASCO)
Lack of affordable prescription glasses and compliance with wear	1. Dispense glasses at school 2. Involve teachers in encouraging the wearing of prescribed glasses 3. Provide two pairs of subsidized glasses 4. Ensure that broken and lost glasses are replaced promptly	• Centers for Medicare & Medicaid Services • Health insurance companies • DHHS • National eye care professional associations (AAOpt, AAOphth, AAPOS) • Industry and glasses manufacturers

	What Can Be Done?	Who Can Help?
	5. Offer no-cost glasses 6. Allow children to choose their glasses 7. Ensure that esthetics of glasses appeal to children 8. Engage in public education to improve awareness and vision health literacy	• National Center for Children's Vision and Eye Health and other national associations that support public education programming • Foundations and Not-for-Profit Agencies (SightSavers, Onesight EssilorLuxottica, VisionSpring, etc)
Lack of consensus on guidelines for comprehensive eye exams by professional organizations	1. Consensus building to develop standardized guidelines for comprehensive eye exams for myopia 2. Economic evaluations to determine cost-effectiveness of models of universal comprehensive eye exams to inform consensus building	• National professional associations (AAP, AOA, AAFP, AAOpt, AAOphth, AAPOS, NMA, AMA) • USPSTF • Local, state, and national funding agencies (NIH, AHRQ, CDC, RPB, etc.) • Researchers (health economists, health services and others)

NOTE: AAFP = American Academy of Family Physicians; AAOpt = American Academy of Optometry; AAOphth = American Academy of Ophthalmology; AAP = American Academy of Pediatrics; AAPOS = American Academy of Pediatric Ophthalmology and Strabismus; AHRQ = Agency for Healthcare Research and Quality; AMA = American Medical Association; AOA = American Optometric Association; APHA = American Public Health Association; ASCO = Association of Schools and Colleges of Optometry; CDC = Centers for Disease Control and Prevention; CMS = The Centers for Medicare & Medicaid Services; DHHS = Department of Health and Human Services; NACHW = National Association of Community Health Workers; NASN = National Association of School Nurses; NIH = National Institute of Health; NMA = National Medical Association; PCORI = Patient-Centered Outcomes Research Institute; RPB = Research to Prevent Blindness; USPSFT = United States Preventive Services Taskforce.
SOURCE: Committee generated.

TABLE 8-8 Summary of Individual-Level Barriers, Potential Actors and Strategies to Overcome Barriers to Vision Screening, Comprehensive Eye Exams and Treatment for Myopia and Other Refractive Errors in Children

Barrier	What Can Be Done?	Who Can Help?
Predisposing Characteristics Age Race, Ethnicity Sex Special healthcare needs Social determinants of health	1. Funding for vision care services within community health centers and federally qualified health centers 2. Funding for local programs to address barriers to access for vision care in medically underserved populations 3. Public education to improve awareness and vision health literacy	• DHHS • Research to Prevent Blindness (RPB) (National Center for Children's Vision and Eye Health) and other nonprofit eye care organizations • APHA • National eye care professional associations (AAOpt, AOA AAOphth, AAPOS)

Factor	Intervention	Organizations
Parental health beliefs	Public education to improve awareness and vision health literacy by patient navigators and peer ambassadors from local communities who understand the culture and social context of parents' beliefs	• National eye care professional associations (AAOpt, AOA AAOphth, AAPOS) • APHA • RPB's National Center for Children's Vision and Eye Health and other nonprofit eye care organizations
Parent mistrust and misconceptions	Public education to improve awareness and vision health literacy by patient navigators and peer ambassadors from local communities who understand the culture and social context of parent's beliefs	• National eye care professional associations (AAOpt, AOA AAOphth, AAPOS) • APHA • RPB's National Center for Children's Vision and Eye Health and other nonprofit eye care organizations
Parent mental and physical disabilities	Funding for local programs to address barriers to access for vision care in medically underserved and health-disparity populations	• DHHS • RPB and other nonprofit eye care organizations
Enabling Factors Type and lack of health insurance Household income Transportation Household structure	1. Funding for local programs to address barriers to access for vision care in medically underserved populations 2. No-cost eye exams 3. Transportation assistance	• DHHS • RPB's National Center for Children's Vision and Eye Health and other nonprofit eye care organizations • State departments of education • Local, state, and national funding agencies (NIH, AHRQ, CDC, RPB, etc.)
Need Factors False positive and negative tests	1. Public education to improve awareness and vision health literacy 2. More accurate screening tests	• National eye care professional associations (AAOpt, AOA, AAOphth, AAPOS) • APHA • RPB (National Center for Children's Vision and Eye Health) and other non-profit eye care organizations • Industry and device manufacturers • Local, state, and national funding agencies (NIH, AHRQ, CDC, RPB, etc.)

Barrier	What Can Be Done?	Who Can Help?
Lack of priority setting for eye and vision care	Public education to improve awareness and vision health literacy provided by patient navigators and peer ambassadors from local communities who understand the culture and social context of parental beliefs	• Researchers (biomedical informatics, engineering, digital health and others) • National eye care professional associations (AAOpt, AOA, AAOphth., AAPOS) • APHA • RPB's National Center for Children's Vision and Eye Health and other nonprofit eye care organizations
Mistrust of vision screening results	Public education to improve awareness and vision health literacy by patient navigators and peer ambassadors from local communities who understand the culture and social context of parental beliefs	• National eye care professional associations (AAOpt, AAOphth, AAPOS) • RPB's National Center for Children's Vision and Eye Health and other non-profit eye care organizations • APHA

NOTES: AAFP = American Academy of Family Physicians; AAOphth= American Academy of Ophthalmology; AAOpt = American Academy of Optometry; AAPOS = American Academy of Pediatric Ophthalmology and Strabismus; AHRQ = Agency for Healthcare Research and Quality; AOA= American Optometric Association; APHA = American Public Health Association; CMS = The Centers for Medicare & Medicaid Services; DHHS = Department of Health and Human Services; NACHW = National Association of Community Health Workers; NASN = National Association of School Nurses; NIH = National Institute of Health; NMA = National Medical Association; RPB = Research to Prevent Blindness; USPSFT = United States Preventive Services Taskforce.
SOURCE: Committee generated.

TABLE 8-9 Summary of Research Barriers, Potential Actors and Strategies to Overcome Barriers to Vision Screening, Comprehensive Eye Exams and Treatment for Myopia and Other Refractive Errors in Children

Barrier	What Can Be Done?	Who Can Help?
Poor data collection for surveillance	National, standardized guidelines for vision screening and the collection of sociodemographic factors such as race vs ethnicity, and sex vs. gender.	• DHHS • State departments of education • National professional associations (AAP, AAFP, AAOpt, AOA, AAOphth, AAPOS, NMA, AMA) • USPSTF • CDC (Vision Health Initiative)
Limited funding to conduct research	Funding institutions to prioritize research for randomized trials to determine the efficacy of	• Research funding organizations (NIH NEI, AHRQ, CDC, RPB and others)

Ethical concerns about randomized trials	• interventions to improve access to vision care for children • Public education on the importance and safety of randomized trials; timely evaluation of treatment outcomes as it relates to standard of care and research	• Researchers • Institutional IRBs • University research departments • State departments of health • Local, state, and national funding agencies (NIH, AHRQ, RPB, etc.)
Poor representation of minoritized populations in research	• Research on the genetic predisposition to myopia development and progression in racial and ethnic minoritized populations • Collaborative efforts with community groups • Local champions to support recruitment efforts • Recruitment strategies that are intentional in diversifying the sample populations for RCTs • Improved design of RCTs	• Research funding organizations (NIH, AHRQ, RPB and others) • Researchers (geneticists, community-based participatory research, and others) • Indian Health Service • Indian tribes or tribal organization • Urban Indian organizations

NOTES: AAP = American Academy of Pediatrics; AAFP = American Academy of Family Physicians; AAOpt = American Academy of Optometry; AAOphth = American Academy of Ophthalmology; AAPOS = American Academy of Pediatric Ophthalmology and Strabismus; AHRQ = Agency for Healthcare Research and Quality; AOA = American Optometric Association; CDC = Centers for Disease Control and Prevention; DHHS = Department of Health and Human Services; IRB = Institutional Review Board; NEI = National Eye Institute; NIH = National Institutes of Health; NMA = National Medical Association; RPB = Research to Prevent Blindness; USPSTF = United States Preventive Services Task Force.

SOURCE: Committee generated.

CONCLUSIONS

Several common themes emerged from the analysis of barriers to myopia detection and treatment. Those barriers are described here in three conclusions that inform the recommendations that follow.

Conclusion 8-1: Multiple barriers to vision care for children exist. The most significant barriers are an uneven awareness of the importance of checking children's vision health, parents' difficulties in gaining access to an eye care professional, and barriers to compliance with prescribed treatments.

Conclusion 8-2: Vision screening is important in identifying children with vision impairment and facilitating access to treatment, but many children are not receiving vision screening and, when they do receive it, often do not receive any recommended referral. One model that has been used successfully is to provide vision screening to all children in congregate locations (schools, fairs, etc.). An alternative that has been successful when resources are scarce is to offer vision screening to targeted groups at increased risk of vision problems or of not receiving treatment (e.g., medically underserved communities, rural communities). For children with lower socioeconomic status and from medically underserved populations, vision screenings within community health centers and federally qualified health centers are an excellent way to provide access to vision care. School boards can also take advantage of Medicaid dollars provided through the Healthy Schools Campaign.

Conclusion 8-3: Vision screening is ineffective without receipt of follow-up eye care for children that need it. Therefore, it is critical that vision screening programs provide effective strategies to ensure that children identified with potential vision impairment receive a comprehensive eye exam by an eye care professional (skilled in providing vision care to children) to diagnose vision disorders and provide treatment. Comprehensive eye exams by eye care professionals, along with facilitators such as social workers or community health workers as patient navigators who assist caregivers with scheduling comprehensive eye exams and provide frequent reminders to attend appointments, have been shown to be effective in increasing follow-up compliance. However, myopia is a lifelong condition requiring follow-up eye examinations and, when needed, replacement of lost or broken glasses. The same barriers to the initial detection of children's vision problems impact continuing care, underscoring a need for an eye care home.

RECOMMENDATIONS

Considering the findings of this consensus report, the committee makes the following recommendations to improve detection and treatment of myopia in children and to address the disparities in accessing vision care.

Recommendation 8-1: The U.S. Department of Health and Human Services, in collaboration with departments of education at the state level, should take measures to ensure that children receive a vision screening before first grade and a comprehensive eye exam, when needed. To facilitate this:

- **Federal agencies such as the Centers for Disease Control and Prevention and other agencies that support public health programming should encourage the implementation of effective vision care programs for children by providing funding or other incentives for vision health care systems that follow the 12 Components of a Strong Vision Health System of Care provided by the National Center for Children's Vision and Eye Health. Priority should be given to programs targeting high-risk groups (i.e., children with lower socioeconomic status, of younger ages [under 6 years], with disabilities, with parents who have low health literacy, or from racial or ethnic minority groups [specifically, Hispanic, non-Hispanic Black, Asian, American Indian, Alaskan Natives, and Pacific Islanders], and children living in medically underserved communities [e.g., rural]).**

- **The Department of Health and Human Services should oversee the provision of cost-effective, standardized, evidence-based national vision screening guidelines to detect refractive errors, amblyopia, and other vision conditions. These guidelines should include a consensus on the ideal target age for screening, screening frequency, the need for re-screening, types of screening tests, tools, and referral criteria.**

- **For children under age 7, the referral criteria for instrument-based screening should include any amount of myopia or a family history of myopia based on the evidence that these predict likely progression to significant myopia.**

- **The Association of Schools and Colleges of Optometry, the National Medical Association, and the American Medical Association should use innovative means to encourage optometric and medical graduates of all backgrounds to pursue residencies in pediatric optometry and residents to pursue fellowships in pediatric ophthalmology. This should be done using innovative strategies such as pipeline and incentive programs to improve the vision care workforce, especially the workforce in rural and low-income communities. Continuing education should be provided for practicing optometrists and ophthalmologists to encourage them to include young children in their practice.**

Recommendation 8-2: An integrated, national data surveillance system is needed to collect state-level data on vision screening, referrals to eye care providers, sociodemographics (age, race, ethnicity, sex, and geographic location) and outcomes of referrals. This data system would not only enhance care integration and communication, but also enable monitoring to ensure that follow-up care is received, especially in high-risk populations. A surveillance system would also support the Department of Health and Human Services' Office of Disease Prevention and Health Promotion's Healthy People 2030 goal of increasing the proportion of children who get vision screening. To facilitate the creation of this system:

- The Centers for Medicare & Medicaid Services should include vision screening in the Core Set of Children's Health Care Quality Measures that are reported annually by all states.
- The Centers for Medicare & Medicaid Services should require reimbursement for vision screening to not be bundled into the global code of well-child visits.
- Professional associations such as the American Academy of Optometry, American Optometric Association, and American Academy of Ophthalmology should work with device manufacturers to create a national database of eye care providers that provide care to children, especially children under the age of 6 years, and the types of health insurance they accept. This database should be in a format that is easily accessible by caregivers and the general public.
- The National Institutes of Health "All of US" Research Program and the Healthy Brain and Child Development Study should include additional measures of adult and child vision disorders.

Recommendation 8-3: The National Institutes of Health, Agency for Healthcare Research and Quality, as well as foundations, nonprofits, and industry and other organizations that support research, such as Research to Prevent Blindness, should seek and encourage opportunities to fund work supporting continued efforts by vision researchers to determine:

- Genetic predisposition to myopia development and progression in racial and ethnic minoritized populations;
- The implementation, effectiveness, and cost-effectiveness of existing and novel interventions in real-world settings to improve access to vision screening, adherence with referrals to eye care providers, and coordination of care across providers compared to standard of care, especially for populations at high risk for vision impairment.
- The prevalence of myopia, referrals to eye care providers, completion of comprehensive eye exams, and treatment in children, especially those from high-risk populations
- Differences in reimbursement processes (e.g., bundled vs. unbundled with global code for well-child visits), reimbursement rates (for vision screening, new and ongoing care by eye care providers) and coverage for prescription glasses across states and health insurance plans; and the influence of those differences on vision health outcomes, especially as it relates to children from high-risk populations; and
- Strategies for promoting adherence with referrals, follow-up care, compliance with wearing prescribed glasses, and improved public awareness of and health education on vision and eye health in children, especially those from high-risk populations.

Recommendation 8-4: Global organizations, such as the World Health Organization and the International Myopia Institute, should identity and inventory best practices for improving access to vision care for medically underserved populations. Where

culturally appropriate, these practices can be generalized to and from the United States.

Recommendation 8-5: Myopia should be classified as a disease and therefore a medical diagnosis by The Centers for Medicare & Medicaid Services. This reclassification is to ensure efforts not only to treat blurry vision resulting from uncorrected or under-corrected refractive error, but also to ensure that the prevention and management of the progression of myopia gets the warranted attention from stakeholders such as federal and state agencies, professional associations, patients, and caregivers. Myopia is a disease with increasing worldwide prevalence and severity, and recognition of the impact of its downstream complications needs to be taken seriously.

REFERENCES

Abdus, S., & Selden, T. M. (2022). Well-child visit adherence. *JAMA Pediatrics, 176*(11), 1143–1145. https://doi.org/10.1001/jamapediatrics.2022.2954

Aday, L. A., & Andersen, R. (1974). A framework for the study of access to medical care. *Health Services Research, 9*(3), 208–220. https://www.ncbi.nlm.nih.gov/pmc/articles/PMC1071804/

Aday, L. A., & Andersen, R. M. (1981). Equity of access to medical care: A conceptual and empirical overview. *Medical Care, 19*(12), 4–27. https://pubmed.ncbi.nlm.nih.gov/11643688/

Adler, N. E., Boyce, T., Chesney, M. A., Cohen, S., Folkman, S., Kahn, R. L., & Syme, S. L. (1994). Socioeconomic status and health: The challenge of the gradient. *The American Psychologist, 49*(1), 15–24. https://doi.org/10.1037//0003-066x.49.1.15

Adler, N. E., & Ostrove, J. M. (1999). Socioeconomic status and health: What we know and what we don't. *Annals of the New York Academy of Sciences, 896*(1), 3–15. https://doi.org/10.1111/j.1749-6632.1999.tb08101.x

Ambrosino, C., Dai, X., Antonio Aguirre, B., & Collins, M. E. (2023). Pediatric and school-age vision screening in the United States: Rationale, components, and future directions. *Children (Basel), 10*(3). https://doi.org/10.3390/children10030490

American Academy of Family Physicians. (n.d.). Clinical preventive service recommendation: Visual difficulties and impairment. https://www.aafp.org/family-physician/patient-care/clinical-recommendations/all-clinical-recommendations/visual.html

American Academy of Ophthalmology. (2018). Preferred Practice Pattern Guidelines. American Academy of Ophthalmology Pediatric Ophthalmology/Strabismus Panel. www.aao.org/ppp.eith.

___. (2022). Vision screening for infants and children. https://www.aao.org/Assets/660a518b-66d6-435d-a614-99b21853626d/638006528877300000/vision-screening-for-infants-and-children-2022-pdf

American Academy of Optometry. (2016). American Academy of Optometry policy statement: Childhood vision screening. https://aaopt.org/position-paper/

American Association for Pediatric Ophthalmology and Strabismus. (n.d.). Vision screening recommendations. https://higherlogicdownload.s3.amazonaws.com/AAPOS/159c8d7c-f577-4c85-bf77-ac8e4f0865bd/UploadedImages/Documents/vision_screening_rec.pdf

American Optometric Association. (2017). Comprehensive Pediatric Eye and Vision Examination. https://www.aoa.org/AOA/Documents/Practice%20Management/Clinical%20Guidelines/EBO%20Guidelines/Comprehensive%20Pediatric%20Eye%20and%20Vision%20Exam.pdf

American Optometric Association, & Cary, D. (2018). *AOA Advocacy Tool Kit.* https://www.aoa.org/AOA/Documents/Advocacy/AOA%20Children%27s%20Vision%20Advocacy%20Toolkit%20MASTER%201.30.18.pdf

Andersen, R. A. (1968). *A behavioral model of families' use of health services*. Center for Health Administration Studies, University of Chicago.

Andersen, R. M. (1995). Revisiting the behavioral model and access to medical care: Does it matter? *Journal of Health and Social Behavior, 36*(1), 1–10. https://doi.org/10.2307/2137284

Andersen, R. M., & Davidson, P. L. (2007). Improving access to care in America: Individual and contextual indicators. In R. M. Andersen, T. H. Rice, & G. F. Kominski (Eds.), *Changing the U.S. Health Care System: Key Issues in Health Services Policy and Management* (3rd ed., pp. 3–31). Jossey-Bass.

Antonio-Aguirre, B., Block, S. S., Asare, A. O., Baldanado, K., Ciner, E. B., Coulter, R. A., DeCarlo, D. K., Drews-Botsch, C., Fishman, D., Hartmann, E. E., Killeen, O. J., Yuen, J., & Collins, M. E. (2024). Association of sociodemographic characteristics with pediatric vision screening and eye care: An analysis of the 2021 National Survey of Children's Health. *Ophthalmology, 131*(5), 611–621. https://doi.org/10.1016/j.ophtha.2023.12.005

Anzeljc, S., Ziemnik, L., Koscher, S., Klein, W., Bridge, C., & Van Horn, A. (2019). Preschool vision screening collaborative: Successful uptake of guidelines in primary care. *Pediatric Quality & Safety, 4*(6), e241. https://doi.org/10.1097/pq9.0000000000000241

Arnold, R. W., Arnold, A. W., Hunt-Smith, T. T., Grendahl, R. L., & Winkle, R. K. (2018a). The positive predictive value of smartphone photoscreening in pediatric practices. *Journal of Pediatric Ophthalmology and Strabismus, 55*(6), 393–396. https://doi.org/10.3928/01913913-20180710-01

Arnold, R. W., Donahue, S. P., Silbert, D. I., Longmuir, S. Q., Bradford, G. E., Peterseim, M. M. W., Hutchinson, A. K., O'Neil, J. W., de Alba Campomanes, A. G., Pineles, S. L., & AAPOS Vision Screening and Research Committees. (2022). AAPOS uniform guidelines for instrument-based pediatric vision screen validation 2021. *Journal of American Association for Pediatric Ophthalmology and Strabismus, 26*(1), e1–e6. https://doi.org/10.1016/j.jaapos.2021.09.009

Arnold, R. W., O'Neil, J. W., Cooper, K. L., Silbert, D. I., & Donahue, S. P. (2018b). Evaluation of a smartphone photoscreening app to detect refractive amblyopia risk factors in children aged 1-6 years. *Clinical Ophthalmology, 12*, 1533–1537. https://doi.org/10.2147/OPTH.S171935

Asare, A. O., Malvankar-Mehta, M. S., & Makar, I. (2017). Community vision screening in preschoolers: initial experience using the Plusoptix S12C automated photoscreening camera. Canadian Journal of *Ophthalmology, 52*(5), 480–485. https://doi.org/10.1016/j.jcjo.2017.02.002

Asare, A. O., Maurer, D., Wong, A. M. F., Ungar, W. J., & Saunders, N. (2022). Socioeconomic status and vision care services in Ontario, Canada: A population-based cohort study. *The Journal of Pediatrics, 241*, 212–220.. https://doi.org/10.1016/j.jpeds.2021.10.020

Bastawrous, A., Rono, H. K., Livingstone, I. A., Weiss, H. A., Jordan, S., Kuper, H., & Burton, M. J. (2015). Development and Validation of a smartphone-based visual acuity test (peek acuity) for clinical practice and community-based fieldwork. *JAMA Ophthalmology, 133*(8), 930–937. https://doi.org/10.1001/jamaophthalmol.2015.1468

Bastawrous, A. & Peek Vision. (n.d.). *Making the invisible, visible*. https://peekvision.org/wp-content/uploads/2023/11/Peek-Vision-Brochure.pdf

Berkowitz, S. T., Finn, A. P., Parikh, R., Kuriyan, A. E., & Patel, S. (2024). Ophthalmology workforce projections in the United States, 2020 to 2035. *Ophthalmology, 131*(2), 133–139. https://doi.org/10.1016/j.ophtha.2023.09.018

Berntsen, D. A., & Walline, J. J. (2023). Delaying the onset of nearsightedness. *JAMA. 329*(6):465–466. doi:10.1001/jama.2022.24386

Bhaskaran, A., Babu, M., Abhilash, B., Sudhakar, N. A., & Dixitha, V. (2022). Comparison of smartphone application-based visual acuity with traditional visual acuity chart for use in tele-ophthalmology. *Taiwan Journal of Ophthalmology, 12*(2), 155–163. https://doi.org/10.4103/tjo.tjo_7_22

Biviji, R., Vora, N., Thomas, N., Sheridan, D., Reynolds, C. M., Kyaruzi, F., & Reddy, S. (2024). Evaluating the network adequacy of vision care services for children in Arizona: A cross-sectional study. *AIMS Public Health, 11*(1), 141–159. https://doi.org/10.3934/publichealth.2024007

Blanchard, J., Ogle, K., Thomas, O., Lung, D., Asplin, B., & Lurie, N. (2008). Access to appointments based on insurance status in Washington, D.C. *Journal of Health Care for the Poor and Underserved, 19*(3), 687–696. https://doi.org/10.1353/hpu.0.0036

Bodack, M. I., Chung, I., & Krumholtz, I. (2010). An analysis of vision screening data from New York City public schools. *Optometry, 81*(9), 476–484. https://doi.org/10.1016/j.optm.2010.05.006

Brener, N. D., Wheeler, L., Wolfe, L. C., Vernon-Smiley, M., & Caldart-Olson, L. (2007). Health services: Results from the School Health Policies and Programs Study 2006. *Journal of School Health, 77*(7), 464–485. https://doi.org/10.1111/j.1746-1561.2007.00230.x

Bright Futures, & American Academy of Pediatrics. (2022). *Recommendations for preventive pediatric health care.* https://downloads.aap.org/AAP/PDF/periodicity_schedule.pdf

Brody, B. L., Roch-Levecq, A. C., Klonoff-Cohen, H. S., & Brown, S. I. (2007). Refractive errors in low-income preschoolers. *Ophthalmic Epidemiology, 14*(4), 223–229. https://doi.org/10.1080/01658100701486822

Bullimore, M. A., & Brennan, N. A. (2019). Myopia control: Why each diopter matters. *Optometry and Vision Science, 96*(6), 463–465. https://doi.org/10.1097/opx.0000000000001367

Bullimore, M. A., Brennan, N. A., & Flitcroft, D. I. (2023). The future of clinical trials of myopia control. *Ophthalmic & Physiological Optics: The Journal of the British College of Ophthalmic Opticians (Optometrists), 43*(3), 525–533. https://doi.org/10.1111/opo.13120

Burn, H., Hamm, L., Black, J., Burnett, A., Harwood, M., Burton, M. J., Evans, J. R., & Ramke, J. (2021). Eye care delivery models to improve access to eye care for Indigenous peoples in high-income countries: A scoping review. *BMJ Global Health, 6*(3), e005208. https://doi.org/10.1136/bmjgh-2020-004484

Burton, M. J., Ramke, J., Marques, A. P., Bourne, R. R. A., Congdon, N., Jones, I., Ah Tong, B. A. M., Arunga, S., Bachani, D., Bascaran, C., Bastawrous, A., Blanchet, K., Braithwaite, T., Buchan, J. C., Cairns, J., Cama, A., Chagunda, M., Chuluunkhuu, C., Cooper, A., Crofts-Lawrence, J., … Faal, H. B. (2021). The Lancet Global Health Commission on Global Eye Health: Vision beyond 2020. *The Lancet Global Health Commission, 9*(4), e489–e551. https://doi.org/10.1016/S2214-109X(20)30488-5

Centers for Medicare & Medicaid Services. (n.d.a). Early and periodic screening, diagnostic, and treatment. https://www.medicaid.gov/medicaid/benefits/early-and-periodic-screening-diagnostic-and-treatment/index.html

___. (n.d.b). Information on Essential Health Benefits (EHB) benchmark plans. https://www.cms.gov/marketplace/resources/data/essential-health-benefits

___. (2024). *2024 mandatory core set of children's health care quality measures for Medicaid and CHIP (Child Core Set).* https://www.medicaid.gov/sites/default/files/2023-08/2024-child-core-set_0.pdf

Chamberlain, P., Lazon de la Jara, P., Arumugam, B., & Bullimore, M. A. (2021). Axial length targets for myopia control. *Ophthalmic & Physiological Optics: The Journal of the British College of Ophthalmic Opticians (Optometrists), 41*(3), 523–531. https://doi.org/10.1111/opo.12812

Chaplin, P. K., & Bradford, G. E. (2011). A historical review of distance vision screening eye charts: What to toss, what to keep, and what to replace. *NASN School Nurse, 26*(4), 221–228. https://doi.org/10.1177/1942602x11411094

Chen, A. H., Abu Bakar, N. F., & Arthur, P. (2019). Comparison of the pediatric vision screening program in 18 countries across five continents. *Journal of Current Ophthalmology, 31*(4), 357–365. https://doi.org/10.1016/j.joco.2019.07.006

Child and Adolescent Health Measurement Initiative. (2018-2019). *National Survey of Children's Health (NSCH) data query.* Data Resource Center for Child and Adolescent Health supported by the U.S. Department of Health and Human Services, Health Resources and Services Administration (HRSA), Maternal and Child Health Bureau (MCHB). www.childhealthdata.org

Chu, R., Huang, K., Barnhardt, C., & Chen, A. (2015). The effect of an on-site vision examination on adherence to vision screening recommendations. *Journal of School Nursing, 31*(2), 84–90. https://doi.org/10.1177/1059840514524599

Ciner, E., Cotter, S., Kulp, M., Hatch, S., Jackson, K., Moore, B., Mutti, D., & Summers, A. (2016). *Childhood Vision Screening.* https://aaopt.org/position-paper/

Collins, M. E., Guo, X., Mudie, L. I., Slavin, R. E., Madden, N., Chang, D., Owoeye, J., Repka, M. X., & Friedman, D. S. (2022a). Baseline vision results from the Baltimore Reading and Eye Disease Study. *Canadian Journal of Ophthalmology, 57*(1), 29–35. https://doi.org/10.1016/j.jcjo.2021.02.014

Collins, M. E., Guo, X., Repka, M. X., Neitzel, A. J., & Friedman, D. S. (2022b). Lessons learned from school-based delivery of vision care in Baltimore, Maryland. *Asia-Pacific Journal of Ophthalmology, 11*(1), 6–11. https://doi.org/10.1097/apo.0000000000000488

Committee on Practice and Ambulatory Medicine, Section on Ophthalmology. American Association of Certified Orthoptists, American Association for Pediatric Ophthalmology and Strabismus, & American Academy of Ophthalmology. (2003). Eye examination in infants, children, and young adults by pediatricians. *Pediatrics, 111*(4 Pt 1), 902–907. https://pubmed.ncbi.nlm.nih.gov/12671132/

Committee on Practice and Ambulatory Medicine, Section on Ophthalmology, American Association of Certified Orthoptists, American Association for Pediatric Ophthalmology and Strabismus, American Academy of Ophthalmology, Simon, G. R., Boudreau, A. D. A., Baker, C. N., Barden, G. A., Hackell, J. M., Hardin, A. P., Meade, K. E., Moore, S. B., Richerson, J., Lehman, S. S., Granet, D. B., Bradford, G. E., Rubin, S. E., Siatkowski, R. M., & Suh, D. W. (2016). Visual System Assessment in Infants, Children, and Young Adults by Pediatricians. *Pediatrics, 137*(1), 28–30. https://doi.org/10.1542/peds.2015-3596

Congdon, N., Zheng, M., Sharma, A., Choi, K., Song, Y., Zhang, M., Wang, M., Zhou, Z., Li, L., Liu, X., Liu, X., & Lam, D. S. C. (2008). Prevalence and Determinants of spectacle nonwear among rural Chinese secondary schoolchildren. *Archives of Ophthalmology, 126*(12), 1717–1723. https://doi.org/10.1001/archopht.126.12.1717

Cotter, S. A., Cyert, L. A., Miller, J. M., & Quinn, G. E. for the National Expert Panel to the National Center for Children's Vision and Eye Health. (2015). Vision screening for children 36 to <72 months: Recommended practices. *Optometry and Vision Science, 92*(1), 6–16. https://doi.org/10.1097%2FOPX.0000000000000429

Couser, N. L., & Smith-Marshall, J. (2011). The Washington Metropolitan Pediatric Vision Screening Quality Control Assessment. *ISRN Ophthalmology, 2011,* 1–5. https://doi.org/10.5402/2011/801957

Davara, N. D., Chintoju, R., Manchikanti, N., Thinley, C., Vaddavalli, P. K., Rani, P. K., & Satgunam, P. (2022). Feasibility study for measuring patients' visual acuity at home by their caregivers. *Indian Journal of Ophthalmology, 70*(6), 2125–2130. https://doi.org/10.4103/ijo.IJO_3085_21

Davidson, S. L., O'Hara, M., & Wagner, R. S. (2016). Management of progressive myopia. *Journal of Pediatric Ophthalmology & Strabismus, 53*(3), 134–136. https://doi.org/10.3928/01913913-20160418-01

De Samanta, A., Mauntana, S., Barsi, Z., Yarlagadda, B., & Nelson, P. C. (2023). Is your vision blurry? A systematic review of home-based visual acuity for telemedicine. *Journal of Telemedicine and Telecare, 29*(2), 81–90. https://doi.org/10.1177/1357633X20970398

de Venecia, B., Bradfield, Y., Trane, R. M., Bareiro, A., & Scalamogna, M. (2018). Validation of Peek Acuity application in pediatric screening programs in Paraguay. *International Journal of Ophthalmology, 11*(8), 1384–1389. https://doi.org/10.18240/ijo.2018.08.21

Department of Health and Human Services. (2023). *Medicaid Program and CHIP mandatory Medicaid and Children's Health Insurance Program (CHIP) core set reporting 2023.* https://www.govinfo.gov/content/pkg/FR-2023-08-31/pdf/2023-18669.pdf

Detty, A. M. R. (2012). School-Based survey Participation: Oral health and BMI survey of Ohio third graders. *Maternal and Child Health Journal, 17*(7), 1208–1214. https://doi.org/10.1007/s10995-012-1107-7

Dhirar, N., Dudeja, S., Duggal, M., Gupta, P. C., Jaiswal, N., Singh, M., & Ram, J. (2020). Compliance to spectacle use in children with refractive errors—A systematic review and meta-analysis. *BMC Ophthalmology, 20*(1), 71. https://doi.org/10.1186/s12886-020-01345-9

Diao, W., Patel, J., Snitzer, M., Pond, M., Rabinowitz, M. P., Ceron, G., Bagley, K., Dennis, K., Weiner, R., Martinez-Helfman, S., Maria, K. S., Burke, B., Aultman, W. B., & Levin, A. V. (2016). The effectiveness of a mobile clinic in improving follow-up eye care for at-risk children. *Journal of Pediatric Ophthalmology & Strabismus, 53*(6), 344–348. https://doi.org/10.3928/01913913-20160629-04

Donahue, S. P., Arthur, B., Neely, D. E., Arnold, R. W., Silbert, D., Ruben, J. B., & POS Vision Screening Committee (2013). Guidelines for automated preschool vision screening: a 10-year, evidence-based update. *Journal of AAPOS, 17*(1), 4–8. https://doi.org/10.1016/j.jaapos.2012.09.012

Donahue, S. P., Baker, C. N., Committee on Practice and Ambulatory Medicine, Section on Ophthalmology, American Association of Certified Orthoptists, American Association for Pediatric Ophthalmology and Strabismus, American Academy of Ophthalmology, Simon, G. R., Boudreau, A. D. A., Barden, G. A., 3rd, Hackell, J. M., Hardin, A. P., Meade, K. E., Moore, S. B., Richerson, J., Lehman, S. S., Granet, D. B., Bradford, G. E., Rubin, S. E., Siatkowski, M., & Suh, D. W. (2016). Procedures for the evaluation of the visual system by pediatricians. *Pediatrics, 137*(1). https://doi.org/10.1542/peds.2015-3597

Donahue, S. P., Baker, J. D., Scott, W. E., Rychwalski, P., Neely, D. E., Tong, P., Bergsma, D., Lenahan, D., Rush, D., Heinlein, K., Walkenbach, R., & Johnson, T. M. (2006). Lions Clubs International Foundation core four photoscreening: Results from 17 programs and 400,000 preschool children. *Journal of AAPOS, 10*(1), 44–48. https://doi.org/10.1016/j.jaapos.2005.08.007

Donahue, S. P., & Nixon, C. N. (2016). Visual system assessment in infants, children, and young adults by pediatricians. *Pediatrics, 137*(1), 28–30. https://doi.org/10.1542/peds.2015-3596

Donahue, S. P., Ruben, J. B., American Academy of Ophthalmology, American Academy of Pediatrics, Ophthalmology Section, American Association for Pediatric Ophthalmology and Strabismus, Children's Eye Foundation, & American Association of Certified Orthoptists (2011). US Preventive Services Task Force vision screening recommendations. *Pediatrics, 127*(3), 569–570. https://doi.org/10.1542/peds.2011-0020

Dotan, G., Truong, B., Snitzer, M., McCauley, C., Martinez-Helfman, S., Santa Maria, K., & Levin, A. V. (2015). Outcomes of an inner-city vision outreach program: Give kids sight day. *JAMA Ophthalmology, 133*(5), 527–532. https://doi.org/10.1001/jamaophthalmol.2015.8

Drescher, J., & Domingue, B. W. (2023). The distribution of child physicians and early academic achievement. *Health Services Research, 58*(Suppl 2), 165–174. https://doi.org/10.1111/1475-6773.14188

Dudovitz, R. N., Izadpanah, N., Chung, P. J., & Slusser, W. (2015). Parent, teacher, and student perspectives on how corrective lenses improve child wellbeing and school function. *Maternal and Child Health Journal, 20*(5), 974–983. https://doi.org/10.1007/s10995-015-1882-z

Dutton, D. B., & Levine, S. (1989). Socioeconomic status and health: Overview, methodological critique, and reformulation. In J. P. Bunker, D. S. Gomby, & B. H. Kehrer (Eds.), *Pathways to Health: The Role of Social Factors* (pp. 29–69). The Henry J. Kaiser Family Foundation.

Ekdawi, N., Kipp, M. A., & Kipp, M. P. (2021). Mandated kindergarten eye examinations in a US suburban clinic: Is it worth the cost? *Clinical Ophthalmology, 15*, 1331–1337. https://doi.org/10.2147/OPTH.S300725

Elam, A. R., Tseng, V. L., Rodriguez, T. M., Mike, E. V., Warren, A. K., Coleman, A. L., & American Academy of Ophthalmology Taskforce on Disparities in Eye Care (2022). Disparities in vision health and eye care. *Ophthalmology, 129*(10), e89–e113. https://doi.org/10.1016/j.ophtha.2022.07.010

Ethan, D., Basch, C. E., Platt, R., Bogen, E., & Zybert, P. (2010). Implementing and evaluating a school-based program to improve childhood vision. *The Journal of School Health, 80*(7), 340–370. https://doi.org/10.1111/j.1746-1561.2010.00511.x

Fairbrother, G., Siegel, M. J., Friedman, S., Kory, P. D., & Butts, G. C. (2001). Impact of financial incentives on documented immunization rates in the inner city: results of a randomized controlled trial. *Ambulatory Pediatrics, 1*(4), 206–212. https://doi.org/10.1367/1539-4409(2001)001<0206:iofiod>2.0.co;2

Feng, P. W., Ahluwalia, A., Feng, H., & Adelman, R. A. (2020). National trends in the United States eye care workforce from 1995 to 2017. *American Journal of Ophthalmology, 218*, 128–135. https://doi.org/10.1016/j.ajo.2020.05.018

Flitcroft, D. I., He, M., Jonas, J. B., Jong, M., Naidoo, K., Ohno-Matsui, K., Rahi, J., Resnikoff, S., Vitale, S., & Yannuzzi, L. (2019) IMI – Defining and classifying myopia: A proposed set of standards for clinical and epidemiologic studies. *Investigative Ophthalmology & Visual Science, 60*(3), M20–M30. https://doi.org/10.1167/iovs.18-25957

Foe, G., & Larson, E. L. (2016). Reading level and comprehension of research consent forms: An integrative review. *Journal of Empirical Research on Human Research Ethics, 11*(1), 31–46. https://doi.org/10.1177/1556264616637483

Frazier, M., Garces, I., Scarinci, I., & Marsh-Tootle, W. (2009). Seeking eye care for children: perceptions among Hispanic immigrant parents. *Journal of Immigrant and Minority Health, 11*(3), 215–221. https://doi.org/10.1007/s10903-008-9160-4

Furtado, J. M., Fernandes, A. G., Silva, J. C., Del Pino, S., & Hommes, C. (2023). Indigenous eye health in the Americas: The burden of vision impairment and ocular diseases. *International Journal of Environmental Research and Public Health, 20*(5). https://doi.org/10.3390%2Fijerph20053820

Guo, X., Nguyen, A. M., Vongsachang, H., Kretz, A. M., Mukherjee, M. R., Neitzel, A. J., Shakarchi, A. F., Friedman, D. S., Repka, M. X., & Collins, M. E. (2022). Refractive error findings in students who failed school-based vision screening. *Ophthalmic Epidemiology, 29*(4), 426–434. https://doi.org/10.1080/09286586.2021.1954664Haller, K., Stolfi, A., & Duby, J. (2022). Comparison of unmet health care needs in children with intellectual disability, autism spectrum disorder and both disorders combined. *Journal of Intellectual Disability Research, 66*(7), 617–627. https://doi.org/10.1111/jir.12932

Hamm, L. M., Yashadhana, A., Burn, H., Black, J., Grey, C., Harwood, M., Peiris-John, R., Burton, M. J., Evans, J. R., & Ramke, J. (2021). Interventions to promote access to eyecare for non-dominant ethnic groups in high-income countries: A scoping review. *BMJ Global Health, 6*(9), e006188. https://doi.org/10.1136/bmjgh-2021-006188

Harewood, J. H, Contreras, M. C., Huang, K. H., Leach, S. L., & Wang, J. (2024). [Access to myopia care—A scoping review]. Paper commissioned by the Committee on Focus on Myopia: Pathogenesis and Rising Incidence.

Hariton, E., & Locascio, J. J. (2018). Randomised controlled trials—The gold standard for effectiveness research: Study design: Randomised controlled trials. *BJOG: An International Journal of Obstetrics and Gynaecology, 125*(13), 1716. https://doi.org/10.1111/1471-0528.15199

Hark, L. A., Shiuey, E., Yu, M., Tran, E., Mayro, E. L., Zhan, T., Pond, M., Tran, J., Siam, L., & Levin, A. V. (2018). Efficacy and outcomes of a summer-based pediatric vision screening program. *Journal of AAPOS, 22*(4), 309.e1–309.e7. https://doi.org/10.1016/j.jaapos.2018.04.006

Harris, N., Roche, E., Lee, P., Asper, L., Wiseman, N., Keel, R., Duffy, S., & Sofija, E. (2023). Vision screening outcomes of 4-5 year-olds reflect the social gradient. *Clinical & Experimental Optometry, 106*(6), 640–644. https://doi.org/10.1080/08164622.2022.2109947

Hartmann, E. E., Block, S. S., Wallace, D. K., & National Expert Panel to the National Center for Children's Vision and Eye Health. (2015). Vision and eye health in children 36 to <72 months: proposed data system. *Optometry and Vision Science, 92*(1), 24–30. https://doi.org/10.1097%2FOPX.0000000000000445

Hartmann, E. E., Bradford, G. E., Chaplin, P. K., Johnson, T., Kemper, A. R., Kim, S., Marsh-Tootle, W., & PUPVS Panel for the American Academy of Pediatrics. (2006). Project Universal Preschool Vision Screening: A demonstration project. *Pediatrics, 117*(2), e226–e237. https://doi.org/10.1542/peds.2004-2809

Healthy People 2030. (n.d.). Social determinants of health. https://health.gov/healthypeople/priority-areas/social-determinants-health

Hendler, K., Mehravaran, S., Lu, X., Brown, S. I., Mondino, B. J., & Coleman, A. L. (2016). Refractive errors and amblyopia in the UCLA Preschool Vision Program: First year results. *American Journal of Ophthalmology, 172*, 80–86. https://doi.org/10.1016/j.ajo.2016.09.010

Henstenburg, J., Thau, A., Markovitz, M., Plumb, J., & Markovitz, B. (2019). Visual impairment and ocular pathology among the urban American homeless. *Journal of Health Care for the Poor and Underserved, 30*(3), 940–950. https://doi.org/10.1353/hpu.2019.0066

Hered, R. W., & Wood, D. L. (2013). Preschool vision screening in primary care pediatric practice. *Public Health Reports, 128*(3), 189–197. https://doi.org/10.1177/003335491312800309

Heslin, K. C., Casey, R., Shaheen, M. A., Cardenas, F., & Baker, R. S. (2006). Racial and ethnic differences in unmet need for vision care among children with special health care needs. *Archives of Ophthalmology, 124*(6), 895–902. https://doi.org/10.1001/archopht.124.6.895

Hillrom. (2020). *Reimbursement guide for instrument-based vision screening.* https://www.hillrom.com/content/dam/hillrom-aem/us/en/marketing/products/spot-vision-screener/documents/APR101102-EN-R1_Spot-Vision-Screener-Reimbursement-Guide_LR.pdf

Holmes, J. M., & Levi, D. M. (2018). Treatment of amblyopia as a function of age. *Vision Neuroscience, 35*, E015. https://doi.org/10.1017/S0952523817000220

Hoover, K., Di Guglielmo, M. D., & Perry, B. (2023). Disparities in vision screening in primary care for young children with autism spectrum disorder. *Pediatrics, 151*(4). https://doi.org/10.1542/peds.2022-059998

Hou, W., Norton, T. T., Hyman, L., Gwiazda, J., & COMET Group (2018). Axial elongation in myopic children and its association with myopia progression in the correction of myopia evaluatin trial. *Eye & Contact Lens, 44*(4), 248–259. https://doi.org/10.1097/ICL.0000000000000505

Huang, A. H., Guo, X., Mudie, L. I., Wolf, R., Owoeye, J., Repka, M. X., Friedman, D. S., Slavin, R. E., & Collins, M. E. (2019). Baltimore Reading and Eye Disease Study (BREDS): Compliance and satisfaction with glasses usage. *Journal of AAPOS, 23*(4), 207.e1–207.e6. https://doi.org/10.1016/j.jaapos.2019.01.018

Hunter, D. G. (2013). Targeting treatable disease—not just risk factors—in pediatric vision screening. *Journal of AAPOS, 17*(1), 2–3. https://doi.org/10.1016/j.jaapos.2012.10.009

Hutchinson, A. K., Morse, C. L., Hercinovic, A., Cruz, O. A., Sprunger, D. T., Repka, M. X., Lambert, S. R., Wallace, D. K., & American Academy of Ophthalmology Preferred Practice Pattern Pediatric Ophthalmology/Strabismus Panel. (2023). Pediatric eye evaluations preferred practice pattern. *Ophthalmology, 130*(3), P222–P270. https://doi.org/10.1016/j.ophtha.2022.10.030

Illinois State Board of Education (2024). Data & accountability: Health requirements/student health data.

Ji, P., Flay, B., Dubois, D., Patton, V., & Day, J. (2006). Consent form return rates for third-grade urban elementary students. *American Journal of Health Behavior, 30*(5), 467–474. https://doi.org/10.5555/ajhb.2006.30.5.467

Jin, Y. P., & Trope, G. E. (2011). Eye care utilization in Canada: disparity in the publicly funded health care system. *Canadian Journal of Ophthalmology. Journal Canadien D'ophtalmologie, 46*(2), 133–138. https://doi.org/10.3129/i10-120

Jonas, D. E., Amick, H. R., Wallace, I. F., Feltner, C., Vander Schaaf, E. B., Brown, C. L., & Baker, C. (2017). Vision screening in children aged 6 months to 5 years: Evidence report and systematic review for the US Preventive Services Task Force. *JAMA, 318*(9), 845–858. https://doi.org/10.1001/jama.2017.9900

Jones-Jordan, L. A., Sinnott, L. T., Manny, R. E., Cotter, S. A., Kleinstein, R. N., Mutti, D. O., Twelker, J. D., Zadnik, K., & Collaborative Longitudinal Evaluation of Ethnicity and Refractive Error (CLEERE) Study Group. (2010). Early childhood refractive error and parental history of myopia as predictors of myopia. *Investigative Ophthalmology & Visual Science, 51*(1), 115–121. https://doi.org/10.1167/iovs.08-3210

Jong, M., Jonas, J. B., Wolffsohn, J. S., Berntsen, D. A., Cho, P., Clarkson-Townsend, D., Flitcroft, D. I., Gifford, K. L., Haarman, A. E. G., Pardue, M. T., Richdale, K., Sankaridurg, P., Tedja, M. S., Wildsoet, C. F., Bailey-Wilson, J. E., Guggenheim, J. A., Hammond, C. J., Kaprio, J., MacGregor, S., & Smith, E. L., 3rd. (2021). IMI 2021 Yearly Digest. *Investigative Ophthalmology & Visual Science*, *62*(5), 7. https://doi.org/10.1167/iovs.62.5.7

Kemper, A. R., & Clark, S. J. (2006). Preschool vision screening in pediatric practices. *Clinical Pediatrics*, *45*(3), 263–266. https://doi.org/10.1177/000992280604500309

Kemper, A. R., Bruckman, D., & Freed, G. L. (2003). Receipt of specialty eye care by children. *Ambulatory Pediatrics*, *3*(5), 270–274. https://doi.org/10.1367/1539-4409(2003)003<0270:ROSECB>2.0.CO;2

Kemper, A. R., Uren, R. L., & Clark, S. J. (2006). Barriers to follow-up eye care after preschool vision screening in the primary care setting: findings from a pilot study. *Journal of AAPOS*, *10*(5), 476–478. https://doi.org/10.1016/j.jaapos.2006.07.009

Kentucky Department of Education. (2024). *Student health services: Student health data.* https://www.education.ky.gov/districts/SHS/Pages/Student-Health-Data.aspx

Killeen, O. J., Cho, J., Newman-Casey, P. A., Kana, L., & Woodward, M. A. (2021). Barriers and facilitators to obtaining eyeglasses for vulnerable patients in a Michigan free clinic. *Optometry and Vision Science*, *98*(3), 243–249. https://doi.org/10.1097/opx.0000000000001661

Killeen, O. J., Choi, H., Kannan, N. S., Asare, A. O., Stagg, B. C., & Ehrlich, J. R. (2023). Association between health insurance and primary care vision testing among children and adolescents. *JAMA Ophthalmology*, *141*(9), 909–911. https://doi.org/10.1001/jamaophthalmol.2023.3644

Kim, P., Daly, J. M., Berkowitz, S., & Levy, B. T. (2020). Use of the Fluoride Varnish Billing Code in a Tertiary Care Center Setting. *Journal of Primary Care & Community Health*, *11*. https://doi.org/10.1177/2150132720913736

Kimel, L. S. (2006). Lack of follow-up exams after failed school vision screenings: An investigation of contributing factors. *The Journal of School Nursing*, *22*(3), 156–162. https://doi.org/10.1177/10598405060220030601

Kindle, T., & Spencer, T. (2019). A review of childhood vision screening laws and programs across the United States. *South Dakota Medicine*, *72*(7), 299–302. https://pubmed.ncbi.nlm.nih.gov/31461584/

Kleinstein, R. N., Mutti, D. O., Sinnott, L. T., Jones-Jordan, L. A., Cotter, S. A., Manny, R. E., Twelker, J. D., Zadnik, K., & Collaborative Longitudinal Evaluation of Ethnicity and Refractive Error Study Group. (2021). Uncorrected refractive error and distance visual acuity in children aged 6 to 14 years. *Optometry and Vision Science*, *98*(1), 3–12. https://doi.org/10.1097/opx.0000000000001630

Kleinstein, R. N., Sinnott, L. T., Jones-Jordan, L. A., Sims, J., Zadnik, K., & Collaborative Longitudinal Evaluation of Ethnicity and Refractive Error Study Group. (2012). New cases of myopia in children. *Archives of Ophthalmology*, *130*(10), 1274–1279. https://doi.org/10.1001/archophthalmol.2012.1449

Kodjebacheva, G., Brown, E. R., Estrada, L., Yu, F., & Coleman, A. L. (2011). Uncorrected refractive error among first-grade students of different racial/ethnic groups in southern California: Results a year after school-mandated vision screening. *Journal of Public Health Management and Practice*, *17*(6), 499–505. https://doi.org/10.1097/PHH.0b013e3182113891

Kodjebacheva, G. D., Maliski, S., & Coleman, A. L. (2015). Use of eyeglasses among children in elementary school: Perceptions, behaviors, and interventions discussed by parents, school nurses, and teachers during focus groups. *American Journal of Health Promotion*, *29*(5), 324–331. https://doi.org/10.4278/ajhp.120315-QUAL-140

Kodjebacheva, G., Brown, E. R., Estrada, L., Yu, F., & Coleman, A. L. (2011). Uncorrected refractive error among first-grade students of different racial/ethnic groups in southern California: results a year after school-mandated vision screening. *Journal of Public Health Management and Practice*, *17*(6), 499-505. doi:10.1097/PHH.0b013e3182113891

Kruszewski, K., May, C., & Silverstein, E. (2023). Evaluation of a combined school-based vision screening and mobile clinic program. *Journal of AAPOS, 27*(2), 91.e1–91.e5. https://doi.org/10.1016/j.jaapos.2023.01.010

Kulp, M. T., & Group, V. I. P. S. (2009). Findings from the Vision in Preschoolers (VIP) Study. *Optometry and Vision Science, 86*(6), 619–623. https://doi.org/10.1097/OPX.0b013e3181a59bf5

Kulp, M. T., Ciner, E., Maguire, M., Moore, B., Pentimonti, J., Pistilli, M., Cyert, L., Candy, T. R., Quinn, G., & Ying, G. (2016). Uncorrected hyperopia and preschool early literacy. *Ophthalmology, 123*(4), 681–689. https://doi.org/10.1016/j.ophtha.2015.11.023

Kulp, M. T., Ciner, E., Ying, G. S., Candy, T. R., Moore, B. D., Orel-Bixler, D., & VIP Study Group, and the VIP-HIP Study Group. (2022). Vision screening, vision disorders, and impacts of hyperopia in young children: Outcomes of the Vision in Preschoolers (VIP) and Vision in Preschoolers - Hyperopia in Preschoolers (VIP-HIP) studies. *Asia-Pacific Journal of Ophthalmology, 11*(1), 52–58. https://doi.org/10.1097/APO.0000000000000483

Lalor, S. J. H., Formankiewicz, M. A., & Waugh, S. J. (2016). Crowding and visual acuity measured in adults using paediatric test letters, pictures and symbols. *Vision Research, 121*, 31–38. https://doi.org/10.1016/j.visres.2016.01.007

Lam, M., & Grasse, N. (2019). Community health centers (CHCs) under environmental uncertainty: An examination of the Affordable Care Act of 2010 and early Medicaid expansion on CHC margin. *Nonprofit Policy Forum, 10*(2). https://doi.org/10.1515/npf-2019-0016

Law, M. X., Pimentel, M. F., Oldenburg, C. E., & de Alba Campomanes, A. G. (2020). Positive predictive value and screening performance of GoCheck Kids in a primary care university clinic. *Journal of AAPOS, 24*(1), 17.e1–17.e5. https://doi.org/10.1016/j.jaapos.2019.11.006

Lee, K. E., Sussberg, J. A., Nelson, L. B., & Thuma, T. B. (2023). What we learned about the economic and workforce issues in pediatric ophthalmology: Access to eye care and possible solutions. *Journal of Pediatric Ophthalmology & Strabismus, 60*(5), 323–329. https://doi.org/10.3928/01913913-20230620-02

Lee, P. P., Hoskins, H. D., & Parke, D. W. (2007). Access to care: Eye care provider workforce considerations in 2020. *Archives of Ophthalmology, 125*(3), 406–410. https://doi.org/10.1001/archopht.125.3.406

Lee, P. P., West, S. K., Block, S. S., Clayton, J., Cotch, M. F., Flynn, C., Geiss, L. S., Klein, R., Olsen, T. W., Owsley, C., Primo, S. A., Rubin, G. S., Ryskulova, A., Sharma, S., Friedman, D. S., Zhang, X., Crews, J. E., & Saaddine, J. B. (2012). Surveillance of disparities in vision and eye health in the United States: An expert panel's opinions. *American Journal of Ophthalmology, 154*(6 Suppl), S3–S7. https://doi.org/10.1016/j.ajo.2012.09.006

Lee, Y. H., Chen, A. X., Varadaraj, V., Hong, G. H., Chen, Y., Friedman, D. S., Stein, J. D., Kourgialis, N., & Ehrlich, J. R. (2018). Comparison of access to eye care appointments between patients with Medicaid and those with private health care insurance. *JAMA Ophthalmology, 136*(6), 622–629. https://doi.org/10.1001/jamaophthalmol.2018.0813

Levinson, D. R. (2010). Most Medicaid children in nine states are not receiving all required preventive screening services. *Office of Inspector General, U.S. Department of Health and Human Services.* https://oig.hhs.gov/oei/reports/oei-05-08-00520.pdf

Lillvis, J. H., Lillvis, D. F., Towle-Miller, L. M., Wilding, G. E., & Kuo, D. Z. (2020). Association of state vision screening requirements with parent-reported vision testing in young children. *Journal of AAPOS, 24*(5), 291.e1–291.e6. https://doi.org/10.1016/j.jaapos.2020.04.015

Lipson, M. J., Boland, B., & McAlinden, C. (2022). Vision-related quality of life with myopia management: A review. *Contact Lens & Anterior Eye: The Journal of the British Contact Lens Association, 45*(3), 101538. https://doi.org/10.1016/j.clae.2021.101538

Loh, A. R., & Chiang, M. F. (2018). Pediatric vision screening. *Pediatrics in Review, 39*(5), 225–234. https://doi.org/10.1542/pir.2016-0191

Lowry, E. A., & de Alba Campomanes, A. G. (2016). Cost-effectiveness of school-based eye examinations in preschoolers referred for follow-up from visual screening. *JAMA Ophthalmology*, *134*(6), 658–664. https://doi.org/10.1001/jamaophthalmol.2016.0619

Lyons, S. A., Johnson, C., & Majzoub, K. (2011). School based vision centers: Striving to optimize learning. *Work*, *39*(1), 15–19. https://doi.org/10.3233/wor-2011-1146

Ma, X., Zhou, Z., Yi, H., Pang, X., Shi, Y., Chen, Q., Meltzer, M. E., le Cessie, S., He, M., Rozelle, S., Liu, Y., & Congdon, N. (2014). Effect of providing free glasses on children's educational outcomes in China: Cluster randomized controlled trial. *BMJ (Clinical research ed.)*, *349*, g5740. https://doi.org/10.1136/bmj.g5740

Maguire, M. G., & Vision in Preschoolers Study Group. (2007). Children unable to perform screening tests in vision in preschoolers study: Proportion with ocular conditions and impact on measures of test accuracy. *Investigative Ophthalmology & Visual Science*, *48*(1), 83–87. https://doi.org/10.1167/iovs.06-0384

Manny, R. E., Sinnott, L. T., Jones-Jordan, L. A., Messer, D., Twelker, J. D., Cotter, S. A., Kleinstein, R. N., Crescioni, M., & CLEERE Study Group. (2012). Predictors of adequate correction following vision screening failure. *Optometry and Vision Science*, *89*(6), 892–900. https://doi.org/10.1097/OPX.0b013e318255da73

Marsh-Tootle, W. L., Frazier, M. G., Kohler, C. L., Dillard, C. M., Davis, K., Schoenberger, Y. M., & Wall, T. C. (2012). Exploring pre-school vision screening in primary care offices in Alabama. *Optometry and Vision*, *89*(10), 1521–1531. https://doi.org/10.1097/OPX.0b013e318269ca9f

Marsh-Tootle, W. L., Funkhouser, E., Frazier, M. G., Crenshaw, K., & Wall, T. C. (2010). Knowledge, attitudes, and environment: What primary care providers say about pre-school vision screening. *Optometry and Vision Science*, *87*(2), 104–111. https://doi.org/10.1097/OPX.0b013e3181cc8d7c

Marzolf, A. L., Peterseim, M. M., Forcina, B. D., Papa, C., Wilson, M. E., Cheeseman, E. W., & Trivedi, R. H. (2017). Use of the Spot Vision Screener for patients with developmental disability. *Journal of AAPOS*, *21*(4), 313–315.e1. https://doi.org/10.1016/j.jaapos.2017.04.008

McCurry, T. C., Lawrence, L. M., Wilson, M. E., & Mayo, L. (2013). The plusoptiX S08 photoscreener as a vision screening tool for children with autism. *Journal of AAPOS*, *17*(4), 374–377. https://doi.org/10.1016/j.jaapos.2013.05.006

McNamara, N. A., & Polse, K. A. (2019). Community health centers: A model for integrating eye care services with the practice of primary care medicine. *Optometry and Vision Science*, *96*(12), 905–909. https://doi.org/10.1097/OPX.0000000000001458

Medicine, I. O. (2012). *Essential health benefits*. National Academies Press. https://doi.org/10.17226/13234

Messer, D. H., Mitchell, G. L., Twelker, J. D., Crescioni, M., & CLEERE Study Group. (2012). Spectacle wear in children given spectacles through a school-based program. *Optometry and Vision Science*, *89*(1), 19–26. https://doi.org/10.1097/OPX.0b013e3182357f8c

Miller, J. M., Lessin, H. R., American Academy of Pediatrics Section on Ophthalmology, Committee on Practice and Ambulatory Medicine, American Academy of Ophthalmology, American Association for Pediatric Ophthalmology and Strabismus, & American Association of Certified Orthoptists. (2012). Instrument-based pediatric vision screening policy statement. *Pediatrics*, *130*(5), 983–986. https://doi.org/10.1542/peds.2012-2548

Modest, J. R., Majzoub, K. M., Moore, B., Bhambhani, V., McLaughlin, S. R., & Vernacchio, L. (2017). Implementation of instrument-based vision screening for preschool-age children in primary care. *Pediatrics*, *140*(1), e20163745. https://doi.org/10.1542/peds.2016-3745Morrison, A. S. (1998). Screening. In K. J. Rothman & S. Greenland (Eds.), *Modern Epidemiology* (2nd ed., p. 510). Lippincott Williams & Wilkins.

Mu, Y., Bi, H., Ekure, E., Ding, G., Wei, N., Hua, N., Qian, X., & Li, X. (2016). Performance of spot photoscreener in detecting amblyopia risk factors in Chinese pre-school and school age children attending an eye clinic. *PloS One, 11*(2), e0149561. https://doi.org/10.1371/journal.pone.0149561

Muhammad, M., & Tumin, D. (2022). Unmet needs for vision care among children with gaps in health insurance coverage. *Journal of AAPOS, 26*(2), 63.e1–63.e4. https://doi.org/10.1016/j.jaapos.2021.12.005

Musch, D. C., Andrews, C. A., Schumann, R. A., & Baker, J. D. (2022). A comparative study of two photoscreening devices with manual vision screening involving preschool children. *Journal of Pediatric Ophthalmology & Strabismus, 59*(1), 46–52. https://doi.org/10.3928/01913913-20210610-01

National Academies of Sciences, Engineering, and Medicine. (2016). Making eye health a population health imperative: Vision for tomorrow. *The National Academies Press.* https://doi.org/10.17226/23471

National Center for Children's Vision and Eye Health. (2016). Vision screening guidelines by age. https://nationalcenter.preventblindness.org/vision-screening-guidelines-by-age/

National Center for Education Statistics. (n.d.). *Number and percentage of public school students eligible for free or reduced-price lunch, by state: Selected school years, 2000-01 through 2021-22.* https://nces.ed.gov/programs/digest/d22/tables/dt22_204.10.asp

Nebraska Legislature, *State ex rel. Shineman v. Board of Education,* 152 Neb. 644, 42 N.W.2d 168 (1950).

Newacheck, P. W., Hughes, D. C., & Stoddard, J. J. (1996). Children's access to primary care: differences by race, income, and insurance status. *Pediatrics, 97*(1), 26–32.

Nishimura, M., Wong, A., Cohen, A., Thorpe, K., & Maurer, D. (2019). Choosing appropriate tools and referral criteria for vision screening of children aged 4-5 years in Canada: a quantitative analysis. *British Medical Journal Open, 9*(9), e032138. https://doi.org/10.1136/bmjopen-2019-032138

Nishimura, M., Wong, A., Dimaris, H., & Maurer, D. (2020). Feasibility of a school-based vision screening program to detect undiagnosed visual problems in kindergarten children in Ontario. *Canadian Medical Association Journal, 192*(29), E822–E831. https://doi.org/10.1503/cmaj.191085

Nishimura, M., Wong, A., & Maurer, D. (2024). Continued care and provision of glasses are necessary to improve visual and academic outcomes in children: Experience from a cluster-randomized controlled trial of school-based vision screening. *Canadian Journal of Public Health.* https://doi.org/10.17269/s41997-024-00884-8

Nowroozzadeh, M. H. (2016). School-based myopia prevention effort. *JAMA, 315*(8), 819–820. https://jamanetwork.com/journals/jama/fullarticle/2492866

O'Colmain, U., Low, L., Gilmour, C., & MacEwen, C. J. (2016). Vision screening in children: A retrospective study of social and demographic factors with regards to visual outcomes. *British Journal of Ophthalmology, 100*(8), 1109–1113. https://doi.org/10.1136/bjophthalmol-2015-307206

O'Donnell, L., Duran, R., San Doval, A., Breslin, M., & Juhn, G. (1997). Obtaining written parent permission for school-based health surveys of urban young adolescents. *Journal of Adolescent Health, 21*, 376–383. https://doi.org/10.1016/S1054-139X(97)00110-3

O'Hara, M. A. (2016). Instrument-based pediatric vision screening. *Current Opinion in Ophthalmology, 27*(5), 398–401. https://doi.org/10.1097/icu.0000000000000289

Oke, I., Lutz, S. M., Hunter, D. G., & Galbraith, A. A. (2023). Vision screening among children with private insurance: 2010–2019. *Pediatrics, 152*(3), e2023062114. https://doi.org/10.1542/peds.2023-062114

Painter, S., Ramm, L., Wadlow, L., O'Connor, M., & Sond, B. (2021). Parental home vision testing of children during COVID-19 pandemic. *British and Irish Orthoptic Journal, 17*(1), 13–19. https://doi.org/10.22599/bioj.157

Payerols, A., Eliaou, C., Trezeguet, V., Villain, M., & Daien, V. (2016). Accuracy of PlusOptix A09 distance refraction in pediatric myopia and hyperopia. *BMC Ophthalmology, 16*, 72. https://doi.org/10.1186/s12886-016-0247-8

Perez, S., Sabharwal, S., Nakayoshi, A., & de Alba Campomanes, A. G. (2022). Parental perspectives on factors influencing eyeglass wear compliance in preschoolers from low-income families in San Francisco. *Journal of AAPOS, 26*(4), 183.e1–183.e6. https://doi.org/10.1016/j.jaapos.2022.05.004

Peterseim, M. M. W., Papa, C. E., Wilson, M. E., Cheeseman, E. W., Wolf, B. J., Davidson, J. D., & Trivedi, R. H. (2014). Photoscreeners in the pediatric eye office: Compared testability and refractions on high-risk children. *American Journal of Ophthalmology, 158*, 932–938. https://doi.org/10.1016%2Fj.ajo.2014.07.041

Peterseim, M. M., Papa, C. E., Parades, C., Davidson, J., Sturges, A., Oslin, C., Merritt, I., & Morrison, M. (2015). Combining automated vision screening with on-site examinations in 23 schools: ReFocus on Children Program 2012 to 2013. *Journal of Pediatric Ophthalmology and Strabismus, 52*(1), 20–24. https://doi.org/10.3928/01913913-20141124-01

Pirindhavellie, G. P., Yong, A. C., Mashige, K. P., Naidoo, K. S., & Chan, V. F. (2023). The impact of spectacle correction on the well-being of children with vision impairment due to uncorrected refractive error: a systematic review. *BMC Public Health, 23*(1), 1575. https://doi.org/10.1186/s12889-023-16484-z

Pober, J. S., Neuhauser, C. S., & Pober, J. M. (2001). Obstacles facing translational research in academic medical centers. *FASEB Journal, 15*(13), 2303–2313. https://doi.org/10.1096/fj.01-0540lsf

Prevent Blindness. (2020). Pediatric vision benefits available under the Affordable Care Act. https://preventblindness.org/pediatric-vision-benefits-available-under-the-affordable-care-act/

___. (2022). *Analysis of School-Age Vision Screening by State.* https://preventblindness.org/vision-screening-requirements-by-state/

Qian, X., Li, Y., Ding, G., Li, J., Lv, H., Hua, N., Wei, N., He, L., Wei, L., Li, X., & Wang, J. (2019). Compared performance of Spot and SW800 photoscreeners on Chinese children. *The British Journal of Ophthalmology, 103*(4), 517–522. https://doi.org/10.1136/bjophthalmol-2018-311885

Rajalakshmi, A. R., & Rajeshwari, M. (2019). Efficacy of bruckner's test for screening of refractive errors by non-ophthalmologist versus ophthalmologist: A comparative study. *Middle East African Journal of Ophthalmology, 26*(4), 185–188. https://doi.org/10.4103%2Fmeajo.MEAJO_121_19

Rajesh, A. E., Davidson, O., Lacy, M., Chandramohan, A., Lee, A. Y., Lee, C. S., Tarczy-Hornoch, K., & IRIS® Registry Analytic Center Consortium. (2023). Race, Ethnicity, Insurance, and Population Density Associations with Pediatric Strabismus and Strabismic Amblyopia in the IRIS® Registry. *Ophthalmology, 130*(10), 1090–1098. https://doi.org/10.1016/j.ophtha.2023.06.008Register, S. J. (2010). Visual acuity and stereopsis screening results in an underserved community. *Optometry, 81*(4), 200–204. https://doi.org/10.1016/j.optm.2009.11.002

Rein, D. B., Wittenborn, J. S., Phillips, E. A., Saaddine, J. B., & Vision and Eye Health Surveillance System Study Group. (2018). Establishing a vision and eye health surveillance system for the nation: A status update on the vision and eye health surveillance system. *Ophthalmology, 125*(4), 471–473. https://doi.org/10.1016/j.ophtha.2017.10.014

Repka, M. X., Li, C., & Lum, F. (2023). Multivariable analyses of amblyopia treatment outcomes from a clinical data registry. *Ophthalmology, 130*(2), 164–166. https://doi.org/10.1016/j.ophtha.2022.09.005

Robert Wood Johnson Foundation Commission to Build a Healthier America. (2009). *Race and socioeconomic factors affect opportunities for better health* (Issue Brief No. 5). https://folio.iupui.edu/bitstream/handle/10244/659/commission2009issuebrief5.pdf?sequence=2

Rono, H. K., Bastawrous, A., Macleod, D. A. I., Wanjala, E., Di Tanna, G. L., Weiss, H. A., & MJ, B. (2018). Smartphone-based screening for visual impairment in Kenyan school children: A cluster randomised controlled trial. *Lancet Global Health, 6*, 924–932. https://doi.org/10.1016/s2214-109x(18)30244-4

Ross, E. L., & Stein, J. D. (2016). Enhancing the Value of Preschool Vision Screenings. *JAMA Ophthalmology, 134*(6):664–665. doi:10.1001/jamaophthalmol.2016.0822

Sabharwal, S., Nakayoshi, A., Lees, C. R., *Perez*, S., & de Alba Campomanes, A. G. (2021). Prevalence and factors associated with eyeglass wear compliance among preschoolers from low-income families in San Francisco, California. *JAMA Ophthalmology, 139*(4), 433–440. https://doi.org/10.1001/jamaophthalmol.2020.7053

Sankaridurg, P., Berntsen, D. A., Bullimore, M. A., Cho, P., Flitcroft, I., Gawne, T. J., Gifford, K. L., Jong, M., Kang, P., Ostrin, L. A., Santodomingo-Rubido, J., Wildsoet, C., & Wolffsohn, J. S. (2023). IMI 2023 Digest. *Investigative Ophthalmology & Visual Science, 64*(6), 7. https://doi.org/10.1167/iovs.64.6.7

Saxena, R., Sharma, P., & Pediatric Ophthalmology Expert Group. (2020). National consensus statement regarding pediatric eye examination, refraction, and amblyopia management. *Indian Journal of Ophthalmology, 68*(2), 325–332. https://doi.org/10.4103/ijo.IJO_471_19

Saydah, S. H., Gerzoff, R. B., Saaddine, J. B., Zhang, X., & Cotch, M. F. (2020). Eye care among US adults at high risk for vision loss in the United States in 2002 and 2017. *JAMA Ophthalmology, 138*(5), 479–489. https://doi.org/10.1001/jamaophthalmol.2020.0273

Scheive, M., Rowe, L. W., Tso, H. L., Wurster, P., Kalafatis, N. E., Camp, D. A., & Yung, C. W. R. (2022). Assessment of patient follow-up from student-run free eye clinic to county ophthalmology clinic. *Scientific Reports, 12*(1). https://doi.org/10.1038/s41598-022-05033-0

Secor-Turner, M., Sieving, R., Widome, R., Plowman, S., & Vanden Berk, E. (2010). Active parent consent for health surveys with urban middle school students: Processes and outcomes. *Journal of School Health, 80*(2), 73–79. https://doi.org/10.1111/j.1746-1561.2009.00468.x

Shakarchi, A. F., & Collins, M. E. (2019). Referral to community care from school-based eye care programs in the United States. *Survey of Ophthalmology, 64*(6), 858–867. https://doi.org/10.1016/j.survophthal.2019.04.003

Sharma, A., Wong, A. M., Colpa, L., Chow, A. H., & Jin, Y. P. (2016). Socioeconomic status and utilization of amblyopia services at a tertiary pediatric hospital in Canada. *Canadian Journal of Ophthalmology, 51*(6), 452–458. https://doi.org/10.1016/j.jcjo.2016.05.001

Shin, P., & Finnegan, B. (2009). Assessing the need for on-site eye care professionals in community health centers. Policy brief (George Washington University Center for Health Services Research and Policy), 1–23. https://hsrc.himmelfarb.gwu.edu/cgi/viewcontent.cgi?article=1021&context=sphhs_policy_briefs

Shipman, S. A., Lan, J., Chang, C. H., & Goodman, D. C. (2011). Geographic maldistribution of primary care for children. *Pediatrics, 127*(1), 19–27. https://doi.org/10.1542/peds.2010-0150

Siegler, N. E., Walsh, H. L., & Cavuoto, K. M. (2024). Access to pediatric eye care by practitioner type, geographic distribution, and US population demographics. *JAMA Ophthalmology, 142*(5), 454–461. https://doi.org/10.1001/jamaophthalmol.2024.0612

Sight Savers America. (2020). *2019–2020 Biennial Report*. https://sightsaversamerica.org/wp-content/uploads/2021/08/2019-2020-Biennial-Report.pdf

Silverstein, M., Scharf, K., Mayro, E. L., Hark, L. A., Snitzer, M., Anhalt, J., Pond, M., Siam, L., Tran, J., Hill-Bennett, T., Zhan, T., & Levin, A. V. (2021). Referral outcomes from a vision screening program for school-aged children. *Canadian Journal of Ophthalmology, 56*(1), 43–48. https://doi.org/10.1016/j.jcjo.2020.07.009

Simon, G. R., Boudreau, A. D. A., Baker, C. N., Barden, G. A., Hackell, J. M., Hardin, A. P., Meade, K. E., Moore, S. B., Richerson, J., Lehman, S. S., Granet, D. B., Bradford, G. E., Rubin, S. E., Siatkowski, R. M., Suh, D. W., & Granet, D. B. (2016). Visual system assessment in infants, children, and young adults by pediatricians. *Pediatrics, 137*(1). https://doi.org/10.1542/peds.2015-3596

Simon, J. W., Bradfield, Y., Smith, J., Ahn, E., & France, T. D. (2007). Recruitment and manpower in pediatric ophthalmology and strabismus. *Journal of AAPOS, 11*(4), 336–340. https://doi.org/10.1016/j.jaapos.2007.04.004

Singman, E., Matta, N., Fairward, A., & Silbert, D. (2013). Evaluation of PlusoptiX photoscreening during examinations of children with autism. *Strabismus, 21*(2), 103-105. https://doi.org/10.3109/09273972.2013.786736

Sopeyin, A., Young, B. K., & Howard, M. A. A. (2021). 2020 evaluation of portable vision screening instruments. *Yale Journal of Biology and Medicine, 94*, 107–114. https://pubmed.ncbi.nlm.nih.gov/33795987/

State of Alabama. (2024). *State of Alabama Executive Budget fiscal year 2024.* https://budget.alabama.gov/wp-content/uploads/2023/03/State-of-Alabama-Budget-Report-2024-FINAL-Updated.pdf

State of Illinois. (2024). *State of Illinois eye examination report.* http://www.idph.state.il.us/HealthWellness/EyeExamReport.pdf

Stein, J. D., Andrews, C., Musch, D. C., Green, C., & Lee, P. P. (2016). Sight-threatening ocular diseases remain underdiagnosed among children of less affluent families. *Health affairs (Project Hope), 35*(8), 1359–1366. https://doi.org/10.1377/hlthaff.2015.1007

Stults, C. D., Liang, S. Y., Wilcox, J., & Nyong'o, O. L. (2024). Amblyopia care trends following widespread photoscreener adoption. *JAMA Ophthalmology, 142*(3), 188–197. https://doi.org/10.1001/jamaophthalmol.2023.6434

Sung, N. S., Crowley, W. F., Jr, Genel, M., Salber, P., Sandy, L., Sherwood, L. M., Johnson, S. B., Catanese, V., Tilson, H., Getz, K., Larson, E. L., Scheinberg, D., Reece, E. A., Slavkin, H., Dobs, A., Grebb, J., Martinez, R. A., Korn, A., & Rimoin, D. (2003). Central challenges facing the national clinical research enterprise. *JAMA, 289*(10), 1278–1287. https://doi.org/10.1001/jama.289.10.1278

Swanson, M. W., Lee, S. D., Frazier, M. G., Bade, A., & Coulter, R. A. (2020). Vision screening among children with autism spectrum disorder. *Optometry and Vision Science, 97*(11), 917–928. https://doi.org/10.1097/opx.0000000000001593

Syed, S. T., Gerber, B. S., & Sharp, L. K. (2013). Traveling towards disease: Transportation barriers to health care access. *Journal of Community Health, 38*(5), 976–993. https://doi.org/10.1007/s10900-013-9681-1

Thirunavukarasu, A. J., Hassan, R., Limonard, A., & Savant, S. V. (2023). Accuracy and reliability of self-administered visual acuity tests: Systematic review of pragmatic trials. *PLoS One, 18*(6), e0281847. https://doi.org/10.1371/journal.pone.0281847

Tigges B. B. (2003). Parental consent and adolescent risk behavior research. *Journal of Nursing Scholarship, 35*(3), 283–289. https://doi.org/10.1111/j.1547-5069.2003.00283.x

United States Department of Health and Human Services. (2024). Social Determinants of Health. https://health.gov/healthypeople/priority-areas/social-determinants-health

United States Preventive Services Task Force. (2024). AAFP Clinical Preventive Services Recommendations. https://www.aafp.org/family-physician/patient-care/clinical-recommendations/aafp-cps.html

U.S. Census Bureau. (2023, September 28). *NSCH Datasets.* Census.gov. https://www.census.gov/programs-surveys/nsch/data/datasets.html

U.S. Preventive Services Task Force, Grossman, D. C., Curry, S. J., Owens, D. K., Barry, M. J., Davidson, K. W., Doubeni, C. A., Epling, J. W., Jr, Kemper, A. R., Krist, A. H., Kurth, A. E., Landefeld, C. S., Mangione, C. M., Phipps, M. G., Silverstein, M., Simon, M. A., & Tseng, C. W. (2017). Vision screening in children aged 6 months to 5 years: US Preventive Services Task Force recommendation statement. *JAMA, 318*(9), 836–844. https://doi.org/10.1001/jama.2017.11260

U.S. Preventive Services Task Force, Loh, A. R., Chiang, M. F., Donahue, S. P., Baker, C. N., Committee on Practice and Ambulatory Medicine, section on Ophthalmology, American Association of Certified Orthoptists, American Association for Pediatric Ophthalmology and Strabismus, American Academy of Ophthalmology, Child Vision Collaborative, UNMC College of Public Health, Omaha Public Schools, Hospital, C., Center, M., Kerkman, J., & Dingman, H. (2022). *VISION SCREENING GUIDE.* https://www.education.ne.gov/wp-content/uploads/2023/06/VisionScreeningGuide-2022-2-1.pdf

Varadaraj, V., Frick, K. D., Saaddine, J. B., Friedman, D. S., & Swenor, B. K. (2019). Trends in eye care use and eyeglasses affordability: The US National Health Interview Survey, 2008-2016. *JAMA Ophthalmology, 137*(4), 391–398. https://doi.org/10.1001/jamaophthalmol.2018.6799

Varma, R., Tarczy-Hornoch, K., & Jiang, X. (2017). Visual impairment in preschool children in the United States: Demographic and geographic variations from 2015 to 2060. *JAMA Ophthalmology*, *135*(6), 610–616. https://doi.org/10.1001/jamaophthalmol.2017.1021

Vaughan, J. M., Wheeler, D., & Summers, A. (2010) Lay vision screening: Can the Plusoptix vision screener replace the LEA symbol chart and random dot stereotest? *Investigative Ophthalmology & Visual Science*, *51*, 2341. https://iovs.arvojournals.org/article.aspx?articleid=2371008

Vitale, S., Ellwein, L., Cotch, M. F., Ferris, F. L., 3rd, & Sperduto, R. (2008). Prevalence of refractive error in the United States, 1999–2004. *Archives of Ophthalmology*, *126*(8), 1111–1119. https://doi.org/10.1001/archopht.126.8.1111

Vongsachang, H., Friedman, D. S., Inns, A., Kretz, A. M., Mukherjee, M. R., Callan, J., Wahl, M., Repka, M. X., & Collins, M. E. (2020). Parent and Teacher Perspectives on Factors Decreasing Participation in School-Based Vision Programs. *Ophthalmic Epidemiology*, *27*(3), 226–236. https://doi.org/10.1080/09286586.2020.1730910

Wahl, M. D., Fishman, D., Block, S. S., Baldonado, K. N., Friedman, D. S., Repka, M. X., & Collins, M. E. (2021). A comprehensive review of state vision screening mandates for schoolchildren in the United States. *Optometry and Vision Science*, *98*(5), 490–499. https://doi.org/10.1097/OPX.0000000000001686

Wall, T. C., Marsh-Tootle, W., Evans, H. H., Fargason, C. A., Ashworth, C. S., & Hardin, J. M. (2002). Compliance with vision-screening guidelines among a national sample of pediatricians. *Ambulatory Pediatrics*, *2*(6), 449–455. https://doi.org/10.1367/1539-4409(2002)002<0449:CWVSGA>2.0.CO;2

Wallace, D. K., Morse, C. L., Melia, M., Sprunger, D. T., Repka, M. X., Lee, K. A., Christiansen, S. P., & American Academy of Ophthalmology Preferred Practice Pattern Pediatric Ophthalmology/Strabismus Panel. (2018). Pediatric Eye Evaluations Preferred Practice Pattern®: I. Vision screening in the primary care and community setting; II. Comprehensive ophthalmic examination. *Ophthalmology*, *125*(1), P184–P227. https://doi.org/10.1016/j.ophtha.2017.09.032.

Walsh, H. L., Parrish, A., Hucko, L., Sridhar, J., & Cavuoto, K. M. (2023). Access to pediatric ophthalmological care by geographic distribution and US population demographic characteristics in 2022. *JAMA Ophthalmology*, *141*(3), 242–249. https://doi.org/10.1001/jamaophthalmol.2022.6010

Wang, J., Xie, H., Morgan, I., Chen, J., Yao, C., Zhu, J., Zou, H., Liu, K., Xu, X., & He, X. (2022). How to Conduct School Myopia Screening: Comparison Among Myopia Screening Tests and Determination of Associated Cutoffs. *Asia Pac J Ophthalmol (Phila)*, *11*(1), 12-18. https://doi.org/10.1097/APO.0000000000000487

Wang, P., Bianchet, S., Carter, M., Hopman, W., & Law, C. (2023). Utilization and barriers to eye care following school-wide pediatric vision screening. *Canadian Journal of Ophthalmology, 58*(5), 465-471. https://doi.org/10.1016/j.jcjo.2022.04.009

Wang, X., Congdon, N., Ma, Y., Hu, M., Zhou, Y., Liao, W., Jin, L., Xiao, B., Wu, X., Ni, M., Yi, H., Huang, Y., Varga, B., Zhang, H., Cun, Y., Li, X., Yang, L., Liang, C., Huang, W., . . . Ma, X. (2017). Cluster-randomized controlled trial of the effects of free glasses on purchase of children's glasses in China: The PRICE (Potentiating Rural Investment in Children's Eyecare) study. *PLoS One, 12*(11), e0187808. https://doi.org/10.1371/journal.pone.0187808

Williams, M. J., & Eberhardt, J. L. (2008). Biological conceptions of race and the motivation to cross racial boundaries. *Journal of Personality and Social Psychology, 94*(6), 1033–1047. https://doi.org/10.1037/0022-3514.94.6.1033

Williams, S., Wajda, B. N., Alvi, R., McCauley, C., Martinez-Helfman, S., & Levin, A. V. (2013). The challenges to ophthalmologic follow-up care in at-risk pediatric populations. *Journal of AAPOS*, *17*(2), 140–143.

Williams, S., Wajda, B. N., Alvi, R., McCauley, C., Martinez-Helfman, S., & Levin, A. V. (2013). The challenges to ophthalmologic follow-up care in at-risk pediatric populations. *Journal of AAPOS*, *17*(2), 140-143. doi:10.1016/j.jaapos.2012.11.021

Wolf, E. R., Donahue, E., Sabo, R. T., Nelson, B. B., & Krist, A. H. (2021). Barriers to Attendance of Prenatal and Well-Child Visits. *Academic Pediatrics, 21*(6), 955-960. doi:10.1016/j.acap.2020.11.025

Wolfenden, L., Kypri, K., Freund, M., & Hodder, R. (2009). Obtaining active parental consent for school-based research: A guide for researchers. *Australian and New Zealand Journal of Public Health, 33,* 270-5. https://doi.org/10.1111/j.1753-6405.2009.00387.x

Wolffsohn, J. S., Flitcroft, D. I., Gifford, K. L., Jong, M., Jones, L., Klaver, C. C. W., Logan, N. S., Naidoo, K., Resnikoff, S., Sankaridurg, P., Smith, E. L., 3rd, Troilo, D., & Wildsoet, C. F. (2019). IMI - Myopia Control Reports Overview and Introduction. *Investigative Ophthalmology & Visual Science, 60*(3), M1–M19. https://www.ncbi.nlm.nih.gov/pmc/articles/PMC6735780/

Woodward, M. A., Hicks, P. M., Harris-Nwanyanwu, K., Modjtahedi, B., Chan, R. V. P., Vogt, E. L., Lu, M. C., Newman-Casey, P. A., & American Academy of Ophthalmology Taskforce on Ophthalmology and Community Health Centers (2024). Eye care in federally qualified health centers. *Ophthalmology.* https://doi.org/10.1016/j.ophtha.2024.04.019

World Health Organization (WHO). (2007). *Global initiative for the elimination of avoidable blindness: Action plan 2006-2011.* WHO Press. https://apps.who.int/iris/handle/10665/43754

___. (2019, May 30). Social determinants of health. https://www.who.int/health-topics/social-determinants-of-health#tab=tab_1

___. (2024). *Vision and eye screening implementation handbook.* WHO Press.

Wu, L., Feng, J., & Zhang, M. (2023). Implementing interventions to promote spectacle wearing among children with refractive errors: A systematic review and meta-analysis. *Frontiers in Public Health, 11.* https://doi.org/10.3389/fpubh.2023.1053206

Xiao, O., Morgan, I. G., Ellwein, L. B., He, M., & Refractive Error Study in Children Study Group (2015). Prevalence of amblyopia in school-aged children and variations by age, gender, and ethnicity in a multi-country refractive error study. *Ophthalmology, 122*(9), 1924–1931. https://doi.org/10.1016/j.ophtha.2015.05.034

Yan, X. R., Jiao, W. Z., Li, Z. W., Xu, W. W., Li, F. J., & Wang, L. H. (2015). Performance of the Plusoptix A09 photoscreener in detecting amblyopia risk factors in Chinese children attending an eye clinic. *PloS One, 10*(6), e0126052. https://doi.org/10.1371/journal.pone.0126052

Yashadhana, A., Fields, T., Blitner, G., Stanley, R., & Zwi, A. B. (2020). Trust, culture and communication: Determinants of eye health and care among Indigenous people with diabetes in Australia. *BMJ Global Health, 5*(1), e001999. https://doi.org/10.1136/bmjgh-2019-001999

Zadnik, K., Sinnott, L. T., Cotter, S. A., Jones-Jordan, L. A., Kleinstein, R. N., Manny, R. E., Twelker, J. D., Mutti, D. O., & Collaborative Longitudinal Evaluation of Ethnicity and Refractive Error (CLEERE) Study Group (2015). Prediction of juvenile-onset myopia. *JAMA Ophthalmology, 133*(6), 683–689. https://doi.org/10.1001/jamaophthalmol.2015.0471

Zhang, X., Elliott, M. N., Saaddine, J. B., Berry, J. G., Cuccaro, P., Tortolero, S., Franklin, F., Barker, L. E., & Schuster, M. A. (2012). Unmet eye care needs among U.S. 5th-grade students. *American Journal of Preventive Medicine, 43*(1), 55–58. https://doi.org/10.1016/j.amepre.2012.01.032

Zhang, X., Wang, J., Li, Y., & Jiang, B. (2019). Diagnostic test accuracy of Spot and Plusoptix photoscreeners in detecting amblyogenic risk factors in children: A systemic review and meta-analysis. *Ophthalmic and Physiological Optics: Journal of the College of Optometrists, 39*(4), 260–271. https://doi.org/10.1111/opo.12628

Zhou, Y., Chia, M. A., Wagner, S. K., Ayhan, M. S., Williamson, D. J., Struyven, R. R., Liu, T., Xu, M., Lozano, M. G., Woodward-Court, P., Kihara, Y., Allen, N., Gallacher, J. E. J., Littlejohns, T., Aslam, T., Bishop, P., Black, G., Sergouniotis, P., Atan, D., . . . Keane, P. A. (2023). A foundation model for generalizable disease detection from retinal images. *Nature, 622*(7981), 156–163. https://doi.org/10.1038/s41586-023-06555-x

9

Implications for Stakeholders and an Agenda for Future Research

This report has summarized what is known about the current prevalence of myopia, how prevalence has changed in the past several decades, techniques for diagnosing and assessing myopia, factors that contribute to the onset and progression of myopia, the biological mechanisms involved in the development and progression of myopia, options for treating myopia, barriers to the diagnosis and treatment of myopia, and strategies to mitigate these barriers. Across all of these topics, the committee has identified knowledge gaps and made recommendations for future actions to further develop the knowledge base related to myopia and to reduce the incidence and negative consequences of the disease.

This chapter presents implications for stakeholders who would have critical roles in carrying out the recommendations, which are also presented at the end of each chapter where they are organized by topic. Here they are organized by stakeholder group, including eye care professionals; parents and caregivers; policy-making agencies and organizations at the local, state, federal, and global levels; payors; industry partners; and researchers and funding agencies. Some information may be repetitive; this is intentional and aims to facilitate stakeholders from each facet to read a limited number of sections if their preference is to remain focused on how they and their finite resources can affect change. The final section targeted toward researchers and funding agencies proposes an agenda for future research.

OPHTHALMOLOGISTS, OPTOMETRISTS, OTHER CLINICIANS, AND PROFESSIONAL SOCIETIES

While a variety of assessment and diagnostic technologies are clinically available to identify and characterize the myopic eye, there is no consensus on what the mandatory assessment and diagnostic components of a clinical examination of the myopic patient should be, aside from clinical standards for routine and comprehensive examinations in general. This lack of standardization creates variability in clinical care and affects the availability of data for downstream analyses, such as for population studies and artificial intelligence efforts. To address these issues, ophthalmologists, optometrists, and other professionals who conduct vision examinations or screenings, organizations representing them (such as the American Academy of Pediatrics, American Academy of Pediatric Ophthalmology and Strabismus, American Academy of Optometry, and American Academy of Ophthalmology), researchers, and other stakeholders in the field of myopia should discuss and develop consensus standards for the assessments and diagnostics that they deem most important for population-level studies.

Ophthalmologists and optometrists should utilize cycloplegia both for refraction and for visualizing the fundus exam in patients with myopia, particularly for younger patients who have large accommodative and pupil constriction ability. Fundus imaging is valuable for assessing posterior eye pathologies associated with myopia, as it records color views of the retina. If possible and available, other objective structural measurements of the eye should be obtained, including measurements of axial length and the use of optical coherence tomography.

Vision screening is ineffective without receipt of follow-up eye care for children that need it. Therefore, it is critical that vision screening programs provide effective strategies to ensure that children identified with potential vision impairment receive a comprehensive eye exam by an eye care professional (skilled in providing vision care to children) to diagnose vision disorders and provide treatment. Comprehensive eye exams by eye care professionals, along with facilitators such as social workers or community health workers as patient navigators who assist caregivers with scheduling comprehensive eye exams and provide frequent reminders to attend appointments, have been shown to be effective in increasing follow-up compliance. However, myopia is a lifelong condition requiring follow-up eye examinations and, when needed, replacement of lost or broken glasses. The same barriers to the initial detection of children's vision problems impact continuing care, underscoring a need for an eye care home.

Treatment options for myopia progression have increased in the last 20 years, with clinical trials showing that axial growth of the human eye can be slowed down with optical and pharmaceutical intervention. Current treatments for myopia progression include multifocal optical corrections (orthokeratology, soft multi- and dual-focal contact lenses, peripheral refractive error spectacles) and atropine eye drops. Atropine is the only pharmacological treatment for myopia progression widely available and used across the globe. Stronger concentrations of atropine produce better treatment effects but more side effects, including rebound effect. Atropine 0.01% is the mostly widely used, although its treatment effects appear limited. Overall, treatments for myopia progression have limited effects. The largest treatment effect of any published treatment option remains under 0.75 diopters (D) over 2 years, based on recent systematic reviews of myopia treatment options. Some treatment options are effective in the first year and less effective in subsequent years.

A majority of counties in the United States do not have a pediatric eye care specialist. The Association of Schools and Colleges of Optometry, the National Medical Association, and the American Medical Association should use innovative means to encourage optometric and medical graduates of all backgrounds to pursue residencies in pediatric optometry, and residents to pursue fellowships in pediatric ophthalmology. Additionally, eye doctors who have no formal training in pediatrics should be encouraged to pursue continuing education to enhance vision care of the child. Innovative strategies that create direct collaboration patterns and incentive programs to improve the vision care workforce, especially the workforce in medically underserved communities, are likely to foster increased access to care.

Professional associations such as the American Academy of Optometry, American Optometric Association, and American Academy of Ophthalmology should create a national database of eye care providers that provide care to children, especially children under the age of 6 years, and the types of health insurance they accept. This database should be in a format that is easily accessible by caregivers and the general public.

INDIVIDUALS WITH MYOPIA AND PARENTS/CAREGIVERS OF CHILDREN WITH OR AT RISK OF DEVELOPING MYOPIA

Time outdoors is consistently reported to protect against myopia, especially in the younger years. Exact recommendations for exposure time and time of day are yet to be developed, but existing evidence shows that time outdoors for children during daylight can delay (or may even prevent) the onset of myopia. This is a significant finding, as children whose onset of myopia occurs at a young age are more likely to develop a higher amount of eventual myopia than children with onset at older ages. It is also important to ensure that outdoor time is safe for the skin by using sunscreen, and hats or sunglasses should be worn to protect the eyes against short-wavelength exposure.

As discussed in Chapter 8, children ages 12 months to 3 years should receive instrument-based screening to detect disorders of the eye that may lead to vision impairment from amblyopia, and children should receive visual acuity screening at ages 3, 4, 5, 6, 8, 10, 12, and 15 years. Instrument-based screening is recommended as an alternative to visual acuity assessments for children ages 3 to 5 years who are unable or unwilling to complete visual acuity screening or who have developmental delays or neurodevelopmental disorders such as attention deficit hyperactivity disorder (ADHD) or autism spectrum disorder (ASD). If any component of the vision screening is abnormal, the parent or caregiver should receive a referral to take the child to an eye care provider for a comprehensive eye examination. As myopia is a lifelong condition that worsens throughout childhood, it is important to establish an eye care home and adhere to treatment long-term, including replacement of corrective glasses if broken or lost.

POLICY-MAKING AGENCIES AND ORGANIZATIONS AT THE STATE AND LOCAL, FEDERAL, AND GLOBAL LEVELS

Local and State Departments of Health and Departments of Education

Vision screening is important in identifying children with vision impairment and facilitating access to treatment, but many children are not receiving vision screening and, when they do, they often do not make it to the eye doctor or get the needed glasses. One model that has been used successfully is to provide vision screening to all children in congregate locations (schools, fairs, etc.). An alternative that has been successful when resources are scarce is to offer vision screening to targeted groups at increased risk of vision problems or of not receiving treatment. For underserviced populations, vision screenings held at community health centers and federally qualified health centers are an excellent way to provide access to vision care. To expand universal screening programs, school boards can also take advantage of Medicaid dollars provided through the Healthy Schools Campaign.

Vision screening is ineffective without receipt of follow-up eye care for the children who need it. Therefore, it is critical that vision screening programs provide effective strategies to ensure that children identified with potential vision impairment receive a comprehensive eye exam by an eye care professional (skilled in providing vision care to children) to diagnose vision disorders and provide treatment. These strategies should involve deliberate and collaborative efforts between eye care providers, public health units, health insurance plans (Medicaid and the Children's Health Insurance Program), early-intervention and school-based services, and other stakeholder institutions and agencies.

Onsite comprehensive eye exams by eye care professionals, in conjunction with facilitators such as social workers or community health workers who assist caregivers with scheduling comprehensive eye exams and provide frequent reminders to attend appointments, have been shown to be effective. Strategies to ensure compliance with treatment and receipt of follow-up eye care should extend beyond the initial comprehensive eye exam to support the replacement of broken or lost glasses and ongoing comprehensive eye care and the establishment of an eye care home. Future coordinated care should follow "Best Practices and Policy: 12 Components of a Strong Visual Health System of Care" provided by the National Center for Children's Vision and Health, especially as myopia is a lifelong condition requiring regular intervention.

Federal Agencies

Myopia is a disease with increasing worldwide prevalence and severity, and the impact of its downstream complications needs to be taken seriously. Federal agencies have an important role to play in promoting behaviors that may be protective against myopia, as well as promoting the screening, diagnosis, and treatment of myopia. An important first step is for the Centers for Medicare & Medicaid Services to classify myopia as a disease and therefore a medical diagnosis. This reclassification is needed to ensure that efforts not only to treat blurry vision resulting from uncorrected or undercorrected refractive error, but also to prevent and manage the progression of myopia. This may help get the warranted attention from stakeholders such as federal and state agencies, professional associations, patients, and caregivers, thus increasing feasibility of care for the public beyond a simple pair of glasses.

The Centers for Disease Control should produce guidelines, supported by departments of education and healthcare providers, promoting more time outdoors for children. Consideration should be given to ensure that outdoor time is safe for the skin and eye by using sunscreen and other protection against short-wavelength exposure. These guidelines should include children across the age range of 3 to at least 16 years.

The U.S. Department of Health and Human Services, in collaboration with departments of education at the state level, should take measures to ensure that children receive a vision screening before first grade and a comprehensive eye exam when needed. To facilitate this:

- Federal agencies, such as the Centers for Disease Control and Prevention, and other agencies that support public health programming should encourage the implementation of effective vision care programs for children by providing funding or other incentives for vision health care systems that follow the 12 Components of a Strong Vision Health System of Care provided by the National Center for Children's Vision and Eye Health.
- The Department of Health and Human Services (DHHS) should oversee the provision of cost-effective, standardized, evidence-based national vision screening guidelines to detect refractive errors, amblyopia, and other vision conditions. These guidelines should include a consensus on the ideal target age for screening, screening frequency, types of screening tests, tools, and referral criteria.
- For children under age 7, the referral criteria for instrument-based screening should include any amount of myopia or a family history of myopia based on the evidence that these predict likely progression to significant myopia.

- The Centers for Medicare & Medicaid Services should require reimbursement for vision screening to not be bundled into the global code of well-child visits.

An integrated, national data surveillance system for collecting data on vision screening, referrals to eye care providers, and outcomes of referrals at the state level is also needed. This data system would not only enhance care integration and communication, but also enable monitoring to ensure that follow-up care is received. A surveillance system would also support the DHHS Office of Disease Prevention and Health Promotion's (OASH) Healthy People 2030 goal of increasing the proportion of children who get vision screening. To facilitate the creation of this system:

- The Centers for Medicare & Medicaid Services should include vision screening in the Core Set of Children's Health Care Quality Measures that are reported annually by all states.
- The National Institutes of Health's All of US Research Program and Healthy Brain and Child Development Study should include additional measures of adult and child vision disorders.

Global Organizations

Global organizations such as the World Health Organization and the International Myopia Institute should collect best practices for improving access to vision care for medically underserved populations.

The Centers for Disease Control and Prevention should coordinate with the World Health Organization so that both organizations are using consistent, harmonized definitions and monitoring methods. Data subsequently collected should then consistently follow these methods so that future worldwide comparisons can be used to identify the influence of economic development, lifestyle, and ethnicity on the prevalence of refractive error.

International and national entities (e.g., International Myopia Institute, National Eye Institute, and similar) should collaborate to further efforts to develop a consortium/network repository for myopia-related clinical data. This would be beneficial for standardization not only for clinical care but also for research, particularly with artificial intelligence efforts.

PAYORS

As mentioned above, for patients with myopia, particularly for younger patients who have accommodative ability, clinicians should utilize cycloplegia both for refraction and for visualizing the fundus. Clinicians should also obtain other objective assessments of the eye, including more robust structural measurements such as axial length and optical coherence tomography. Health and vision insurance providers and other payors should reimburse for evaluation of these tests that may help identify disease elements of myopia, in addition to the determination of refractive error. Such examinations and tests should be covered at least annually to allow for longitudinal, cohesive care.

INDUSTRY PARTNERS

Children are most at risk for progression of myopia, and designing assessment and diagnostic technologies tailored to children enhances the description of their myopic eyes. This may allow for more precise treatment for this critical population. Developers of assessment and diagnostic technologies should consider the ability to use the technology in multiple age groups and settings as a major design criterion. This includes making the technology time-efficient to perform and "child-friendly." Technologies that are portable and cost-effective for the end user are also more likely to increase accessibility and have broader adoption.

Researchers and developers of assessment and diagnostic technologies should design assessments and tests to better understand the myopic eye, its development, and its environment (the visual diet). In addition to identifying eyes that are already myopic, there is a need to also identify eyes at risk of myopia (i.e., pre-myopic state in childhood) or other key events (e.g., pre-pathologic myopia state in adulthood). Other diagnostic technologies to support these goals include, for example, biometric and functional measurements to develop individualized eye modeling, improved choroidal imaging, and imaging technologies to measure 3D eye shape and assess the refractive state across the entire retina.

Technologies to better capture and quantify the visual experience of children and animals included in studies of myopia are also needed. Industry partners have an important role in providing:

- Comprehensive quantification of the features of the visual diet of preschool and school-age children; and
- Sensors that can be used by researchers to accurately monitor the visual diet of children including time outdoors, working distance, and screen time.

Developers of electronic devices should collaborate with academic scientists to conduct research on the visual consequences of the use of electronic devices, especially in children at risk of developing myopia.

RESEARCHERS AND FUNDING AGENCIES

The committee identified many gaps in the knowledge base related to myopia. This section presents an agenda for data collection and research organized by topic area, including prevalence, factors that contribute to the onset and progression of myopia, mechanisms involved in myopia pathogenesis, treatment strategies and barriers to detection and treatment of myopia.

Myopia Prevalence

While there is evidence that myopia is increasing worldwide, there are scant data for the current prevalence in the United States, and existing data are not sufficient to precisely quantify the increase in prevalence (see Chapter 3). One major limitation of the research on prevalence is inconsistency in what is used as the threshold for determining myopia; in reviewing the literature, the committee encountered studies that used a range of cut points (0.25, 0.50, 0.75, and 1.00 D); measurement techniques and the age of assessment also vary across studies. The manner in which myopia is determined is also heterogenic including automated measures, lensometry, self-report, and others. Large-scale surveillance studies with representative populations have not been funded in more than 20 years. To improve data on prevalence in the United States:

- The Centers for Disease Control and Prevention and state health departments should collect consistent data on the prevalence of myopia in the United States, prioritizing surveillance on myopia prevalence in children and using standardized procedures. A central repository should be created so that consistent data can be uploaded into a central data base.
  - For such population statistics, the data should comprise objective measures at various ages, collected longitudinally from an early age, and repeated cross-sectional measurements using consistent methodology.
  - The data should include the entire distribution of refractive errors, not just the mean and the age of onset. Otherwise, a shift in part of the distribution (e.g., high myopia) or age of onset (e.g., starting before age six) that would suggest the need for different policy/practice responses could be obscured.
- Researchers investigating myopia prevalence should use standardized procedures and upload data into a central database. The data should comprise objective measures at various ages, collected longitudinally from an early age or by repeated cross-sectional measurements using constant methodology. The data should include the entire distribution of refractive errors, not just the mean and the age of onset. New data-gathering efforts should place U.S. data in the context of worldwide trends to allow for comparisons to formulate novel hypotheses about etiology and treatment development especially related to national education policies and practices, urban development, and outdoor lifestyle tendencies.
- The National Institutes of Health's All of US Research Program and its Healthy Brain and Child Development Study should include additional measures of adult and child vision disorders that would generate valuable data across the country that will inform research questions and eye care policies.

Factors that Contribute to the Onset and Progression of Myopia

The environmental variable with the highest level of evidence contributing to myopia is the protective effect of time outdoors (see Chapter 5). The implication is that the prevalence of myopia is increasing, at least in part, because of inadequate time spent outdoors by recent generations of children. Of the features of the outdoor environment that may be beneficial in delaying the onset of myopia, the strongest evidence is for increased luminance (i.e., brightness), which likely works, at least in part, through dopaminergic signaling. However, studies addressing other salient differences between the indoor and outdoor environments, such as the spectral composition of light (i.e., light at different wavelengths), have yet to be tested widely in humans. Furthermore, the data supporting the roles of near work and electronic devices in myopia is limited or inconclusive, even though these factors are often stated as the cause for myopia. (See Chapter 5 for discussion of the research on near work and electronic devices.)

The National Institutes of Health and other funders, including private foundations, should solicit and fund research to investigate novel questions about the genetic and environmental mechanisms contributing to myopia, with special emphasis on the following topics:

- Identification of specific features of the indoor and outdoor visual diet that cause or inhibit myopia development, including luminance levels and spectral characteristics of different light sources.
- The "ON/OFF imbalance hypothesis" which potentially links many salient visual differences between the outdoor and indoor environments with retinal pathways that have been implicated in myopigenesis, including dopaminergic amacrine cells and intrinsically photosensitive retinal ganglion cells (ipRGCs).
- The role of near work in causing myopia, versus other factors in the environment while engaging in near work which emphasize:
  - Preschool children as well as school-aged children, with special attention to the ages at which children are first exposed to these visual stimuli
  - Children at risk for the development of myopia
- Longitudinal studies of environmental risk factors for myopia that incorporate technologies for data capture of working distance, temporal properties of near activities, and the spectral characteristics of indoor and outdoor activities.
- Studies to further develop and validate promising diagnostic biomarkers (e.g., axial elongation and choroidal thickness changes, ocular shape, optical aberrations) and technologies that may be useful for myopia diagnostics, management, and understanding of the disease.
- Studies to assess both genetic factors—including polygenic scores—and environmental factors to account for confounding and interactive effects.
- Studies in animal models to better understand the mechanisms through which genetic and environmental influences lead to myopia.

Mechanisms Involved in Myopia Pathogenesis

While retinal signaling has been shown to be fundamental to emmetropization and myopia development, as opposed to higher order brain processing, the precise causal mechanisms that underlie this process have remained elusive (see Chapter 6). Importantly, the entire retina, not only the fovea, plays a critical role in regulating eye growth. Two potential mechanisms include, the 'luminance network" and a closed feedback loop for homeostasis of eye growth.

The 'luminance network' of the retina has been proposed as a mechanistic link between the reduced time today's child spends outdoors and the increased incidence of myopia. This network encodes light intensity and includes dopaminergic amacrine cells and melanopsin-expressing intrinsically photosensitive retinal ganglion cells, and is uniquely dependent on some subset of channels within the retinal ON pathways. However, a gap in knowledge exists as to how this system controls refractive eye growth. Closed-loop feedback is hypothesized to be essential for achieving precise homeostasis of eye growth. However, the exact roles of candidate retinal image properties—such as defocus, blur, contrast (spatial, spectral and temporal) and chromaticity—responsible for fine-tuning this process are currently unknown, and so are the specific mechanisms through which these features are encoded by the retinoscleral signaling cascade. More research is needed to determine how the retina encodes these image features and links them to refractive growth signals.

Funding agencies, including the National Institutes of Health, the National Science Foundation, the Department of Defense, and private foundations, as well as industry, should seek to fund proposals across disciplines for both human and animal studies to investigate the biological and optical mechanisms of emmetropization and myopia. These studies should include:

- determining the visual environments stimulating ON pathways,
- molecular contributions to refractive eye growth,
- modeling studies to determine the interaction of contributing ocular and environmental elements,
- identification of candidates for retinoscleral signaling and retinal neurons that detect the sign of defocus,
- elucidating the role of the choroid in regulating eye growth,
- the changes in the sclera that lead to axial elongation,
- the influence of gene–environment interactions of myopia susceptibility,
- and the development of in-vitro experimental models to probe causal mechanisms on a cellular and subcellular level.

To accomplish this, funding agencies should target audacious proposals to foster the innovative, multi-disciplinary research that is needed to fully harmonize our understanding of visual information processing by the retina that leads to changes in scleral remodeling. Particular gaps in knowledge include the roles of the visual environment, ocular optics, retinal circuits, and signaling proteins involved in retinoscleral signaling, particularly the luminance pathway.

Experimental evidence from animal models indicates that the fovea is not necessary for emmetropization and myopia development. Thus, the field of myopia research should adopt a retinocentric—in contrast to a foveocentric—approach. Specifically:

- basic researchers should develop eye models that can be readily tailored to individual variation ("personalized models") to link the visual diet to image formation across the entire retina.
- clinical researchers should propose optical treatments with a full understanding of the consequences for the peripheral retinal image.

Screening, Diagnosis, and Treatment

While treatment options for myopia progression have increased in the last 20 years, current optical treatments and the use of the only pharmacological treatment widely available, have limited effects (see Chapter 7). Time outdoors, an emerging treatment strategy is consistently reported to have protective effects. The current state of knowledge on treatment options reflects our limited understanding of the fundamental mechanisms of eye length regulations.

Current literature suggests that combination therapy shows minimal to no additive impact. However, studies have only used the minimally effective 0.01% concentration of atropine in combination with other treatments. Combination therapy should be studied using higher concentrations.

Clinical trials for myopia treatments have provided important insights into the progression of myopia. Predictors of myopia progression include a child's existing refractive error, age, sex, and ethnic identity. Past myopia progression does not predict future progression.

Myopia tends to progress faster when onset is at younger ages, which may suggest early treatment of myopia in the preschool years. It is unclear whether treatments known to be effective for low to moderate myopia in school-aged children are effective in preschool-aged children, and also unclear whether treatments for low to moderate myopia in school-aged children are effective in children with high myopia or myopia associated with genetic and systemic disorders.

Funding agencies and other funders, including the National Institutes of Health, Research to Prevent Blindness, and others, need to support research to develop new treatment strategies for myopia, and to determine mechanisms for current treatments. Progress in this area needs intentionally integrated, multidisciplinary basic and clinical vision science research. Areas of urgent focus are listed here.

- Develop fundamental studies—potentially including animal models—of the mechanisms by which existing and new therapies affect eye growth.
- Perform research on the mechanisms of atropine to determine the causes of treatment effects and side effects, thereby providing opportunities to optimize the treatment efficacy in children or to develop novel pharmaceuticals with fewer side effects.
- Design studies to identify the ideal dosing characteristics, including concentration and cadence, for more specific pharmaceuticals to slow eye growth.
- Develop new pharmaceutical options to provide structural scleral reinforcement, without creating dose-dependent side effects. Further research is needed to identify and develop pharmacological agents that are more effective and have fewer adverse effects than current options.
- Determine optimal parameters for time outdoors, including duration per day, chromatic elements, time of day, and needed safety measures, in order to prevent or delay myopia onset. Such studies may create the opportunity to develop treatments for myopia that can be used indoors, independently of time outdoors.
- Develop rigorous investigations of combination therapies.
- Conduct longer-term studies or assessments in adulthood to weigh the costs of myopia treatment against it benefits in terms of the ultimate amount of myopia and effects on ocular health.
- Combine bench and eye model studies of visual optics including the spectral composition of light, peripheral refractive characterization, and contrast to develop optical corrections for best visual performance and optical quality.
- Identify biomarkers of the pre-myopic, myopic, and treated eye to reveal novel pathways that can delay or prevent onset of myopia, to identify when to start treatments, and to monitor the effects of imposed treatments. A short-term biomarker that could reliably predict longer-term treatment outcomes is required.

It seems likely that myopia control treatments are to be used throughout childhood and perhaps through young adulthood, so the safety of any treatment is paramount. Scientists should focus on developing strategies to minimize short-term and long-term side effects.

Funding for multi-center randomized clinical trials should be directed toward longer-term human studies starting at earlier ages, on treatment and off treatment, to determine the long-term benefit with respect to ultimate refractive error and ocular health.

Barriers to Detection and Treatment of Myopia

While myopia can be identified through vision screening and comprehensive eye exams, multiple barriers exist to identifying and treatment myopia (see Chapter 8). Myopia starts at an early age when children are not able to communicate, or even realize, that they have blurry distance vision. Further, it is necessary that vision screening is followed by comprehensive eye exams and treatment. There are significant barriers to conducting research on these factors, including poor data collection for surveillance, limited funding to conduct research, ethical concerns about randomized trials, and poor representation of minoritized populations in research. The following recommendations focus on research areas that could facilitate removal of these barriers.

The National Institutes of Health, Agency for Healthcare Research and Quality, and other organizations that support research, such as Research to Prevent Blindness, should seek and encourage opportunities to fund work that will support continued efforts to determine:

- The effectiveness, cost-effectiveness, and implementation of novel interventions to improve access to vision screening and completed referrals to eye care providers compared to standard of care, especially for underserved populations that typically experience inequities in accessing care;
- The prevalence of myopia, referrals to eye care providers, completion of comprehensive eye exams, and treatment in children;
- Differences in reimbursement processes (e.g., bundled vs. unbundled with global code for well-child visits), reimbursement rates for various vision care services, and coverage for prescription glasses across the states; and
- Strategies for promoting completed referrals, follow-up care, compliance with wearing prescribed glasses, and improved public awareness on vision and eye health in children.

SUMMARY

Despite decades of research in myopia, there is much to be learned. The preponderance of evidence suggests that myopia should be treated beyond simply correcting blurry vision. It is a disease that can affect long-term visual health. Effectively treating myopia will require audacious research that translates vision and animal science to clinical practice patterns. Care of the myopic child who becomes the myopic adult will require intentional integration and coordinated strategic policies as the local, state, national, and global levels. Myopia is no longer just for eye doctors.

Appendix A
Committee Biosketches

K. DAVINA FRICK (*Co-Chair*, she/her/hers) is a health economist and professor at the Johns Hopkins Carey Business School who began her career at and maintains joint appointments in the Johns Hopkins Bloomberg School of Public Health. She also holds a joint appointment in the Department of Ophthalmology at the Johns Hopkins School of Medicine. Frick has done substantial work on the burden of blindness and the cost-effectiveness of various interventions aimed at preventing blindness. She participated in organizing and delivering a Health Economics and Outcomes Research on-demand workshop for the Association for Research in Vision and Ophthalmology (ARVO) and has presented her work at the ARVO annual meeting, the World Health Organization, and the European Society for International Ophthalmology. Frick's research and teaching extend beyond only vision and eye issues and cost-effectiveness as she has worked in women's health, oncology, and a variety of nursing areas as well as teaching about the United States healthcare system, about economics more generally, and about values-based business leadership. She received her Ph.D. in economics and health services organization and policy from the University of Michigan.

TERRI L. YOUNG (*Co-Chair*, she/her/hers) is the Peter A. Duehr Professor and chairwoman of the Department of Ophthalmology and Visual Sciences at the University of Wisconsin-Madison (UW). She has secondary UW appointments in the Departments of Pediatrics and Medical Genetics. Young is a pediatric ophthalmologist and clinician-scientist with expertise in ophthalmic genetics and genomics in the areas of refractive errors -particularly myopia, ocular development, and childhood glaucoma. She has multiple service years to the National Eye Institute as a member of its Board of Scientific Counselors and multiple permanent member study sections. Young has served in multiple leadership roles for the Association for Research in Vision and Ophthalmology (ARVO) and was appointed a Gold Fellow in 2015. After serving on the ARVO Foundation Board, she now serves as an elected member of the ARVO Board of Trustees. Young also serves on the Board of Directors of the Wisconsin Council of the Blind and Visually Disabled; and Board of Directors for the Heed Ophthalmic Foundation. Additionally, she serves on the Board of Trustees of the Association of University Professors in Ophthalmology (and is currently President-Elect). She serves on the journal editorial boards of *Experimental Eye Research* and *Investigative Ophthalmology* and *Visual Science*; and is an associate editor of the *Journal of the American Association of Pediatric Ophthalmology and Strabismus.* She was an Industry Consultant for Aerpio Pharmaceuticals, Inc. Young received her M.D. from Harvard Medical School and her M.B.A. from Duke University.

AFUA O. ASARE (she/her/hers) is a research assistant professor in the Department of Ophthalmology & Visual Sciences at the John A. Moran Eye Center, University of Utah and adjunct assistant professor at the Department of Population Health Sciences, University of Utah.

Her research concerns the early identification of vision impairment in young children through the development and implementation of evidence-based health interventions using a health equity lens. A particular area of interest has been the use of user centered design to develop and implement provider-facing clinical decision support tools in Electronic Health Record Systems to improve the uptake of vision screening in pediatric primary care and referrals to eye care providers. Asare is a member of the Advisory Committee and co-Secretary of the Children's Vision Equity Alliance in the National Center for Children's Vision and Eye Health. She is also a member of Health Equity and Communications Task Force in the Center for Vision and Population Health. She received her Doctor of Optometry (O.D.) from the Department of Optometry & Visual Science at the Kwame Nkrumah University of Science and Technology in Kumasi, Ghana, Master in Public Health (MPH) from the Harvard T.H. Chan School of Public Health at Harvard University, Master in Vision Science (MSc) from the University of Waterloo School of Optometry and Vision Science in Waterloo, Canada and her Ph.D. from the Institute of Health Policy, Management and Evaluation at the University of Toronto, Canada. Asare completed a postdoctoral fellowship at the University of Utah John A. Moran Eye Center.

DAVID BERSON (he/him/his) is a professor and past chair in the Department of Neuroscience at Brown University. His research concerns the structural and functional organization of the mammalian retina. A particular focus has been the intrinsically photosensitive retinal ganglion cells, a special class of retinal output neuron that responds directly to light, as rods and cones do. These neurons encode information about light intensity and exert wide-ranging effects in the retina and brain. They may contribute to the reduced risk of myopia among those spending more time outdoors. Berson is a fellow of the American Association for the Advancement of Science and a recipient of the Friedenwald Award from Association for Research in Vision and Ophthalmology. He received his bachelor's degree in psychology at Brown University and his Ph.D. in neuroanatomy from Massachusetts Institute of Technology. Berson completed postdoctoral stints at Brown and at the Schepens Eye Research Institute.

RICHARD T. BORN (he/him/his) is a professor of neurobiology at Harvard Medical School (HMS) and former director of the Harvard Ph.D. program in neuroscience. He was a postdoctoral fellow in the Hubel/Livingstone lab, undertook a second postdoc with William Newsome at Stanford and then returned to HMS as an assistant professor in the Department of Neurobiology. Born's laboratory studies has studied cortical visual processing vision in nonhuman primates, with a particular focus on mechanisms of visual motion processing and the computational role of cortico-cortical feedback. His scientific work has been recognized with fellowships from the Klingenstein, Whitehall, Kirsch and Lefler Foundations and the Jesse L. Sigelman Award for Innovation and Excellence. Born has also received the Harvard Division of Medical Sciences Award for Exceptional Leadership in Graduate Education in recognition of his efforts to promote quantitative literacy among students in the biological sciences. He received his M.D. from Harvard Medical School.

JING CHEN (she/her/hers) is an assistant professor of human factors and human-computer interaction in the Department of Psychological Sciences at Rice University. She has conducted research on the fundamental principles of human performance and decision-making, and their application to solving human-automation interaction problems in application domains such as autonomous driving, cybersecurity, uncrewed aerial systems, and healthcare. With a keen interest in understanding the perceptual and cognitive processes of individuals with disabilities, particularly those with visual impairments, Chen is passionate about designing systems and environments that meet their specific needs. She is a recipient of the Earl Alluisi Award for Early Career Achievement from the American Psychological Association, the Rising Star Award from the Association for Psychological Science, and the George E. Briggs Dissertation Award from the American Psychological Association. Chen is a fellow of the American Psychological Association and the Psychonomic Society. She received a M.S. in industrial engineering and her Ph.D. in psychology from Purdue University.

JEREMY A. GUGGENHEIM (he/him/his) is a professor in the School of Optometry & Vision Sciences, Cardiff University (United Kingdom [UK]). He was formerly an associate professor and associate head in the School of Optometry at Hong Kong Polytechnic University (Hong Kong). Guggenheim's research addresses the causes of nearsightedness (myopia), applying methods from a range of disciplines, including genetics, epidemiology and animal studies. He is a member of the international myopia genetics Consortium for Refractive Error and Myopia, the UK Biobank Eye and Vision Consortium, and the International Myopia Institute. He serves on the editorial boards of the academic journals *Investigative Ophthalmology & Visual Science* (associate editor), *Ophthalmic & Physiological Optics* and *Translational Vision Science & Technology* and is on the Scientific Advisory Board of the Fight for Sight (UK) charity. He was awarded the Biennial Arthur Bennett Prize for Outstanding Research Anywhere in the World, by the UK College of Optometrists. He received his Ph.D. from Cardiff University.

ANTHONY N. KUO (he/him/his) is an associate professor of ophthalmology at the Duke University School of Medicine with a secondary appointment in biomedical engineering at Duke University. He is a clinician-scientist with both an active clinical practice as well as laboratory program. Clinically, Kuo is a board-certified ophthalmologist with additional sub-specialty fellowship training in cornea and refractive surgery. His research focuses on development and translation of ophthalmic imaging technologies. This includes work to use a clinical ophthalmic imaging technique (optical coherence tomography) to characterize the shape of the eye in myopia. His laboratory work has been supported by research program grants from the National Institutes of Health (NIH). Kuo is also a standing member on a NIH study section and has served on an American Academy of Ophthalmology (AAOphth) committee to assess ophthalmic technologies. He has been the recipient of the Alcon Young Investigator's Award and Research to Prevent Blindness's Physician-Scientist Award. He received his M.D. from Vanderbilt University.

DAPHNE MAURER (she/her/hers) is a Distinguished University Professor in the Department of Psychology, Neuroscience and Behaviour at McMaster University in Canada and a professor (status-only) in the Institute of Health Policy, Management and Evaluation of the University of Toronto. She has published over 200 peer-reviewed papers during her 50 years doing laboratory research on the development of vision in babies and children, including work on the effects of congenital cataracts after surgical removal. Maurer has done extensive field studies on the methods and utility of screening the vision of kindergarten children in schools and advised the Ontario government on this topic. For her lifetime's work she received the Donald O. Hebb Distinguished Contribution Award of the Canadian Society for Brain, Behaviour and Cognitive

Science. She is a fellow of the Royal Society of Canada and of the Association for Psychological Science. She received a Ph.D. in child development from the University of Minnesota.

J. ANTHONY MOVSHON (he/him/his) is University Professor and Silver Professor in the Center for Neural Science at New York University (NYU). He is also founding director of NYU's Center for Neural Science. Movshon's lab studies vision and visual perception, using a multidisciplinary approach that combines biology, behavior, and theory. His work explores the way that the neural networks in the brain compute and represent the form and motion of objects and scenes; the way that these networks contribute to perception and to the control of visually guided action; and the way that visual experience influences brain development in early life. Among his honors are the Young Investigator Award from the Society for Neuroscience, the Rank Prize in Optoelectronics, the António Champalimaud Vision Award, the Golden Brain Award from the Minerva Foundation, and the Karl Spencer Lashley Award from the American Philosophical Society. Movshon received his Ph.D. in experimental psychology from Cambridge University. He is a member of the National Academy of Sciences, and a fellow of the American Academy of Arts and Sciences, of the American Association for the Advancement of Science, and of the Association for Psychological Science.

DONALD O. MUTTI (he/him/his) is the E.F. Wildermuth Foundation Professor in Optometry at The Ohio State University College of Optometry. His current research projects are the Bifocal Lenses in Nearsighted Kids (BLINK and BLINK2) studies, National Eye Institute (NEI)-funded evaluations of childhood myopia progression with multifocal soft contact lenses. Mutti began his research career in the contact lens industry with CooperVision Ophthalmic Products after which he entered academia to pursue studies of refractive error development. He was a co-investigator on the NEI-funded Collaborative Longitudinal Evaluation of Ethnicity and Refractive Error study, a 21-year investigation of ocular component development and risk factors for myopia. Mutti was also the principal investigator of the NEI-funded Berkeley Infant Biometry Study, an eight-year investigation of ocular component development and emmetropization in infancy. Additionally, he reported receiving nonfinancial support from Bausch + Lomb during the conduct of the BLINK study. Mutti also served as the principal investigator for a recent study with Lentechs LLC, which developed a multifocal contact lens for presbyopia. He has received research funding from Johnson & Johnson, and he served on the advisory board for Welch Allyn. His research accomplishments have been recognized with the Irvin M. and Beatrice Borish Award and the Glenn A. Fry Award from the American Optometric Foundation. He is a fellow of the American Academy of Optometry and a silver fellow of the Association for Research in Vision and Ophthalmology. He received his O.D. degree and his Ph.D. from the School of Optometry at the University of California, Berkeley.

MACHELLE T. PARDUE (she/her/hers) is a professor and vice chair of research in the Department of Ophthalmology at Emory University and a senior research career scientist at the Atlanta VA Healthcare System. She is elucidating the retinal mechanisms of myopia by leveraging the power of mouse models. Pardue's lab has investigated the contributions of several retinal pathways and retinal signaling molecules in myopic eye growth using transgenic mouse models. She has been named a gold fellow for the Association for Research in Vision and Ophthalmology and a fellow of the American Institute of Medical and Biological Engineers. Pardue received her doctorate in vision science and biology at the University of Waterloo. Her post-doctorate training was in visual electrophysiology at Loyola School of Medicine and Hines VA Hospital in Chicago.

RAMKUMAR SABESAN (he/him/his) is an associate professor and director of basic and translational science at the University of Washington (UW), Department of Ophthalmology. He holds adjunct appointments in the departments of UW Bioengineering and of Biological Structure and is a member of the Graduate program in Neuroscience and University of Washington Institute for Neuroengineering. The Sabesan lab studies functional mechanisms by which retinal photoreceptors and their ensuing visual pathways mediate the most fundamental aspects of vision. This is enabled by paradigms of ophthalmic adaptive optics and optoretinography that provide in vivo cellular scale access to the visual system for physiological and psychophysical assays. Sabesan has received several awards including the Burroughs Wellcome Fund Careers at the Scientific Interfaces Award, Research to Prevent Blindness Career Development Award, Alcon Research Institute Young Investigator Award, and being named a Kavli fellow by the National Academy of Sciences. He earned his Ph.D. in optics at the Institute of Optics and Center for Visual Science at the University of Rochester. He did a postdoctoral fellowship at the School of Optometry at University of California, Berkeley before joining UW as faculty.

JODY ANN SUMMERS (she/her/hers) is a professor and vice chair of research in the Department of Cell Biology at the University of Oklahoma Health Sciences Center. After completing a post-doctoral fellowship at the University of Pittsburgh, she obtained her first National Institutes of Health R01 grant entitled, "Regulation of Scleral Growth and Remodeling in Myopia" which she still holds today. The primary objective of Summers' research is to understand, at the molecular level, the mechanism by which the visual environment controls the postnatal growth of the eye. Her research was initiated when little was known about the molecular composition of the sclera and the role of the sclera in regulating eye size and the development of myopia. Since then, Summers has clearly demonstrated in several animal models that the sclera is a dynamic tissue, capable of rapidly altering its molecular composition in response to changes in the visual environment to regulate ocular size and refraction. Based on these studies, she has directed her research toward identification of intraocular growth regulators as targets for the potential treatment and prevention of myopia. Summers received her Ph.D. in anatomy and cell biology from the University of North Dakota.

KATHERINE K. WEISE (she/her/hers) is a professor of optometry at the University of Alabama at Birmingham (UAB). After studying the safety and tolerability of pirenzepine in the late 90's, she became co-investigator for the Correction of Myopia Evaluation Trial at UAB. Weise co-chaired the Myopia Treatment Study 1 for the Pediatric Eye Disease Investigator Group (PEDIG) and was lead co-author of the main outcome paper on low-dose atropine. In addition to National Institutes of Health-funded trials on strabismus, amblyopia, and vision-related concussion care, she investigates in two industry-sponsored myopia studies: MiSight post-approval study and CHAPERONE study of micro-dose dispensing of low-dose atropine. Weise earned the UAB President's Award for Excellence in Teaching, and the Hero for Sight Award to honor individuals whose impact on children's eyecare in the state of Alabama has been both lasting and profound. She will serve as network co-chair for PEDIG from through 2024–

2028. Weise received her O.D. from the Illinois College of Optometry and her M.B.A. from the University of Alabama at Birmingham.

Appendix B
Disclosure of Unavoidable Conflict of Interest

The conflict of interest policy of the National Academies of Sciences, Engineering, and Medicine (http://www.nationalacademies.org/coi) prohibits the appointment of an individual to a committee authoring a Consensus Study Report if the individual has a conflict of interest that is relevant to the task to be performed. An exception to this prohibition is permitted if the National Academies determines that the conflict is unavoidable and the conflict is publicly disclosed. A determination of a conflict of interest for an individual is not an assessment of that individual's actual behavior or character or ability to act objectively despite the conflicting interest.

Donald Mutti has a financial conflict of interest in relation to the Committee on Focus on Myopia—Pathogenesis and Rising Incidence because he is a consultant for Vyluma, a company developing pharmaceuticals for myopia control, and also for Ocular Services on Demand.

The National Academies has concluded that, for this committee to accomplish the tasks for which it was established, its membership must include at least one individual with current experience and expertise in exploring the biological and environmental factors that could explain myopia's increasing incidence, including in the clinical use of the results of research advances in emmetropization. As described in his biographical summary, Dr. Mutti has extensive experience researching and developing personal monitoring technology to determine the effect of light exposure on myopia progression, and he has played a key role in establishing current views of the protective effects of time outdoors and the limited influence of near work on the risk of myopia onset and progression.

The National Academies has determined that the experience and expertise of Dr. Mutti is needed for the committee to accomplish the task for which it has been established. The National Academies could not find another available individual with the equivalent expertise and experience who does not have a conflict of interest. Therefore, the National Academies has concluded that the conflict is unavoidable.

The National Academies believes that Dr. Mutti can serve effectively as a member of the committee, and the committee can produce an objective report, taking into account the composition of the committee, the work to be performed, and the procedures to be followed in completing the study.

Appendix C
Glossary

Accommodation of the eye Refers to the eye's ability to adjust its focus to see objects clearly at different distances. This is achieved by changing the shape and curvature of the eye's natural lens to bring images into sharp focus on the retina.

Agonist A molecule that binds to a receptor and initiates a response. Receptors often behave like switches; agonists turn the switch "on." Agonists can be natural substances such as hormones or neurotransmitters, or they can be synthetic. Many drugs are agonists. See also "antagonist."

Allele One of two or more versions of a DNA sequence (a single base or a segment of bases) at a given genomic location. An individual inherits two alleles, one from each parent, for any given genomic location where such variation exists. If the two alleles are the same, the individual is homozygous for that allele. If not, the individual is heterozygous.

Anisometropia The presence of asymmetric refraction between the two eyes, typically defined by a difference of 1 or more diopter.

Antagonist A molecule that binds to a receptor but does not initiate a response. Receptors often behave like switches; antagonists turn the switch "off" by blocking the receptor binding site. Many drugs are antagonists. See also "agonist."

Axial length In layman's language, this is the distance in millimeters from the front of the eye to the back of the eye. Technically, axial length is measured along the optical axis from the corneal apex to the front surface of the retina. The axial length of the eye in an emmetropic human adult is approximately 23 mm.

Blur A loss of sharpness in an image, especially the image on the retina. Blur can be caused by defocus, by optical aberrations other than those that lead to defocus, or by a motion of the image.

Cerebral cortex or cortical brain Outermost layer of tissue in the brain. The cerebral cortex, also referred to as gray matter, covers the cerebrum, which is the largest portion of the brain. The cerebral cortex is responsible for integrating sensory impulses, directing motor activity, and controlling higher intellectual functions.

Choroid A layer of tissue lying beneath the retina that has a very rich blood supply. A key role of the choroid is to provide nutrients and oxygen for the retina.

Ciliary body A part of the middle layer of the wall of the eye. The ciliary body is found behind the iris and includes the ring-shaped muscle that changes the shape of the lens when the eye focuses. It also produced the clear fluid that fills the space between the cornea and the iris.

Cones (or cone cells) *See Photoreceptors.*

Cost-effective measure Informally, a preventive measure or treatment that provides good value for money spent; sometimes simply "cost-saving" or "less expensive." More formally, a preventive measure or treatment that leads to improved outcomes at lower costs or one that costs less than a threshold monetary level per improved outcome. The U.S. government does not use such thresholds; some other countries do.

Cost-effectiveness analysis Informally, a study looking at both resources used and outcomes for a preventive measure or intervention. More formally, an analysis in which the costs and effects of two or more interventions are compared. If one is more effective and less expensive it is said to "dominate;" in turn, the one that is more expensive and less effective is "dominated." In general, one is interested in the amount of resources that need to be spent for improved outcomes; in the United States this is expressed in dollars spent for each unit of change in outcome. The ratio is called an "incremental cost-effectiveness ratio."

Cross-sectional study A type of research study in which a group of people is observed, or certain information is collected, at a single point in time or over a short period of time.

Cycloplegia The paralysis of the ciliary muscle of the eye resulting in dilatation of the pupil and paralysis of accommodation. This can be achieved by instilling cycloplegic agents such as atropine, cyclopentolate, or tropicamide eye drops.

Defocus In optics, defocus is the aberration in which an image is out of focus. This aberration causes loss of sharpness and contrast. It will be familiar to anyone who has used a camera, video-camera, microscope, telescope, or binoculars. Optically, defocus refers to a translation of the focus along the optical axis away from the detection surface.

Degenerative myopia Also known as *malignant, pathological,* or *progressive* myopia, is characterized by marked fundus changes, such as posterior staphyloma, and associated with a high refractive error and subnormal visual acuity after correction. This form of myopia gets progressively worse over time. Degenerative myopia has been reported as one of the main causes of visual impairment.

Direct cost A cost that actually involves the exchange of money, which may occur electronically. This is in contrast to indirect or productivity or time costs, which in analyzing vision care costs are used with the recognition that treatments and intervention require time for the patient (and often caregiver) that could be used to produce economic output (even within the home) and that changes in educational attainment that are related to being able to see better can also lead to changes in economic output (even within the home).

Dopamine Also known as DA, an abbreviation for 3,4-dihydroxyphenethylamine, dopamine is a neuromodulatory molecule that plays several important roles in cells. An organic chemical of the catecholamine and phenethylamine families, it constitutes about 80% of the catecholamine content in the brain. In the brain, dopamine functions as a neurotransmitter—a chemical released by neurons (nerve cells) to send signals to other nerve cells. Neurotransmitters are synthesized in specific regions of the brain but affect many regions systemically. The brain includes several distinct dopamine pathways, one of which plays a major role in the motivational component of reward-motivated behavior.

Ecologic (or ecological) study An epidemiology study design in which the unit of observation is the population or community. Ecologic studies of geographical associations between disease prevalence and risk factor levels may provide a broader range of exposure to the risk factor than within-population studies.

Emmetropization The developmental process that matches the eye's optical power to its axial length so that the unaccommodated eye is focused at distance. This is a process whereby the refractive components and the axial length of the eye come into balance during postnatal development in order to induce *emmetropia* (vision with no refractive error). A person with emmetropia may be referred to as an *emmetrope*.

Epidemiology The study of the determinants, occurrence, and distribution of health and disease in a defined population.

Epigenetics The study of how changes in behavior and the environment cause changes in gene expression. Unlike genetic changes, epigenetic changes are reversible and do not change a person's DNA sequence, but they do change how the body reads a DNA sequence.

Federally qualified health centers (FHQCs) and rural health clinics (RHCs) Safety-net providers that deliver prevention and primary services in an outpatient clinic setting.

Form deprivation myopia Myopia that occurs when the eye is deprived of clear vision by light scattering, not because of a focusing error. In a young human or animal whose eyes are still in their growth phase, form deprivation acts as a strong signal for the eye to grow and become myopic.

Fovea Short for *fovea centralis*, it is a small, central pit located in the macula lutea, at the back of the retina, and is composed of closely packed cone cells.

Genome wide association study (GWAS) A test of hundreds of thousands of genetic variants across many participants to find those statistically associated with a specific trait or disease. This methodology has generated a myriad of robust associations for a range of traits and diseases, and the number of associated variants is expected to grow steadily as GWAS sample sizes increase. GWAS results have a range of applications, such as gaining insight into a phenotype's underlying biology, estimating its heritability, calculating genetic correlations, making clinical risk predictions, informing drug development programs and inferring potential causal relationships between risk factors and health outcomes.

Glutamate An amino acid and also acts as a neurotransmitter in the central nervous system.

Glutamatergic   Refers to neurons or synapses that release glutamate as a neurotransmitter. These neurons play crucial roles in many cognitive functions and are involved in various neurological disorders.

Glutamine   A conditionally essential amino acid that performs many functions in the body. Glutamine is essential for the homeostasis of glutamatergic neurotransmission. Glutamine is also the most abundant extracellular amino acid in the body. Glutamine is a precursor to glutamate, which acts as a neurotransmitter in glutamatergic signaling pathways in the brain and nervous system.

Glutaminergic   Refers to neurons or synapses that use glutamine as a precursor to synthesize glutamate. Glutaminergic neurons convert glutamine into glutamate through the enzyme glutaminase.

Glutaminergic amacrine cells (GACs) Glutaminergic amacrine cells are specialized neurons found in the retina, part of the eye's neural network that processes visual information. These cells are called "glutaminergic" because they use glutamine, which can be converted into glutamate, to mediate their functions.

Glycosaminoglycan (GAG) Also known as mucopolysaccharides, are negatively-charged polysaccharide compounds. They are long, unbranched polysaccharide molecules composed of repeating disaccharide units that are present in every mammalian tissue.

High myopia   This is generally defined as nearsightedness requiring a glasses correction of 6.00 diopters or more and is sometimes referred to as *degenerative myopia* or *pathological myopia*.

Hyperopia   Farsightedness, that is, the condition of the eyes in which light from distant objects is brought to a focus behind the retina when accommodation is relaxed. In older individuals this leads to blurry vision, but in children and young adults it often leaves them able to see clearly by accommodative focusing of the crystalline lens. Hyperopia occurs because the eye is too short relative to the focusing power of its optical elements.

Intraocular pressure Similar to blood pressure, the eye maintains a stable pressure. The intraocular pressure helps ensure that the eye retains its correct shape. Intraocular pressure is measured in units of mm Hg. Commonly abbreviated to "IOP".

Intrinsically photosensitive retinal ganglion cells (ipRGCs) Also called *photosensitive retinal ganglion cells (pRGC),* or *melanopsin-containing retinal ganglion cells (mRGCs)*, ipRGCs are a type of neuron in the retina of the mammalian eye. These are photoreceptor cells that are particularly sensitive to the absorption of short-wavelength (blue) visible light. They communicate information directly to the area of the brain called the suprachiasmatic nucleus, also known as the central "body clock," in mammals.

Lateral geniculate nucleus (LGN) Also called the *lateral geniculate body* or *lateral geniculate complex*, it is a structure in the thalamus and a key component of the mammalian visual pathway. It is a small, ovoid, ventral projection of the thalamus where the thalamus connects with the optic nerve.

Mendelian randomization (MR) A term that applies to the use of genetic variation to address causal questions about how modifiable exposures influence different outcomes. The principles of MR are based on Mendel's laws of inheritance and instrumental variable estimation methods, which enable the inference of causal effects in the presence of unobserved confounding.

Melanopsin A type of photopigment belonging to a larger family of light-sensitive retinal proteins called *opsins* and encoded by the gene Opn4. In the mammalian retina, there are two additional categories of opsins, both involved in the formation of visual images: rhodopsin and photopsin (types I, II, and III) in the rod and cone photoreceptor cells, respectively. In humans, melanopsin is found in intrinsically photosensitive retinal ganglion cells (ipRGCs). It is also found in the iris of mice and primates. Melanopsin plays an important non-image-forming role in the setting of circadian rhythms as well as other functions.

Muscarinic acetylcholine receptors, or mAChRs Acetylcholine receptors that form G protein-coupled receptor complexes in the cell membranes of certain neurons and other cells. They play several roles, including acting as the main end-receptor stimulated by acetylcholine released from postganglionic fibers in the parasympathetic nervous system.

Myopia A type of refractive error of the eye characterized by blurry distance vision, yet sharp near vision (nearsightedness).

Oblate and prolate spheroid shapes If an ellipse is rotated about its major axis, the result is a *prolate* spheroid, elongated like a rugby ball (less pointy than an American football). If an ellipse is rotated about its minor axis, the result is an *oblate* spheroid, flattened like a lentil or a plain M&M candy piece.

Opsin *See Melanopsin*

Orthokeratology A modality of contact lens wear that serves as an alternative to spectacles, to provide clear vision for patients with myopia. By contrast to conventional contact lenses that are worn during the daytime, orthokeratology contact lenses are worn overnight and not in the daytime. During overnight wear, the shape of the orthokeratology contact lens and the pressure of the eyelid re-mold the front surface of the cornea, such that the refractive error of the eye becomes less myopic. The contact lenses need to be worn every night. Also known as "ortho-K."

Photopic vision Vision in lighting conditions as bright as ordinary room illumination or outdoors during daylight.

Photoreceptors Specialized cells for detecting light. Two types of photoreceptors reside in the retina: cones and rods. The cones are responsible for daytime vision, while the rods respond under dark conditions. The cones come in three varieties that each responds to a different portion of the visible spectrum, allowing for color vision: L, M, and S types (for long, middle, and short wavelength). Rods have a spectral sensitivity that differs from that of cones.

Plus or minus lenses Types of lenses include (A) converging (convex or plus) lenses, and (B) diverging (concave or minus) lenses. The focal point of a plus lens occurs where parallel light rays that have passed through the lens converge to form an image. The focal point of a minus lens occurs where parallel light rays entering the lens appear to diverge.

Prolate shape *See Oblate and prolate spheroid shapes*

Randomized controlled trial (RCT) A study in which the participants are divided by chance into separate groups to compare different treatments or other interventions. A randomized controlled trial is a form of scientific experiment used to control factors not under direct experimental control. Examples of RCTs are clinical trials that compare the effects of drugs, surgical techniques, medical devices, diagnostic procedures, or other medical treatments.

Refractive error A type of vision problem that makes it hard to see clearly. Such an error happens when the shape of the eye keeps light from focusing correctly on the *retina* (see below). Refractive errors are the most common type of vision problem. The most common refractive errors are myopia (near-sightedness), hyperopia (far-sightedness), astigmatism, and presbyopia (difficulty reading up close due to lens stiffness, which most commonly affects individuals above the age of 40 years).

Refractive surger Any surgical procedure that corrects the refractive error of the eye.

Retina A layer of photoreceptor cells and glial cells within the eye that captures incoming light and transmits signals representing (primarily) color and luminance along neuronal pathways as both electrical and chemical signals for the brain to perceive a visual picture.

Retinitis pigmentosa An inherited retinal disease, also known as an inherited retinal dystrophy, characterized by progressive loss of peripheral (side) vision. The condition often occurs in families. Inheritance can follow different pattern in different families, depending on which gene is affected.

Rods *See Photoreceptors*

Sclera an opaque, tough layer of tissue that forms the outer shell of the middle and back of the eye. The tissue of the sclera is continuous with the cornea. The sclera largely determines the size and shape of the eye.

Scleral collagen Collagen is a protein that forms long, strong fibers. The fibers are woven together to form tough yet pliable tissues known as "connective tissue." Examples of connective tissue include tendon, skin, and the sclera.

Scotopic vision Vision in very dim lighting conditions.

Vision screening Vision screening uses a limited set of procedures designed to detect problems with the eye or vision that can then be diagnosed and treated through a comprehensive eye examination.

Visual field Similar to field of view, the visual field is the angular extent that can be seen by the eye. Because the retinal image is an inverted picture of the world, the visual field is seen by the opposite retina (e.g., objects in the temporal visual field of the right eye are seen by that eye's nasal retina).